A Practical Manual of
PEDIATRIC CARDIAC INTENSIVE CARE

T0074140

A Practical Manual of
PEDIATRIC CARDIAC INTENSIVE CARE

Editors

Rakhi Balachandran
MD (Anesthesia) PDCC (Cardiac Anesthesia)
Professor
Department of Cardiac Anesthesia
Amrita Institute of Medical Sciences and Research Centre
Amrita Vishwa Vidyapeetham
Kochi, Kerala, India

Aveek Jayant
MD (Anesthesia) DM (Cardiac Anesthesia)
Professor and Head
Department of Cardiac Anesthesia
Amrita Institute of Medical Sciences and
Research Centre
Amrita Vishwa Vidyapeetham
Kochi, Kerala, India

R Krishna Kumar
MD DM (Cardiology) FAHA
Professor and Head
Department of Pediatric Cardiology
Amrita Institute of Medical Sciences and
Research Centre
Amrita Vishwa Vidyapeetham
Kochi, Kerala, India

Foreword

Stephen J Roth

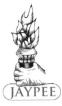

JAYPEE BROTHERS MEDICAL PUBLISHERS
The Health Sciences Publisher
New Delhi | London

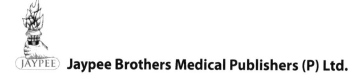

Jaypee Brothers Medical Publishers (P) Ltd.

Headquarters
Jaypee Brothers Medical Publishers (P) Ltd
EMCA House, 23/23-B
Ansari Road, Daryaganj
New Delhi 110 002, India
Landline: +91-11-23272143, +91-11-23272703
+91-11-23282021, +91-11-23245672
Email: jaypee@jaypeebrothers.com

Corporate Office
Jaypee Brothers Medical Publishers (P) Ltd
4838/24, Ansari Road, Daryaganj
New Delhi 110 002, India
Phone: +91-11-43574357
Fax: +91-11-43574314
Email: jaypee@jaypeebrothers.com

Overseas Office
J.P. Medical Ltd
83 Victoria Street, London
SW1H 0HW (UK)
Phone: +44 20 3170 8910
Fax: +44 (0)20 3008 6180
Email: info@jpmedpub.com

Website: www.jaypeebrothers.com
Website: www.jaypeedigital.com

A Practical Manual of Pediatric Cardiac Intensive Care

First Edition: 2022

ISBN: 978-93-90595-63-1

Printed at Repro India Limited

CONTRIBUTORS

PRINCIPAL CONTRIBUTORS

Current and Former Members of the Pediatric Heart Program of the Amrita Institute of Medical Sciences, Amrita Vishwa Vidyapeetham, Medical Campus, Kochi

Rakhi Balachandran
MD (Anesthesia) PDCC (Cardiac Anesthesia)
Professor
Department of Cardiac Anesthesia
Amrita Institute of Medical Sciences and
Research Centre
Amrita Vishwa Vidyapeetham
Kochi, Kerala, India

Praveen Reddy Bayya
MS MCh (CVTS) FPCS
Assistant Professor
Department of Cardiovascular and
Thoracic Surgery
(Division of Pediatric Cardiac Surgery)
Amrita Institute of Medical Sciences and
Research Centre
Amrita Vishwa Vidyapeetham
Kochi, Kerala, India

Aveek Jayant
MD (Anesthesia) DM (Cardiac Anesthesia)
Professor and Head
Department of Cardiac Anesthesia
Amrita Institute of Medical Sciences and
Research Centre
Amrita Vishwa Vidyapeetham
Kochi, Kerala, India

Jessin P Jayashankar
MD (Anesthesia) FCA (Cardiac Anesthesia)
Associate Professor
Department of Cardiac Anesthesia
Amrita Institute of Medical Sciences and
Research Centre
Amrita Vishwa Vidyapeetham
Kochi, Kerala, India

Mahesh Kappanayil
DCH DNB (Pediatrics) FNB (Pediatric Cardiology)
Professor
Department of Pediatric Cardiology
Amrita Institute of Medical Sciences and
Research Centre, Amrita Vishwa Vidyapeetham
Kochi, Kerala, India

Balaganesh Karmegaraj
MD (Pediatrics) DM (Pediatric Cardiology)
Assistant Professor
Department of Pediatric Cardiology
Amrita Institute of Medical Sciences and
Research Centre, Amrita Vishwa Vidyapeetham
Kochi, Kerala, India

Pragnatha Komaravolu MBBS MRCPH
Assistant Professor
Department of Rheumatology
Amrita Institute of Medical Sciences and
Research Centre, Amrita Vishwa Vidyapeetham
Kochi, Kerala, India

Brijesh P Kottayil MS MCh (CVTS)
Associate Professor
Department of Cardiovascular and
Thoracic Surgery
Head (Division of Pediatric Cardiac Surgery)
Amrita Institute of Medical Sciences and
Research Centre, Amrita Vishwa Vidyapeetham
Kochi, Kerala, India

Mani Ram Krishna
DNB (Pediatrics) FNB (Pediatric Cardiology)
Assistant Professor
Department of Pediatric Cardiology
Amrita Institute of Medical Sciences and
Research Centre, Amrita Vishwa Vidyapeetham
Kochi, Kerala, India

R Krishna Kumar
MD DM (Cardiology) FAHA
Professor and Head
Department of Pediatric Cardiology
Amrita Institute of Medical Sciences and
Research Centre
Amrita Vishwa Vidyapeetham
Kochi, Kerala, India

Sreelakshmi P Leeladharan
MD (Anesthesia) DM (Cardiac Anesthesia)
Assistant Professor
Department of Cardiac Anesthesia
Amrita Institute of Medical Sciences and
Research Centre, Amrita Vishwa Vidyapeetham
Kochi, Kerala, India

Thushara Madathil
MD (Anesthesia) DM (Cardiac Anesthesia)
Assistant Professor
Department of Cardiac Anesthesia
Amrita Institute of Medical Sciences and
Research Centre, Amrita Vishwa Vidyapeetham
Kochi, Kerala, India

Suresh G Nair
MD DA (Anesthesia) FIACTA (Hon) FTEE (Hon)
Lead Consultant
Anesthesia and Critical Care
Aster Medcity
Kochi, Kerala, India

Amitabh C Sen
DNB (Anesthesia) PDCC (Cardiac Anesthesia)
Consultant Anesthesiologist
Sultan Qaboos University Hospital
Muscat, Oman

Balaji Srimurugan MS MCh (CVTS) FPCS
Assistant Professor
Department of Cardiovascular and Thoracic
Surgery (Division of Pediatric Cardiac Surgery)
Amrita Institute of Medical Sciences and
Research Centre, Amrita Vishwa Vidyapeetham
Kochi, Kerala, India

Balu Vaidyanathan
MD (Pediatrics) DM (Cardiology)
Professor
Department of Pediatric Cardiology
Head (Fetal Cardiology Division)
Amrita Institute of Medical Sciences and
Research Centre, Amrita Vishwa Vidyapeetham
Kochi, Kerala, India

Sudheer Babu Vanga
MD (Anesthesia) FCA DM (Cardiac Anesthesia)
Testamur in American Society of Echocardiography
Assistant Professor
Department of Cardiac Anesthesia
Amrita Institute of Medical Sciences and
Research Centre, Amrita Vishwa Vidyapeetham
Kochi, Kerala, India

ADDITIONAL CONTRIBUTORS

Co-Authors of reproduced manuscript

Andrew C Argent
MBBCh MMed MD (Pediatrics) FRCPCH FCPaeds (SA)
Professor Emeritus
Department of Pediatrics and Child Health
University of Cape Town
Cape Town, South Africa

Amina Khan RN RM BSCN NCLEX RN
Critical Care Nurse
Intensive Care Unit
El Campo Memorial Hospital
Texas, USA

FOREWORD

The vast majority of children with congenital heart disease (CHD) are born and live in low- and middle-income countries (LMICs). As progress in human development in LMICs proceeds over the next 20–30 years, and communicable diseases cause less childhood mortality, we can anticipate that CHD, a leading birth defect throughout the world, will become more visible and prominent as a pediatric disease. Recognizing this demographic transition, leaders in pediatric health care, governments, and private organizations in many LMICs have begun to develop the human and technical resources to establish pediatric cardiovascular programs capable of delivering high-quality surgical outcomes – centers of excellence.

In India, the pediatric cardiovascular program at the Amrita Institute of Medical Sciences (AIMS) in Kochi, Kerala, is an excellent example of this possibility. The program at AIMS was established in 1998 with Dr R Krishna Kumar as one of its founding members. The program's development has been aided by sustained partnerships with Children's HeartLink (CHL) plus several faculties and staff from Boston Children's Hospital and Lucile Packard Children's Hospital, Stanford. Dr Kumar and his surgical, anesthesia, and nursing colleagues recognized the importance of establishing excellence in the provision of cardiac intensive care for their surgical patients, and they thus focused on building both a high-performing, multidisciplinary team and a dedicated pediatric cardiac intensive care unit (PCICU) at AIMS. I had the privilege of assisting the team at AIMS with this effort, and between 2000 and 2008, I participated in five visits to Kochi that were sponsored by CHL. Physicians and nurses from the PCICU at AIMS also visited Boston and Palo Alto during this time to observe clinical practice and learn about the structure and governance of our units and programs. Today, AIMS has a 24-bed dedicated PCICU that supports the intensive care of 650–700 cardiac surgical patients per year. The team has achieved excellent clinical outcomes, and their program is now regarded as among the best in India, with patients referred from throughout India, South Asia, and Africa with it for cardiac care. In 2012, Children's HeartLink designated AIMS as the first Children's HeartLink Center of Excellence in pediatric cardiac care and training.

This manual represents the collective knowledge and clinical experience of the AIMS pediatric cardiac team, and it has been created by them to serve as a practical bedside resource for physician trainees, nurses, and other frontline care-providers in the PCICU. Unlike existing handbooks developed at programs in high-resource settings, it presents key clinical information about specific defects, problems, and clinical management approaches within the context of 20 years of practice in a resource-constrained setting. For example, one chapter is devoted to perioperative nutritional rehabilitation; in India, as in other LMICs, it is common for younger cardiac patients presenting for surgery late and to have severe failure to thrive at hospital admission. And while a chapter on the use of extracorporeal membrane oxygenation is included, there is no discussion of the clinical details of mechanical circulatory support with ventricular assist devices or cardiac transplantation for terminal heart failure, too costly and complex therapies. One chapter is also offered on the most important considerations for establishing a PCICU in a limited-resource environment.

In addition to providing key information about cardiac intensive care for CHD patients, this manual promotes the practice of critical thinking at the bedside. Successful intensive care depends in part on vigilance – the "eyes and ears" at the bedside looking and listening for signals that could represent early indications of clinical decompensation. Building critical thinking skills among care team members is the best way to expand the scope of vigilance to include "minds" as well as "eyes and ears", and this manual will assist those who embrace it in those fundamental skills.

Stephen J Roth MD MPH
Professor of Pediatrics (Cardiology)
Stanford University School of Medicine
Attending Physician, Cardiovascular Intensive Care
Lucile Packard Children's Hospital, Stanford
Palo Alto, California, USA

This manual of cardiac intensive care seeks to serve as a ready reckoner to nurses and resident doctors involved in the perioperative intensive care of patients with congenital heart disease. Much of what is written here has been distilled over two decades of institutional experience in caring for children with congenital heart disease.

The essence of pediatric cardiac intensive care is coordinated multidisciplinary teamwork involving nurses, pediatric cardiologists, surgeons, anesthesiologists, pediatricians and intensivists. Much of the care is finally delivered via the bedside nurse. The role of supporting personnel that includes respiratory therapists, care assistants, clinical pharmacists, nutrition specialists, medical social workers, and biomedical technicians is equally critical.

The pediatric heart program at Amrita Institute of Medical Sciences has been established in 1998 and has evolved over the past two decades. The program performs 650–700 cases annually and has accumulated substantial expertise in providing comprehensive care for neonates, infants and children with congenital heart disease. The surgical team has achieved excellence in performing all the complex congenital heart lesions in infants and adult patients alike. We strongly believe that the results achieved is largely a reflection of the multidisciplinary team approach that we have all passionately embraced.

This manual has attempted to incorporate some of the key aspects of the general postoperative care of patients undergoing congenital heart surgery, special considerations in each type of congenital heart disease, the expected postoperative complications and their management. Though we have attempted to touch upon some of the pertinent aspects of pediatric cardiac intensive care, we are cognizant of the fact that this book is by no means complete. We also recognize that institutional protocols may vary substantially and there be more than one way to take care of specific situations. Thus, rather than serving as a comprehensive reference, it aims to provide bedside solutions to common problems encountered in postoperative cardiac critical care.

This book looks to specifically assist care-providers in pediatric heart programs encountered in low and middle-income countries. Therefore, there are chapters that are specially devoted to issues that are of particular significance in low resource environments. There are chapters devoted to nutrition, pulmonary hypertension, and healthcare-associated infections. The final chapter of the book is devoted to special considerations in establishing a pediatric cardiac intensive care unit in a limited resource environment.

We would sincerely solicit feedback on the manual from its readership and hope to make this a work in progress that improves with time.

Rakhi Balachandran
Aveek Jayant
R Krishna Kumar

ACKNOWLEDGMENTS

This book has been a collective effort of past and present members of the pediatric heart program at the Amrita Institute of Medical Sciences (AIMS), Kochi, Kerala, India. Firstly, we wish to thank all the contributors who have dedicated their valuable time and knowledge in preparing the individual chapters of this manual. We sincerely acknowledge Dr Suresh G Nair, former Professor and Head, Cardiac Anesthesia and Cardiac Intensive Care Services for laying down an administrative and training framework that stands us in good stead to this day. We also thank Dr Suresh G Rao, Dr Krishnanaik Shivaprakasha and Dr Sunil GS, former pediatric cardiac surgeons whose unparalleled surgical expertise laid the foundation of excellent surgical outcomes and many unit policies related to the care of children undergoing surgical correction of heart defects.

Excellence in nursing care is paramount in facilitating good surgical outcomes. We wish to place on record our deep gratitude to our past and present nursing staff for dedicating long and stressful hours in the passionate care of critically ill children with heart disease. We specifically acknowledge the efforts of Ms Sreeja Mohan, our former Nurse In-Charge, whose impeccable clinical acumen and leadership skills facilitated training of her junior colleagues and implementation of unit policies and protocols to perfection. We specially acknowledge Ms Saibala, Director of Nursing Services, for her leadership and wholehearted support of the pediatric heart program.

The junior doctors and postgraduate residents form the main workforce of the unit for delivering uninterrupted care for sick children before and after heart surgery. Their enthusiasm and desire to learn have enabled the senior faculty to keep abreast with the latest developments in the sub-specialty and inspired them to deliver the best possible outcomes. We sincerely thank all our past and present resident doctors and faculties for contributing to the clinical work in the intensive care unit. We also thank all the supporting clinical staff of the pediatric heart program including respiratory therapists, perfusionists, technicians, physiotherapists, nutrition specialists, pharmacists, medical social workers, care assistants, biomedical engineers, members of the electrical department, and secretarial staff.

A number of developments in our intensive care program have been specifically facilitated by our decades-long association with Children's HeartLink (*www.childrensheartlink.org*), a non-governmental organization based in Minneapolis, USA. They helped foster the vision of multidisciplinary postoperative care and contributed greatly to the development of a cohesive team of caregivers. They have enabled training exchanges with experts at various stages of the program development and have facilitated short-term training of our faculty at centers of excellence in the United States. Their support has greatly helped in skill development and training of our nurses, infection control and a number of quality improvement initiatives.

We must specifically acknowledge those who have, in the past, visited our program regularly to enhance the quality of care. Dr Stephen Roth, Professor of Pediatrics (Cardiology)

Stanford University School of Medicine was instrumental in laying the foundations of pediatric cardiac intensive care at AIMS. Dr VM Reddy, Professor, Pediatric Cardiothoracic and Vascular Surgery, UCSF, USA has taken a special interest in training our team to perform surgery for complex heart defects and for preterm infants. Sandra Staveski, RN, PhD, Assistant Professor, Family Health Care Nursing, School of Nursing, UCSF has a long and extremely fruitful association with the AIMS pediatric heart program. She has contributed greatly to elevating the quality of our nursing in the ICU and has helped establish our nurse residency program.

Our intensive care unit has embraced a commitment to continuous quality improvement right from its inception. We joined the International Quality Improvement Collaborative (IQIC) for Congenital Heart Disease (*https://iqic.chboston.org/*), a global project to improve outcomes in children undergoing congenital heart surgery. The introspection of data and annual benchmarking facilitated by this project enabled us to continuously strive towards achieving better standards. Here, we specially acknowledge the efforts of Mr Abish Sudhakar, Research Assistant, Pediatric Cardiology in maintaining a robust database and facilitating the annual international audit of this data.

Sustaining a successful pediatric heart program requires the unconditional support of the administrative leadership. We sincerely thank Dr Prem Nair, Medical Director, for his wholehearted support of the pediatric heart program. We also acknowledge the efforts of Dr Sanjeev K Singh, Medical Administrator, Amrita Institute for his contributions towards spearheading continuous quality improvement and infection control initiatives in the pediatric cardiac intensive care unit.

Additionally, Dr Balaji Srimurugan and Dr Praveen Reddy have made all the illustrations in this manual despite their hectic schedule.

Above all we are also blessed by the divine persona of Her Holiness Mata Amritanandamayi for Her graceful oversight of the pediatric heart program and unconditional support.

We acknowledge the strong support of our family members who have stood by us during the thick and thin of our professional life and withstood the challenges that resulted from our long periods of absence.

Finally, we must express our deep and heartfelt gratitude to our patients and their families for giving us the opportunity to trust us with their health and the opportunity to at once, serve and learn from them.

CONTENTS

SECTION 2

CARDIAC LESION SPECIFIC POSTOPERATIVE MANAGEMENT

SECTION 3

COMMON POSTOPERATIVE COMPLICATIONS

SECTION

General Considerations

Preoperative Stabilization and Transportation Guidelines in Infants with Heart Disease

Mahesh Kappanayil

Reviewed by: R Krishna Kumar

■ INTRODUCTION

Pediatric cardiac programs in tertiary care hospitals receive neonates and infants from other healthcare facilities such as pediatric units, pediatric intensive care units (PICU) and neonatal intensive care units (NICU) elsewhere. These babies are referred with suspected or confirmed diagnosis of congenital heart disease (CHD). Most of these patients, can be categorized as "critical" CHD and are transferred on mechanical ventilation, inotropes, and prostaglandin E1 (PGE1) infusion support, requiring urgent surgical or catheter intervention for survival. An increasing number of newborn heart surgeries are now being done in many Indian institutions with encouraging outcomes. Pediatric heart surgery has now become relatively safe, due to relentless efforts at improving expertise, technique, infrastructure, technology and establishing quality control initiatives. Additionally, with increasing awareness and funding from government as well as philanthropic organizations, funding for surgery is now available for an increasing number of families.

An analysis of the outcomes of 1,028 consecutive infants operated at Amrita Institute of Medical Sciences (AIMS) Kochi, published in 2015, showed that the preoperative clinical condition of infants and neonates has profound impact on their eventual surgical outcomes. Preoperative sepsis, intensive care unit (ICU) stay, and ventilation were shown to be adversely associated with postoperative mortality and morbidity.[1] Therefore, to further improve the outcomes of infant heart surgery, it is essential to review and optimize the preoperative status of these critically ill patients.

▌ RATIONALE FOR ENSURING SAFE TRANSPORTATION

In a recent study at AIMS, Kochi, on newborn transfers with CHD, we found that majority of these patients are transported in ambulances as emergency.[2] Unfortunately systems for patient transport, are not well-established in India and other low- and middle-income countries (LMIC). Systems for communication, transmission of vital clinical information and real time monitoring of the condition of the baby during transport are virtually non-existent. Referrals often happen through direct personal communication between clinicians at either end, often with inadequate documentation of clinical details. Transportation is often carried out by, generic ambulance service personnel, with little or no training on the management of neonates/infants with heart disease. Moreover, majority of the babies are transported without an accompanying pediatrician or pediatric trained nurse with insufficient monitoring.

GOALS OF SAFE TRANSPORTATION AND PREOPERATIVE STABILIZATION

In order to ensure the best possible post-operative outcomes for neonates and infants with congenital heart disease, it is important to address the following:

1. Ensuring clear communication, discussion and documentation of issues pertaining to the patient between referring and receiving clinical teams.
2. Optimizing the clinical status of the baby (as much as possible) prior to transport.
3. Ensuring safe, well-monitored transport.
4. Ensuring safe receipt of the baby at receiving hospital.
5. Appropriate preoperative stabilization of clinical status prior to the surgery.

STEP-WISE APPROACH

Suspecting CHD in the Newborn or Infant

Nearly 250,000 children are born every year in India with CHD.[3,4] It is important to suspect and diagnose "critical" CHD as early as possible, since most require urgent intervention.

Nearly 100,000 children are born with critical CHD every year in India. These include: duct-dependent pulmonary circulation (DDPC), duct-dependent systemic circulation (DDSC), total anomalous pulmonary venous connection (TAPVC), d-transposition of great arteries (dTGA), tetralogy of Fallot (TOF), and anomalous origin of left coronary artery from pulmonary artery.

All neonates and infants must be thoroughly assessed to rule out critical/major CHD as part of newborn examination including pulse oximetry. In babies with cyanosis and low oxygen saturation, hyperoxia test can be considered to differentiate cyanosis due to CHD from other causes in controlled environment such as ICU. Chest X-ray (CXR) and electrocardiography (ECG) may provide additional clues to the presence of CHD. Echocardiogram performed by skilled personnel is ideal for confirmation of the diagnosis, however, it is not readily available in all healthcare settings.

What is the Course of Action Once a Major Heart Disease is Suspected?

Understand Underlying Physiology

- *Decreased pulmonary blood flow*: This is typically identified by the combination of significant desaturations (<85%) together with dark lung fields on the CXR. There is limited response to administering oxygen, sometimes none at all.
  - *Duct-dependent pulmonary circulation*: This is a distinct subset within the category of decreased pulmonary blood flow. Here the ductus arteriosus is responsible for all or almost all pulmonary blood flow.
- *Increased pulmonary blood flow*: These babies are seldom significantly hypoxic (with the exception of transposition) and have features of heart failure in the form of tachypnea, labored breathing, pulsatile precordium and, hepatomegaly. The CXR shows a large heart size and increased lung vasculature. Oxygen administration has the potential of worsening the status of these patients by increasing pulmonary blood flow at the expense of systemic blood flow.
  - *Duct dependent systemic blood flow*: The ductus arteriosus is responsible for all of the aortic flow (ascending and descending) or descending aortic flow alone. Often the pulmonary blood flow is in competition with the systemic circulation. The overall pulmonary blood flow tends to be

increased because of the relatively lower pulmonary vascular resistance.

- *Transposition physiology*: Here the oxygen rich pulmonary venous blood is sent back to the lungs and poorly oxygenated blood returning via systemic veins [superior vena cava (SVC) and inferior vena cava (IVC)] is routed to the aorta resulting in severe desaturation. Survival is only possible through communications that allows mixing of pulmonary and systemic venous blood.
- *Pulmonary venous obstruction*: Pulmonary venous congestion with pulmonary arteriolar vasoconstriction result in elevation in pulmonary vascular resistance that translates into reduced pulmonary blood flow and increased cyanosis. Examples include obstructed total anomalous pulmonary venous connection, cor triatriatum, congenital mitral stenosis, mitral atresia with restrictive atrial septal defect (ASD) and pulmonary venous stenosis.
- *Ventricular dysfunction*: Ventricular dysfunction and heart failure can occur as a result of obstructive lesions (critical coarctation, severe aortic stenosis) or other causes that include anomalous left coronary artery from pulmonary artery, myocarditis, persistent tachyarrhythmia, and metabolic causes such as hypocalcemia. The physiological consequence is that of low cardiac output often with pulmonary venous hypertension.

OPTIMIZE CLINICAL CONDITION IN ACCORDANCE WITH UNDERLYING PHYSIOLOGY

General Measures

- Secure at least two intravenous access. The second access serves as a backup especially when critical medication such as PGE1 is on flow.

- Prevention of hypothermia and maintain normal body temperature.
- Maintain fluid and electrolyte balance and prevent hypoglycemia.
- Monitoring and maintenance of vital parameters [heart rate, blood pressure, respiratory rate, oxygen saturation (SaO_2)].
- Monitoring and optimization of metabolic parameters and end organ functions (blood sugar, liver function tests, coagulation, renal function tests, lactates).
- Identification of sepsis and appropriate management.

Specific Conditions

Reduced Pulmonary Blood Flow

Duct dependent pulmonary circulation: All lesions that are accompanied by pulmonary atresia, or critically reduced pulmonary blood flow

- Ensure adequate hydration
- Reliable vascular access
- *PGE1 infusion*: Start at 0.05 μg/kg/min and titrate according to SaO_2 (target SaO_2 80–85%); this can often be brought down to 0.01 μg/kg/min after initial stabilization.[5,6]

Increased Pulmonary Blood Flow/ Congestive Heart Failure

Large left-to-right shunt lesions: Truncus arteriosus, aortopulmonary window, ventricular septal defect (VSD) with coarctation, single ventricle lesions without pulmonary stenosis.

- Restricted fluid intake (two-thirds restriction)
- Decongestive medications as needed
  - *Diuretics*: Furosemide bolus/infusion
  - *Afterload reducing agents*: Dobutamine/milrinone/enalapril
- *If ventilated*: Room air or low fraction of inspired oxygen (FiO_2), with permissive

hypercapnia (arterial PCO_2 45–50 mm Hg)—this is done deliberately to avoid pulmonary overcirculation.

Parallel Circulation with Poor Mixing

- Maintain good hydration for adequate circulatory volumes
- PGE1 infusion if SaO_2 poor (<70%)
- Mechanical ventilation need not be instituted on the basis of saturation thresholds. If the baby is blue with saturations ~70%, it is often not necessary to ventilate if there is no significant respiratory distress.

Duct-dependent Systemic Circulation

- Start PGE1 infusion at 0.05–0.1 µg/kg/min with monitoring of lower limb pulses and perfusion, renal/liver/gut functions.
- Oxygen inhalation should be avoided as far as possible; this lowers pulmonary vascular resistance and worsens the physiological consequences of the lesion.
- *If ventilated*: Room air/low FiO_2 ventilation, with permissive hypercapnia (arterial PCO_2 45–50 mm Hg) is preferred. It is critically important not to ventilate overzealously. Oxygen saturations in the low 80s are far more acceptable than systemic underperfusion from systemic steal as a result of a lowered pulmonary vascular resistance.

Obstructed TAPVC

- Restricted fluid (50–75%) in view of congested lungs
- *If ventilated*: FiO_2 may be targeted to maintain saturation >70%; however, this may not always be possible especially in severe cases.

Special Instructions in All Patients with Critical CHD

- In a baby expected to need a cardiac intervention, avoid femoral arterial/venous punctures

- Preserve and maintain vascular access sites diligently
- Ventilation/fluid management should *always* be customized to the physiology (as detailed above).
- Meticulous adherence to standard infection control practices at all times while handling the baby, access sites and surroundings.

ARRANGING TRANSFER TO TERTIARY CARE HOSPITAL

Initial Communication

Pediatric cardiac unit (PCU) at the tertiary care hospital may be informed through phone. Contact number should be shared.

Transfer of Clinical Summary of the Patient to the Receiving Hospital

Checklist of essential information to be provided to the receiving hospital:

- Demographics and basic information
  - Name
  - Age including date and time of birth
  - Gender
  - Gestational age
  - Birth weight
  - Current weight
  - Neonatal resuscitation score (APGAR)
  - Presumed or confirmed cardiac diagnosis
  - *Information on parents*: Whether accompanying the baby or not
- Cardiac and hemodynamic status
  - Heart rate
  - Blood pressure and perfusion
  - All peripheral pulses
  - Temperature
  - Respiration
  - Oxygen saturation
  - Heart sounds/murmurs
- Comorbidities
  - *Sepsis*: Blood counts, C-reactive protein, blood culture, blood gas, blood glucose

- *Organ functions*: Central nervous system, hepatic, renal, respiratory status
- Genetic syndromes/dysmorphology
- Others (Any other surgery, etc.)
- Ongoing medications (with dose/route/frequency/duration)
  - Decongestives
  - Antibiotics
  - Inotropes
  - Prostaglandin E1
  - Other major medications
- Ventilation
  - Spontaneous
  - *Mechanical ventilation*: Mode, rate, FiO_2, peak inspiratory pressure (PIP), positive end-expiratory pressure (PEEP)
  - *ABG/VBG*: pH, PO_2, PCO_2, lactate
- Family
  - Relevant social history
  - Current family situation
  - Specific parental preferences, if any.

Reply to the Referring Hospital

Once above information is transmitted to the PCU at tertiary hospital, the following decisions should be conveyed back to the referring unit:

- Suitability for transfer to receiving hospital for further management
- Need, and approximate time required for ensuring availability of ICU bed to receive the baby
- Overall outlook for the cardiac condition and future outcomes
- Funding source [registration under Rashtriya Bal Swasthya Karyakram (RBSK), government funding schemes, etc.].

Referring team must share above information with the parents/caregivers of the patient, and obtain their willingness for transfer to receiving hospital.

Organizing Transport

Transport may be arranged through one of the following three means:

1. Ambulance services of the referring hospital
2. Ambulance services of the receiving hospital
3. Other ambulance service providers.

Where available, a transport application may be utilized (see *www.neoport.org*).

■ THE PROCESS OF TRANSPORT

The following information must be recorded and documented at *initiation* of transport (*in addition* to the previously mentioned checklist):

1. *Personnel accompanying*: Doctor/nurse/paramedics/parents
2. *Vitals*: Heart rate, blood pressure, pulses, temperature, SaO_2
3. *Metabolic parameters*: Lactate, blood sugar
4. *Vascular access sites*: Location and functioning
5. *IV drugs on flow*: Route, dose, dilution, rate of flow
6. *Endotracheal tube*: Size and length secured
7. *Ventilator settings*.

Checklist of parameters to be recorded in transit, with frequency:

- For example, HR continuous, noninvasive blood pressure (NIBP) every 30 minutes, temperature every 30 minutes, random blood sugar every 60 minutes, etc.

It is important to inform the team at receiving hospital once the transport begins from the referring institution. If possible, continue contact with the transporting team during transit.

■ POST TRANSPORT

- Once the baby is received at tertiary hospital, the team should stabilize the child and perform a thorough general and cardiac assessment. A detailed feedback should be provided to the referring unit as soon as possible.

- As per the clinical condition of the baby, the referring team should provide periodic updates on the further treatment and outcomes of the referred patient.

■ CONCLUSION

This chapter summarizes the process of enabling optimal stabilization and safe transport of a baby with congenital heart disease. This is the vital first step that often goes wrong in low resource environments. Attention to basic details listed here can go a long way in improving overall outcomes.

REFERENCES

1. Reddy NS, Kappanayil M, Balachandran R, Jenkins KJ, Sudhakar A, Sunil GS, et al. Preoperative determinants of outcomes of infant heart surgery in a limited-resource setting. Semin Thorac Cardiovasc Surg. 2015;27(3):331-8.
2. Karmegaraj B, Mahesh K, Sudhakar A, Kumar RK. Impact of transport on arrival status and outcomes in newborns with heart disease: a low- middle income country perspective. Cardiol Young. 2020;30(7):1001-8.
3. Saxena A. Congenital heart disease in India: a status report. Indian Pediatr. 2018;55:1075-82.
4. Kumar RK. Universal heart coverage for children with heart disease in India. Ann Pediatr Card. 2015;8:177-83.
5. Ramnarayan P, Intikhab Z, Spencely N, Iliopoulos I, Duff A, Millar J. Interhospital transport of the child with critical cardiac disease. Cardiol Young. 2017;27:S40-46.
6. Browning Carmo KA, Barr P, West M, Hopper NW, White JP, Badawi N. Transporting newborn infants with suspected duct dependent congenital; heart disease on low-dose prostaglandin E1 without routine mechanical ventilation. Arch Dis Child Fetal Neonatal Ed. 2007;92:117-9.

Transfer of Patients from Operating Room to Pediatric Cardiac Intensive Care Unit after Congenital Heart Surgery

Rakhi Balachandran, Aveek Jayant

■ INTRODUCTION

Transfer of a postoperative patient after congenital heart surgery from operating room (OR) to postoperative intensive care unit (ICU) is a high-risk procedure.[1,2] The critically ill patient, along with devices in situ and monitoring equipment, adds to the stress and dynamics of transfer. Yet still, some children might have precarious hemodynamics, the transfer process might itself trigger instability (from sedation lightening, fluid shifts, and so on) and a small minority would have an open sternum or a shift on extended extracorporeal circulation. This process is also fraught with probability of human or mechanical errors, which can pose further threats to the safety of these critically ill patients. Historically, the handoff process has been streamlined to a large extent by imbibing lessons from aviation and motor racing industry.[3] In a prospective interventional study observing 50 postsurgery patient handovers, Catchpole et al. had demonstrated that the implementation of a multidisciplinary handover protocol successfully reduced mean number of technical errors, information handover omissions, and duration of handoff process.[3] Hence, it is imperative that the pediatric cardiac team should have a predefined handoff policy and each individual of the multidisciplinary team possess a comprehensive understanding of the procedures involved in transfer of these patients. In this chapter, we have summarized the steps employed at our center for facilitating a streamlined transfer of the pediatric cardiac surgical patient from OR to the postoperative pediatric cardiac intensive care unit (PCICU).

■ SEQUENCE OF VARIOUS EVENTS INVOLVED IN THE TRANSFER

Pre-handover Phase

Step 1: Sending the OR to PCICU transfer sheet

This step initiates the process of transfer of patients from OR to PCICU and includes the dispatch of a completed OR to ICU transfer chart by the anesthesiologist in OR. A suggested model of OR to PCICU transfer chart is depicted in **Annexure 1**. This chart incorporates details of anticipated ventilator settings, endotracheal tube (ETT) size and level of fixture, location of invasive intravascular monitoring catheters, infusion rate/dose/dilution of inotropes and other medicine infusions, specific complications anticipated, and expected plan for postoperative ventilation. Typically, this step is done as soon as the patient is successfully weaned off bypass and deemed hemodynamically stable in the OR.

Step 2: PCICU postoperative bed setup

Personnel: The bedside nurse and the PCICU nursing assistant/technician are responsible

Annexure 1: OT to ICU transfer chart.

Department of Anesthesiology
OT to ICU Transfer Details

Surgery:	*Weight:*	*BSA:*
Ventilator settings		*ET TUBE*
Mode:	Size:	
TV:	Oral/Nasal:	
RR:	Tube length:	
I.E:		
FiO$_2$		

Lines	*Drugs*	*Dose/rate*
Peripheral venous:	1.	
	2.	
Artery:	3.	
	4.	
Central venous:	5.	
	6.	

Monitoring parameters:

Blood products required:

Plan:

Comments:

Anesthesiologists' Receiving Notes

Date of surgery:

Preop diagnosis:

Surgical procedure:

Significant events during anesthesia and surgery

Supports:

Dopamine:	....	μg/kg/min
NTG:	....	μg/kg/min
Adrenaline:	....	μg/kg/min
SNP:	....	μg/kg/min
Dobutamine:	....	μg/kg/min
Noradrenaline:	....	μg/kg/min
Milrinone:	....	μg/kg/min
Others:	....	

IABP: ....

Hemodynamics:

HR:	.... /min ....
Rhythm:	....
SpO$_2$:	....
BP:	....
CVP:	....
PA:	....
RA:	....
PCWP:	....
Peripheries:	.... Warm .... Cool

Chest:

Air entry: ....

ABG: ....

Remarks/Issues:

Plan:

Signature of Doctor: ....

for set up of postoperative bed and equipment in the PCICU.

Equipment

- Warmer bed or bassinet with monitor shelf
- Transport IV pole with smooth rolling wheels
- Transport monitor with adequate battery back up
- *Cables*: Electrocardiogram (ECG) cables with five leads, one composite module with two pressure cables, and SpO_2 cable with sensor. The cables should be placed in a clean tray on the bed
- Oxygen cylinder with adequate supply
- Manual resuscitation bag of appropriate size for the age of the patient. This should be checked for the integrity of various parts and valves by the team leader or intensivist and kept in a clean cover on the bed
- A container of chlorhexidine hand sanitizer to ensure hand hygiene of the personnel involved in the transfer.

Step 3: Setting up of the PCICU ventilator

- The bedside nurse/respiratory therapist (RT) should be responsible for the setting up of ventilator. The type of ventilator is likely to vary from institution to institution. At our institution, this is the Engstrom Carestation™ (GE Healthcare, USA). Sterilized tubing should be used for each new patient while assembling the circuitry and for checking out the ventilator. This will be replaced with the patients' circuit from the OR upon arrival. Breathing circuit with transparent/semitransparent inspiratory and expiratory tubing should be used while setting up the circuit. This is to facilitate easy detection of the presence of circuit condensate.
- Heated water humidifiers are used for all children <30 kg and for patients weighing >30 kg, a heat and moisture exchanger should be attached to the end of ETT.

- A heat and moisture exchanger should also be used at the expiratory port of the ventilator.
- The ventilator settings should correspond to the prescribed settings suggested in the transfer sheet.
- Appropriate alarm limits should be set in accordance with the prescribed ventilator settings.

Step 4: Preparing physician order sets

The anesthesiologist on call/pediatric cardiac intensivist should document all the medication orders appropriate for the patient in the physician order sheet. The physician orders should include recommended daily maintenance fluid allowance, type of maintenance fluid required, perioperative antibiotic orders, pain and sedation medications, H_2-receptor blocking agents (ranitidine), inotrope infusion orders, diuretics, and anticoagulants (if indicated).

Step 5: Informing the PCICU about anticipated arrival time

The anesthesiologist in the OR should inform the expected arrival time of the patient to the PCICU team. This is to ensure the presence of all stakeholders in the postoperative care process to receive the patient. This typically includes, on call PCICU physician, pediatric cardiology team, bedside nurse, and medical social worker who should be available when the patient reaches the PCICU.

Handover Phase

Patient and Technology Transfer

This involves transfer of patient and monitoring technology to the ICU bed and transport monitor, respectively. All personnel engaged in the handoff process should perform hand hygiene with chlorhexidine sanitizer before touching the patient or the bed. "Sign out" part of the safe surgical list should be completed by the circulating nurse in OR before initiating

Annexure 2: Safe surgical checklist.

Congenital Heart Surgery Perioperative Checklist

Before Induction Sign In	Before Skin Incision Time Out	Before Patient Leaves OR Sign Out
Have the circulator and anesthesiologist together confirmed:	**Have all team members introduced themselves by name and role?**	**Have the surgeon and circulator together confirmed:**
☐ Patient identity?	**Has the surgeon verbally confirmed to team:**	☐ Surgical procedure(s) performed?
☐ Operative site (s)?		☐ Instrument, sponge, and needle counts?
☐ Procedure(s) to be performed and informed consent obtained?	☐ Correct patient, site, and procedure(s) and consent?	☐ Second dose of antibiotic administered?
☐ Medication allergies?	☐ Relevant imaging and studies reviewed?	**Surgical Safety Bundle (Mandatory)**
☐ Active warming in place?	☐ Need for implants or other prosthetics?	☐ Preoperative skin preparation
☐ Need for external defibrillator paddles/temporary pacing?	☐ Need for circulatory arrest/ selective cerebral perfusion?	☐ Clippers used
☐ Availability of blood products/ irradiated blood products?	**Has the anesthesiologist verbally confirmed:**	☐ Antibiotic prophylaxis
Has the anesthesiologist confirmed:	☐ Antibiotics given within 60 minutes of incision?	☐ Blood glucose level was normal throughout surgery
☐ IV access available?		
☐ Possibility of difficult airway/ aspiration?		
☐ Preoperative medicine/ antibiotics?		
Has the perfusionist verbally confirmed:	**Each Team Member must Verbalize They have No Concerns with Proceeding** 🛑 **STOP**	
☐ Readiness of CPB circuit?		

Anesthesiologist   **Surgeon**

Name: ....   Signature: ....   Name: ....   Signature: ....

Filled by: ....   Designation: ....   Signature: ....

---

the transfer. A prototype of the safe surgical checklist is depicted in **Annexure 2**.

Preparing for transfer: The primary responsibility of handling the physiological status of the patient in the vulnerable postoperative phase vests on the anesthesiologist. Hence, in most OR to ICU handoffs, anesthesiologist is deemed the transport and transition team leader. The anesthesiologist should be in command of the patient, monitoring system, and ventilation. The transport and transition leader should possess essential skill sets relating to teamwork, effective communication, and critical management of the patient in the event of a crisis. The following checklist has to be ensured before transfer to ICU bed:

- The patient should be examined for ETT position and stability, central line, and arterial line fixation.
- All three ways on infusion lines should be reassessed to ensure that essential drugs are running.
- Battery backup of all syringe infusion pumps should be verified.
- All nonessential drugs for transfer period should be turned off with the syringe pumps either put off or in the stand-by mode.
- Endotracheal suctioning is not generally encouraged at this point of time unless very essential.
- The central venous pressure (CVP) and arterial line transducers should be taped on to transducer holder or cardboard box.

- Two 20 mL syringes containing blood, fresh frozen plasma, or colloid should be kept ready as volume for replacement, if there is a need for rapid intravenous administration as in hypovolemia.
- Emergency drugs preloaded in syringes should be kept in a sterile tray (Inj. adrenaline 20 µg/mL, Inj. calcium gluconate 100 mg/mL, Inj. atropine 0.1 mg/mL, Inj. ephedrine 3 mg/mL, Inj. 2% lignocaine, preservative free (Xylocard) 2 mg/mL, Inj. 7.5% sodium bicarbonate 20 mL).
- A dual-chamber pacemaker with battery back up and cables should be available on the transport bed.

Coordinating the transfer: The anesthesia team (anesthesiologist and anesthesia technician) should ensure the following transition items.

- Remove the OR ECG leads from the patient and attach the ECG leads from the transport monitor.
- The arterial pressure cable in the OR monitor should be disconnected from the transducer and replaced with that of the transport monitor. The transducer should then be rezeroed.
- The CVP cable should be exchanged for the cable from the transport monitor.
- The pressure bag should be removed from the transducer flushes and the stopcock to the transducer should be closed.
- The SpO_2 cable with sensor from the transport monitor has to be attached to the patient.
- Battery back up of syringe pumps containing the inotrope infusions has to be ensured.
- All the required syringe pumps should be transferred to the transfer IV pole.
- The pacemaker with appropriate cables should be taped to the bed, if the patient is being paced.

- The prepared agent for volume transfusion and emergency drugs should be kept in a sterile tray, which is accessible to the anesthetist during transfer.

The operating department technician should check the following action items:

- The warmer bed should be moved into the OR
- The chest tubes should be secured using appropriate adhesives prior to transfer
- The cautery plate used during surgery should be removed from the patient
- Assist in shifting the patient on to the transport bed
- Ensure that the oxygen supply from the cylinder is turned on when the patient is hand ventilated using Ambu bag after shifting to the bed.

Once all the monitoring cables are transferred to the transport monitor and the chest tubes clamped, the patient is ready to be transferred to the bed.

The anesthesiologist stabilizes the ETT and the head of the patient during transfer to the ICU bed. Care should be taken that the infusion lines/drains are not stretched or entangled during transfer. The intercostal drainage bottles should be suspended in such a way that they remain at a lower level than the patient.

The ventilation will be taken over by the anesthesiologist using the Ambu bag once the baby is on the transport bed. The patient should be covered by a sterile sheet/towel to prevent hypothermia during transfer.

The bed should be moved to the PCICU by the anesthesiologist, OR technician, and the anesthesia technician.

A surgeon and a nurse who assisted in the surgical procedure should accompany the patient during transfer.

Receiving the patient in the PCICU: The bedside nurse, team leader, buffer nurse, PCICU technician, PCICU anesthesiologist/physician, respiratory therapist, pediatric cardiologist on call physician, and medical social worker should be available to receive the patient.

The following action items should be completed within first 2 minutes:

- Anesthesiologist should connect the patient to the PCICU ventilator. He should also check the ETT stability, bilateral air entry, and the appropriateness of the ventilator settings.
- The OR technician should ensure that intercostal drainage bottles are safely placed below the patient and appropriate negative suction pressure (-10 cmH$_2$O) is maintained from the wall suction outlet.
- RT should cross check the ventilator settings and ensure bilateral air entry. The RT should be ready to assist in ETT suctioning, if required emergently.
- Bedside nurse should check whether all the infusion pumps are turned on and the power cords plugged in. If the patient is being paced, verify whether pacemaker is functioning appropriately and note down the settings.
- PCICU technician should first transfer the SpO$_2$ cable onto the ICU monitor. This is followed by the transfer of the pressure module to the ICU monitor. At least one monitoring modality should be available at any point of time during the process of transferring the modules. If the pressure cables are tangled it should be reconnected one at a time. Alternatively, the monitoring module can also be transferred en bloc to the PCICU monitor.

The 2-minute checklist should be read out by the team leader or buffer nurse once the pressure cables are transferred and hemodynamic parameters are available on the ICU monitor. A suggested model of the 2-minute checklist is depicted in **Annexure 3**.

Information Handover

Once the patient is safely transferred to ICU bed and monitoring equipment, the OR team should handover the critical information pertaining to the patient, to the ICU team. This exchange of information should be attended by the anesthesiologist from OR, intensivist on call in PCICU, a member of the surgical team, bedside nurse and on-call pediatric cardiologist. Several studies have shown that a streamlined handoff process or use of a preformed handoff tool can minimize information omissions and improve communication with minimal errors.[4–6]

The information exchange should summarize the cardiac diagnosis, significant preoperative issues (requirement of ventilator/inotropic support/concerns of infection), details of intubation, intravascular lines, surgical procedure, cardiopulmonary bypass time, cross-clamp time, intraoperative concerns and significant hemodynamic events, bleeding issues, blood product usage, inotropes and other infusions, concerns with regard to ventilation, plan for extubation, indication for pacing, if being paced and the settings, expected concerns in the immediate postoperative period, and the timing of last dose of paralysis/sedation/antibiotic. The accompanying surgeon should handover the details of surgical procedure to the PCICU team, and share information on problems that are likely to be anticipated in the immediate postoperative period. Procedural notes should be promptly written thereafter.

Post-handover Phase

Post-handover phase demands continuing vigil by the ICU intensivist and the bedside nurse.

Annexure 3: Postoperative and post-sternal closure checklist.

S. No	2 Minutes checklist	Yes	No	Remarks
1.	**Ventilator parameters:**			
A	Has the patient been connected to the ventilator and humidifier is on?			
B	Is the chest expansion adequate?			
C	Air entry equal on both sides?			
D	Has the appropriate FiO_2 been set?			
2.	**Infusion pumps:**			
A	Power codes connected and switched on?			
B	Infusion pumps running as per the rate and dose specified in OT shifting chart			
C	All the three-way taps are tight and online			
3.	**Pacemaker:**			
A	Is the patient being paced?			
B	Is the set pacing rate corresponding to monitor rate?			
4.	Is the radiant warmer/Bair Hugger on?			
5.	Is the ICD suction on?			

S. No	5 Minutes checklist			
1.	**Monitor:**			
A	Arterial transducer zeroed and online			
B	Venous transducer zeroed and online			
C	Is the transducer in proper position			
D	Monitor for appropriate ECG leads			
E	Pacemaker functioning			
F	Pulse oximeter connected			
G	Temperature probe in place			
H	Is the patient being warmed			
2.	**Ventilator parameters:**			
A	Is the chest expansion adequate?			
B	Has the appropriate rate and tidal volume set?			
C	Has the appropriate PEEP and PS set?			
D	Is the peak airway pressure normal?			
3.	**Infusion pumps:**			
A	Are all pumps running on main power supply?			
B	Drug concentration checked according to the weight of the patient			
C	Syringe pump pressure limits set to level 3/4			
D	All three-way taps opened and online			
E	Is the injection port connected			

Contd…

Contd...

4.	**Chest tubes**
A	Clamps on chest tubes removed
B	Is the low suction connected and switched on?
5.	**Invasive line site:**
A	Proper dressing
B	Oozing
C	Edema/discoloration
6.	Is there any oozing from the surgical site
7.	Are there any signs of pressure sore
8.	Are there any blister/burns
9.	Urinary catheter – Any kinks/disconnection

Name: ....   **Name of the Staff checked:** ....

MRD NO: ....   **Date and Time:** ....

The bedside nurse should assess the following critical points

- Assess perfusion by noting pedal pulses
- Assess breath sounds and heart sounds
- Check inotropes and other infusions as well as confirm the drug dose and rate
- Check all lines for air and patency
- If the patient is being paced, the settings have to be documented
- Ensure that the temperature probe is in situ and that the overhead warmer is functioning (especially in infants and neonates).

The buffer nurse should ensure the following action items:

- Ensure that low suction is applied to all chest tubes (except in open sternum cases)
- Obtain vital signs and record on flow sheet
- Record the level of drainage and the urine output on the flow sheet
- Record the inotrope infusions and their rates on the flow sheet when read out by the bedside nurse
- Send the initial arterial blood gas (ABG) and laboratory tests

- Administer the prescribed medications and document the same.
- Request for a chest X-ray.

The 5-minute checklist should be completed once the patient is settled **(Annexure 3)**. The anesthesiologist on duty in the PCICU should remain at the bedside till the arrival of the first ABG and the patient deemed hemodynamically stable. Appropriate adjustments to ventilator settings should be made after the assessment of the first ABG.

This completes the process of transfer into the PCICU.

■ SUMMARY

Transfer of a patient after congenital heart surgery from OR to postoperative ICU, is a complex process that has to be executed with meticulous precision. To streamline the transfer and to minimize errors as well as information omissions during the process, the task is generally divided among a multidisciplinary team with allocation of specific roles to each member. The entire team of PCICU should be involved in the information handover following the physical transfer of the patient, so that key concerns and anticipated complications are clear to all the stakeholders.

■ REFERENCES

1. Joy BF, Elliot E, Hardy C, Sullivan C, Backer CL, Kane MJ. Standardised multidisciplinary protocol improves handover of cardiac surgery patients to the intensive care unit. Pediatr Crit Care Med. 2011;12:304-8.
2. Roth SJ. Postoperative care. In: Chang AC, Hanley FL, Wernovsky G, Wessel DL (Eds). Pediatric Cardiac Intensive Care. Baltimore: Williams and Wilkins; 1998. pp. 163-88.
3. Catchpole KR, De Leval MR, Mcewan A, Pigott N, Elliott MJ, Mcquillan A, et al. Patient handover from surgery to intensive care: Using Formula 1 pit stop and aviation models to improve safety and quality. Pediatr Anaesth. 2007;17:470-8.
4. Chenault K, Moga MA, Shin M, Petersen E, Backer C, De Oliveira GS Jr, et al. Sustainability of protocolised handover of pediatric cardiac surgery patients to the intensive care unit. Pediatr Anaesth. 2016;26:488-94.
5. Gleicher Y, Mosko JD, Mc Ghee I. Improving cardiac operating room to intensive care unit hand over using a standardized process. BMJ Open Qual. 2017;6:e000076.
6. Zavalkoff SR, Razack SI, Lavoie J, Dancea AB. Handover after pediatric heart surgery: a simple tool improves information exchange. Pediatr Crit Care Med. 2011;12:309-13.

Invasive Arterial Blood Pressure Monitoring and Care of Arterial Lines

Rakhi Balachandran, Amitabh C Sen

Reviewed by: Amitabh C Sen

■ INTRODUCTION

Invasive arterial blood pressure monitoring is routinely performed in all patients undergoing repair of congenital heart disease. Intra-arterial lines facilitate real time monitoring of arterial blood pressure as well as periodic arterial blood gas (ABG) analysis in critically ill patients after congenital heart surgery. A comprehensive understanding of various aspects of invasive arterial blood pressure monitoring is essential for members of pediatric cardiac team for efficient monitoring, and for maintaining the lines without complications in the postoperative period.

GOALS OF INVASIVE ARTERIAL BLOOD PRESSURE MONITORING

- For continuous hemodynamic monitoring of arterial blood pressure, and waveform.
- To obtain samples for blood gas analysis, and laboratory tests.
- To monitor the effects of vasoactive medications.

■ CHOICE OF SITE

Any peripheral arterial site can be chosen for monitoring based on the following facts:
- The vessel should be large enough to reflect the true systemic arterial pressure.
- Adequate collateral flow exists to the distal tissues perfused by the vessel.
- The nature of the cardiac defect and the site, and side of the lesion (e.g., repair

of coarctation of aorta, Blalock-Taussig shunt).

Frequently cannulated sites in pediatric cardiac surgical patients are discussed here:
- *Radial artery*: This is a commonly used site of cannulation as it is peripherally located, easy to access and maintain, and has the least incidence of complications.[1,2] However, access may be challenging in low birthweight and preterm infants. Additionally, it may not provide a true reflection of the central aortic pressure at the time of weaning off cardiopulmonary bypass (CPB) due to effects of CPB on the vascular tone.[3] The choice of side depends on whether the blood flow to the arm is likely to be interrupted during surgery, e.g., Blalock-Taussig shunt, coarctation of aorta repair with subclavian flap plasty, etc.
- *Femoral artery*: This site may be used in situations where radial access is difficult or lower limb blood pressures need to be specifically monitored (e.g., coarctation repair), and in complex congenital heart surgeries where femoral arterial pressure monitoring may be more accurate after separation from CPB. An important consideration in patients with congenital heart disease is maintaining the patency of the vessel for future cardiac catheterizations as there is likelihood of thrombosis when there is prolonged residence of the catheter inside the artery. Femoral arterial cannulation is also

avoided if there is a need to preserve the artery for cannulation during CPB particularly in reoperative cardiac surgery. Compared to radial arterial cannulae, this line is more susceptible to accidental displacements in the postoperative period, due to patient movement.

- *Dorsalis pedis and posterior tibial arteries*: These are less frequently used sites for arterial cannulation. Systolic and pulse pressure recordings in dorsalis pedis are higher than radial or brachial pressures in children and hence should be interpreted with caution.[1] Proper fixation and use of stabilizing splints might be useful to avoid accidental displacements.

- *Axillary artery*: Though not a routine site for arterial cannulation, axillary artery may be used if there is need to monitor upper limb blood pressure when radial access is difficult. This arterial distribution has rich collateral supply through subclavian artery. Extreme caution should be taken to avoid accidental flushing of air bubbles into this line. Proximity of the catheter tip to aortic arch might increase the risk of air bubbles reaching the cerebral circulation in the event of arterial air embolism. Adequate precautions should be taken to avoid injury to brachial plexus during positioning of the arm or while performing the arterial puncture.

- *Brachial artery*: Brachial artery monitoring gives a better representation of the aortic pressure as compared to radial artery pressure,[4] but this artery is rarely cannulated because of lack of collateral supply and increased risk of ischemic complications. However, recent studies show safety and accuracy of brachial artery pressure monitoring comparable to that of radial artery.[4,5] Convincing data is sparse in pediatric population, though a study has shown safety in 200 cannulations in neonates undergoing cardiac surgery.[6] Ideally brachial artery cannulation, using a proper size catheter, may be reserved for only those patients who are extremely difficult to cannulate, to avoid arterial cut down, and extreme caution has to be maintained for monitoring ischemic complications.

ARTICLES FOR ARTERIAL LINE INSERTION

- Gown pack with sterile towel
- Sterile gloves
- Arterial line tray/suture removal set
- Chlorhexidine tincture
- Alcohol swab
- 1 cc syringe with 2% xylocaine for local anesthesia, dose diluted as per weight of child
- Catheter (BD Insyte™ of appropriate size- 24G, 22G or 20G)
- Pediatric guidewire
- No. 11 surgical blade
- Suture material (3-0 Nylon)
- Sterile transparent dressing
- 5 cm extension line with three-way
- 5 cc syringe
- Normal saline (heparinized saline flush systems are not recommended)
- Pressure monitoring tubing with flush system
- Arterial line transducer kit
- Pressure bag
- Splints
- Ultrasound machine with linear probe (5–13 MHz). Sterile ultrasound probe cover and jelly.

ARTERIAL PRESSURE MONITORING SETUP[7]

- Prepare the continuous flush system using normal saline, with the transducer, and make sure the system is devoid of air bubbles.

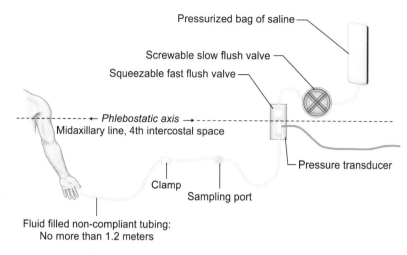

Fig.1: Continuous flush system and phlebostatic axis.
Source: www.derangedphysiology.com

- Attach the transducer cables to the monitor.
- Connect the catheter to the monitoring system once the catheter is placed intra-arterially.
- Level the transducer at the phlebostatic axis (4th intercostal space-mid axillary line and transducer should be taped to the bed) **(Fig. 1)**.
- Zero calibrate the transducer (choose the appropriate scale to get the best waveform and set appropriate alarm limits).
- Observe the arterial waveform **(Fig. 2)**. Obtain the pressure reading, and document on the flow sheet.
- Label date, and time on the pressure bag and tubing.
- In case of patients returning from operating room (OR), transducer and tubing with flush system will be provided from the OR.
- Apply secure dressing and label with date and time of insertion.

INSERTION CARE

The arterial line should be inserted under all aseptic precautions. Sterile equipment, gloves, and field should be used for the procedure. If guidewire exchange is anticipated, gown, and drapes should be used. Strict aseptic precautions should be emphasized by the bedside nurse using a checklist. The patient should be monitored for hemodynamic and airway instability during the procedure. The catheter should be securely fixed or sutured.

MAINTENANCE OF ARTERIAL LINES: NURSING CONSIDERATIONS

- Assess the pulse, color, warmth, capillary refill, movement and sensation of the distal extremity every hour.
- Assess the insertion site, and surrounding area for leaking, discharge, swelling or discoloration.
- Dressing changes are typically indicated once in every 7 days when transparent dressing is used.[8] However, if there is blood contamination under the transparent dressing or when the occlusive seal is broken, or when the dressing is dampened or soiled, it should be changed immediately. The date of dressing change should be documented.

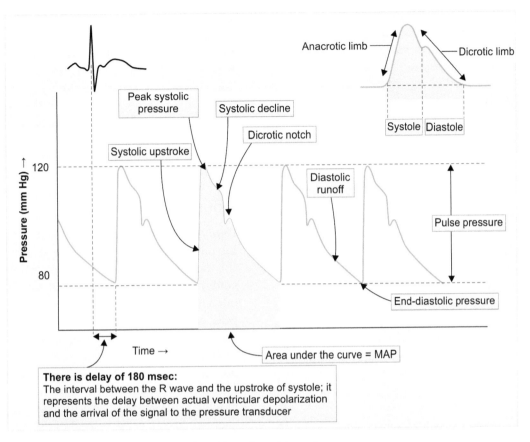

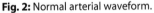

Fig. 2: Normal arterial waveform.

(MAP: mean arterial pressure)

Source: www.derangedphysiology.com

- Follow strict aseptic precautions while handling the access ports for sampling or flushing.
- Close observation of the monitoring system for the presence of any air bubbles and blood clots.
- Ensure that the pressure bag is inflated to 300 mm Hg and flush solutions are not exhausted.
- Monitor the extremities with the indwelling line for impaired perfusion or localized absence of peripheral pulses.
- Zero calibrate the transducer once every shift, or in case of any disconnections.

- Set appropriate scales and alarm limits for the monitoring system.
- Cross check with cuff pressures maintained at 300 mm Hg, at least once a shift and document in the flow sheet. If using a syringe pump for continuous flow, maintain a rate of 3 mL/h.[9]

CHANGE OF DRESSING AND INSERTION SITE CARE[7]

A dressing change is indicated if the existing dressing is saturated with blood, drainage or intravenous fluid or if the dressing or tape is loosened and the line is no longer secure.

- *Articles required*: Sterile transparent dressing, alcohol swabs, chlorhexidine solution, sterile gauze, dressing tray and sterile gloves.
- Two nurses are required to change the dressing. One person stabilizes the extremity and line while the other changes the dressing.
- Perform hand hygiene, and wear clean gloves.
- Remove the old dressing after securing the line.
- Observe the insertion site for signs of infection, redness, swelling, drainage or skin damage.
- Remove gloves, perform hand hygiene, and wear sterile gloves.
- Clean the insertion site with chlorhexidine solution. The strokes should be from center to outer aspect or in a circular fashion from insertion site outwards.
- Clean the catheter from insertion site to hub, being careful not to dislodge the catheter.
- Allow the chlorhexidine solution to dry completely.
- Apply transparent dressing.
- Observe the waveform for optimal position.
- Immobilize the extremity with appropriate sized splints.
- Remove gloves and perform hand hygiene.
- Label the dressing with date of insertion and date of dressing.

PROCEDURE FOR ARTERIAL BLOOD GAS SAMPLING

- Perform hand hygiene with alcohol solution, and wear hand care/sterile gloves.
- Wipe the sampling port with spirit or alcohol swab.
- Place a 2 × 2 gauze under the port, and attach a 2 mL syringe. Draw approximately 1 mL blood to minimize dilution. Then attach the heparinized 1 cc syringe to the port, and draw 0.3 mL blood for ABG. The initially aspirated blood is reinfused. The catheter is then flushed to clear blood remaining in the lumen.
- Flush the sampling port and the tubing completely free of blood by pulling the fast flush valve of the transducer. Clean the sampling port once again with spirit swab before applying the stopper to the port.

TROUBLESHOOTING

- *Dampened/absent waveform*: Make sure the patient is stable before manipulating the arterial line system. Only after confirming the hemodynamic stability by other monitors such as pulse oximetry and ECG, causes of damped system should be explored. Causes of dampened waveform include loose connections, clots or air bubbles in the line. Check pulse and cuff pressures. Make sure that there are no air bubbles in the system. Check for any loose connections. Check for distal perfusion, and blanching of extremity. If no evidence of spasm or impaired distal perfusion, reposition the extremity and re-tape it. Aspirate for blood return and flush with 0.3 mL of saline to improve waveform. If resistance is felt, do not flush forcefully.
- *Back bleed into the pressure monitoring lines*: This may be due to loose connections or partially opened stopcocks or damaged parts in the pressure monitoring system. If the site of loose connections is not obvious, then systematically check each part of the pressure monitoring system, and identify the site of problem.
- *False reading*: This can be due to improper zeroing or calibration. For values that are grossly out of range, it is worthwhile to confirm correct measurements by rezeroing, and calibrating.

COMPLICATIONS: DETECTION AND MANAGEMENT

- *Bleeding from insertion site*: This may occur in coagulopathy, misplacement of the catheter, disconnections in the system or if the insertion site was dilated too much. If excessive bleeding is detected, check for misplacement of the catheter or any loose connections in the monitoring system. Prompt application of pressure dressing and correction of coagulopathy can help reduce the bleeding around the insertion site.
- *Infection*: The risk of bacteremia becomes significant when the catheter has been present for long time (>1 week). Change the site of insertion when the line has remained in situ for more than 1 week. Monitor the insertion site for discharge, leaking or discoloration. Change the dressings when indicated. Use aseptic precautions while accessing the arterial line. The tubing, flush systems, and transducer are changed under strict aseptic precautions every 48 hours. Maintain a closed system always. All three-ways and ports should be properly closed after sampling, and zeroing of the transducer.
- *Thrombosis and distal ischemia*: The risk of thrombosis increases with prolonged cannulation. The size of the catheter should suit the size of the vessel. At our center, a 24G Insyte™/cannula is used for all infants less than 5 kg for radial artery cannulation. A larger 22G Insyte™/cannula may be used for the femoral artery catheterization in patients weighing less than 5 kg. Older children, above 10 kg, may accept a 20G catheter in the femoral artery. Accidental injection of hyperosmolar solutions into the catheter can predispose to thrombosis. Improper maintenance of the flush system and lack of clearance of blood after sampling can also lead to clot formation.

Precautions:
- Monitor the adequacy of flush system.
- Ensure that the tubings are completely cleared of blood after sampling.
- Carefully observe the arterial tracing for loss of amplitude.
- Inspect the distal extremity for signs of poor peripheral perfusion (capillary refill, skin temperature, color, movement and sensation).
- If poor perfusion is detected the catheter should be removed.
- If the catheter is suspected to be blocked do not flush forcibly as this might dislodge a clot. Aspirate blood back into a syringe to remove possible clots rather than pushing them into the artery. The aspirated blood should then be discarded.
- *Vasospasm*: This will manifest as dampening of the arterial waveform, blanching of the extremity, and sometimes pain. Vasospasm can be induced by cold, rapid forcible flushing or accidental injection of hypertonic solutions through the line. 2 mL of 1% xylocaine injected through the extension port may minimize spasm. Rewarming after CPB may also improve vasospasm.
- *Accidental injection*: This is a technical error. Arterial lines should be labeled. No drug should be injected through the arterial line. If accidental intra-arterial injection occurs, the catheter should not be immediately removed as it can be used to administer therapeutic agents such as preservative free lignocaine or papaverine to prevent reflex vasospasm. It is important to maintain a close vigil for signs of ischemia in the affected limb. Sympatholysis with stellate ganglion block or caudal block may also be beneficial

to reduce vasoconstriction and improve peripheral perfusion.

- *Air embolism*: Air bubbles can be readily introduced into arterial catheters because of the transit of fluid from the flush system, loose connections or during sampling, and flushing of the line. The bedside nurse should perform strict air-checks every hour while recording vital signs. Monitor for loss of amplitude of the waveform, which may indicate air in the line.

REMOVAL OF ARTERIAL LINE

The decision to remove arterial line is taken when it is no longer required for the post-operative care. Early removal of all invasive lines is recommended to prevent the development of complications and avoid catheter related bloodstream infections.

Articles

Suture removal set, sterile gloves, hand sanitizer, alcohol swabs, chlorhexidine solution, gauze pieces, and adhesive tape.

Procedure

- Obtain physician orders for removal of arterial line
- Perform hand hygiene, do skin preparation with chlorhexidine solution, close the three-way
- Remove sutures for central arterial lines
- Hold gauze and remove catheter
- Apply pressure for 5 minutes
- Apply dressing
- Remove gloves
- Perform hand hygiene
- Document date and time of removal on flow sheet.

SUMMARY

Invasive arterial blood pressure monitoring is part of the standard hemodynamic monitoring after congenital heart surgery. Careful

attention is warranted during insertion, and maintenance of lines to prevent complications; and ensure patency of line during use, in critically ill patients. Early removal of line is advocated as soon as the line is nonessential for postoperative care to minimize catheter related complications.

REFERENCES

1. Lake CL, Edmonds HL. Monitoring of the pediatric cardiac patient. In: Lake CL, Booker PD (Eds). Pediatric Cardiac Anesthesia, 4th edition. Philadelphia: Lippincott Williams and Wilkins; 2005. pp. 190-227.
2. Adatia I, Cox PN. Invasive and noninvasive monitoring. In: Chang AC, Hanley FL, Wernovsky G, Wessel DL (Eds). Pediatric Cardiac Intensive Care. Baltimore: Lippincott Williams and Wilkins; 1998. pp. 137-47.
3. Chauhan S, Saxena N, Mehrotra S, Rao BH, Sahu M. Femoral artery pressure are more reliable than radial artery pressures on initiation of cardiopulmonary bypass. J Cardiothorac Vasc Anaesth. 2000;14:274-6.
4. Singh A, Bahadorani B, Wakefield BJ, Makarova N, Kumar PA, Zhen-Yu Tong M, et al. Brachial arterial pressure monitoring during cardiac surgery rarely causes complications. Anesthesiology. 2017;126:1065-76.
5. Lakhal K, Robert-Edan V. Invasive monitoring of blood pressure: a radiant future for brachial artery as an alternative to radial artery catheterisation? J Thorac Dis. 2017;9(12):4812-6.
6. Schindler E, Kowald B, Suess H, Niehaus-Borquez B, Tausch B, Brecher A. Catheterization of the radial or brachial artery in neonates and infants. Paediatr Anaesth. 2005;15(8):677-82.
7. Stanford University. LPCH Intensive Care Protocols. [online] Available from: https://med.stanford.edu/peds/rotations/core/picu.html. [Last Accessed February; 2021].
8. Centers for Disease Control and Prevention. CDC guidelines for prevention of intravascular catheter related infections, 2011. [online] Available from: https://www.cdc.gov/infectioncontrol/pdf/guidelines/bsi-guidelines-H.pdf. [Last Accessed February; 2021].
9. Robertson-Malt S, Malt GN, Farquhar V, Greer W. Heparin versus normal saline for patency of arterial lines. Cochrane Database Syst Rev. 2014;2014(5):CD007364.

Central Venous Catheters in Pediatric Cardiac Patients

Rakhi Balachandran
Reviewed by: Aveek Jayant

■ INTRODUCTION

Central venous catheters (CVCs) are often placed in pediatric cardiac surgical patients to facilitate hemodynamic monitoring, to administer intravenous fluids or medications and occasionally for postoperative parenteral nutrition.[1,2] In our practice, CVCs are placed most often in the operating room (OR) under anesthesia and sometimes in the pediatric cardiac intensive care unit (PCICU) or in cardiac catheterization laboratory. CVC insertion and its maintenance in critically ill children have its own share of complications which can occur either during insertion or due to its long-term residence in a central vein.[3] With the near universal use of ultrasound in our practice the mechanical complications during catheter insertion have become rare; the infectious complications of an invasive device in the bloodstream have arguably come to the fore. This chapter intends to provide an overview of management of CVCs in pediatric cardiac surgical patients.

▌ DEFINITION AND SITE OF CANNULATION

Central venous access is defined as placement of a catheter such that the catheter is inserted into one of the venous great vessels, namely superior vena cava (SVC), inferior vena cava (IVC), brachiocephalic vein, internal jugular vein (IJV), subclavian vein, iliac vein or common femoral vein. For the purpose of central venous pressure (CVP) monitoring, the tip of the CVC should be placed in the distal SVC, SVC/right atrium (RA) junction, or in the IVC, at or above the level of the diaphragm. These are the largest veins with the highest flow rate in the venous system. Infusion of cytotoxic, hypertonic, hypotonic, acidic or alkaline solutions in these locations minimizes the risk of venous thrombosis, drug infiltration or extravasation, and vessel perforation.

Typically for pediatric cardiac surgery, the favored sites of CVC insertion are the IJV, subclavian vein or femoral vein. Though the subclavian vein site is recommended for short-term non-tunneled CVCs to lower infection risk in adult patients, there has been no guidelines in pediatric age group.[4] The choice of site also depends upon anatomical considerations such as the presence of dextrocardia, bilateral SVC and surgical considerations such as Glenn shunt/Fontan procedure where jugular venous pressure may not reflect the true CVP. Ultrasound guided cannulation technique has become a popular aid in CVC insertion, facilitating the ease of insertion as well as limiting complications.[5]

The right IJV is the most common route for central venous access in most congenital heart repairs as the vein follows a straight course to the RA and is easily accessible with the landmark method.[6] Left IJV is generally avoided since it may sometimes connect to a persistent left sided superior vena cava (LSVC) draining into an unroofed coronary sinus. Additionally there is the potential risk of chylothorax due to accidental injury to the thoracic duct or venous thrombosis.[7,8] Subclavian route is not usually preferred since the catheter can get kinked during the placement of sternal retractors during cardiac surgery although intensive care groups caring for neonates are exploring the use of ultrasound-guided supraclavicular or confluence access in small neonates with high success. It is rational to avoid cannulating femoral vein as there is likelihood of thrombosis due to higher catheter-lumen ratio in small infants and to preserve venous patency for future cardiac catheterizations or interventional procedures. However in patients with univentricular physiology undergoing cavopulmonary connections, femoral site is often preferred by clinicians to minimize the incidence of SVC thrombosis. A peripherally inserted central catheter (PICC) may be considered in patients who require longer duration of central venous lines for administration of medications or for parenteral nutrition.[9]

A suggested protocol for CVC cannulation in PCICU is described here.

ARTICLES REQUIRED FOR CVC CANNULATION

- Sterile gown pack with a hand towel
- Sterile gloves
- 2.5% chlorhexidine gluconate with alcohol solution (chlorhexidine tincture)
- Linen pack
- Central line tray with a fenestrated sterile drape (Hole towel)
- CVC—4Fr double lumen/5.5Fr triple lumen
- BD Insytes™—24G, 22G
- *Surgical blade*: No. 11
- Normal saline
- 1 mL syringe with 1% lignocaine for local anesthesia
- 5 mL syringe
- *Sterile gauze pieces*: 2 cm × 2 cm
- 3-way with stopcock
- *Suture material*: 3-0 Nylon
- Sterile transparent dressing
- Pressure monitoring tubing with continuous flush system
- Transducer kit with cables
- Pressure bag
- Sterile plastic cover for ultrasound probe
- Ultrasound machine with linear probe.

CATHETER CHARACTERISTICS

Polyurethane/Teflon (Polytetraflouroethylene) catheters are preferred over polyvinyl chloride (PVC) or polyethylene catheters due to fewer infectious complications.[4]

The size of the catheter is determined by age of the patient and the size of the vein. A 4 Fr double lumen 5 cm catheter is preferred in neonates and young infants weighing <5 kg. 5.5 Fr triple lumen catheters are preferred in older children. In order to minimize the risk of bloodstream infection, it is reasonable to use a catheter with minimum number of ports or lumens essential for management of the patient.

PREINSERTION PROCEDURE

- Explain the procedure to the patient, and family as appropriate, and obtain written consent.
- Follow nil per os (NPO) instructions in nonventilated patients for procedural sedation if required.
- Ensure that coagulopathies are corrected before the procedure.

- Assemble all the essential supplies by the bedside before the commencement of the procedure.
- Ensure that appropriate monitors are in place—ECG, SPO$_2$, NIBP/invasive arterial pressure, and temperature monitoring.
- Emergency resuscitation drugs and equipment (Pediatric crash cart, defibrillator, and temporary pacemaker) should be available at the bedside to manage any hemodynamic complications that might occur during the procedure.
- Bedside nurse should read the central line insertion checklist before the commencement of the insertion. A model of central line insertion bundle checklist is shown in **Figure 1**.

■ INSERTION CARE

- 3 minutes hand washing with chlorhexidine scrub solution should be done by the inserting physician.

- CVC should be inserted aseptically using maximal sterile barrier precautions. The bedside nurse should monitor the inserting practitioner for breach in sterile precautions. Physician must wear cap, mask, sterile gown, sterile gloves, and maintain strict aseptic technique throughout the procedure.
- Prepare skin with 2.5% chlorhexidine gluconate tincture (30 seconds scrub) before CVC insertion. Though the use of chlorhexidine gluconate for skin preparation has not been approved for neonates, several centers are using this agent without major adverse effects. (If chlorhexidine is contraindicated due to previous hypersensitivity reactions povidone-iodine solution can be used. Allow 2 minutes contact time for skin disinfection if povidone-iodine solution is used). Allow the antiseptic to dry prior to insertion.

AIMS: INSERTION BUNDLE CHECKLIST Dept. of Infection Control				
Name:			Dr./Dept:	
Central line insertion date:		Date of U. Catheterization:	Date of intubation:	
Inserted by:		Inserted by:	Intubated by:	
CENTRAL LINE BUNDLE CHECKLIST		U. CATHETER BUNDLE CHECKLIST	INTUBATION CHECKLIST	
☐	Hand hygiene performed before catheter insertion and manipulating the catheter	☐ Hand hygiene performed before catheter insertion	☐	Hand hygiene performed before intubation
☐	Maximal barrier precautions followed (gown, gloves, mask, etc.)	☐ Aseptic technique followed/ sterile equipment used	☐	Aseptic technique followed
☐	Chlorhexidine skin antisepsis done	☐	☐	Sterile/disinfected equipment used
☐	Optimal catheter site selection (preferrably subclavian)	☐ Proper disinfection of insertion site done	☐	Maximal barrier precautions followed (gloves, mask, cap, etc.)
☐	Catheter insertion is documented/ labeled (date, time, and personnel)	☐ Application of lubricant or anesthetic gel	☐	Oral suction done before insertion
☐	Antiseptic dressing done	☐ Catheter gently inserted	☐	ET-tube gently inserted
Comments if any:		☐ Replace if a break in asepsis occurs	☐	Used sterile suction catheter and gloves for each ET-suctioning
		☐ Proper securing of catheter in the bladder	☐	Checked cuff pressure and dislocation of ET-tube done
		☐ Catheterization is documented/ labeled (date, time, and personnel)	☐	Proper securing of ET-tube done

Fig. 1: A prototype of bundle checklist.

- The patient should be monitored for airway and hemodynamic compromise during the procedure.
- Ultrasound guidance is recommended if equipment is available to reduce the number of cannulation attempts and prevent mechanical complications.
- After insertion, location of the tip of the catheter should be confirmed from the waveform and pressure recording.
- All catheters should be sutured in place with 3-0 Nylon to prevent migration and inadvertent removal. The catheter tip location should be verified immediately after insertion with the help of a chest X-ray.
- Use sterile transparent dressing to cover the insertion site. The transparent dressing permits visual inspection of the exit site and minimizes the need for frequent dressing changes. However if, the insertion site is oozing/bleeding, gauze and tape dressing can be used till this resolves.
- Do not use any topical antibiotic at the insertion site.
- The date and time of catheter placement should be documented on the top of the dressing.

CVC MONITORING SYSTEM AND TRANSDUCER SETUP

- Prepare the continuous flush system with the transducer and make sure the system is devoid of air bubbles. Normal saline is used as continuous flush for CVCs.
- Attach the transducer cables to the monitor.
- Connect the catheter to the monitoring system once the catheter tip is located in the SVC-RA junction.
- Level the transducer at the phlebostatic axis (i.e., 4th intercostal space in the mid axillary line). Transducer is typically taped to the patient bed.
- Zero—calibrate the transducer (choose the appropriate scale to get the best waveform and set appropriate alarm limits).
- Obtain the pressure reading, and document on the flow sheet.
- Label date, and time on the pressure bag and tubing.
- In case of patients returning from OR, transducer and tubing with flush system will be provided from the OR.

NORMAL CVP WAVEFORM

The normal CVP waveform is depicted in **Figure 2**.

CVC COMPLICATIONS

Monitor the patient for probable complications of central venous catheterization[10] during and after the insertion.

Immediate

- *Inadvertent arterial puncture with hematoma formation*: Accidental arterial puncture is a frequent complication following CVC insertion.[11] Ultrasound-guided techniques are generally preferred to minimize this complication and to ensure high success rates.[12] In the event of a hematoma, local compression of the site with gauze dressing will usually control the bleeding, and limit hematoma formation. The bedside nurse should also monitor the neck, arm or shoulder area for any swelling which may appear after the insertion.
- *Pneumothorax*: This is a potential complication which can occur after subclavian vein cannulation. This can be identified clinically by low oxygen saturations, reduced air entry/breath sounds in the ipsilateral hemithorax, increased air leak from chest drains, and occasionally subcutaneous emphysema. In a nonventilated patient, there may be a sudden onset tachypnea, and

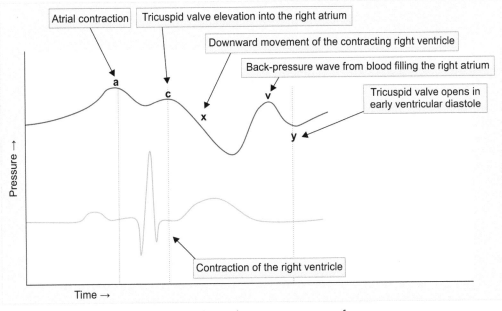

Fig. 2: Normal central venous pressure waveform.
Source: www.derangedphysiology.com

desaturation. A tension pneumothorax can also cause hemodynamic instability. It is reasonable to obtain a chest X-ray after central line insertion in the ICU to confirm the position of the catheter tip, and to rule out pneumothorax.

- *Arrhythmias:* Transient atrial or ventricular arrhythmias can occur during the passage of guidewire during central line insertion. This can be minimized by limiting the depth of guidewire insertion. ECG waveform should be carefully monitored for the occurrence of arrhythmias.

- *Air embolism:* This can occur when there is a negative pressure in the venous system or due to accidental flushing of air bubbles into the catheter. Paradoxical air embolism can occur if the patient has a patent foramen ovale or an intracardiac shunt. Entry of air bubbles into the coronary system can produce ST elevation in ECG waveform, tachycardia, and hemodynamic instability. Air embolism into the cerebral circulation can be one of

potential causes for postoperative stroke or seizures after congenital heart surgery.

- *Hemothorax:* Injury to a major blood vessel or RA/right ventricle (RV) perforation with nonflexible guidewires can rarely occur leading to bleeding, and hemothorax. It is usually identified by hemodynamic instability or increased bleeding from the intercostal drains.

Late Complications

Infectious Complications

- A *localized infection* at the catheter site can manifest as redness, swelling or oozing from the site. Patient may sometimes develop fever or tachycardia and the bedside nurse should vigilantly monitor for these clinical signs.

- *Central Line Associated Bloodstream Infection (CLABSI):* This is an important cause of morbidity in critically ill children in pediatric intensive care units.[13] A CLABSI is a primary bloodstream infection (BSI) in a patient who had a central line within 48 hours of the development of the BSI and is not related to an infection at another site.[14] This is not the same as catheter related BSI, which is a clinical definition that is used when diagnosing and treating patients, and requires specific laboratory testing that identifies catheter as the source of infection. Common causative organisms include gram positive organisms such as *Staphylococcus aureus, Coagulase-negative staphylococci (CoNS), Enterococcus, etc. and gram negative organisms such as Klebsiella pneumoniae, Escherichia coli and Pseudomonas aeruginosa*. A more specific diagnosis of catheter related bloodstream infection (CRBSI) follows from either demonstrating earlier time to positivity or colony count >10^5 colony forming units per mL from two specimens: one from the catheter and another from a peripheral venous site.

- *Occlusion*: Resistance to flow of infusion when attempting to flush a catheter may indicate occlusion. Aspiration with syringe may demonstrate inability to draw blood samples from the catheter. This can happen due to thrombosis or inadvertent kinking of the catheter. It can rarely be caused by precipitation of any medications or solution incompatibilities. Thrombosis is one of the dreaded complications after pediatric cardiac surgery. Neonates, patients with low oxygen saturation (<85%), use of deep hypothermic circulatory arrest, longer cumulative times of central lines, previous thrombosis, heart transplantation, and use of extracorporeal membrane oxygenation (ECMO) has been associated with postoperative thrombosis after pediatric cardiac surgery.[15] Thrombosis can be decreased by using a continuous flush system that ensures the patency of the catheter. Several centers prophylactically use a continuous heparin drip to prevent venous thrombosis in neonates and small infants with indwelling CVCs though there is no strong evidence in favor of heparin flushes when compared to normal saline for periodic flushing of the catheter. Precipitation occluding the catheter can also be limited to a large extent by taking care not to allow mixing of medications or solutions with known incompatibilities (e.g., calcium and bicarbonate). A collective team effort to remove CVC at the earliest possible window, seems to be the best strategy to prevent significant venous thrombosis.

CVC INSERTION SITE CARE AND DRESSING POLICY[16]

Transparent dressings are preferred as it offers visibility of the catheter insertion site while monitoring for signs of infection or bleeding. Transparent dressings should be changed every 7 days or sooner if it becomes loose or soiled. If gauze is used under the dressing, then the sterile dressings should be changed every 48 hours or sooner if it is soiled or loose. Assess and change gauze dressing as needed. Change to transparent dressing as soon as possible.

CVC DRESSING CHANGE

Articles: Sterile transparent dressing, alcohol swabs, chlorhexidine solution, sterile gauze pieces, dressing tray, sterile gloves.
- Two nurses are required to change the dressing. One person stabilizes the patient and limits movement, while the other changes the dressing.
- Perform hand hygiene and wear clean gloves.
- Remove the old dressing and the tape, while securing the catheter.
- Observe the insertion site for signs of infection, redness, swelling, discharge and skin damage.

- Remove gloves, perform hand hygiene, and wear sterile gloves.
- Clean the catheter site with chlorhexidine solution. The strokes should be from the center to outer aspect or in a circular fashion from insertion site outwards.
- Clean the catheter if soiled from insertion site to hub, being careful not to dislodge the catheter.
- Allow the cleansing solution to dry completely.
- Apply sterile transparent dressing.
- Observe the CVP waveform for optimal position.

CVC MONITORING AND MAINTENANCE[16]

Monitoring Guidelines

- Central venous lines should be continuously monitored for waveform, and pressure.
- Appropriate alarm limits should be set.
- Transducers are to be taped to the bed, and leveled at the phlebostatic axis.
- A continuous flush system with pressure infuser to be used at 300 mm Hg.
- Zero calibrate the transducers at least once a shift and with position changes.
- If using multilumen catheters, designate each lumen for a specific infusion or purpose. Use the distal lumen for CVP monitoring and blood sampling. Inotropes should be infused through a dedicated lumen. All infusions should be labeled at the proximal and distal ends of the extension lines.
- Use minimum number of three ways required for administering drugs or infusions through the central lines to decrease infectious complications.
- An injection port should be connected at the proximal access port for administering stat drugs which need to be given through the central line.

- CVC access ports should not be kept open. It should be closed with sterile end caps or needleless connectors.
- Monitor the system continuously for presence of air bubbles. Ensure that all air bubbles are removed after accessing the catheter or changing the IV tubing.
- Monitor the system for any backflow of blood into the extension lines. If noted to have any backflow, look for any loose connections or emptying of the continuous flush solution bag. The lines should then be flushed free of any traces of blood.
- Flush the catheters using push-pause technique to increase turbulence and more effectively clear the lumen. Ensure that all air bubbles are displaced from the lumens after accessing the catheter.
- All connections must be luer locked, to minimize catheter or tubing disconnection.

Catheter Maintenance

One of the key quality improvement interventions that has successfully brought down CLABSI have been the use of central line bundle checklists.[17] This refers to the systematic use of a group of evidence-based practices to prevent central line associated BSIs by all members of the health care team by the utilization of a prevention bundle checklist. Typically the bundle checklist action items should be monitored while maintaining the catheter in PCICU. A prototype of a composite bundle checklist for preventing hospital acquired infections that is utilized at our center is provided as **Figure 3**. In patients with CVC in PCICU ensure the following points:

- Follow the central line bundle checklist for maintenance of the catheter.
- The duration for which the catheter is maintained in the postoperative period, is dictated by the clinical need and assessed daily during multidisciplinary rounds.

Pt. Name:	MRD No.	Dr./Dept	ICU

CENTRAL LINE BUNDLE FOLLOW-UP

CENTRAL LINE REMOVED ON: DONE BY:

	DAY 1			DAY 2			DAY 3			DAY 4			DAY 5			DAY 6			DAY 7		
	Shift 1	Shift 2	Shift 3	Shift 1	Shift 2	Shift 3	Shift 1	Shift 2	Shift 3	Shift 1	Shift 2	Shift 3	Shift 1	Shift 2	Shift 3	Shift 1	Shift 2	Shift 3	Shift 1	Shift 2	Shift 3
Hand hygiene performed before and after manipulating the catheter																					
Hub cleaning done before accessing the catheter																					
Daily review of catheter insertion site																					

U. CATHETER BUNDLE FOLLOW-UP

FOLEY'S CATHETER REMOVED ON: DONE BY:

	Shift 1	Shift 2	Shift 3	Shift 1	Shift 2	Shift 3	Shift 1	Shift 2	Shift 3	Shift 1	Shift 2	Shift 3	Shift 1	Shift 2	Shift 3	Shift 1	Shift 2	Shift 3	Shift 1	Shift 2	Shift 3
Proper fixing of catheter on thigh																					
Urobag not touching the floor																					
Urine flow should remain unobstructed																					
Perform routine hygienic metal care																					
Hand washing done after catheter/urobag manipulation																					
Maintaining closed drainage system																					
Uro bag emptied every 6 hours																					
Proper disinfection of sample collection site																					
Urine aspirated for culture using sterile needle and syringe																					
Specimen transported to lab within 2 hours of collection																					
Sterility maintained throughout the procedure																					
Hand washing done after removal of gloves																					

VENTILATOR BUNDLE FOLLOW-UP

DATE OF EXTUBATION: DONE BY:

	Shift 1	Shift 2	Shift 3	Shift 1	Shift 2	Shift 3	Shift 1	Shift 2	Shift 3	Shift 1	Shift 2	Shift 3	Shift 1	Shift 2	Shift 3	Shift 1	Shift 2	Shift 3	Shift 1	Shift 2	Shift 3
Head elevation (30–45°C)																					
Antiseptic oral care																					
Daily sedation vacation																					
PUD prophylaxis																					
DVT prophylaxis																					
Assessment of readiness to extubate																					

Instructions: If "Yes" place "√" or "x" if "No"/Please write comment (if any) in the respective box.

Fig. 3: A prototype of maintenance bundle checklist.

- The catheter should be promptly removed as soon as it is not essential for patient care.
- The catheter site should be monitored regularly for any evidence of infection and leaking.
- If the catheter is suspected as a source of infection, it should be promptly removed.

Accessing the Catheter for Injection

- Minimize the number of manipulations, and entries into the catheter. Combine the tasks to decrease the risk of contamination.
- Perform hand hygiene using antiseptic soap and water or chlorhexidine hand rub before and after handling the catheters and IV system.
- Wear sterile gloves.
- The injection port should be wiped with chlorhexidine swab for 15 seconds. Attach the medication syringe or IV tubing to the port, taking care not to introduce air bubbles, and infuse the medication. After the medication is infused, remove air bubbles if any, and flush the catheter with normal saline by pulling the fast flush valve of the transducer.
- Flush and discard volumes may be less for fluid sensitive patients (<3 kg), and more for patients with larger catheters, but should be at least three times the catheter lumens' priming volume.
- Perform hand hygiene after accessing the catheter.

Blood Drawing

- Perform hand hygiene and wear clean gloves.
- Turn off all infusions briefly and clamp lumens not used for blood sampling before drawing blood.
- Draw the sample from the largest or the most distal lumen if possible.
- Place a 2 × 2 cm gauze piece under the sampling port.

- Clean the sampling port and aspirate 5 mL blood from the larger lumen. Then withdraw the amount of blood required for laboratories and inject into appropriate vacuette®. Reinfuse the initially aspirated 5 mL blood after drawing the samples for laboratories without any air bubbles.
- Flush the catheter and hub with normal saline and restart previously stopped infusions.
- If no medication is to be given, close with a fresh stopper/injection port.

REMOVAL OF CENTRAL LINE IN THE ICU

Articles: Suture removal set, sterile gloves, hand rub, alcohol swabs, chlorhexidine solution, No. 11 surgical blade, gauze pieces, and adhesive tape.
- Central lines should be removed when no longer essential, and early deintensification should be encouraged to minimize colonization and occurrence of catheter related BSI.
- The decision to remove the CVC should be taken based on the hemodynamic status of the child, requirement of inotropic supports, need for frequent sampling of blood and need for parenteral nutrition.
- Obtain confirmation from ICU physician.
- Two staff nurses are required, one to stabilize the patient, and another to remove the line.
- Stop infusions, and close the T-connector or three-way.
- Perform hand hygiene, and wear clean gloves.
- Remove the dressing.
- Skin preparation should be done with chlorhexidine solution.
- Stabilize the catheter, and remove sutures using the No. 11 surgical blade.
- Withdraw the catheter slowly.

- Apply manual pressure with gauze for at least 5 minutes, until bleeding is controlled.
- If bleeding is controlled, apply occlusive dressing to prevent air embolism through skin tract. Otherwise apply pressure for 5 minutes followed by pressure dressing and close monitoring.
- Inspect the catheter and make sure it is intact.
- Remove gloves.
- Perform hand hygiene.
- Document on flow sheet the date of removal, condition of catheter, and any associated complications during removal.

■ SUMMARY

Central venous pressure monitoring and use of CVCs are routine practices in postoperative period after congenital heart surgery. CVC can be associated with complications during insertion, and maintenance. Institution of care bundles helps to improve standard of care, and minimizes catheter-related complications. Prolonged duration of an indwelling CVC increases morbidity, and the team should collectively decide on catheter removal at the earliest.

■ REFERENCES

1. Heitmiller ES, Wetzel RC. Hemodynamic monitoring considerations in pediatric critical care. In: Rogers MC, Nicholas DG (Eds). Text Book of Pediatric Intensive Care. Baltimore: Williams and Wilkins; 1996. pp. 607-41.
2. Lake CL, Edmonds HL. Monitoring of the pediatric cardiac patient. In: Lake CL, Booker PD (Eds). Pediatric Cardiac Anesthesia, 4th edition. Philadelphia: Lippincott Williams and Wilkins; 2005. pp. 190-227.
3. Karapinar B, Cura A. Complications of central venous catheterisation in critically ill children. Pediatr Int. 2007;49:593-9.
4. Centers for Disease Control and Prevention. CDC guidelines for prevention of intravascular catheter related infections, 2011. [online] Available from: https://www.cdc.gov/infectioncontrol/pdf/guidelines/bsi-guidelines-H.pdf. [Last accessed February; 2021].
5. He C, Vieira R, Marin JR. Utility of ultrasound guidance for central venous access in children. Pediatr Emer Care. 2017;33:359-64.
6. Trieschman U, Kruessel M, Udink ten F Cate, Sreeram N. Central venous catheters in children and neonates (Part 2)—access via the internal jugular vein. Images Pediatr Cardiol. 2008;10:1-7.
7. Jadhav AP, Stahlheber C, Hofmann H. Traumatic chyle leak. A rare complication of left internal jugular vein cannulation. Am J Med Sci. 2011;341:238-9.
8. Saxena P, Shankar S, Kumar V, Naithani N. Bilateral chylothorax as a complication of internal jugular vein cannulation. Lung India. 2015;32:370-4.
9. Scott Warren VL, Morley RB. Pediatric vascular Access. BJA Educ. 2015;15:199-206.
10. Kusminsky R. Complications of central venous catheterisation. J Am Coll Surg. 2007;204:681-96.
11. Casado Flores J, Barja J, Martino R, Serrano A, Valdivieslo A. Complications of central venous catheterization in critically ill children. Pediatr Crit Care Med. 2001;2:57-62.
12. Lau CS, Chamberlain RS. Ultrasound guided central venous catheter placement increases success rates in pediatric patients: a meta-analysis. Pediatr Res. 2016;80:178-84.
13. Yogaraj JS, Elward AM, Fraser VJ. Rate, risk factors and outcomes of nosocomial primary bloodstream infections in pediatric intensive care unit patients. Pediatrics. 2002;110:481-5.
14. Centers for Disease Control and Prevention. (2020). NHSN Patient Safety Component Manual. [online] Available from: https://www.cdc.gov/nhsn/pdfs/pscmanual/pcsmanual_current.pdf. [Last accessed February; 2021].
15. Manlhiot C, Menjak IB, Brandao LR, Greunwald CE, Schwartz SM, Sivarajan B, et al. Risk, clinical features, and outcomes of thrombosis associated with pediatric cardiac surgery. Circulation. 2011;124:1511-99.
16. Packard L. Children's Hospital protocols (resource material). California: Stanford University; 2013.
17. Tang HJ, Lin HL, Lin HY, Lieung PO, Chuang YC, Lai CC. The impact of central line insertion bundle on central line-associated bloodstream infection. BMC Infect Dis. 2014;14:356-62.

Transthoracic Intracardiac Lines in Pediatric Cardiac Surgical Patients

Rakhi Balachandran, Brijesh P Kottayil

Illustration: Balaji Srimurugan

Reviewed by: Praveen Reddy Bayya

■ INTRODUCTION

Transthoracically placed intracardiac catheters have an established role in the perioperative hemodynamic management of patients undergoing congenital heart surgery. An increase in the complexity of congenital cardiac repairs and early corrective surgery for critical congenital heart diseases have resulted in increased utilization of these catheters in the perioperative period after congenital heart surgery.[1] Additionally, transthoracically placed right atrial lines form an important alternate route for venous access in very small neonates and infants (especially those undergoing single ventricle palliations) who are at risk for upper body venous thrombosis when neck veins are cannulated. Hemodynamic data derived from intracardiac lines help to assess the critical determinants of cardiac output namely preload, afterload, contractility as well as the transpulmonary gradients in cavopulmonary shunts. The waveform monitoring from these catheters can also give valuable information about rhythm disturbances and function of atrioventricular valves. However, the use of these lines have also been fraught with concomitant risks such as bleeding, need for reintervention, thrombosis and infection.[1,2] The commonly used intracardiac lines are right atrial lines, pulmonary artery lines and left atrial lines. Typically these lines are placed intraoperatively into their respective site and reinforced by a double purse string technique before separation from cardiopulmonary bypass under direct visualization. The intracardiac catheters are exteriorized by passing through a hollow needle brought out through a dependent and lateral location to the sternotomy wound so that it does not cross the midline and fixing the catheter to the skin with the aid of sutures. This chapter provides an overview of the different intracardiac catheters used in pediatric cardiac surgery and its management in the pediatric cardiac intensive care unit (PCICU).

■ TYPES OF TRANSTHORACIC INTRACARDIAC LINES

Pulmonary Artery Line

Though flow directed pulmonary artery catheters are available for adult patients for cardiac output monitoring, the utility in pediatric patients is limited due to small patient size and non-availability of suitable catheters in the very young patients. In neonates and children, a single lumen catheter inserted per operatively by direct puncture of the main pulmonary artery or placed through right atrium across the tricuspid valve, right ventricle and into the pulmonary artery, functions as the pulmonary artery (PA) catheter. When inserted through the right atrium the purported risk of bleeding at the time of the removal is lower since the entry point of the catheter is through the low pressure right atrium.[3] PA lines are brought out transcutaneously and sutured to the skin. PA lines should be transduced continuously and PA pressures monitored. Though generally transthoracic monitoring lines are removed in first 48–72 hours after surgery, in patients with labile pulmonary vascular resistance it is reasonable to leave them for a longer duration for optimizing hemodynamic management.

Common Indications

Pulmonary artery pressure monitoring is employed in children with high propensity for developing postoperative pulmonary hypertension, e.g., total anomalous pulmonary venous connection, truncus arteriosus, complete atrioventricular canal defects, large ventricular septal defect (VSD) with severe pulmonary hypertension, and for children undergoing pulmonary artery banding (to assess the appropriateness of the size of the band).

Hemodynamic Utility of PA Lines

- *Continuous monitoring of PA pressure and waveforms*: In patients with pulmonary hypertension, PA pressure has to be interpreted in relation to the systemic blood pressure.[4] Most consistently accepted definition of pulmonary hypertension is a mean PA pressure >25 mm Hg. A PA systolic pressure more than ½ systemic systolic pressure merits concern. It is also important to monitor the trends in PA pressure when an indwelling line allows continuous pressure monitoring in the postoperative period. Increase in PA pressure to systemic arterial pressure along with hypotension and desaturation is suggestive of pulmonary hypertensive crisis.

- *Monitoring of mixed venous oxygen saturation*: Mixed venous oxygen saturation measured from blood gas analysis of a sample obtained from PA line is a surrogate measure of adequacy of peripheral circulation and tissue oxygen delivery. A low cardiac output state results in increased tissue oxygen extraction and reduces the oxygen saturation of venous blood returning to heart. A value >70% in two ventricle physiology and a value >55% in single ventricle physiology is suggestive of adequate cardiac output.

- *Detection of residual intracardiac shunts*: An absolute PA oxygen saturation >80% at an FIO_2 <0.5 is indicative of a residual left to right shunt at ventricular level in patients who have undergone a VSD or tetralogy of Fallot (TOF) repair.[4]

- Administration of vasoactive medications if no other access is available.

- Change in pressures recorded on "pull back" of the PA catheter into the right ventricle can provide accurate information about the right ventricular outflow tract pressure gradients in TOF repair.[2]

Left Atrial Lines

Left atrial (LA) lines are single lumen catheters inserted per operatively through purse string sutures in the left atrial appendage or guided through the right superior pulmonary vein into the left atrium. The waveform monitoring provides guidance for appropriate placement of the line. This line is brought out percutaneously through the left side of the anterior chest wall and fixed to the skin with sutures.

Common Indications of LA Line

LA lines are usually inserted in patients who are likely to develop postoperative left ventricular dysfunction (e.g., repair of anomalous origin of left coronary artery from pulmonary artery, complex two ventricular conversion, etc.) and to monitor left atrial or common atrium filling pressures or transpulmonary gradients in patients with Glenn or total cavopulmonary connections.[3]

Hemodynamic Utility of LA Line

- *Left atrial pressure and waveform monitoring*: Typically, mean left atrial pressure (LAP) varies between 4 and 12 mm Hg and is often 1–2 mm Hg higher than right atrial pressure.
- Any LAP >14 mm Hg merits prompt evaluation. Common causes of elevated LAP include decreased ventricular function, poor left ventricular compliance, left ventricular hypoplasia, mitral valve stenosis or regurgitation, or cardiac tamponade. LAP is decreased in low intravascular volume status reflecting inadequate preload.
- To understand left ventricular function, preload and afterload.
- To detect left atrioventricular valve regurgitation and mitral valve function.
- To estimate the transpulmonary gradient, which is the driving force for pulmonary blood flow in patients after Fontan operation and thus guide postoperative hemodynamic management. Transpulmonary gradient is calculated as difference between central venous pressure (CVP) and LAP [Transpulmonary gradient (TPG) = CVP–LAP]. In patients undergoing Fontan, CVP measured via a catheter in the femoral vein is used for calculating transpulmonary gradient. This helps to differentiate various causes of low cardiac output in patients with Fontan physiology. Inadequate preload is indicated by a low CVP and low LA

TABLE 1: Causes of low cardiac output state (LCOS) in total cavopulmonary connections.[4]

Cause of LCOS	CVP	LAP
Hypovolemia (decreased preload)	Low	Low
Increased PVR	High	Low
Ventricular dysfunction (pump failure)	High	High
Fontan pathway obstruction	High	Low

(CVP: central venous pressure; LAP: left atrial pressure; PVR: pulmonary vascular resistance)

pressure. Elevated pulmonary vascular resistance is indicated by an elevated CVP and a low LAP. Pump failure is indicated by simultaneous elevation of both CVP and LAP. Anatomic obstruction of the systemic venous pathway is also indicated by a high CVP and a low LAP.[4] The trouble shooting of causes of low cardiac output state in total cavopulmonary connection or post-Fontan state is given in **Table 1**.

Right Atrial Lines

Transthoracic right atrial lines are inserted per operatively through a purse string in the right atrial appendage and brought out percutaneously through the right side of anterior chest wall. These lines are also used to provide important vascular access in extremely low weight infants less than 2.5 kg to avoid cannulating small neck veins and avert the potential risk of thrombosis. These lines are also used in some centers in patients with single ventricle physiology for ensuring patency of neck veins and preserve the integrity of superior vena cava for future single ventricle palliations. Additionally transthoracic right atrial lines may be resorted to in situations of difficult central venous access.

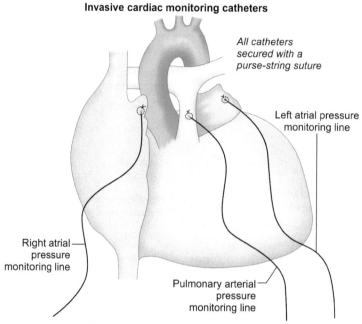

Invasive cardiac monitoring catheters

All catheters secured with a purse-string suture

Left atrial pressure monitoring line

Right atrial pressure monitoring line

Pulmonary arterial pressure monitoring line

Fig. 1: Intracardiac catheters in postoperative pediatric cardiac patient.

Uses

- Monitoring of right atrial pressures, which indicates right ventricular (RV) preload and function.
- Right atrial waveform monitoring: This gives valuable clinical clues in diagnosis of arrhythmias and atrioventricular valve function.
- Administration of vasoactive medications.
- For obtaining blood samples.
- For provision of total parenteral nutrition.

A diagrammatic representation of various intracardiac monitoring lines is provided in **Figure 1**.

GENERAL NURSING GUIDELINES FOR INTRACARDIAC TRANSTHORACIC LINES[5]

- All the lines should be labeled carefully, close to the catheter stopcock and near the transducer.
- Secure all the lines to the child. This is usually sutured onto the chest wall.
- Transparent dressing used at the exit site may be changed every 7 days.
- All the lines should be continuously transduced with proper alarm limits.
- All the lines should be zeroed with every shift and with every position change of the patient.
- All the lines should have continuous flush system with saline.
- All lines should be monitored for accidental disconnections, loss of waveforms and dislodgement.
- Close observation, to avoid air bubbles in all transthoracic lines.
- Chest tubes are generally maintained in patients with transthoracic lines in situ.
- All lines, which are inserted for monitoring purpose, can be used to administer drugs in an emergency situation when no other access is available. However, LA lines

should be cautiously used due to risk of embolism.

- The use of heparin drip at 1 unit/hour is reasonable to mitigate the risk of thrombosis.[3] When heparin drip is used, it should be stopped 4 hours before anticipated removal.

Though transthoracic catheters have been used for decades in pediatric cardiac surgery, there are wide practice variations in the nursing care management of these lines across institutions. Based on a multi-institutional survey transthoracic lines were utilized for accessing blood samples (68%), for administration of medications (75–93%) and for parenteral nutrition (58%).[6] Standard concentration of heparin (1 unit/mL of saline) for maintaining patency was used in 84% institutions and transthoracic lines were removed in ICU in 98% of institutions. Dressings are changed once every 7 days in most institutions (65%). 95% of nurses reported that the catheters were used for 3 days or more. In institutions, which allowed the lines to remain longer than 5 days, the catheter is more likely to be used for wider practices such as sampling and administration of medications and blood products.[6]

GUIDELINES FOR REMOVAL OF TRANSTHORACIC LINES

Timing

Transthoracic lines are usually removed in the ICU as soon as they are not essential for patient care. The removal of intracardiac lines is practically a blind procedure if the sternum is closed and may occasionally result in bleeding and major hemodynamic disturbances. If the transthoracic lines are present in open sternum patients they are removed at the time of sternal closure if they are no longer needed. This is to enable

immediate surgical intervention in the case of a serious adverse event during removal. If the lines need to be retained for longer duration for monitoring purposes they are not removed until at least 5 days postoperatively. Preferably the lines should be removed when intercostal drains (ICD) are in situ. The removal of an intracardiac line is typically performed by a member of the surgical team.

General Guidelines

- Transthoracic line removal should be done in the ICU only.
- Check recent coagulation parameters and hemoglobin concentration. Coagulation profile has to be normalized before removal. Preferably platelet count should be greater than $70,000/mm^3$, international normalized ratio (INR) < 1.6, fibrinogen level > 1 g/L.
- Transthoracic lines should be removed only in the presence of the ICU physician or cardiac anesthesiologist.
- Ensure nil per oral (NPO) status for procedural sedation if required.

Preparation

Preparation should focus on assembling necessary drugs and equipment. The following items should be arranged by the patient's bedside:

- *Drugs*: Anesthesia drugs (midazolam, ketamine, fentanyl, glycopyrrolate) and emergency drugs (adrenaline, atropine, calcium gluconate, 2% lignocaine and sodium bicarbonate)
- Crash cart
- Equipment for emergency intubation
- Ambu bag with appropriate size mask
- Oxygen mask or nasal cannula
- Packed red cells/ blood components should be arranged and readily available

if significant bleeding occurs during line removal.

Procedure

- Attach ECG monitor, SPO$_2$ and NIBP.
- Obtain adequate intravenous (IV) access if not already in place. Check the patency and function of an existing IV line.
- Sedative medications are administered in a titrated manner to obtain a quiescent state. Hypertension resulting from agitation or crying can predispose to bleeding during line removal.

Post Removal

- Document vital signs every 15 minutes for 1 hour and every 30 minutes for second hour.
- If ICD is in situ, monitor for drainage.
- Asses the child for evidence of bleeding and tamponade. This is identified by tachycardia, hypotension, pallor, respiratory distress, presence of blood in chest tubes if any, and altered mental status.
- Obtain a hematocrit 1 hour post removal or sooner if bleeding is suspected.
- If there is an evidence of bleeding or tamponade, notify the surgical team immediately. Prepare for resuscitation, emergent intubation and chest reopening.
- If uneventful, ensure that the child wakes up as the sedation wears off.
- Do not leave the patient unattended at least for 2 hours after the removal.
- Obtain a chest X-ray and ECG.
- Screening bedside echo to assess ventricular function and effusion.
- Patient should be shifted to ward only after ensuring adequate level of consciousness, hemodynamic stability and absence of bleeding confirmed by clinical evaluation and relevant imaging.

COMPLICATIONS OF TRANSTHORACIC LINES

Complications Occurring during Residence of Catheter

- *Catheter nonfunction*: Catheters are considered non-functional when there is dampened or absent waveform. It may also be associated with inability to aspirate blood or transfuse infusions through the catheter. This can be either due to catheter migration, kinking or thrombus formation. Catheter nonfunction should be reported to the surgical team and investigated systematically. Sometimes this may necessitate prompt removal of catheter.
- *Thrombus formation*: The known risk factors for thrombus formation are young age, prematurity and prolonged catheter use.[1] This will manifest as loss of waveform or inability to aspirate/infuse the line. An echocardiography can rule out thrombus in cardiac chambers or great vessels.
- *Catheter associated infection*: This is a potential complication which can increase postoperative morbidity. The risk factors for central line associated bloodstream infection in pediatric ICU include longer duration of use and presence of more than one central venous catheter.[7] In patients with transthoracic lines, open sternum was identified to be a risk factor for infection.[1] In a recent retrospective review of 2,736 central lines and risk factors for development of catheter associated bloodstream infections, right atrial lines and internal jugular lines had a lower rate of infection compared to peripherally inserted central venous catheters.[8] This highlights the

utility of right atrial lines in patients who need long-term central venous access in the postoperative period and in whom it is important to preserve venous patency for future interventions.

- *Air embolism*: Accidental injection of air into the transthoracic lines during access or flushing the catheter can cause air embolism.

Complications during Removal

- *Bleeding*: This is the most devastating complication associated with transthoracic line removal. Bleeding may manifest as increased chest tube drainage, hemodynamic instability or cardiac tamponade. Meticulous monitoring is required in the post removal period to detect this complication. This complication may require emergent return to operating room (OR) for surgical intervention. In a large study of 6,690 catheters, the overall bleeding rate was 0.22%.[2] However, the bleeding in this study was defined by chest tube drainage of 10–20 mL/kg, need for transfusion, cardiac tamponade or need for reintervention. Incidence of bleeding also varies with the type of transthoracic lines. Gold et al.[2] identified PA catheters to be more associated with hemodynamically important bleeding compared to RA and LA catheters. A subsequent study by Flori et al.[1] showed overall bleeding rate of 35%, however hemodynamic compromise was noted in only 2.6% of catheter removals. Though they encountered more bleeding with LA catheter removal, it was attributed to catheter placement technique and suturing. A more recent study concluded a higher bleeding rate with RA catheters attributing it to the thinner wall and higher fragility of right atrium.[9]

- *Catheter retention*: This is indicated by inability to physically remove the catheter at the time desired. This may occur due to knotting, migration or entrapment by fascial closure sutures. These patients require surgical intervention for successful removal. Fractured or embolized catheter tips may require intervention in cardiac catheterization laboratory for retrieval.

- *Need for reintervention*: Reintervention is often necessitated by bleeding, hemodynamic instability, catheter retention or fragmentation of the catheter tip.

■ SUMMARY

Transthoracic lines are frequently used for perioperative management in pediatric cardiac surgical patients as they provide valuable data on the critical determinants of cardiac output. Transthoracic lines are associated with a small but definite risk for complications such as bleeding, thrombosis, nonfunction and infection. However, with continued experience in use and establishment of well-defined protocols for monitoring and removal, transthoracic lines can be utilized with minor risks.[10] Meticulous nursing care and vigilant monitoring during its removal in the postoperative period are required to avert major complications. In centers, less experienced with the use of these lines, the risk benefit ratio has to be considered while utilizing these catheters in postoperative management of pediatric cardiac surgical patients.

■ REFERENCES

1. Flori HR, Johnson LD, Hanley FL, Fineman JR. Transthoracic intracardiac catheters in pediatric patients recovering from congenital heart surgery: associated complications and outcomes. Crit Care. 2000;28:2997-3001.
2. Gold JP, Jonas RA, Lang P, Elixson EM, Mayer JE, Castaneda AR. Transthoracic intracardiac

monitoring lines in pediatric surgical patients: a ten-year experience. Ann Thorac Surg. 1986;42(2):185-91.

3. Beham K, Dave H, Kelly J, Frey B, Hug MI, Brotschi B. Transthoracic intracardiac catheters in pediatric cardiac patients: a single center experience. Pediatr Anaesth. 2017;27:918-26.

4. Roth SJ. Post-operative care. In: Chang AC, Hanley FL (Eds). Pediatric Cardiac Intensive Care. Philadelphia: Lippincott Williams & Wilkins; 1998. pp. 151-87.

5. Stanford University. LPCH protocols (Resource Material). [online] Available from: http://med.stanford.edu/pedcriticalcare/patient-care/PICU.html. [Last Accessed March, 2021].

6. Lisanti AJ, Fitzgerald J, Helman S, Dean S, Sorbello A, Griffis H. Nursing practice with transthoracic intracardiac catheters in children: international benchmarking study. Am J Crit Care. 2019;28:174-81.

7. Ferreira La Torre FP, Baldanzi G, Troster EJ. Risk factors for vascular catheter associated blood stream infections in pediatric intensive care units. Rev Bras Ter Intensiva. 2018;30:436-42.

8. Garcia X, Pye S, Tang X, Gossett J, Prodhan P, Bhutta A. Catheter associated blood stream infections in intracardiac lines. J Pediatr Intensive Care. 2017;6:159-64.

9. Pratap H, Millar J, Butt W, d'Udekem Y. Complications of intrathoracic lines placed during cardiac surgery. J Thorac Cardiovasc Surg. 2015;149:1212-3.

10. Stein ML, Quinonez LG, Dinardo JA, Brown ML. Complications of intracardiac and central venous lines in neonates undergoing cardiac surgery. Pediatr Cardiol. 2019;40:733-7.

Fluid and Electrolyte Management in Pediatric Cardiac Intensive Care Unit

Rakhi Balachandran
Reviewed by: Aveek Jayant

◼ INTRODUCTION

Fluid handling and management of intravascular volume is crucial for optimizing tissue perfusion and hence oxygen delivery in the postoperative period after pediatric cardiac surgery. Both hypovolemia and hypervolemia can generate potential harm in these critically ill patients. The optimal fluid regimen is still unclear. The evaluation of the right amount, choice of fluids, and tailoring fluid strategies to suit the appropriate cardiovascular physiology are key challenges that intensivists face in pediatric cardiac critical care. Though "goal directed" fluid-management strategies have been proposed for individualizing fluid management in adult critically ill patients, techniques for accurately assessing fluid status and fluid responsiveness are not well-established in infants and children.

◼ PHYSIOLOGICAL CONSIDERATIONS

Two important physiological considerations that need to be understood are the distribution of total body water (TBW) and regulation of extracellular fluid volume. TBW is divided into extracellular (one-third) and intracellular (two-third) compartments. Extracellular fluid is distributed between the intravascular (one-fourth) and interstitial (three-fourths) compartments. The intravascular volume constitutes the effective circulating volume that maintains the perfusion of the tissues. This is the key fraction that can be manipulated through perioperative interventions. Though the intravascular and interstitial compartments are separated by capillary membranes, several physiological forces determine potential fluid shifts between these two compartments. Recent advances show that the integrity of the glycocalyx layer coating the vascular endothelium may be challenged by pathological processes involved in systemic inflammation, and hormonal changes resulting from excessive volume resuscitation, further aggravating the fluid shifts between compartments resulting in tissue edema.[1] This concept becomes particularly relevant in the context of systemic inflammatory response syndrome that occurs as a sequel to cardiopulmonary bypass (CPB) in patients undergoing cardiac surgery.

The percentage of TBW varies with age. In adults, TBW comprises 60% of lean body weight. TBW is 75–80% in newborns and its percentage decreases with age. The higher composition of TBW in the younger population compared to adults was attributed to the reduced fat content and increased muscle mass proportion.[2] The distribution of sodium critically affects water homeostasis, as it forms the most abundant extracellular cation. This is physiologically controlled by the hypothalamus and the juxtaglomerular

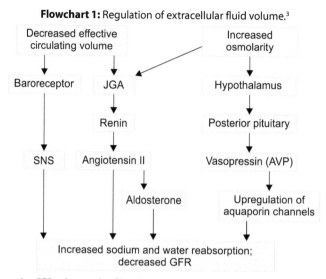

Flowchart 1: Regulation of extracellular fluid volume.[3]

(AVP: arginine vasopressin; GFR: glomerular filtration rate; JGA: juxtaglomerular apparatus; SNS: sympathetic nervous system)

apparatus of the kidney through a feedback loop. Hyperosmolarity sensed by the osmoreceptors in hypothalamus leads to upregulation of aquaporin channels in collecting duct in the kidney. Osmoreceptors in the kidney detect changes in the solute delivery as well as the volume status and promote water and sodium retention via the renin-angiotensin-aldosterone axis. The regulation of extracellular fluid volume[3] is shown in **Flowchart 1**. The higher percentage of the body weight in TBW and immature osmoregulatory mechanisms subject neonates and young infants to a higher risk of hemodynamic compromise in situations of volume depletion.[3]

SPECIFIC CHALLENGES IN PEDIATRIC CARDIAC PATIENTS

Patients who have undergone repair of congenital heart disease pose specific challenges. CPB and systemic inflammatory response is closely linked to fluid shifts that occur between osmotic compartments in the body. The impact of CPB is overwhelming due to its effect on hemodilution related to circuit prime and the systemic inflammatory response triggered by the exposure of the patients' blood to nonphysiological extracorporeal circuits. Additionally surgical losses, degree of hypothermia during CPB affecting vascular tone, use of diuretics and osmotic agents in the perioperative period, and cardiac dysfunction substantially impact fluid status and management.[4] The varying age of the pediatric cardiac surgical population and the diverse cardiac pathophysiology involved in each type of congenital heart disease necessitate an individualized fluid management strategy tailored to the patient profile.

Fluid overload (FO) is a well-recognized physiological disturbance associated with congenital heart surgery under CPB occurring in nearly 30% of infants.[5] Systemic inflammatory response, capillary leak syndrome, fluid resuscitation, and influence of the high volumes of CPB prime with hemodilution have been the common proposed mechanisms. In addition to this, several perioperative processes also lead to increased release of

Flowchart 2: Mechanisms for sodium and water disturbance after cardiopulmonary bypass.

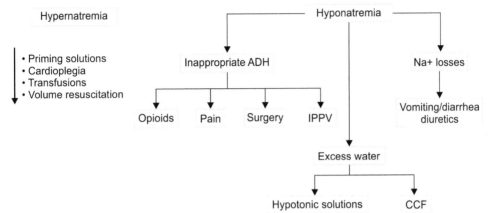

(CCF: congestive cardiac failure; IPPV: intermittent positive pressure ventilation; ADH: antidiuretic hormone)

antidiuretic hormone (ADH).[6] Disturbances in sodium homeostasis affect water balance resulting in postoperative salt and water overload after pediatric cardiac surgery (**Flowchart 2**). Excessive FO is being increasingly identified to be a major factor contributing to adverse perioperative outcomes by prolonging ventilation, delaying chest closure in neonates, increasing length of stay, limiting nutritional intake, and promoting acute kidney injury.[7] In a prospective study of 98 patients undergoing CPB, a fluid balance of 5% above preoperative bodyweight was associated with longer hospital stays, increased ventilation hours, prolonged inotropic requirement, and higher rates of acute kidney injury.[8] Hence, it is rational that perioperative fluid management strategies after congenital heart repairs have taken a paradigm shift from "volume liberal" strategy to "volume restricted" management to minimize FO and to expedite the postoperative recovery of patients.

In this chapter, based on available evidence and common clinical practice scenarios, we have attempted to summarize the current fluid management strategies in pediatric cardiac surgical patients.

GOALS OF POSTOPERATIVE FLUID THERAPY

The goals of postoperative fluid therapy are as follows:
- Maintain effective circulating volume to optimize organ perfusion and tissue oxygen delivery
- Avoid electrolyte imbalances
- Avoid FO, so as to minimize lung water/tissue edema.

POSTOPERATIVE FLUID REQUIREMENTS

Postoperative fluid needs can be classified into maintenance fluid requirements and replacement volume needed to compensate for perioperative losses. Maintenance fluid therapy should meet the fluid and electrolyte requirements needed by an average individual with normal intracellular and extracellular fluid volumes over a 24-hour period.

Maintenance fluid therapy:
- This meets the 24-hour requirement of fluid and electrolytes
- Accounts for insensible losses (evaporative loss)
- Accounts for urinary loss.

Replacement fluid therapy:

- This meets the ongoing abnormal fluid losses
- Replacement for blood loss
- Replacement for third space losses like chest tube output, peritoneal drains, etc.

Maintenance Fluid Requirement

Maintenance fluid requirements can be calculated using either the body surface area method (1,500–1,700 mL/m²/day) or the caloric expenditure method [100 mL/kg/day (<10 kg) + 50 mL/kg/day (10–20 kg) + 20 mL/kg/day (>20 kg)].[9,10]

In most units, the maintenance fluid requirements are calculated using the body surface area method. This method typically provides 50% of the estimated average daily requirement for a normal pediatric patient on the first two postoperative days. However, when it reaches 1,500 mL/m²/day it is almost equal to the expected daily requirement in normal pediatric patients with a weight of less than 5 kg. However, in general, considering the increased salt and water retention attributed to CPB, maintenance fluid requirements are reduced to one-half to one-third of the normal requirements in the early postoperative period (<72 hours) to facilitate extubation and deintensification. A suggested postoperative maintenance fluid strategy is provided in **Tables 1 and 2**. Caloric expenditure method may be followed in nonsurgical pediatric patients who may require intensive care in the pediatric cardiac intensive care unit (PCICU) (**Table 3**). Daily maintenance electrolyte requirements are depicted in **Table 4**.

Subsequent to the first day after surgery, fluid intake should be adjusted according to the clinical and laboratory evaluation of the patient's hydration and biochemical status. In the absence of systemic or pulmonary edema,

TABLE 1: Daily maintenance fluid allowance in pediatric cardiac patients undergoing surgery with CPB.

Day	Fluid-mL/m²/day	Comments
Day of surgery	500	Constitutes 50% maintenance compared to nonsurgical patients
POD 1	750	Can be increased in older children who are fast tracked
POD 2	1,000	However, in situations where fluids are to be further restricted the increments in fluid can be adjusted according to the discretion of intensivist
POD 3	1,250	
POD 4	1,500	

(CPB: cardiopulmonary bypass; POD: postoperative day)

TABLE 2: Fluid strategy in patients undergoing cardiac surgery without CPB (e.g., Blalock-Taussig shunts, patent ductus arteriosus ligation, coarctation of aorta).

Days	Fluid (mL/kg/day)	
DOS	60	
POD 1	70	Full maintenance requirements can be achieved over 3–5 days period in most stable infants
POD 2	80	
POD 3–4	(90–100)	

(CPB: cardiopulmonary bypass; DOS: day of surgery; POD: postoperative day)

TABLE 3: Caloric expenditure method (nonsurgical patients).

Weight	Fluid allowance
<10 kg	100 mL/kg/day
10–20 kg	1,000 mL + 50 mL/kg for each kg between 11 and 20
>20 kg	1,500 mL + 20 mL/kg for each kg > 20 kg

TABLE 4: Daily maintenance requirements of electrolytes for pediatric patients.

Electrolyte	Daily maintenance dose
Sodium	2–5 mEq/kg
Potassium	2–4 mEq/kg
Calcium	50–200 mg/kg
Phosphorus	0.5–1.5 mmol/kg
Magnesium	0.25–1 mEq/kg

fluid intake may be gradually increased to achieve full maintenance requirements over a 2–5 day period.

Special situations, which merits alterations in the standard maintenance fluid rate include:

- Systemic to pulmonary shunts to decrease the risk of shunt thrombosis from hemoconcentration.
- Cavopulmonary anastomosis—to provide adequate preload for nonpulsatile blood flow.
- Presence of postoperative pyrexia increases fluid requirement. A practical guide is to allow an increase in water intake by about 10% for each degree rise in temperature above 37.5°C.
- Severely malnourished infants in the recovery phase to permit adequate nutritional intake for catch up growth.

In these patients, the fluid allowance is tailored to the clinical status of the patient.

In patients weighing > 15 kg, maintenance fluid rates are initiated at 1–1.5 mL/kg/h in the first 24–48 hours and increased to 2 mL/kg/h from second postoperative day.

Choice of Maintenance Fluid

Traditionally, hypotonic fluids have been prescribed to perioperative pediatric patients. However, this strategy has resulted in an increase in the incidence of hyponatremia after surgery.[11-13] Hyponatremia had been linked to adverse neurological outcomes in pediatric patients who have been administered hypotonic fluids.[14] Hyponatremia facilitates translocation of free water from extracellular to intracellular compartments predominantly affecting the brain. Pediatric patients are vulnerable to the consequences of water translocation due to high-brain intracellular sodium levels (27% more than adults) and decreased Na^+–K^+ ATPase activity

creating a substrate for cerebral edema. This along with high brain/skull ratio facilitates rapid development of brain edema due to free-water movement into the brain cells.[6] A landmark review by Bailey et al., has brought to light the adverse effects of hyponatremia and hypernatremia in pediatric surgical patients challenging the long-favored tradition of administering hypotonic IV fluids like one-fourth normal saline in children.[6] Surgery under CPB is associated with the risk of both hypernatremia and hyponatremia.[15] The mechanisms for sodium disturbances after pediatric cardiac surgery have been previously elucidated in **Flowchart 2**. We also need to consider the increased requirement of glucose in neonatal population who are vulnerable to hypoglycemia while optimizing the composition of maintenance fluid. Normoglycemia during fasting cannot be maintained in neonates as reduced liver mass (glycogen stores) and muscle mass (protein stores) results in impaired glycogenolysis and gluconeogenesis.

Common fluids available for perioperative fluid therapy include crystalloids and colloids. The crystalloids include normal saline, 5% dextrose, dextrose normal saline, ringer lactate, and plasmalyte A, the last two being balanced crystalloids isosmotic with plasma. The most common isotonic fluid, normal saline is an unbalanced crystalloid and is known to produce hyperchloremic acidosis. In a recent pediatric trial in patients undergoing major surgery, patients who received normal saline had worse outcomes in terms of mortality, renal failure needing dialysis and acidosis along with other complications, compared to patients receiving a balanced crystalloid solution.[16] In a recent review by Rizza et al. the authors caution against the possibility of renal damage and acidosis while administering unbalanced crystalloids and favor a balanced crystalloid solution for maintenance fluid therapy in the pediatric cardiac surgical patient.[17]

Though, there is no high-quality evidence, current fluid recommendations suggest administration of a dextrose-added balanced crystalloid solution for maintenance therapy. Hypotonic fluids should be preferably avoided. Therefore, we suggest dextrose-added Ringer lactate solution or plasmalyte A for perioperative fluid therapy. The concentration of dextrose is dictated by the age of the patient. Neonates and young infants who are vulnerable for hypoglycemia may be prescribed 2.5–10% dextrose-added solutions to maintain blood glucose levels as well as to provide fluid and electrolyte requirements needed for metabolism.

Replacement Fluid Therapy

Replacement therapy targets replacement of ongoing abnormal fluid losses. This also includes the third space losses (chest tube output, peritoneal drains, etc.). Volume replacement in most pediatric units is typically provided by colloids, crystalloids, blood products, or human albumin. There are no established guidelines for ideal replacement fluids. Crystalloids do not remain in the intravascular compartment and are known to migrate to extravascular spaces leading to tissue edema. The common colloids in clinical use include human albumin, hydroxyethyl starches (HES), and gelatin. Human albumin is a frequently used colloid for volume replacement in many established cardiac surgical settings, even though a definite outcome benefit compared to other resuscitation fluids is not yet well-established. Though, its use in CPB prime had been supported by evidence suggesting a reduced positive fluid balance and lesser postoperative weight gain,[18] the data suggesting

superiority over other replacement fluids are lacking in postoperative pediatric cardiac surgical patients. Additionally, its efficacy in post-CPB inflammatory states or sepsis is also questionable as albumin leaks out of the intravascular compartment due to increased capillary permeability in these settings adding to tissue edema. The other disadvantages worth mentioning include infection risk and allergic reactions. Moreover, the use of albumin in low-middle income countries is limited due to prohibitive costs and the availability of cost effective alternatives such as HES. HES are synthetic colloids. The earlier generation of HES has been linked to coagulation abnormalities contributing to postoperative bleeding and worsening of renal function induced by renal tubular swelling due to these solutions.[19] The safety in neonates is also not well-established. Though, the earlier generation of HES have the above mentioned side effects the newer generation of low-molecular weight, low molar substitution ratio, 6% HES (e.g., Voluven®- MW 130/MS 0.4) seems to have a better safety profile in some pediatric trials with less impact on postoperative bleeding and renal complications. In a propensity matched analysis in 1,495 patients undergoing pediatric cardiac surgery use of newer generation HES (Voluven® 130/0.4) was associated with less-positive fluid balance, decreased blood product use and no increased renal morbidity compared to human albumin.[20] Due to the lack of high-quality evidence, synthetic colloids should be used with caution in pediatric patients especially neonates and adherence to the manufacturer specified ceiling dose should be meticulously followed.

Blood loss in the postoperative period may warrant packed red blood cells (PRBC) transfusion for volume resuscitation.

RBC transfusion in children has been associated with poor clinical outcomes.[21] Use of blood and blood components should be dictated by hemoglobin level and clinical markers of tissue perfusion. The ideal hemoglobin level is not clear. The two strategies that are commonly debated are a restrictive transfusion strategy and a liberal transfusion strategy. The various pediatric intensive care trials have chosen a range of 7–9.5 g/dL in the restrictive group and 9.5–13 g/dL in the liberal group. A landmark trial, TRIPICU (Transfusion Requirements in Pediatric Intensive Care) study, compared the outcome of new onset organ failure in hemodynamically stable critically ill children between groups, which are liberally transfused (Hb target <9.5 g/dL) and a restrictive group (Hb target <7 g/dL).[22] The restrictive group was not inferior in outcomes to the liberal group. A subgroup analysis of children undergoing cardiac surgery also demonstrated no worse outcomes in terms of organ dysfunction in the restrictive group. A prospective randomized trial that included single ventricle patients undergoing cavopulmonary connections (a subset that is likely to receive more blood transfusions in ICU) compared transfusion for hemoglobin < 9 g/dL with clinical indications (restrictive) and liberal, <13 g/dL irrespective of clinical indicators.[23] The mean hemoglobin levels were lower in the restrictive group with fewer transfusions and donor exposures. The restrictive group did not have any worse outcomes of tissue perfusion indicated by the difference in lactate levels or arteriovenous oxygen content or arteriocerebral oxygen content. This suggests that even children after single ventricle palliations can tolerate lower hemoglobin levels without compromising tissue perfusion. While comparing outcomes in children undergoing palliative procedures or biventricular repair for congenital heart disease using restrictive versus liberal targets (i.e., 7 g vs. 9 g/dL, respectively with clinical indicators for biventricular repairs and 9.5 and 12 g/dL, respectively for palliative procedures), there have been lower mean hemoglobin levels and fewer transfusions in the restrictive group. There was also no increase in peak/mean lactate levels, arteriovenous oxygen content difference or other adverse postoperative outcomes in the restrictive groups.[24]

Based on this evidence, children undergoing two ventricle corrections may be able to tolerate hemoglobin levels as low as 7 g/dL and those with single ventricle palliations can accommodate hemoglobin levels up to 9 g/dL.[25] However, rather than targeting a specific numerical threshold, attention to clinical indicators also merits consideration while choosing the hemoglobin trigger.

▌ HOW TO MONITOR FLUID STATUS AND INTRAVASCULAR VOLUME?

A thorough clinical evaluation will offer valuable clues to the fluid status and adequacy of perfusion in the postoperative patients. The common clinical indicators are listed below:

- *Clinical methods*:
  - Skin temperature (Warm extremities)
  - Adequacy and volume of peripheral pulses
  - Capillary refill time < 2S
  - Skin turgor/state of mucous membrane for assessment of hydration
  - Lung auscultation/cardiac evaluation
  - Mental status examination
  - Vital signs (HR, blood pressure, SaO_2)
  - Urine output
  - Fluid balance
  - Daily weight.
- *Laboratory parameters*: Electrolytes/arterial blood gas (ABG), blood urea nitrogen (BUN)/serum creatinine, hematocrit, urine analysis.

- *Surrogates of oxygen delivery*:
  - Central venous oxygen saturation (SVO_2 >70% in two ventricle physiology and >55% in single ventricle physiology)
  - Serum lactate levels < 2 mmol/L.

Assessment of Fluid Responsiveness

Fluid responsiveness implies that a bolus of fluid infusion produces an augmentation of cardiac output and a meaningful improvement in tissue perfusion. This can be assessed in intensive care setting by assessment of static variables or dynamic variables.

Static Variables

- Heart rate
- Systolic arterial blood pressure
- Mean arterial pressure
- *Preload pressures*: This include central venous pressure (CVP), pulmonary artery occlusion pressure, and left atrial pressure. Though, pulmonary artery catheterization is a gold standard for hemodynamic monitoring and cardiac output measurement in adults, its use in pediatric patients is restricted due to the small size and presence of intracardiac shunts. Left atrial pressure monitoring is used in some congenital heart repairs where ventricular dysfunction is anticipated (e.g., repair of anomalous origin of left coronary artery from pulmonary artery, complex biventricular conversions, etc.). CVP is the commonly available monitor to measure filling pressure in cardiac intensive care units; however, its reliability is challenged by factors which alter the ventricular compliance. In noncompliant stiff heart, CVP will be elevated even if the ventricles are underfilled. External factors like high ventilator pressures and increased intra-abdominal pressure may also influence the reliability of CVP.

Dynamic Variables

- These variables make use of variations in stroke volume and cardiac output resulting from cardiopulmonary interactions during mechanical ventilation. Positive pressure ventilation results in decrease in venous return during inspiration, due to increased intrathoracic pressure. This leads to a decrease in the right ventricular preload and right ventricular output. Subsequently, the left atrial venous return, left ventricular preload, and cardiac output will be reduced. The reverse happens during expiration. This variability becomes more pronounced in volume depleted hearts suggesting preload responsiveness. Stroke volume variation during respiratory cycle of greater than 10–15% indicates that patient is fluid responsive.[17] The changes in stroke volume are also reflected in arterial pressure waveform with pronounced respiratory variations. The disadvantage of this parameter is that the accuracy is questionable in nonventilated or spontaneously breathing patients, patients with open sternum (due to variation in thoracic and lung compliance) and in presence of arrhythmias.
- *Echocardiographic parameters*:
  - Variations in inferior vena cava (IVC) diameter during inspiration of >20% suggest fluid responsiveness. However, the results vary depending on the skills of the echocardiographer. Additionally, this is not a practical option for continuous bedside evaluation.
  - Respiratory variation in aortic blood flow velocity (ΔV peak) has emerged as a reliable predictor of fluid responsiveness in pediatric studies.[26] This technique demands considerable

operator skills and equipment to obtain reliable bedside results. It may also be affected by arryhthmias, ventilator settings, and open sternum situations.

- *Simple bedside clinical markers*: Improvement in heart rate and blood pressure with a passive leg raise/direct pressure on the inferior margin of the liver can be used as a simple bedside test to assess fluid responsiveness. The mechanism is by increasing venous return to the heart and assessing its response on the hemodynamics.

To summarize, in the absence of complex goal-directed monitoring modality, simple clinical assessment, and observation of CVP/left atrial pressure remain the common hemodynamic tools to assess intravascular volume status and preload responsiveness in pediatric cardiac patients.

How to Administer a Fluid Bolus?

Typically, a volume challenge is given by 5–10 mL/kg bolus crystalloid/colloid or blood product. It is safer to deliver this as a continuous infusion over 10–15 minutes, to avoid the consequences of ventricular dilation in patients with poor ventricular compliance. In neonates and young infants, fluid aliquots of 5–10 mL may be slowly administered in syringes carefully observing the CVP, blood pressure, and heart rate. If this produces a favorable response in stroke volume by noting the change in blood pressure and CVP, the full bolus of 5–10 mL/kg may be infused over an hour as continuous infusion.

HOW TO MANAGE FLUID OVERLOAD?

As FO is known to contribute to adverse postoperative outcomes perioperative fluid management strategies should aim at preventing FO and also to facilitate fluid removal, if there is evidence of FO. FO is indicated by generalized edema and evidence of increased lung water with poor lung compliance.

Calculation of Fluid Overload

Fluid overload % can be calculated by two methods given below:

1. $$\frac{Total\ fluid\ in - Total\ fluid\ out \times 100}{Preoperative\ weight}$$

2. $$\frac{Current\ weight - Preoperative\ weight \times 100}{Preoperative\ weight}$$

A fluid overload of 5–10% is considered pathologic.

Prevention of Fluid Overload

The chief strategy is by restrictive administration of fluids and maintaining adequate volume for optimal tissue perfusion as guided by other clinical indices. In fluid sensitive patients, the total volume of other fluids that are given as carriers for drug administration and the volume of catheter flush solutions should be carefully controlled to avoid excessive fluid administration. All syringe pumps should be used at controlled flow rates to avoid excessive fluid administration.

Fluid Removal

This can be done prophylactically, or when there is evidence of FO. The principal strategy followed in pediatric cardiac care settings is by the use of diuretic therapy.[27] The loop diuretic furosemide is the commonly used pharmacological agent. A continuous infusion of furosemide is preferred in early postoperative period while bolus doses of diuretics are likely to precipitate sudden fluid shifts leading to hypovolemia. Combination with agents like metolazone/ethacrynic acid/acetazolamide may have a synergistic effect. In patients with acute kidney injury and oliguria with FO, fluid removal by peritoneal dialysis/continuous renal replacement therapy (CRRT) may be considered.[28]

◼ ELECTROLYTE MANAGEMENT

Sodium Management

Most patients in the post-CPB period are sodium overloaded. Sodium overload results from the electrolyte composition of the crystalloid solutions used to prime the bypass circuit. Hyponatremia in the post-bypass period reflects free-water excess. Serum sodium level < 125 mEq/L may be associated with neurological symptoms and should be managed with water restriction and cautious administration of normal saline solution. Sodium deficit is corrected according to the equation below.[29]

Sodium (Na) deficit =
(Desired Na⁺ – Patient Na⁺) × 0.6 × Weight in kg

Hypernatremia is frequent in early postoperative period. This usually occurs in patients with renal failure or in infants who have received large amounts of sodium bicarbonate or those who have large free-water deficit (due to diuretic therapy). It should be managed with sodium restriction and liberal fluid intake. The amount of fluid that should be given to correct the hypernatremia is as per the formula below.

$$Change\ in\ serum\ Na = \frac{Infusate\ Na^+ - Serum\ Na^+}{TBW}$$

(TBW in liters = Body weight × 0.6).

Estimates the effect of 1 L of any infusate on the serum Na⁺.

The rate of reduction of serum sodium should not preferably exceed 0.5 mmol/L/hr to avoid complications related to cerebral edema and convulsions. It is generally recommended that the reduction in serum Na should not be more than 10 mmol/L in 24 hours.[30]

Potassium Management

Potassium is the most abundant cation in the intracellular fluid. Serum potassium levels after CPB may be influenced by fluid and electrolyte shifts following CPB, pH of blood and tissues, beta agonists, and diuretic therapy. The usual daily requirement of potassium ranges between 2–3 mEq/kg/day in infants and 1–2 mEq/kg/day in children. Disturbances in potassium physiology can precipitate major electrophysiological and hemodynamic consequences and hence demand meticulous monitoring and management.

Monitoring potassium levels:
- Serum potassium is typically monitored every 4 hours by arterial blood sampling in most postoperative ventilated patients. However, more frequent sampling may sometimes be required in clinical situations such as hemodynamically significant arrhythmias with persistent electrolyte imbalances or in patients requiring frequent IV potassium correction in the postoperative period.

Hypokalemia

This is a frequent electrolyte disturbance after congenital heart surgery. This warrants correction to prevent arrhythmias in postoperative period.

Suggested guidelines for intravenous potassium therapy
- *Indication for administration of intravenous potassium:*
  - Potassium is a high-alert medication and has to be handled with utmost care.
  - Intravenous potassium replacement is indicated in patients with documented hypokalemia, i.e., serum potassium < 3.5 mEq/L
- *Calculation of deficit:*
  Potassium deficit (mEq/L) = 0.3 × body weight × (4.0 – observed serum K⁺).
- *Monitoring during potassium administration:*

- Continuous ECG monitoring is indicated while administering intravenous potassium infusion.
- Serum potassium should be monitored within 2 hours after the infusion is complete.
- Monitor and document urine output hourly.
  - *Dosing and administration*:
    - *Potassium prescription*: Written prescription for potassium chloride (KCl) administration has to be obtained from the physician prior to initiation of potassium correction. Verbal orders are not recommended.
    - *Dilution of KCl*: Usually 10 mEq KCl is diluted in 20 mL normal saline (0.5 mEq/mL)
    - Potassium infusions should be administered by syringe pumps only. The syringes should be labeled with the name of drug, dose, and dilution.
    - Intravenous potassium should be administered through a central venous line only.
    - Prior to administration, the dose, dilution, rate of infusion, and the intravenous line through which infusion is to be administered are to be checked by two staff nurses.
    - Potassium infusion rates should not exceed 0.5 mEq/kg/hr. If the calculated deficit is >0.5 mEq/kg/hr, recheck serum potassium by arterial blood gases (ABG) analysis at the end of 1 hour and supplement the remaining deficit only if required.
    - If the patient has coexisting metabolic acidosis, bicarbonate correction should be given after correcting the potassium deficit to avoid further intracellular shifts of potassium.
- Serum potassium levels should be rechecked and documented at the end of 1 hour of potassium correction.

Hyperkalemia

Hyperkalemia may occur in the postoperative period as a result of renal dysfunction, sequelae of low cardiac output syndrome, excessive potassium supplementation in IV fluids, redistribution of K^+ as in acidosis, effects of drugs, and massive blood transfusions.

A serum potassium level >4 mEq/L should be viewed with caution. Serum potassium levels >4.5 mEq/L require immediate treatment.

Treatment of Hyperkalemia

- Stop all potassium containing infusions.
- Calcium gluconate 50–100 mg/kg slow intravenous injection.
- Glucose-insulin bolus constituted by 0.05 unit/kg insulin in 5 mL of 25% dextrose should be given as a slow intravenous injection. This causes intracellular shift of potassium thus lowering serum potassium level.
- Injection furosemide 1 mg/kg IV bolus to facilitate excretion of potassium.
- Administer sodium bicarbonate 1–2 mEq/kg over several minutes to promote alkalosis and intracellular shift of potassium.
- Calcium polystyrene sulfonate (K^+ binding resin) can be added in children with persistent hyperkalemia at the dose of 0.3 g/kg every 6–8 hours administered via the nasogastric tube or as a retention enema.
- Initiate peritoneal dialysis promptly, if coexisting acute kidney injury is suspected.
- Identify and treat the cause of hyperkalemia.

Calcium Management

Routine monitoring of ionized calcium levels is indicated in all postoperative patients. Typically, calcium levels obtained from periodic ABG samples are followed in most centers for perioperative calcium management. Normal serum ionized calcium levels are 1.14–1.30 mmol/L. Calcium is administered in pediatric cardiac settings as an inotrope, as a physiological antagonist against hyperkalemia and in patients who have a substrate for calcium deficiency (Digeorge syndrome). Transfusion of large volumes of citrated anticoagulated blood, loop diuretics, which increases excretion of calcium, and acute respiratory alkalosis, are also likely to precipitate hypocalcemia in the postoperative setting.[9,31]

Guidelines for Calcium Administration

- Serum calcium levels are usually monitored once in every 4–6 hours along with arterial blood gas analysis.
- Ionized calcium levels should be maintained above 1.1 mmol/L.
- Intravenous calcium supplementation can be given by bolus doses of calcium gluconate 50–100 mg/kg every 6–8 hours. If multiple intermittent boluses of calcium are required to maintain normal level, then a continuous infusion of calcium can be used (2–4 mL/kg/day).
- Intravenous calcium supplementation should be given through a central venous line only. Extravasation of calcium can cause tissue necrosis.
- Sodium bicarbonate and calcium should not be administered together through the same intravenous catheter lumen since precipitation is likely.

Magnesium Management

Magnesium is principally an intracellular cation with substantial role in cellular metabolism, enzymatic reactions, and influences the function of excitable tissues such as cardiac muscle.[32]

Perioperative hypomagnesemia is associated with ventricular dysrhythmias such as ventricular tachycardia (VT), ventricular fibrillation (VF), torsades de pointes, etc. A serum magnesium level <0.7–0.8 mmol/L in older children and adults, and <0.6 mmol/L in neonates is suggestive of hypomagnesemia.[9]

Intravenous Magnesium Therapy Guidelines

- *Indications for intravenous administration of magnesium*: IV magnesium sulfate is given for the treatment of documented hypomagnesemia in patients with ventricular arrhythmias and for refractory hypocalcemia.
- Physician order should be obtained for starting magnesium infusion.
- *Dose of intravenous magnesium therapy*: 0.1 mL/kg of 50% $MgSO_4$ (or 25–50 mg/kg) diluted in 15 mL 5% dextrose or normal saline to be administered intravenously over 30 minutes to 1 hour.
- Assess baseline vital signs and level of consciousness before administration because magnesium sulfate is a central nervous system depressant.
- Continuous hemodynamic monitoring should be done while administering IV magnesium sulfate.
- Urine output should be monitored hourly and should be > 1 mL/kg/hr.
- Serum magnesium levels should be monitored 1 hour after administering the medication.
- Watch for signs of toxicity-flushing, hypotension, arrhythmias, heart blocks, central nervous system depression, muscle weakness, respiratory distress, etc.

- Antidote for toxicity is 10% calcium gluconate (100 mg/kg).

SUMMARY

Fluid management of the postoperative pediatric cardiac patient is an integral part of facilitating optimal postoperative recovery. CPB and systemic inflammatory response lead to tremendous fluid shifts and variation in intravascular volume status after cardiac surgery. Practically, clinical indicators and CVP remain the common bedside tools for assessing fluid status. More accurate dynamic variables may be used when expertise and equipment is available. Preventing FO, facilitating fluid removal in case of established FO, and meticulous monitoring of intravascular volume status in the post-operative period are important measures for facilitating better postoperative outcomes.

REFERENCES

1. Chappell D, Westphal M, Jacob M. The impact of glycocalyx on microcirculatory oxygen distribution in critical illness. Curr Opin Anaesthesiol. 2009;22:155-62.
2. Friis-Hansen B. Water distribution in the foetus and newborn infant. Acta Paediatr Scand. 1983;305:7-11.
3. Davidson D, Basu RK, Goldstein SL, Chawla LS. Fluid management in adults and children: Core Curriculum 2014. Am J Kidney Dis. 2014;63:700-12.
4. Schumaker J, Klotz KF. Fluid therapy in cardiac surgery patients. Appl Cardiopulm Pathophysiol. 2009;13:138-42.
5. Hassinger AB, Wald EL, Goodman DM. Early postoperative fluid overload precedes acute kidney injury and is associated with higher morbidity in pediatric cardiac surgery patients. Pediatr Crit Care Med. 2014;15:131-8.
6. Bailey AG, McNaull PP, Jooste E, Tuchman JB. Perioperative crystalloids and colloid fluid management in children: where are we and how did we get here? Anaesth Analg. 2010;110:375-90.
7. Hazle MA, Gajarski RJ, Yu S, Donohue J, Blatt NB. Fluid overload in infants following congenital heart surgery. Pediatr Crit Care Med. 2013;14:44-9.
8. Delpachitra MR, Namachivayam SP, Millar J, Delzoppo C, Butt WW. A case control analysis of postoperative fluid balance and mortality after pediatric cardiac surgery. Pediatr Crit Care Med. 2017;18:614-22.
9. Roth SJ. Post operative care. In: Chang AC, Hanley FL, Wernovsky G, Wessel DL (Eds). Pediatric Cardiac Intensive Care. Philadelphia: Lippincott Williams & Wilkins,1998; pp. 151-87.
10. Kouchukos NT, Blackstone EH, Hanley FL, Kirklin JK. Postoperative care. In: Kirklin Barrat-Boyes Cardiac Surgery. Philadelphia: Elsevier Saunders; 2013. pp. 190-250.
11. Burrows F, Shutack J, Crone R. Inappropriate secretion of antidiuretic hormone in a postsurgical population. Crit Care Med. 1983;11:527-31.
12. Moritz ML, Ayus JC. Hospital acquired hyponatrmia–why are hypotonic parenteral fluids still being used? Nat Clin Pract Nephrol. 2007;3:374-82.
13. Choong K, Kho ME, Menon K, Bohn D. Hypotonic versus isotonic saline in hospitalised children: a systemic review. Arch Dis Child. 2006;91:828-35.
14. Arieff AI. Hyponatremia and death or permanent brain damage in healthy children. BMJ. 1992;304:1218-22.
15. Lee JJ, Kim YS, Jung HH. Acute serum sodium concentration changes in pediatric patients undergoing cardiopulmonary bypass and the association with postoperative outcomes. SpringerPlus. 2015;4:641.
16. Shaw AD, Bagshaw SM, Goldstein SL, Scherer LA, Duan M, Schermer CR, et al. Major complications, mortality and resource utilisation after open abdominal surgery: 0.9% saline compared to plasmalyte. Ann Surg. 2012;255:821-9.
17. Rizza A, Romagnoli S, Ricci Z. Fluid status assessment and management during the perioperative phase in pediatric cardiac surgery patients. J Cardiothorac Vasc Anaesth. 2016;30:1085-93.
18. Russell JA, Navickis RJ, Wilkes MM. Albumin vs crystalloid for pump priming in cardiac surgery: meta-analysis of controlled trials. Crit Care. 2015;19:79.
19. Legendre C, Thervet E, Page B, Percheron A, Noel LH, Kreis H, et al. Hydroxyethyl starch and osmotic-nephrosis-like lesions in kidney transplantation. Lancet. 1993;342:248-9.

20. Van der Linden P, Dumoulin M, Lerberghe CV, Torres CS, Willems A, Faraoni D. Efficacy and safety of 6% hydroxyethyl starch 130/0.4 (voluven) for perioperative volume replacement in children undergoing cardiac surgery: a propensity matched analysis. Crit Care Med. 2015;19:87-97.

21. Willems A, Lerberghe CV, Gonsette K, De Ville A, Melot C, Hardy JF, et al. The indication for perioperative red blood cell transfusions is a predictive risk factor for severe postoperative morbidity and mortality in children undergoing cardiac surgery. Eur J Cardiothorac Surg. 2014;45:1050-7.

22. Lacroix J, Hébert PC, Hutchison JS, Hume HA, Tucci M, Ducruet T, et al; TRIPICU Investigators; Canadian Critical Care Trials Group; Pediatric Acute Lung Injury and Sepsis Investigators Network. Transfusion strategies for patients in pediatric intensive care units. N Engl J Med. 2007;356:1609-19.

23. Cholette JM, Rubenstein JS, Al eris GM, Powers KS, Eaton M, Lerner NB. Children with single-ventricle physiology do not benefit from higher hemoglobin levels post cavopulmonary connection: results of a prospective, randomized, controlled trial of a restrictive versus liberal red-cell transfusion strategy. Pediatr Crit Care Med. 2011;12:39-45.

24. Cholette JM, Swartz MF, Rubenstein J, Henrichs KF, Wang H, Powers KS, et al. Outcomes using a conservative versus liberal red blood cell transfusion strategy in infants requiring cardiac operation. Ann Thorac Surg. 2017;103:206-14.

25. Cholette JM, Faraoni D, Goobie SM, Ferraris V, Hassan M. Patient blood management in pediatric cardiac surgery: a review. Anaesth Analg. 2017;127(4):1002-16.

26. Gan H, Canneson M, Chandler JR, Ansermino JM. Predicting fluid responsiveness in children. A systematic review. Anaesth Analg. 2013;117:1380-92.

27. Favia I, Garisto C, Rossi E, Piccardo S, Ricci Z. Fluid management in pediatric cardiac intensive care. Contrib Nephrol. 2010;164:217-26.

28. Santos CR, Branco PQ, Gaspar A, Bruges M, Anjos R, Goncalves MS, et al. Use of peritoneal dialysis after surgery for congenital heart disease in children. Perit Dial Int. 2012;32:273-9.

29. Meyers RS. Pediatric fluid and electrolyte therapy. J Pediatr Pharmacol Ther. 2009;14:204-11.

30. Adrogue HJ, Madias NE. Hypernatremia. N Engl J Med. 2000;132:1493-9.

31. Booker PD. Postoperative care: General principles. In: Lake CL, Booker PD (Eds). Pediatric Cardiac Anesthesia. Philadelphia: Lippincott Williams & Wilkins; 2005. pp. 633-53.

32. Jahnen-Dechent W, Ketteler M. Magnesium basics. Clin Kidney J. 2012;5:i3-14.

Blood Glucose Management after Pediatric Cardiac Surgery

Rakhi Balachandran

Reviewed by: Aveek Jayant

■ INTRODUCTION

Hyperglycemia is a well-recognized metabolic disturbance after pediatric cardiac surgery.[1-3] The proposed mechanisms include stress response to surgery and cardiopulmonary bypass (CPB) resulting in alterations in counterregulatory hormones (such as cortisol, glucagon and growth hormone) and increased catecholamine secretion.[2] Both these changes will result in increased glycolysis and gluconeogenesis trying to maintain the glucose fuel needed for vital organs during the phase of critical illness. Additionally, prolonged stress response and exogenous factors promote peripheral and hepatic insulin resistance. Patients with cardiovascular failure and hyperglycemia are also prone for pancreatic beta cell dysfunction and an absolute insulin deficiency.[4] Iatrogenic factors such as parenteral nutrition, glucocorticoids administered during surgery and CPB, vasoactive drug infusions, and hypothermia add to the burden of hyperglycemia. There is accumulating evidence that hyperglycemia is associated with adverse outcomes in pediatric intensive care units.[1,3,5,8] Hyperglycemia had been linked to increased rates of hospital acquired infections, renal failure, liver dysfunction and cerebral injury.[3-8] Both intensity and duration of hyperglycemia had been associated with increased morbidity and mortality in infants undergoing congenital heart repairs on CPB.[1] The predominant adverse effects of hyperglycemia are attributed to cellular glucose overload with increased peroxynitrite production which can induce apoptotic changes in cardiomyocytes, renal cells, thymocytes and neurons.[6,7] Increased peroxynitrite can also lead to accelerated consumption of endogenous nitric oxide (NO) resulting in endothelial dysfunction.[2,8] Hyperglycemia also interferes with neutrophil chemotaxis and impairs complement fixation resulting in increased propensity for infections. Therefore, maintaining euglycemia has assumed importance in both adult and pediatric critical care units to prevent complications and to improve outcomes.

SUMMARY OF EVIDENCE FOR BLOOD GLUCOSE MANAGEMENT IN PEDIATRIC INTENSIVE CARE POPULATION

Insulin therapy has been traditionally used for blood glucose control in hyperglycemic patients in critical care settings. Insulin lowers blood glucose levels and prevents the adverse effects of hyperglycemia induced end organ injury. It also corrects the disturbed lipid profile, promotes anabolism and modulates immune function.[9] The beneficial effects of insulin also extend to promotion of vascular endothelial function and antithrombotic effects. A blood glucose level >150 mg/dL is commonly employed to define the threshold for treatment of hyperglycemia in critically ill children including neonates as this seems to have the strongest association with poor outcomes.[9,10] Incidence of hyperglycemia defined by the above threshold in critically ill children ranges from 49 to 72%.[11]

There are no established guidelines for glucose control in pediatric cardiac patients. The two common strategies employed in many randomized controlled studies published in pediatric critically ill patients include, either a tight glucose control or standard/conventional care.[12-16] The summary of major trials in pediatric intensive care population is provided in **Table 1**.

The glucose ranges for standard care suggested by Macrae et al. and Vlaesselers et al. range from 180 to 215 mg/dL. The lower limit of glucose level to stop insulin therapy in standard care was set at 180 mg/dL as it corresponds to the renal threshold for glycosuria.[15] The benefits of intensive insulin therapy in critically ill patients was first recognized following the landmark study of Van den Berghe et al. in adult patients suggesting a mortality benefit with tight glucose control.[12] Subsequently pediatric data emerged via several randomized controlled

TABLE 1: Randomized controlled trials of intensive insulin therapy versus standard care in pediatric critical care patients

Study	Sample size	Age (years)	Patient category	Glucose range (mg/dL)	Outcomes TGC vs. standard
Vlasselaers et al.[13]	700	0–16	75% Cardiac 25% Medical/surgical	<1 year 50–80 vs. >180–215 >1 year 70–100 vs. 180–215	• Shorter ICU stay (5.51 vs. 6.15 days (p = 0.017) • Lower mortality (3% vs 6%, p = 0.038 • Hypoglycemia (25% vs 1%, p < 0.0001 • Lower CRP levels in TGC
Agus et al.[14] (SPECS trial)	980	0–3	Cardiac surgery	80–110 vs. Standard care	• 30-day rate of health care associated infections—number of infections per 1,000 patient days in cardiac ICU (8.6 vs. 9.9, p = 0.67) • Severe hypoglycemia • 3% vs. 1%, p = 0.03
Macrae et al.[15] (CHIP trial)	1369	0–16	61% Cardiac 39% Medical/surgical	72–126 vs. 180–215	• Number of days alive and free of mechanical ventilation (mean between group difference–0.36 days: not significant • Severe hypoglycemia • 7.3% vs. 1.5%, p < 0.001
Agus et al.[16] (HALF-PINT study)	713	0–17	Medical/surgical	80–110 vs. 150–180	• Number of ICU free days • 20 vs. 19.4, p = 0.86 • Healthcare associated infections 3.4% vs. 1.1%, p = 0.04 • Severe hypoglycemia 5.2% vs. 2% p = 0.03

(ICU: intensive care unit; CRP: C-reactive protein; TGC: tight glucose control)

trials (RCTs) comparing tight glycemic control versus standard care (conventional care) focusing pediatric intensive care units.[13-16] Mostly there was marked heterogeneity among the patient population of the trials featuring general pediatric patients, pediatric cardiac surgical patients, patients with septic shock, burns, and those with traumatic brain injury. The creation of a generalized guideline for glycemic control, is unrealistic due to varying patient subsets, different glycemic targets, glucose control algorithms, sampling techniques and implementation logistics which results in inconsistent outcome benefits.

Though the first RCT on pediatric intensive care patients in Leuven including cardiac surgery patients by Vlasselaers et al.[13] showed a mortality benefit with intensive insulin therapy [9 (3%) vs. 20 (6%) p = 0.038], there was an alarming incidence of hypoglycemia in the group with tight glucose control, (25% vs. 1%, p = 0.0001). Subsequent studies employed less rigid glycemic targets for intensive insulin therapy, however none of them have demonstrated a mortality benefit. The only favorable outcome demonstrated in a couple of recent trials is on reduction of acquired infections.[13,17] In the most recent multicenter trial, Heart and Lung Failure Pediatric Insulin Titration (HALF-PINT) study,[16] which excluded cardiac surgical patients, the median number of ICU free days did not differ significantly from the lower target (80–110 mg/dL) to higher target group (150–180 mg/dL), i.e., 20 days versus 19.4 days, p = 0.86. Patients in the lower target group had lower rates of health care associated infections compared to higher target group (1.1% vs. 3.4 %, p = 0.04).

The major deterrent against embracing the tight glucose control strategy in most pediatric critical care settings is the overwhelming burden of hypoglycemia. Hypoglycemia is a common complication after intensive insulin therapy and occurrence of hypoglycemia as a consequence of tight glucose control is linked to adverse outcomes including mortality in cardiac surgery subgroup. In a multicenter randomized trial in 1,369 patients tight glucose control was associated with higher incidence of severe hypoglycemia (7.3% vs. 1.5%, p < 0.001). In a subgroup analysis including cardiac surgical patients, 10.6% of patients who had at least one hypoglycemic episode died compared to those who did not have hypoglycemia (2.1%, p < 0.001).[15] According to a recent review by Srinivasan et al.,[18] the mode of concomitant nutrition support strategy [being early parenteral nutrition (PN) or early enteral nutrition (EN)], should also be factored in while considering the hypoglycemic events in most of these trials. According to this review, it is likely that the delayed PN initiation group might have experienced more hypoglycemia episodes in some of the trials. Early PN is more likely to be associated with hyperglycemia in critical care settings. They conclude that when EN is the favored mode of nutrition support in tight glucose control with intensive insulin therapy, it may be responsible for the worse outcomes associated with hypoglycemia.[18] In standard care insulin therapy, early EN may be complementary in terms of maintaining gut integrity and fewer infections.

◼ A SUGGESTED BLOOD GLUCOSE MANAGEMENT STRATEGY

Based on available evidence, tight glycemic control has not generated superior outcomes in terms of morbidity and mortality in pediatric critical care population. The optimal glycemic target also remains unclear. The stress hyperglycemia after cardiac surgery most often resolves within 24 hours with limitation of stressors, extubation, and resumption of enteral nutrition intake. Though the target of 150 mg% has been accepted to define hyperglycemia in several studies the threshold for initiating insulin therapy may vary as per institutional guidelines of glycemic ranges. The upper limits of blood glucose levels in conventional glucose management strategies ranges from 180 to 215 mg%. We suggest initiating insulin therapy when at least two consecutive blood sugar measurements exceed 215 mg% in two consecutive arterial blood gas (ABG) obtained at 1-hour interval. The following section elaborates the blood glucose management strategy that is followed at our center for pediatric cardiac patients.

Definition of Hyperglycemia

A patient is defined to be hyperglycemic if blood glucose measured by ABG is greater than 150 mg%. Desirable blood glucose target range is 100-150 mg/dL. However, considering the allowance for stress hyperglycemia in the initial 24 hours and return to baseline spontaneously in majority of cases, the threshold for initiating insulin therapy has been set at 215 mg/dL. This also offers a safety margin against the potential harm of inducing hypoglycemia as a sequelae of insulin therapy. The threshold for stopping insulin infusion is a blood glucose level of 180 mg%.

Insulin Therapy in Pediatric Cardiac Intensive Care Unit (PCICU)

Phase 1: *Establishment of hyperglycemic state*
Check blood glucose (BG) on admission and every 4th hourly, if BG levels are within acceptable limits.
1. If BG level is greater than 215 mg% repeat ABG after 1 hour
2. If the two consecutive BG measurements remain > 215 mg% go to Phase 2.

Phase 2: *Initiate insulin treatment if two consecutive blood glucose measurements at 1 hour interval is >215 mg%*
1. Initiate insulin treatment at 0.05 unit/kg/hour. Repeat ABG after 1 hour
2. If the drop in BG level is <25% and BG levels are >250 mg% increase insulin infusion rate by 50% (0.07 unit/kg/hour). Continue at same rate if BG is between 200 and 250 mg%
3. If the drop in BG is >50% decrease insulin infusion by 50%. (0.025 unit/kg/hour)
4. If the drop in BG is between 25 and 50%, continue at 0.05 unit/kg/hour
5. If BG exceeds 300 mg% increase insulin infusion to 0.1 unit/kg/hour. Monitor blood sugar levels hourly. We usually avoid bolus insulin doses to avoid precipitous drop in blood sugar levels and hypokalemia.

% change in glucose is calculated as:

$$\frac{Previous\ value - Current\ value \times 100}{Previous\ value}$$

Phase 3: *Glycemic maintenance in desirable range (100–150 mg%)*
1. Check BG levels with every blood gas.
2. If BG decreases below 180 mg%, stop insulin infusion. Check BG 2 hours after stopping insulin infusion or till it is stabilized within the normal range.
3. If the BG falls below 100 mg%, start 10% glucose containing solution as maintenance fluid.
4. If the BG falls below 60 mg%, notify physician, give a bolus of 2.5 mL/kg 10% dextrose. Monitor BG every hour till BG levels stabilize.

Preparation and Administration of Insulin Solution

Ten units of human insulin should be diluted in 20 mL normal saline. Insulin should always be administered by means of a syringe infusion pump. Insulin should be administered along with a carrier of 0.9% normal saline running at 1 mL/h via a dedicated peripheral venous catheter.[19] Care should be taken to avoid flushing of the IV tubing containing the insulin drip as it may result in delivery of a large bolus and trigger hypoglycemia. Insulin solutions should be replaced every 24 hours. Insulin infusions should be preferably stopped before transport of the patient to a remote location (operating room/Cath lab/Radiology suite). Insulin should also be stopped when there is reduction in caloric intake or when feeding is interrupted.

Side Effects of Insulin Therapy

Two important aspects which should be considered in patients on insulin infusion is the occurrence of hypokalemia and hypoglycemia. These are discussed here.

1. *Control of potassium levels*: Insulin causes intracellular shift of potassium and this can potentially trigger arrhythmias. Meticulous attention to serum potassium levels during blood gas analysis and prompt correction of hypokalemia has to be ensured. Potassium levels should preferably be corrected to 4 mmol/L and has to be measured at least 4th hourly, while on insulin infusion. Also, any metabolic disturbance producing acidosis can cause the shift of potassium back to extravascular compartment and subsequent hyperkalemic episodes have to be carefully sought for. Nurses and intensivists should be mindful of conditions which can promote shifts of potassium between body fluid compartments and modify therapy accordingly.

2. *Diagnosis and management of hypoglycemia*: Hypoglycemia is a serious complication after insulin therapy in pediatric intensive care units. Hypoglycemia has been linked to adverse neurodevelopmental outcomes.[10,20] The vulnerable population for hypoglycemia includes neonates, very low birth weight and small for gestational age (SGA) infants, patients in sepsis, or those with hepatic dysfunction. Persistent or recurrent hypoglycemia may result in long-term visual disturbance, hearing impairment, cognitive dysfunction, secondary epilepsy and central nervous system (CNS) disorders especially in a developing brain.[19] Prevention, detection and prompt treatment of hypoglycemia should be an integral part of insulin treatment algorithms to ensure favorable postoperative outcome. Ideal glucose control algorithms incorporate continuous glucose monitoring and computer guided insulin titration along with well trained nurses and intensive care team.[14-16] The randomized control trial of intensive insulin therapy by Vlasselaers[13] at Leuven PICU had been viewed critically, due to the high incidence of hypoglycemia (<40 mg/dL). However, in the 4-year follow-up study of these patients those who had tight glycemic control did not have a worse measure of intelligence than those who received conventional care.[21] The authors concluded that prompt diagnosis with accurate tools and correction of hypoglycemia judiciously without producing a rebound hyperglycemia may be critical in preventing brain damage.[21]

Definition: Though a wide range of threshold for defining hypoglycemia exist in varying age groups, for simplistic treatment purposes, any blood glucose level less than 60 mg% should be considered as hypoglycemia.

A blood glucose less than 40 mg% should be considered as severe hypoglycemia.

Treatment: If the patient is on insulin infusion it should promptly be stopped. A glucose containing intravenous maintenance infusion should be started. If it is feasible to resume enteral nutrition intake, initiate feeding after physician consultation. Hypoglycemia in neonates and infants are typically treated by administration of 2.5 mL/kg of 10% dextrose (may be repeated) or 2 mL/kg 25% dextrose. Higher concentrations of dextrose >10% should not be administered through a peripheral intravenous line as it is likely to cause thrombophlebitis.

▪ SUMMARY

The current evidence does not support tight glucose control in pediatric cardiac population. In centers practicing conventional glucose control regimes, the usual threshold for initiating insulin treatment ranges from 200 to 215 mg% to prevent adverse effects of prolonged hyperglycemia in pediatric cardiac patients. Meticulous glucose monitoring tools, nurse driven insulin titration algorithms, and prompt recognition of hypoglycemia in vulnerable population is imperative for favorable neurodevelopmental outcomes in critically ill pediatric patients. Attention to modes of nutrition delivery and early enteral nutrition may have a substantial impact on the blood glucose management in pediatric cardiac patient.

▪ REFERENCES

1. Polito A, Thiagarajan R, Laussen PC, Gauvreau K, Agus MS, Scheurer MA, et al. Association between intraoperative and early post-operative glucose levels and adverse outcomes after complex congenital heart surgery. Circulation. 2008;118:2235-42.
2. Ulate KP, Raj S, Rotta AT. Critical illness hyperglycemia in pediatric cardiac surgery. J Diabetes Sci Technol. 2012;6:29-36.
3. Yates AR, Dyke PC 2nd, Taeed R, Hoffman TM, Hayes J, Feltes TF, et al. Hyperglycemia is a marker for poor outcome in the postoperative pediatric cardiac patient. Pediatr Crit Care Med. 2006;7:351-5.
4. Preissig CM, Rigby MR. Hyperglycemia results from beta cell dysfunction in critically ill children with respiratory and cardiovascular failure: a prospective observational study. Crit Care. 2009;13:R27.
5. Falcao G, Ulate K, Kouzekanani K, Bielefeld MR, Morales JM, Rotta AT. Impact of postoperative hyperglycemia following surgical repair of congenital heart defects. Pediatr Cardiol. 2009; 30:1098-104.
6. Arstall MA, Sawyer DB, Fukazawa R, Kelly RA. Cytokine mediated apoptosis in cardiac myocytes: the role of inducible nitric oxide synthase induction and peroxynitrite generation. Circ Res. 1999;85:829-40.
7. Vinas JL, Sola A, Hotter G. Mitochondrial NOS upregulation during renal I/R causes apoptosis in peroxynitrite–dependent manner. Kidney Int. 2006;2006;69:1403-9.
8. Li JM, Shah AM. Endothelial cell superoxide generation: regulation and relevance for cardiovascular pathophysiology. Am J Physiol Regul Integr Comp Physiol. 2004;287:R1014-30.
9. Verbruggen SC, Joosten K, Castillo L, van Goudoever JB. Insulin therapy in the pediatric intensive care unit. Clin Nutrition. 2007; 26:677-80.
10. Arsenault D, Brenn M, Kim S, Gura K, Compher C, Simpser E, et al. ASPEN Clinical guidelines: hyperglycemia and hypoglycemia in the neonate receiving parenteral nutrition. J Parenter Enteral Nutr. 2012;36:81-95.
11. Srinivasan V, Agus MSD. Tight Glucose Control in critically ill children-a systematic review and meta-analysis. Pediatr Diab. 2014;15: 75-83.
12. Van Den Berghe G, Wouters P, Weekers F, Verwaest C, Bruyninckx F, Schetz M, et al. Intensive insulin therapy in critically ill patients. N Engl J Med. 2001;345:1359-67.
13. Vlasselaers D, Milants I, Desmet L, Wouters PJ, Vanhorebeek I, van den Heuvel I, et al. Intensive insulin therapy for patients in pediatric intensive care: a prospective randomized controlled study. Lancet. 2009;373:547-56.
14. Agus MSD, Steil GM, Wypij D, Costello JM, Laussen PC, Langer M, et al. Tight glycemic control versus standard care after pediatric cardiac surgery. N Engl J Med. 2012;367:1208-19.

15. Macrae D, Grieve R, Allen E, Sadique Z, Morris K, Pappachan J, et al. A randomized trial of hyperglycemic control in pediatric cardiac intensive care. N Engl J Med. 2014;370:107-18.

16. Agus MSD, Wypij D, Hirschberg EL, Srinivasan V, Faustino EV, Luckett PM, et al. Tight glycemic control in critically ill children. N Engl J Med. 2017;376:729-41.

17. Jeschke MG, Kulp GA, Kraft R, Finnerty CC, Mlcak R, Lee JO, et al. Intensive insulin therapy in severely burned pediatric patients. A prospective randomized trial. Am J Resp Crit Care Med. 2010;182:351-9.

18. Srinivasan V. Nutrition support and tight glucose control in critically ill children: food for thought. Front Pediatr. 2018;6:340.

19. Gaies MG, Langer M, Alexander J, Steil GM, Ware J, Wypij D, et al Design and rationale of Safe Pediatric Euglycemia after Cardiac surgery (SPECS): a randomized controlled trial of tight glycemic control after pediatric cardiac surgery. Pediatr Crit Care Med. 2013;14: 148-56.

20. Su J, Wang Li. Research advances in neonatal hypoglycemic brain injury. Transl Pediatr. 2012;1:108-15.

21. Mesotten D, Gielen M, Sterken C, Claessens K, Hermans G, Vlasselaers D, et al. Neurocognitive development of children 4 years after critical illness and treatment with tight glucose control. A randomized controlled trial. JAMA. 2012; 308:1641-50.

Pain and Sedation Management in Pediatric Cardiac Intensive Care Unit

Rakhi Balachandran
Reviewed by: Aveek Jayant

■ INTRODUCTION

Pediatric patients require analgesia and sedation to reduce pain, to enable quiescence during mechanical ventilation, and to facilitate postoperative care. Optimal pain and sedation management during the critical period in the intensive care unit (ICU) is also known to impact long-term neurocognitive outcomes of the developing pediatric brain.[1] Some of the admitted patients to pediatric cardiac intensive care units (PCICU) also have marginal hemodynamic status, which could potentially overwhelm standard guidance on sedation and analgesia in pediatric intensive care. Practitioners should strive to maintain a balance between creating hemodynamic perturbance while ensuring comfort and minimizing distress. With sustained improvement in surgical pathways, increasing numbers of patients are also being fast tracked to earlier extubation and discharge from PCICU; titrating perioperative sedation/analgesia to this end point is seen as a new imperative.

Optimizing sedation and pain control, while facilitating early extubation, is a challenging process. PCICUs cater to a heterogeneous population with respect to age, differing developmental stages and varying biological needs. Unlike adults, titrating sedation in nonverbal vulnerable patients is simultaneously an art and a skill. Finally, inadequate attention to sedation and analgesia could also produce delirium, accelerated catabolism, immune dysfunction, and respiratory compromise.[1]

▌ BENEFITS OF ANALGESIA AND SEDATION AFTER PEDIATRIC CARDIAC SURGERY

- Adequate analgesia and sedation after congenital heart surgery can decrease the stress response to cardiac surgery and cardiopulmonary bypass.
- Analgesia decreases the sympathetic response to pain and thus the myocardial work and oxygen demand.
- Adequate sedation is essential to facilitate mechanical ventilation by ensuring patient ventilator synchrony and to prevent inadvertent complications related to patient agitation.
- Postoperatively, patients with pulmonary artery hypertension require tailored analgesia and sedation to prevent occurrence of life-threatening pulmonary hypertensive crisis.
- Painful procedures, which when performed in the postoperative period such as central line placement, intercostal drain insertion, cardioversion, bronchoscopy, and delayed sternal closure requires additional doses of analgesics and sedatives.
- In patients who are having a prolonged ICU stay, ensuring patient comfort augments postoperative recovery by avoiding

respiratory compromise, facilitating anabolism, and preventing complications such as delirium and withdrawal.

GENERAL PRINCIPLES OF PAIN MANAGEMENT

The general dictum is that all patients in a postoperative ICU should be considered as having pain for even the simplest procedure that is performed, and therefore need adequate analgesia. The pain management strategy should encompass the following general principles:

- Regular assessment of pain score using age appropriate scale.
- The level of pain should be promptly documented by the bedside nurse.
- The level of pain reported by the patient must be considered the current standard for analgesia.
- Patients who cannot communicate should be assessed for the presence of pain-related behaviors and physiological indicators of pain.
- A therapeutic plan for analgesia should be established for each patient and regularly reviewed.
- Use of a sedation algorithm when available, helps to standardize care and improve quality metrics.
- Systematically monitor for signs of withdrawal or tolerance in patients who require long-term analgesia and sedation.

ASSESSMENT OF PAIN

Pain is a subjective experience. A patient's reporting of pain is the single most reliable indicator of pain and must be considered the standard to guide analgesic therapy. However, assessment of pain in nonverbal neonates, infants, and small children is a major challenge. A variety of pain scales are available, which make use of facial expression, motor responses, and physiological indices for assessment of

pain in this subset of patients. Autonomic signs such as hypertension, tachycardia, pupillary size, diaphoresis, and tearing can also be used as a guide to pain perception in children. If breathing spontaneously, changes in respiratory pattern like tachypnea, grunting, and splinting of the chest wall may be evident if the patient is experiencing pain.

Pain Assessment Tools

Various age appropriate tools are available for assessment of pain in pediatric patients. Neonatal Pain Agitation and Sedation Scale (N-PASS) as well as Face Legs Activity Cry and Consolability (FLACC) Scale are frequently employed in nonverbal neonates and infants (**Tables 1 and 2**). Older patients can be evaluated using Wong Baker Faces Scale (**Fig. 1**) or 0-10 scale (**Fig. 2**).

Frequency of Assessment

Pain scores should be typically assessed on admission into PCICU and with every vital sign measurement. Additionally, pain needs to be assessed, whenever a patient complains of pain, and within an hour of a pain management intervention.

Who should Perform the Pain Assessment?

Bedside nurse, who is the primary care giver, is the most appropriate person for pain assessment. It is crucial to identify the location of pain along with assessment of pain scores. This has to be appropriately communicated to the attending physician/intensivist and documented in the flowchart.

MODES OF PAIN MANAGEMENT

Current practice patterns of pediatric pain management are multimodal, employing a combination of drugs or techniques that have different modes of action. This enables to provide analgesia while reducing the incidence

TABLE 1: Neonatal Pain Agitation and Sedation Scale (N-PASS) for neonatal age group.[2]

Assessment criteria	Sedation −2	−1	Normal 0	Pain/Agitation 1	2
Crying Irritability	No cry with painful stimuli	Moans or cries minimally with painful stimuli	• Appropriate crying • Not irritable	• Irritable or crying at intervals • Consolable	• High-pitched or Silent-continuous cry • Inconsolable
Behavior state	• No arousal to any stimuli • No spontaneous movement	• Arouses minimally to stimuli • Little spontaneous movement	• Appropriate for gestational age	• Restless, squirming • Awakens frequently	• Arching, kicking • Constantly awake or • Arouses minimally/ no movement(not sedated)
Facial expression	• Mouth is lax • No expression	• Minimal expression with stimuli	• Relaxed • Appropriate	• Any pain expression intermittent	• Any pain expression continual
Extremities tone	• No grasp reflex • Flaccid tone	• Weak grasp reflex • Decreased muscle tone	• Relaxed hands and feet • Normal tone	• Intermittent clenched toes, fists, finger splay • Body is not tense	• Continual clenched toes, fists or finger splay • Body is tense
Vital signs HR, BP, RR, O_2 sats	• No variability with stimuli • Hypoventilation or apnea	Less than 10% variability from baseline with stimuli	Within baseline or normal for gestational age	• Increased 10–20% from baseline • SaO_2 76–85% with stimulation- quick increase	• Increase > 20% from baseline • SaO_2 <75% with stimulation-slow increase • Out of sync with vent

Premature pain assessment:
+3 if <28 weeks gestation/corrected age
+2 if 28–31 weeks gestation/corrected age
+1 if 32–35 weeks gestation/corrected age
Goal of pain treatment/intervention: Score <3
Light sedation: −5 to −2 as goal
Deep sedation: −10 to −5 as goal
Source: Hummel P, Puchalski M, Creech SD, Weiss MG. Clinical reliability and validity of the N-PASS: neonatal pain, agitation and sedation scale with prolonged pain. J Perinatol. 2008;28:55-60.
(BP: blood pressure; HR: heart rate; RR: respiratory rate)

TABLE 2: FLACC behavioral pain assessment scale for nonverbal patients.[3]

	The FLACC behavioral pain assessment scale	
	Scoring	
Categories	0	1	2
---	---	---	---
Face	No particular expression or smile	• Occasional grimace or frown; withdrawn • Disinterested	• Frequent to constant frown, clenched jaw • Quivering chin
Legs	Normal position or relaxed	Uneasy, restless, tense	Kicking or legs drawn up
Activity	Lying quietly, normal position, moves easily	Squirming, shifting back and forth, tense	Arched, rigid, or jerking
Cry	No cry (awake or asleep)	Moans or whimpers, occasional complaint	• Crying steadily, screams, or sobs • Frequent complaints
Consolability	Content, relaxed	Reassured by occasional touching, hugging or being talked to, distractable	Difficult to console or comfort

Each category is scored from 0 to 2 resulting in total score between 0 and 10

Interpreting the behavioral score: 0 = Relaxed and comfortable, 1–3 = Mild discomfort, 4–6 = Moderate pain, 7–10 = Severe discomfort, pain, or both.
Source: Merkel S, Voepel-Lewis T, Malviya S. Pain assessment in infants and young children: the FLACC scale. Am J Nurs. 2002;102:55-8.
(FLACC: face legs activity cry consolability)

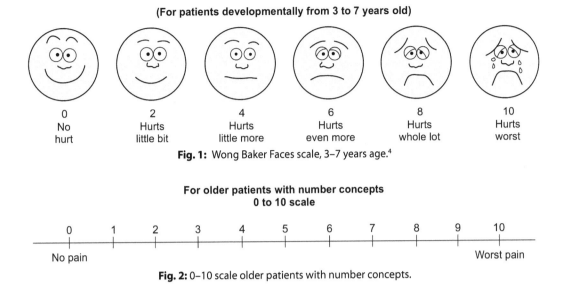

(For patients developmentally from 3 to 7 years old)

| 0 | 2 | 4 | 6 | 8 | 10 |
| No hurt | Hurts little bit | Hurts little more | Hurts even more | Hurts whole lot | Hurts worst |

Fig. 1: Wong Baker Faces scale, 3–7 years age.[4]

**For older patients with number concepts
0 to 10 scale**

0 1 2 3 4 5 6 7 8 9 10

No pain   Worst pain

Fig. 2: 0–10 scale older patients with number concepts.

and severity of side effects of individual drugs.[5] For example, avoid high doses of some drugs like opioids, thus reducing the concerns of withdrawal/dependence.

The choice of appropriate drug in a cardiac surgical patient will also be dictated by the hemodynamic status, presence of pulmonary artery hypertension, level of sedation required, the presence or absence of ventilator support and the need for early extubation and fast tracking.

Pharmacological Methods

Key Definitions

An understanding of the actions of each category of agents is needed while choosing the appropriate agent for pain management or sedation or both.

Analgesics: These are pharmacological agents that *provide pain relief* by acting on various pain pathways. For example, paracetamol, morphine, fentanyl.

Sedatives: These agents allow *reduction in level of consciousness of the patient and induce sleep.* For example, midazolam, lorazepam.

Paralytic agents: These drugs are muscle relaxants, which *produces neuromuscular blockade and results in paralysis.* For example, pancuronium, vecuronium, atracurium, rocuronium.

Paralytic agents should only be used when it is absolutely essential to limit patient movement (e.g., low cardiac output states, pulmonary hypertensive crisis, acute lung injury with severe hypoxia, etc.).

However, there are some pharmacological agents that combine both sedative and analgesic properties. For example, morphine, fentanyl, dexmedetomidine (Dex), ketamine, etc. The secondary properties of the drugs should be judiciously explored while optimizing postoperative care.

Analgesics

Opioids: Opioid analgesia remains the main stay of postoperative analgesia in the pediatric cardiac ICU.[6] The most widely used opioids include fentanyl and morphine. Opioids can be given as intermittent doses or continuous infusion. Continuous infusions are generally preferred, since it produces predictable blood levels, and helps to avoid periods of over sedation and under-medication. Additionally, continuous infusion helps to minimize the respiratory depression, which may be more pronounced with bolus doses. Patients who receive opioids for longer duration are likely to develop tolerance.

- *Morphine*: This is an opioid analgesic, which acts via "μ" opioid receptors in the central nervous system (CNS). Morphine relieves visceral, somatic, and neuropathic pain. It also has a sedative effect, which is beneficial in a postoperative child on ventilator. The "unit" dose of intravenously administered morphine is typically 0.05–0.1 mg/kg. It has also a relatively short half-life (3–4 hours). Hence, continuous infusion of morphine (10–40 µg/kg/h) is advocated to maintain reliable blood levels. The effects of morphine are prolonged in neonates with renal failure and reduced glomerular filtration rate (GFR). It should also be used with caution in hepatic dysfunction and sepsis where there is likely to be a decreased clearance.[7] A notable side effect of morphine is histamine release, which may result in hypotension with bolus injections. Due to wide individual variations in opioid requirements, the dose and timing of the drug should be titrated to the effect. Titration can avoid over sedation as well as maximize pain-free periods. Discontinuation of morphine can produce withdrawal phenomena and hence children should be closely monitored for signs of withdrawal.
- *Fentanyl*: Fentanyl is 100 times more potent than morphine. It has a rapid onset of action within 1 minute and a short duration action of 30–45 minutes. Typical intravenous bolus dose is 1–5 µg/kg. Fentanyl blocks painful stimuli with concomitant hemodynamic stability. Fentanyl causes less histamine release

than morphine and hence associated with less incidence of hypotension. It is usually given as an infusion of 1–5 µg/kg/h. Rapid bolus administration of doses >5 µg/kg may be associated with glottic spasm as well as chest wall rigidity. Because of the favorable hemodynamic profile, fentanyl is generally preferred to morphine in patients with low cardiac output state, neonates with pulmonary hypertension, or in patients with critically balanced (pulmonary to systemic) circulation.

Acetaminophen (Paracetamol): Acetaminophen has analgesic and antipyretic effects, and is effective for mild to moderate pain with good safety margin. Acetaminophen by itself cannot be considered as a sole analgesic agent in the immediate postoperative period. It should always be combined with an opioid/alternative analgesic like Dex. The antipyretic effect is beneficial in children developing postoperative fever as a part of inflammatory response to cardiopulmonary bypass. Typical oral dosing is 10–15 mg/kg every 4–6 hours. A maximum daily dose of 90 mg/kg should not be exceeded. Rectal route of administration can be used in ventilated patients at a dose of 30 mg/kg initially followed by 20 mg/kg every 6 hours. However, the rectal route is slow and has variable absorption. Paracetamol is metabolized by liver and hence dose alteration or discontinuation of the drug may be sometimes required in patients with postoperative hepatic dysfunction.

Nonsteroidal anti-inflammatory drugs (NSAIDs): NSAIDs have profound anti-inflammatory and analgesic effects. They inhibit the enzyme cyclooxygenase (COX) and reduce production of prostaglandins at the site of tissue injury, which is responsible for pain. A variety of drugs are available, but superiority of one drug over another is not proven. They can cause side effects such as gastritis, nephropathy, and platelet dysfunction related to the inhibition of the COX1 enzyme in other regions.[5] Information regarding the safety and efficacy of NSAIDs for analgesia in neonates and young infants is limited. Short-term use of NSAIDs may be tolerated by children with low incidence of side effects. Ketorolac and ibuprofen are the most commonly used agents in multimodal pain management strategies. In a recent randomized trial, intravenous ketorolac at 0.5 mg/kg every 6–8 hours was superior to paracetamol and resulted in less use of rescue opioid doses during postoperative care after congenital heart surgery.[8] Recommended intravenous dose of ketorolac is 0.25–0.5 mg/kg every 6 hours. Ibuprofen is typically administered at doses of 10 mg/kg per oral (PO) every 6–8 hours. These drugs should be used with caution in patients who have active gastrointestinal bleeding or renal dysfunction. Use is generally restricted to patients with lower RACHS-1 (Risk Adjustment for Congenital Heart Surgery-1) categories with stable hemodynamics and as an adjunct to weaning from systemic opioids.

Sedative Agents

Midazolam: The commonly used sedative agent in ICU is midazolam. It belongs to the class of benzodiazepines, and acts by activating inhibitory gamma-aminobutyric acid (GABA) receptors in CNS. Midazolam produces sedation, anterograde amnesia and anxiolysis. Side effects include respiratory depression, hypotension and bradycardia. It may be used as intermittent bolus, or continuous infusion. The duration of action may be prolonged when the drug is used as a continuous infusion. Intermittent bolus is administered at a dose of 0.02–0.1 mg/kg IV if the child is agitated.

Special precautions are as follows:

- *Patients with ventricular dysfunction*: Midazolam should be used with caution in patients with significant ventricular dysfunction as bolus doses can precipitate hypotension.
- *Respiratory depression*: Midazolam can cause respiratory depression, if higher doses are used. Monitor for signs of bradypnea or apnea in an extubated child.
- *Tolerance and withdrawal*: Children who receive midazolam for long duration might develop tolerance. Children who become dependent on midazolam may show signs of withdrawal, when the drug is stopped or reduced.
- It has been recently advocated to completely avoid use in pre-term infants (as it can cause significant hypotension) and, limit use, if at all in term neonates.[9]
- Emerging literature shows that use of benzodiazepine sedation in pediatric intensive care increases the chances of delirium by as much as a factor of three.[10]

Lorazepam: This drug belongs to the class of benzodiazepines and is commonly used as an enteral preparation. It is usually used as an alternative sedative agent for the treatment of withdrawal or tolerance to conventional drugs. Intravenous preparation should be used with caution due to the risk of elevated osmolar gap acidosis and renal toxicity due to presence of polyethylene glycol in the formulation. Typical oral dose is 0.1 mg/kg given at 8–12 hours intervals.

Dexmedetomidine (Dex): This is a centrally acting alpha-2 agonist, which is being increasingly used in PCICU. It acts by inhibiting central sympathetic outflow and stimulating the parasympathetic outflow. It has combined analgesic and sedative properties. It induces natural rapid eye movement (REM) sleep and facilitates easy arousal.[5] Dex offers the advantage of relative preservation of upper airway tone allowing extended use after separation from mechanical ventilation.[11]

It is used as an adjunctive sedation agent in multimodal analgesic regimes. It is emerging as one of the key agents in patients planned for early extubation due to its favorable pharmacological profile. Additionally, heart rate lowering properties of Dex is also being explored in the prophylaxis and treatment of tachyarrythmias like junctional ectopic tachycardia in the postoperative period.[12] Side effects include bradycardia, heart block, sinus arrhythmia, nausea, and vomiting. Notably, the bradycardia that results from use of Dex should not be treated with anticholinergics as it can precipitate severe hypertension.[11] Tolerance has been described in neonates and other age groups.[11] It is predominantly used as a continuous intravenous infusion after an initial bolus of 0.5 µg/kg over 20–30 minutes. Continuous infusion is preferred in the dose of 0.25–0.75 µg/kg/h. Withdrawal symptoms can occur after stopping prolonged infusions.

Clonidine: This is a centrally acting alpha-2 agonist. It has analgesic properties with opioid sparing effect. This drug can be used to treat withdrawal and for drug cycling in patients who has prolonged recovery. Predominant side effects include hypotension and bradycardia. It can be administered via enteral or transdermal route. Typical daily dose is 5 µg/kg/day.

Muscle Relaxants

Neuromuscular blocking agents are used in pediatric ICU to facilitate intubation and mechanical ventilation in patients with limited cardiorespiratory reserve to decrease myocardial work and oxygen demand. Paralysis should always be combined with appropriate pain relief and sedation. Paralysis and deep sedation are particularly important in patients with labile pulmonary hypertension or in patients who require reintubation for upper airway edema to reduce movement. Continuous paralysis is not generally encouraged in the ICU management. Children usually do not "fight ventilators" as long as the ventilator settings are appropriate for the infant and they do not have hypoxia or hypocarbia. Prolonged paralysis is associated with risks of prolonged ventilatory support, development of tolerance to a drug and critical illness polyneuropathy in the postoperative period.[13] Extreme caution should be exerted to avoid situations where children are paralyzed without adequate sedation or pain relief.

Agents that are in routine use include nondepolarizing muscle relaxants such as pancuronium, vecuronium, and atracurium. Depolarizing muscle relaxant succinyl choline is primarily used to facilitate rapid sequence intubation in patients with increased risk of aspiration or in those with anticipated difficult intubation.

Nonpharmacological Methods of Pain Management

Sympathetic nursing and careful attention to simple environmental factors enhances comfort and reduce the requirements of analgesics.

According to the recommendations of "consensus guidelines on sedation and analgesia of critically ill children", any correctable environmental and physical factors causing discomfort should be addressed along with the introduction of pharmacological agents.[14]

Nonnutritive sucking: This has been reported to have a calming effect on children. Pacifiers can induce sleep and decrease crying in extubated neonates and small infants. Appropriate size of the pacifier should be chosen to fit the infant's mouth.

Simple repositioning and swaddling of the infant can facilitate comfort. When infants are well-positioned, hand to mouth activity, proper flexion, and self-soothing behaviors are encouraged. Massage and relaxation techniques, which have been proven beneficial in critically ill adults, can be employed in children too.

Sucrose: This has been used as a technique for management of procedure related pain. Administration of sucrose and non-nutritive sucking has a synergistic effect. Sucrose should be administered at least 2 minutes prior to a painful procedure. It should be given by mouth directly on the tongue or buccal surface to be absorbed by the mucous membranes.

Distraction: Distraction with books, bubbles, musical toys, and counting objects is helpful in older kids. It involves shifting the focus of attention from pain.

Music: Calming or relaxing music is known to have a soothing effect on infants and young children. This may be played on tape players with or without head phones.

Attenuating environmental noise: Average sound pressure levels in pediatric units range from 53 to 73 dB.[15] It is recommended that hospital noise levels should not exceed 45 dB during the day and 35 dB at night.[16] Ear muffs can be used in children to ward off annoying ambient noise and minimize sleep deprivation.

Establishing day night cycles especially in older children help them to cope with longer ICU stays. A normal pattern of sleep should be encouraged as sleep deprivation can have deleterious effects on protein synthesis, healing, pulmonary function, and immune system. A daily activity schedule can be prescribed to the child along with the use of clocks, calendars, and lighting changes to maintain day-night orientation.

Parental presence: Parental presence should be encouraged whenever possible. They should be allowed to interact with children and offer comforting touch after ensuring proper hand hygiene. This will be beneficial for the older children to adjust to the longer ICU stays.

Patient Controlled Analgesia

This mode of analgesia is shown to be safe in children aged 7 years or above. A patient controlled analgesia (PCA) pump is programmed to deliver a preset dose of analgesic drug (morphine or fentanyl) to the patient at the push of an attached button. A lock out period between doses prevents administration of repeated doses in a short-time period. PCA has the advantage of enhanced control by the patient and better nursing efficiency. However, adequate preoperative training of the children to use this device may be needed to optimize this technique. Nurse controlled analgesia may be used in neonates and small infants who cannot push the button themselves.

Procedural Sedation

Pediatric patients are likely to undergo painful procedures in postoperative period such as intercostal drain insertion, cardiac catheterization, pericardiocentesis, sternal wound debridement, bronchoscopy, etc. This may necessitate the use of anesthetic agents with sedative-hypnotic and analgesic properties. Common agents include propofol, ketamine, benzodiazepines, and opioids.

The anesthetic drug propofol is an alkyl phenol derivative, which is commonly used as a sedative agent in adult patients. Safety of propofol in pediatric patients has been questioned by reports of life-threatening propofol infusion syndrome (PRIS) characterized by lactic acidosis, bradycardia, oliguria,

TABLE 3: Essential drugs for procedural sedation in pediatric cardiac intensive care units.	
Drug	**Dilution strength**
Ketamine	5 mg/mL (<10 kg) 10 mg/mL (> 10 kg)
Propofol	5 mg/mL (<10 kg) 10 mg/mL (>10 kg)
Fentanyl	5 µg/mL (<10 kg) 10 µg/mL (>10 kg)
Midazolam	0.25 mg/mL (<5 kg) 0.5 mg/mL (>5 kg)
Glycopyrrolate	10–20 µg/mL

TABLE 4: Richmond Agitation-Sedation Scale.[19]		
Score	**Term**	**Description**
+4	Combative	Overtly combative, violent, immediate danger to staff
+3	Very agitated	Pulls or removes tubes or catheters, aggressive
+2	Agitated	Frequent nonpurposeful movement, fights ventilator
+1	Restless	Anxious, but movements not aggressively vigorous
0	Alert and calm	
−1	Drowsy	Not fully alert, but sustained awakening (eye opening/contact) to voice (>10 seconds)
−2	Light sedation	Briefly awakens to voice with eye contact (<10 seconds)
−3	Moderate sedation	Movement or eye opening to voice (but no eye contact)
−4	Deep sedation	No response to voice/but movement or eye opening to physical stimulation
−5	Unarousable	No response to voice or physical stimulation

rhabdomyolysis and myoglobinuria.[17] This complication is usually associated with use of high doses of propofol, sepsis, cerebral injury, etc. Notwithstanding this, propofol is still being used with caution for procedural sedation in many settings.

Ketamine is another commonly used agent which produces dissociative anesthesia by blocking N-methyl D aspartate (NMDA) receptors resulting in sedation, analgesia, and amnesia. Ketamine increases muscle tone and blood pressure due to its sympathomimetic effect. Side effects include emergence delirium and hence is often combined with a benzodiazepine like midazolam. It also increases oral and respiratory secretions. This may be decreased by simultaneous administration of an antisialogogue like glycopyrrolate. A suggested list of medications and their dilutions, which are useful for procedural sedation, is given in **Table 3**.

In addition to this, emergency resuscitation drugs, drugs needed for emergency intubation, airway equipment, crash cart, and defibrillator should also be readily available at bedside before performing any painful interventions in the postoperative patients.

Sedation Assessment Tools

Titrating sedative drugs is challenging in pediatric patients. Common sedation assessment tools make use of behavioral and physiological measures to assess sedation. It is important to assess sedation levels to titrate the pharmacological agents, so that optimal levels are achieved to ensure patient comfort and to minimize complications.

A sedation tool that has been validated for use in critically ill pediatric patients is Richmond Agitation-Sedation Scale (RASS).[18,19] This scale contains three steps including observation, verbal stimulation, and tactile stimulation of the patient (**Table 4**). This may be used in both mechanically ventilated and spontaneously breathing patients.

Side Effects of Long-term Administration of Analgesics and Sedatives

Tolerance

This refers to decreasing clinical effects to a drug after prolonged exposure to it. This primarily occurs due to desensitization of receptors. Greater degree of tolerance is seen with short-acting agents. Tolerance is typically addressed by using long-acting drugs (e.g., Methadone in case of opioid tolerance) or by dose escalation of a particular drug. However, there may be regional differences in choice of sedative and analgesic agents, subject to availability of the drug locally. Adjunctive agents such as Dex, clonidine, or lorazepam are alternative options, which can be used in the setting of drug tolerance.

Withdrawal Syndrome

Prolonged use of some drugs also results in the development of dependence. Abruptly stopping these drugs may result in altered physiological state resulting in withdrawal syndrome after prolonged use. Withdrawal is poorly monitored in many units and can have serious consequences including long-term neurological sequelae.

Withdrawal syndrome occur typically following the discontinuation of sedative agents particularly opioids or benzodiazepines. The potential for developing withdrawal phenomena should be considered after 7 days of continuous opioid or benzodiazepine therapy. The symptoms occur within few hours of stopping the drug and can include CNS manifestations (agitation, seizures, arterial desaturation, hallucinations, and psychosis) and autonomic features (vomiting, diarrhea, tachycardia, hypertension, and fever). The exact mechanism for the development of withdrawal symptoms is poorly understood. A withdrawal assessment tool, which can be maintained by bedside nurses, can help to identify withdrawal early and institute corrective measures. A withdrawal assessment tool-version 1 (WAT-1)[20] validated in children is given in **Table 5**.

A score > 3 on a 12-point scale is considered to be positive for withdrawal.

How to manage and prevent withdrawal?
Strategies:
- Employment of a WAT to identify signs of withdrawal early.

TABLE 5: Withdrawal assessment tool–version 1.[20]

Assessment	Grading	Score
Information from patient's record (past 12 hours)		
Any loose/watery stools	No = 0, Yes = 1	
Any vomiting/wretching/gagging	No = 0, Yes = 1	
Body temperature > 37.8°C	No = 0, Yes = 1	
2 minutes prestimulus observation		
State	Asleep/awake/calm = 0 Awake/distressed = 1	
Tremor	None/mild = 0, moderate to severe = 1	
Any sweating	No = 0, Yes = 1	
Uncoordinated/repetitive movements	None/mild = 0, moderate to severe = 1	
Yawning/sneezing	None or 1 = 0, > 2 = 1	
1 minute stimulus observation		
Startle to touch	None/mild = 0, moderate to severe = 1	
Muscle tone	Normal = 0, increased = 1	
Post-stimulus recovery		
Time to gain calm state	< 2 minutes = 0 2–5 minutes = 1 > 5 minutes = 2	

- Limit total dose and duration of drugs likely to cause withdrawal.
- Tailor the drug to the needs of the patient by appropriate tools for pain and sedation assessment.
- Tapering drugs, which are likely to cause dependence rather than sudden withdrawal.
- Use of alternative opioid drugs (methadone)/adjunctive medications (Dex/clonidine/oral trichlorphos/lorazepam) while weaning the culprit drug.
- Use of nonpharmacological measures while weaning the drug to ensure reestablishment of better sleep architecture in vulnerable patients, e.g., patients with prolonged ICU stay.

NURSING CONSIDERATIONS IN PAIN MANAGEMENT

- Bedside nurse should perform periodic assessment of the pain using the age appropriate pain scales.
- Document pain and sedation scores hourly in the flow sheet. Assessment should be made when the patient reaches the ICU, or whenever the patient complains of pain or show any signs of pain or after the administration of pain medication.
- The bedside nurse is expected to communicate to the intensivist/attending physician, the pain and sedation score of the patient, and initiate appropriate therapeutic measures, if required.
- Administer the PRN (Pro Re Nata or when necessary) pain medications and ensure the delivery of opioid infusion as prescribed by the physician.
- Provide appropriate nonpharmacological measures/behavioral interventions that suit the age of the patient (e.g., position change for comfort, swaddling, distraction measures with toys or books, music, or lullaby).

- The bedside nurse should be aware of the various pain assessment tools, type, and dose of the pain medications and their possible side effects.
- Assess the effectiveness of pain medications once they are administered and inform the physician.

SUMMARY

Pain assessment and treatment of pain should be given high priority in the postoperative management of pediatric cardiac surgical patients. A single drug is often inadequate to provide most desirable actions expected of an ideal agent. Best results are usually obtained by combining pharmacological and nonpharmacological approaches. Adequate pain relief along with creation of a soothing environment in the postoperative period can minimize adverse cardiorespiratory sequelae to pain perception and hasten overall recovery of these children.

APPENDIX
Dosage Guidelines

The dosage guidelines are given in **Tables 6 and 7**.

TABLE 6: Common analgesics and doses.

Name	Dose	Route
Fentanyl	• 0.5–2 µg/kg/h (infusion) • 0.5–1 µg/kg (bolus)	IV IV
Morphine	• 10–40 µg/kg/h (infusion) • 0.1 mg/kg (bolus)	IV IV
Acetaminophen (Paracetamol)	• 10–15 mg/kg q4–6h • Rectal: 30 mg/kg loading and 20 mg/kg q 6h	PO/NG PR
Ketorolac	0.5 mg/kg q6–8h	IV (not more than 5 days)
Ibuprofen	6–10 mg/kg q6–8h	PO/NG

(IV: intravenous; PO: per oral; NG: nasogastric; PR: per rectal)

TABLE 7: Sedatives (S) and muscle relaxants (R).

Drug	Dose	Route
Midazolam (S)	• 0.025–0.2 mg/kg (bolus) • 0.05–0.12 mg/kg/h (infusion)	IV IV
Dexmedetomidine (S)	• 0.5 µg/kg bolus over 10–20 minutes • 0.25–0.75 µg/kg/h (infusion)	IV
Vecuronium (R)	• 0.1 mg/kg (bolus) • 0.05–0.15 mg/kg/h (infusion)	IV
Pancuronium (R)	0.1–0.2 mg/kg (bolus)	IV
Atracurium (R)	• 0.5 mg/kg (bolus) • 5–10 µg/kg/min (infusion)	IV

(IV: intravenous)

◼ REFERENCES

1. Kudchakar SR, Aljohani OA, Punjabi NM. Sleep of critically ill children in the pediatric intensive care unit. A systematic review. Sleep Med Rev. 2014;18:103-10.
2. Hummel P, Puchalski M, Creech SD, Weiss MG. Clinical reliability and validity of the N-PASS: neonatal pain, agitation and sedation scale with prolonged pain. J Perinatol. 2008;28:55-60.
3. Merkel S, Voepel-Lewis T, Malviya S. Pain assessment in infants and young children: the FLACC scale. Am J Nurs. 2002;102:55-8.
4. Keck JF, Gerkensmeyer JE, Joyce BA, Schade JG. Reliability and validity of the faces and word descriptor scales to measure procedural pain. J Pediatr Nurs. 1996;11:368-74.
5. Wright JA. An update of systemic analgesics in children. Anaesth Intens Care Med. 2016;17:280-5.
6. Wolf AR. Postoperative pain management in the pediatric cardiac patient. In: Lake C, Booker PD (Eds). Pediatric Cardiac Anaesthesia, 4th edition. Philadelphia: Lippincott Williams and Wilkins; 2005. pp. 723-34
7. Zalieckas J, Weldon CW. Sedation and analgesia in the ICU. Sem Pediatr Surg. 2015;24:37-46.
8. Amini S, Mahdavi E, Zirak N, Abbasi Tashnizi M, Vakili V. Efficacy and safety of ketorolac for pain management after congenital heart surgery: a comparison to paracetamol. Arch Crit Care Med. 2016;1:e8278.
9. McPherson C. Premedication for endotracheal intubation in the neonate. Neonatal Network. 2018;37(4):238-47.
10. Mody K, Kaur S, Mauer EA, Gerber LM, Greenwald BM, Silver G, et al. Benzodiazepines and development of delirium in critically ill children: estimating the causal effect. Crit Care Med. 2018;46(9):1486-91.
11. Mahmoud M, Barbi E, Mason KP. Dexmedetomidine: what's new for pediatrics? A narrative review. JCM. 2020;9(9):2724.
12. El Amrousy DM, Elshmaa NS, El-Kashlan M, Hassan S, Elsanosy M, Hablas N, et al. Efficacy of prophylactic dexmedetomidine in preventing post operative junctional ectopic tachycardia after pediatric cardiac surgery. J Am Heart Assoc. 2017;6:e004780.
13. Kukreti V, Shameem M, Khilnani P. Intensive care unit acquired weakness in children. Critical illness polyneuropathy and myopathy. Indian J Crit Care Med. 2014;18:95-101.
14. Playfor S, Jenkins I, Boyles C, Choonara I, Davies G, Haywood T, et al. Consensus guidelines on sedation and analgesia in critically ill children. Intensive Care Med. 2006;32:1125-36.
15. Darbyshire JL, Mueller-Trapet M, Cheer J, Fazi FM, Young JD. Mapping sources of noise in an intensive care unit. Anaesthesia. 2019; 74:1018-25.
16. The US Environmental Protection Agency Office of Noise, Abatement and Control. Information on levels of environmental noise requisite to protect public health and welfare with an adequate safety margin. Washington: The US Environmental Protection Agency; 1974.
17. Hatch DJ. Propofol infusion syndrome in children. Lancet. 1999;353:1117-8.
18. Kerson AG, DeMaria R, Mauer E, Joyce C, Gerber LM, Greenwald BM, et al. Validity of the Richmond Agitation -Sedation Scale in critically ill children. J Intens Care. 2016;4:65.
19. Sessler CN, Gosnel MS, Grap MJ, Brophy GM, O'Neal PV, Keane KA, et al. The Richmond Agitation-Sedation Scale: validity and reliability in adult intensive care unit patients. Am J Respir Crit Care Med. 2002;166:1338-44.
20. Franck LS, Harris SK, Soetenga DJ, Amling JK, Curley MA. The Withdrawal Assessment Tool-Version 1 (WAT-1): an assessment instrument for monitoring opioid and benzodiazepine withdrawal symptoms in pediatric patients. Ped Crit Care Med. 2008;9:573-80.

9

CHAPTER

Conventional Mechanical Ventilation in Pediatric Cardiac Intensive Care Unit

Rakhi Balachandran, Aveek Jayant

Reviewed by: Aveek Jayant

■ INTRODUCTION

Children undergoing congenital heart surgery under cardiopulmonary bypass (CPB) require a variable period of mechanical ventilation in the postoperative period. Preoperative lung disease, alterations in lung compliance after CPB, mechanical constraint on the lung or the airway (e.g., vascular rings and slings and Ebstein anomaly) and, ventilation as an adjunct to cardiac support are the usual justifications. Though, early extubation and fast track cardiac surgery are fast gaining momentum in the current era some patients require longer than anticipated duration of ventilatory support after cardiac surgery. Young age, greater severity of illness at postoperative admission, healthcare associated infections, pulmonary artery hypertension (PAH) causing circulatory impairment, noninfectious pulmonary complications, and need for reinterventions are some of the risk factors, which are known to prolong the duration of mechanical ventilation after cardiac surgery.[1] It is imperative that one should possess a comprehensive understanding of the principles of mechanical ventilation as well as the underlying cardiorespiratory physiology in patients with congenital heart disease (CHD) for facilitating optimal postoperative recovery.[2] At the same time, it is also important to continuously consider feasibility of separation from mechanical ventilation as this prolongs intensive care unit (ICU) stay and is in itself not

risk free. This chapter provides a brief overview of the unique physiological considerations in pediatric patients with respect to mechanical ventilation and ventilator strategies suited to specific postoperative cardiac physiology in patients with CHD. In writing, we would strongly advise that readers use our chapter as a broad overview, as mechanical ventilation is a therapy that is evolving at once and, in its core concepts deep and broad in terms of the demands on practitioners' knowledge and expertise.

ANATOMICAL AND PHYSIOLOGICAL CONSIDERATIONS IN PEDIATRIC PATIENTS

The neonatal nose is critical to airway patency as obligate nasal breathing is the norm: this rule is nearly absolute in early premies though it becomes more flexible as premies grow and in term neonates. As a principle, however, all clinicians should respect the fact that in infants, patency of the nares is a crucial component of airway integrity.

The infant larynx is anterior and superior compared to that of the adult airway. In neonates, epiglottis is large, floppy, and superior, often in contact with soft palate favoring nasal over mouth breathing. Overall, the small absolute sizes of the airway result in higher predilection to processes such as stridor because airway resistance varies disproportionately to the absolute airway diameter. Larynx, trachea, and bronchi are compliant; highly susceptible to collapsing and distending forces. Thus, any upper airway obstruction (edema, laryngospasm, vocal cord palsy, etc.) with forced inspiratory efforts can lead to dynamic airway collapse, aggravating respiratory distress in young infants. Such dynamic expiratory airway collapse typically occurs at the thoracic inlet where the difference between the negative intrathoracic pressure and the atmospheric pressure is maximum. Since, small airway resistance contribute to a larger proportion of total airway resistance in infants (50% vs. 20% in adults), any disease affecting small airways (e.g., airway edema subsequent to CPB, bronchiolitis, etc.) can cause significant symptoms in infants per gradual ramp up of increased extraluminal intrathoracic pressure.[3] A more horizontal alignment and compliant rib cage results in paradoxical inward movement of chest wall during inspiration, mostly evident in infants with upper airway obstruction and also precludes using chest wall assistance in airway patency as in adults. This is the reason there is overwhelming emphasis that in managing airway obstruction in children as opposed to adults, it is important to keep them calm. Exaggerated efforts such as in crying or in anxious children can actually worsen collapse.

Lung development in utero begins at 3 weeks postconception. It passes through embryonic, pseudoglandular, canalicular, terminal sac, and alveolar phases. It is moot to point out that the last two phases span weeks 26–36 and 36 weeks to 3 years, respectively. Therefore, infants lack the full complement of alveoli even at term. Infant lungs are prone for early collapse due to lesser supporting elastic tissue in the septae of underdeveloped alveoli along with highly compliant chest wall resulting in low transpulmonary pressures at end expiration. The inadequate

development of collateral pathways of ventilation between alveoli (namely pores of Kohn and bronchoalveolar canals of Lambert) predisposes to the development of atelectasis in the infant lung. A lower percentage of type I slow muscle fibers in the diaphragm and intercostal muscles decrease efficiency of respiratory muscles, resulting in early onset of respiratory fatigue in pathological conditions. Additionally, immature respiratory control mechanisms in neonates and preterm infants can contribute to irregular breathing pattern and breath-to-breath variability. Preterm infants are particularly prone to develop apnea. There is also blunting of responses to hypercarbia and hypoxia, which can lead to life-threatening complications.[4] Excessive inflation during ventilation may also exaggerate the Hering–Breuer reflex, thereby inhibiting inspiration by increased vagal feedback mechanism.[5] Finally, disproportionate equipment dead space and resistance imposed by small caliber endotracheal tubes (ETTs) also mean awareness of such obligate constraints is essential. Unlike in adults, in most preverbal children separation from mechanical ventilation usually also means extubation of the trachea; this is a prerequisite to patient comfort and, because of the relatively smaller size of ETTs, unassisted ventilation actually can impose significant resistance loads on breathing.

▌ CARDIOPULMONARY INTERACTIONS

Heart and lungs work synergistically to facilitate optimal tissue oxygen delivery. The interventions in one system can significantly impact the other. Change in lung volumes and intrathoracic pressure during mechanical ventilation, can affect the key determinants of cardiac performance namely atrial filling or preload, and impedance to ventricular emptying or afterload.[6]

Systemic venous return depends on the pressure gradient between the extra-thoracic great veins and the right atrial (RA) pressure. Since, the RA is housed in the thorax, right atrial pressure (P_{RA}) is directly affected by the intrathoracic pressure (P_{pl}). Spontaneous respiration decreases the intrathoracic pressure (P_{pl}) and increases the intra-abdominal pressure with inspiratory diaphragmatic descent. This in turn increases the gradient between the extra-thoracic veins and the right atrium, thereby encouraging venous return. Positive pressure ventilation reduces this gradient by directly increasing intrathoracic pressure and thus lowers the right ventricular (RV) preload. Clinical conditions such as hypovolemia, septic shock, and gas trapping with obstructive airway disease can exaggerate this positive pressure ventilation induced reduction in preload, causing significant hemodynamic compromise.[6]

Mechanical ventilation can also impact RV afterload by influencing pulmonary vascular resistance (PVR) through changes in lung volume.[3] PVR depends on the balance in vascular tone of alveolar and extra-alveolar vessels. When the lung is inflated above functional residual capacity (FRC), the compression of alveolar vessels can increase PVR. Conversely, when the inflating volumes are too minimal, there is an increase in PVR produced by the collapse of extra-alveolar vessels, which become tortuous as a result of loss of alveolar volume. This is graphically depicted in **Figure 1**.[7] Also, terminal airway collapse, which occurs at low-lung volumes, can facilitate hypoxic pulmonary vasoconstriction (HPV). Hence, it is evident that maintenance of lungs at FRC, without producing large shifts in lung volume, is ideal for maintaining a stable PVR.

Effect of mechanical ventilation on the left ventricle is predominantly on the afterload.

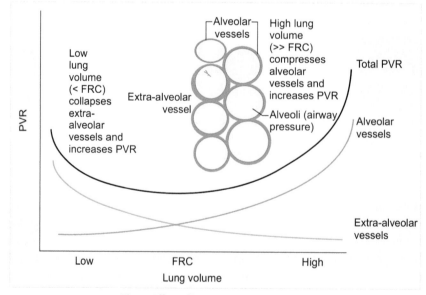

Fig. 1: Effect of lung volumes on PVR.
(FRC: functional residual capacity; PVR: pulmonary vascular resistance)
Source: Balachandran R, Vadlamudi K, Krishna Kumar R. Cyanotic heart disease in a neonate. In: Rajiv PK, Lakshminrusinha S, Vidyasagar D (Eds). Essentials of Neonatal Ventilation, India: Elsevier; 2018.

The primary determinant of left ventricular (LV) afterload is myocardial wall stress, which is a function of LV transmural pressure (i.e., the difference between LV systolic pressure and intrathoracic pressure). Positive pressure ventilation reduces transmural pressure by increasing the intrathoracic pressure and thereby, the pressure differential across the LV wall. Thus, positive pressure ventilation supports myocardial function by decreasing the LV afterload.[6,8]

SPECIAL CHALLENGES WHILE INSTITUTING MECHANICAL VENTILATION IN PEDIATRIC CARDIAC PATIENTS

- Heterogeneity in age and size of the patients undergoing congenital heart surgery necessitates a thorough understanding of developmental organ physiology while optimizing mechanical ventilator settings.
- The ventilator strategy also needs to be tailored to the cardiovascular pathophysiology that is unique to each type of CHD.
- Respiratory physiology and gas exchange are often affected by CPB and the systemic inflammatory response associated with it (e.g., increased extravascular lung water, fluid overload states, poor lung compliance).
- Exaggeration of cardiopulmonary interactions in patients with cardiovascular pathology (e.g., left, right or biventricular dysfunction or at risk ventricular status such as in pulmonary hypertension).
- Some patients with CHD have airway abnormalities such as tracheobronchomalacia, tracheal stenosis, or vascular rings that pose additional ventilation challenges in infants and children (e.g., tetralogy of Fallot with absent pulmonary valve, double aortic arch).
- Presence of genetic syndromes such as Down syndrome, DiGeorge syndrome, etc., with a predisposition to associated airway problems.
- Concomitant severe malnutrition associated with CHD often poses significant challenges to weaning and extubation.
- Poor preoperative states like preoperative pneumonia and mechanical ventilation can impact postoperative ventilatory outcomes.
- In the current era of fast track cardiac surgery, the cardiac intensivists have to strike a balance between facilitating early extubation and preventing extubation failure in these critically ill patients.

EQUIPMENT REQUIRED FOR MECHANICAL VENTILATION IN PCICU

- *Mechanical ventilators*: Most modern mechanical ventilators available today are capable of ventilating neonates and infants with tidal volumes as low as 5–10 mL. Specific neonatal ventilators are also available. If a single summary was to be provided about equipment considerations, do remember that tidal volumes measured at the level of the flow valve of the ventilator (convenient as it is because it does not add to wires, clutter, or weight to the breathing circuit) completely misses compression or compliance losses and only approximates corrections for heating and humidification of the cold dry air. It is therefore routine to use additional sensing elements for small patients; the guidance on the "when" and "how" can be found in the manufacturer specific manuals that all users must familiarize with themselves.
- Disposable pediatric breathing circuit with 22 mm male connector and 15 mm female connector on Y-piece.
- Heated water humidifiers are used for all children <30 kg.

- A heat and moisture exchanger (HME) filter should be attached to the ETT end of the breathing circuit in patients weighing >30 kg. HME filters can increase dead space and work of breathing in smaller children.

■ SETTING UP THE VENTILATOR

Broadly, the therapeutic targets of mechanical ventilation should be, to obtain adequate oxygenation with the lowest feasible fraction of inspired oxygen (FiO_2), normalize alveolar ventilation (maintain PCO_2 within acceptable range, given the cardiovascular physiology), minimize dead space ventilation (by preventing over distension of alveoli), and to facilitate recovery of postoperative cardiorespiratory function.[9] Setting up the ventilator is the responsibility of the bedside nurse, respiratory therapist, and the ICU technician. On arrival of the operating room to intensive care unit (OR-ICU) shifting chart, the ventilator is set up with the prescribed settings in the transfer chart.

Choosing the Mode

Any mode of ventilation can be selected, based on the age, weight, and the cardiorespiratory physiology of the patient. The commonly used modes of mechanical ventilation include volume controlled ventilation (VCV), pressure controlled ventilation (PCV), pressure regulated volume control mode (PRVC), pressure support ventilation (PSV), and volume support ventilation (VSV), the last two being weaning modes. Traditionally, neonates were ventilated almost universally with time cycled, continuous flow, and pressure limited ventilation. Newer evidence from the Cochrane Collaboration[10] suggests that volume targeted modes cause less lung injury, less brain damage as assessed on ultrasound, shorter ventilation times,

and less complications such as a pneumothorax. As we point out below the Pressure Regulated Volume Control mode (PRVC™) or comparable modes such as Pressure Control Ventilation-Volume Guarantee (PCV-VG™) and Volume Guarantee (VG™) tend to bridge the rhetorical sharp divide (though not necessarily proven) between volume and pressure targeted ventilation. As an aside, it is also important that as ventilators evolve and differ little between each other in terms of capability or performance, the expansion of modes, and the names associated with them also pitch for all users to read ventilator manuals before treating patients.

In VCV, the operator can set a prefixed tidal volume, which will be typically delivered in a square wave pattern. In this mode, constant flows are maintained throughout inspiration while the peak inspiratory and mean airway pressure will vary depending on the patients' lung compliance and airway resistance. In PCV mode, the operator sets a constant inspiratory pressure and the flow is delivered in a decelerating waveform pattern. Pressure rapidly builds to a preset value that is maintained throughout inspiration at a constant level, and during exhalation, the pressure is released rapidly allowing passive deflation of the lung to a set positive end expiratory pressure (PEEP) level. This mode avoids the uncontrolled rise in peak airway pressures that may occur with VCV in pathological conditions, preventing further lung injury. In PCV, tidal volume will vary depending on the compliance and resistance of the lung. The rapidity with which the pressure rises to the set level, is operator set, by adjusting the "rise time" on the ventilator. Both VCV and PCV are usually time cycled. PCV is also associated with a more homogeneous gas distribution to alveolar units with varying time constants, thus preventing regional over distension of lungs.[11] While pressure limited

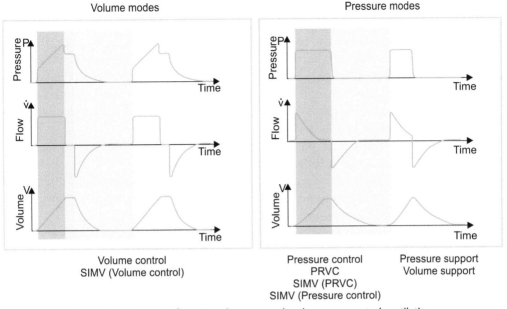

Fig. 2: Ventilator waveforms in volume control and pressure control ventilation.
(SIMV: synchronized intermittent mandatory ventilation; PRVC: pressure regulated volume control)

ventilation offers inherent safety with respect to mechanical complications of ventilation such as pneumothoraces it cannot prevent volutrauma that can occur due to increased patient effort or improved lung compliance or both. The typical waveforms generated during VCV and PCV are depicted in **Figure 2**.

An indexed tidal volume is actually the sum of (1) positive pressure from the ventilator and (2) negative pressure from the patient. As respiratory drive fluctuates usage of these modes allows a more stable tidal volume than otherwise. New modes that combine the advantages of VCV and PCV, while avoiding the disadvantages of each, are the new flavor. The PRVC or PCV-VG, combines the properties of both pressure controlled and volume controlled mode. Though this appears picture perfect it is not, as spontaneous efforts perturb ventilator equilibrium and certain ventilators such as the Draeger Babylog® 8000 plus additionally cycle the ventilators based on an inspiratory tidal volume >30% of the set volume. On the other hand, there is always the counter argument that monotonous tidal volumes are atelectasis prone and the natural fluctuation in tidal volumes in humans otherwise, should also be similarly encouraged on ventilators!

Pressure regulated volume control mode has the combined advantage of a decelerating waveform with lower peak airway pressure, while ventilating alveolar units in a more uniform pattern with guaranteed minute ventilation. Mechanical breaths are in fact pressure controlled; the level of peak inspiratory pressure (PIP) is regulated by a microprocessor on a breath by breath basis to maintain the preset tidal volume. In an earlier study in patients after congenital heart surgery Kocis et al. had demonstrated a 19% reduction in PIP with PRVC mode of ventilation compared to VCV without affecting other hemodynamic or respiratory variables.[12] PRVC or PCV-VG is the most common mode that is used in our institutional practice.

Modern ventilators commonly employ two types of triggering namely pressure trigger or flow trigger to synchronize patient's spontaneous respiratory efforts with that of the ventilator. Pressure trigger senses a drop in circuit pressure by the patients' spontaneous efforts and provides inspiratory pressure support. Flow trigger senses a change in the "bias flow" in the circuit produced by the patient's spontaneous breaths, and provides the appropriate ventilator support. Flow trigger is usually preferred in neonates and young infants due to the decreased work of breathing involved. Various patient triggered spontaneous modes that are used while weaning the patient from the ventilator includes synchronized intermittent mandatory ventilation (SIMV), PSV, and VSV. Weaning from PRVC mode is typically performed through VSV. Here, once the patient starts triggering the ventilator, the patients can be weaned through VSV where each breath is supported to a minimum preset tidal volume.

Pressure Support Ventilation

This is the most common weaning mode used before planning extubation. Each breath is patient triggered and supported by a preset pressure level. The speed of achieving the set pressure support is adjusted by the "rise time". When inspiratory flow declines below a defined threshold value, the ventilator will cycle to expiration. This is usually set as a percentage of inspiratory flow. The tidal volume generated depends on the patients' respiratory efforts, as well as compliance and resistance of the lung.

Common Ventilator Parameters

- *Tidal volume*: Tidal volume should be adjusted while noting the chest wall excursion, exhaled tidal volumes, and airway pressures. Traditionally, large tidal volumes of 10-12 mL/kg were administered to guarantee minute ventilation and prevent atelectasis. However, with increased recognition of ventilator-associated lung injury lower tidal volumes are employed typically in the range of 6-8 mL/kg especially in neonates and young infants.

- As a general rule, tidal volume targets are set as below:
  - 4-5 mL/kg for the typical premie with respiratory distress syndrome
  - 5-6 mL/kg, if <700 g
  - 5-6 mL/kg, if meconium aspiration and air trapping
  - 6 mL/kg, if >2 weeks.

- Though lung protective ventilation strategies employing lower tidal volumes of 4-8 mL/kg and lower inspiratory pressure (plateau pressure of <30 cm H_2O) have been recommended in adult patients with acute respiratory distress syndrome (ARDS),[13] there are no clear guidelines for tidal volume target for lung protection in pediatric patients.[14]

- *Respiratory rate (RR)*: The RR is set according to the age of the patient, by observation of end tidal CO_2 ($ETCO_2$) measurements and blood gas analysis. Ultimately, one should also set ventilator targets to the pH and not to the $ETCO_2$ or its partial pressure reading on a blood gas. When ventilating children below the ranges prescribed usually (as in alkalotic patients) it is worthwhile uptitrating PEEP because hypoventilation can cause loss of alveolar patency when mandatory breaths are readjusted in either volume or frequency to compensate for alkalosis.

- *I:E ratio*: This is the ratio of inspiratory time to expiratory time (I:E ratio). This can vary depending on the inspiratory time and RR that is set. The inspiratory time is generally three times the time constant and expiration, five times the time constant. Most modern ventilators today display the time constants instantaneously. Based on this the inspiratory and expiratory times can be set. Typically, an "I time" of 0.44–0.54 seconds will be optimal for term neonates and 0.25–0.35 seconds for preterm neonates. For patients aged 6–12 months, 0.7–0.8 seconds, and for older patients, 0.8–1.2 seconds will usually suffice.[15] Special attention should be taken to avoid long inspiratory time for infants who are breathing spontaneously. This will limit inspiration by vagal feedback mechanism and may cause patient ventilator asynchrony. The usual I:E ratio setting ranges from 1:2 to 1:2.5. However, in patients with airway obstruction or gas trapping longer expiratory time may be allowed by keeping I:E ratio of 1:3 or 1:4. Typically, the inspiratory times are adjusted based on analysis of the flow time waveform allowing the ventilator just adequate time to achieve the full designated flow before it cycles off. Holding inspiratory times beyond this raises the mean airway pressure (widely regarded as the arbitrator of cardiopulmonary interaction) and increases risks of air leaks. When patients have precarious cardiac status and poor lung compliance it is sometimes possible that practitioners will temporarily use longer inspiratory times to achieve a relatively non-negotiable tidal volume at a lower drive pressure. This often encroaches on expiratory times and if not monitored, the stage is set for auto PEEP and its consequences. It is therefore important that whenever the ventilator settings are manipulated, the absolute times for inspiration and expiration should be checked.

- *Fraction of inspired oxygen (FiO₂)*: The permissible FiO_2 level depends on the specific cardiac physiology in each type of CHD. Typically, in patients with two ventricle physiology FiO_2 is kept at 70–80% on arrival in ICU and subsequently decreased depending on arterial oxygen saturation and evaluation of the first blood gas in the ICU. In patients with Blalock-Taussig shunt, Stage 1 Norwood procedure and pulmonary artery banding, high FiO_2 is particularly avoided to prevent pulmonary over circulation. Generally, a PaO_2 > 60 mm Hg (with the minimum required FiO_2) for biventricular physiology and a PaO_2 > 40 mm Hg (40–55 mm Hg) for single ventricle physiology is reasonable while ventilating postoperative patients. Although, there is scarce evidence in the pediatric population, adult ICU populations seem to be adversely affected with higher than needed levels of dialed oxygen and therefore this caution of using the lowest achievable FiO_2 target is worthwhile.

- *Pressure limit*: This is the upper limit of PIP, whose value should not exceed the set limit during inspiration. Irrespective of the mode of ventilation, the alveolar pressure (plateau pressure during VCV, pressure limit during PRVC, or set pressure during PCV) is typically maintained below 25 cm H_2O. However, in patients with poor lung compliance as in ARDS, higher plateau pressures of 29–32 cm H_2O are allowable.[16] Usually, practitioners would tend to try a pressure limited mode on the riskiest patients first, and use a PIP limit about 3–5 cm H_2O above this limit when transitioning to either dual or volume targeted modes. The PIP is then targeted on a regular basis to keep it no more than 25–30% of the upper limit of the working range of PIP. This is important as the ventilator can provide dangerously high tidal volumes when (1) lung compliance improves, (2) when the proximal sensor is removed such as for nebulizing medications, and (3) when an operator attempts to deliver a manual breath. The PIP alone does not mediate lung injury and as is well known, is a composite measure of both resistance and compliance work. As such, the PIP working ranges and the pressure limit should figure in all periodic assessments of ventilator prescriptions. In essence, while there is a lot of emphasis on PIP adjustments in the higher ranges it is also important to adjust PIP to prevent large tidal volumes periodically in the lower range of prescribed PIP.

- *PEEP*: This is the level of positive pressure provided at the end of expiration to prevent alveolar collapse at end expiration. It promotes alveolar recruitment, expands atelectatic areas, increase lung volume, and improves gas exchange. A PEEP of 5 cm H_2O is provided to all patients. As pointed out PEEP is an individualized prescription that is titrated to achieve lung volumes close to FRC. PEEP can alter cardiac preload, can increase RV afterload when it triggers hyperinflation, and reduce RV afterload when combined with recruitment to treat alveolar collapse. PEEP titration is of special importance in circulations in which pulmonary blood flow is driven by a hydraulic gradient such as the functional single ventricle after a bidirectional Glenn (BDG) shunt or after total cavopulmonary connection. The cessation of PEEP and consequent increase in LV preload can also putatively affect loading conditions in a compromised ventricle and can unmask overt failure on cessation of mechanical ventilation.[17]
- *Alarm limits*: A very important, and often ignored part of ventilator settings, is putting up the appropriate alarm limits

based on expected normal ranges for the set parameters. Ventilator alarms should not be ignored, as they predict important complications such as ETT obstruction, disconnections from ventilator, loss of circuit volume, water in the circuitry, inappropriate FiO_2 delivery, patient ventilator asynchrony, or equipment failure.

COMMON INDICATIONS FOR MECHANICAL VENTILATION IN THE PEDIATRIC CARDIAC INTENSIVE CARE UNIT

- Postoperative phase after congenital heart surgery
- Respiratory failure
- Resuscitation for cardiac arrest in the postoperative period
- Sepsis
- Severe ventricular dysfunction
- Postoperative intervention or ICU procedures.

GOALS OF NURSING CARE FOR A VENTILATED CHILD

Nursing care of mechanically ventilated patients in the ICU can be extremely challenging. The core principles of nursing management include ensuring patient safety and patient comfort.[18-20]

Ensure Patient Safety

This is by careful monitoring and prevention of complications related to mechanical ventilation.

Bedside Safety Measures
- All ventilated patients in PCICU should have a nurse patient ratio of 1:1.
- Do not leave a ventilated child unattended.
- Manual resuscitation bag (Ambu Bag), oxygen tubing, appropriate sized face mask, and suction catheters of appropriate

size, should be available at the bedside at all times.

- Suction equipment should be set up at the suction outlet and checked for proper function.
- A stethoscope should be available at the bedside. Do not transfer stethoscopes from one bedside to next unless thoroughly cleaned.
- Drug tray at the bedside should contain sedative agents (Midazolam 0.5 mg/mL) and muscle relaxants (Vecuronium 1 mg/mL or atracurium 1 mg/mL)
- Crash cart and emergency resuscitation equipment including emergency drugs should be readily accessible.

Monitoring of a Patient on Mechanical Ventilator Support

ICU monitors

- Continuous SPO_2 monitoring.
- $ETCO_2$ monitoring, if available.
- Continuous RR monitoring.
- Continuous ECG monitoring and arterial blood pressure monitoring.
- *Arterial blood gas (ABG) sampling*: An initial ABG is to be done with a FiO_2 of 0.7–0.8 once the patient is settled after arrival in ICU. A repeat sample is done 30 minutes later based on the ventilator changes instituted after the initial ABG. Following this, ABG needs to be done only once in every 4–6 hours, if the ABG values are normal in the second sample.
- *Pain and sedation assessment*: Monitor sedation levels by age appropriate pain scoring tools and sedation scores hourly, and institute appropriate measures to facilitate patient ventilator synchrony.
- Temperature monitoring.

Monitoring: Nursing considerations with respect to mechanical ventilation

- Hourly recording of ventilator settings on the flow sheet.

- Hourly recording of peak airway pressures, plateau pressures, mean airway pressures, and the measured RR. Tidal volumes should be noted every hour especially if infants are on pressure controlled modes of ventilation.
- Check the stability of the ETT and proper fixation. If the tapes are loose or soiled, it should be brought to the notice of the physician and changed.
- Check the patency of the ETT and circuit. If there are secretions in the ETT, which is visible or apparent from auscultation, prompt suctioning should be done. Changes in peak airway pressures can also be used as an indicator of ETT occlusion with secretions. Routine 4th hourly suctioning of ETT is not generally encouraged. Suctioning frequency is dictated by the lung condition, as well as nature and quantity of secretions.
- Monitor the ventilator circuit for the presence of water, which should be removed promptly. Empty the water trap in the expiratory circuit periodically. Maintain ventilator tubings always at a lower level than the patient's mouth to prevent secretions in the tubings draining into the patient.
- Monitor for air leaks especially when uncuffed tubes are used. Air leaks may increase, when the airway edema decreases after the first 24 hours.
- Ventilator tubings should be changed every weekly or when soiled.
- Heated water humidifiers should be used in all pediatric patients.
- Sterile 1 L water bag should be used to fill water in the humidifier. The water level should be checked every hour.
- The temperature of the humidifier should be set at 37°C.
- Constantly assess patient comfort and synchrony with the ventilator. If the

patient appears agitated on the ventilator, the cause should be evaluated and therapeutic measures should be initiated. All patients on ventilator should have baseline analgesia, usually in the form of continuous narcotic infusions. In the absence of any obvious cause, sedation may be given intermittently. Benzodiazepines are typically avoided in the form of continuous infusion. If continuous sedation is required, a short-acting sedative like dexmedetomidine or propofol infusion (in older patients) may be used.

Monitoring for complications
- *Displacement of the ETT*: This can occur due to accidental dislodgement in an agitated child, inadequate securement or inappropriately highly positioned ETT. This can be detected by sudden desaturation, bradycardia, decreased air entry, decreased chest rise or abdominal distension, patient phonating or coughing while on ventilator, loss of ETCO$_2$ tracings, apnea alarm, or loss of waveform on the ventilator interface. When the displacement is obvious, remove the old tube and provide bag mask ventilation with appropriate FiO$_2$. Inform physician on call who should then proceed to reintubate the patient. However, if the patient is comfortable and sustains adequate respiratory efforts with no cardiorespiratory compromise, patient can be provided supplemental oxygen through face mask or noninvasive ventilation as decided by the physician.
- *Obstruction*: This can occur due to retained secretions or kinking or malfunction of the tube. There will be increase in the PIP with activation of peak pressure alarms on the ventilator. Concomitant inability to pass a suction catheter should be looked for, if the tube is totally obstructed. Treatment should depend on the cause and nature of secretions suctioned. If totally obstructed, the tube should be replaced. Kinking of the tube can be prevented by appropriate positioning of the patient and ETT.
- *Pneumothorax*: This is accumulation of air inside the pleural cavity. The clinical signs include desaturation, absent or reduced air entry on the ipsilateral side, decreased chest rise, and increased resonance on percussion. Sometimes subcutaneous emphysema or crepitus may be appreciated. A tension pneumothorax may be accompanied by hemodynamic instability. An ultrasound of the chest will allow rapid diagnosis of pneumothorax. Inform the surgical team emergently. Treatment is by insertion of an intercostal drain and removal of air. Needle aspiration should be considered for tension pneumothorax if expertise for intercostal drain insertion is not immediately available.
- *Barotrauma or volutrauma*: This can occur due to excessive inflation pressures. This may be diagnosed by increased air leak from intercostal drain or development of pneumothorax.
- *Lung collapse*: This can occur if there is a total or partial loss of lung volume. It can be diagnosed by unilateral decreased air entry, desaturation and low PO$_2$ on blood gases. Treatment depends on the cause of lung collapse. Thick mucus plugs, which obstruct the large airways, can be removed by suctioning and chest physiotherapy following saline nebulization.
- *Equipment failure*: Ventilator malfunction can be a potential complication. This can be due to faulty equipment, disconnections or leaks in the circuit, power failure, or failure in gas supply. If there is ventilator failure, Ambu ventilation should be provided. Prompt attention to the cause

or replacement of the equipment is then carried out.

Ensure Patient Comfort

Positioning

Patients should be nursed with head end of bed elevated to 15–30°. Infants and toddlers can be nursed in lateral position with position change in every 2 hours. Pressure points should be appropriately padded or rested on air or water cushions to prevent injury.

Minimizing Patient Stressors

Common stress factors for pediatric patients in intensive care settings includes pain, anxiety from parental separation, hunger, ambient noise and cold environment.

- Pain control measures should be provided with the help of pain assessment tools.
- *Prevention of hypothermia*: Neonates and infants are vulnerable to develop hypothermia. Typically, neonates and infants are nursed in bassinets with overhead warmers. Warming blankets should be provided in older children for minimizing heat loss and decreasing discomfort.
- Enteral feeds should be initiated early. Oral pacifiers to enable non-nutritive sucking may be provided for soothing infants.
- Parental presence may be ensured as soon as feasible in the postoperative period to decrease anxiety.
- General body care may be given at regular intervals to maintain hygiene. Mouth care should be provided in every shift.
- Wound care, dressing changes and catheter care are also given at regular intervals to prevent nosocomial infections.
- *Avoid sleep disturbances*: Alteration in sleep-wakefulness cycles can occur in critically ill patients leading to delirium. Allow periods of uninterrupted sleep as much as possible by clustering care and limiting

stress as much as possible. Prolonged sleep disturbance can also contribute to long-term psychological disturbances.

- Day-night orientation should be facilitated to older patients who are on prolonged ventilation by showing them time on wall clocks, making a daily routine timetable (e.g., brushing teeth/mouth care, feeding time, sleep or rest time) and reducing the intensity of ambient light and noise at night.
- Ear muffs can be used to ward-off ambient noise.
- Music therapy is known to have a soothing effect and decrease stress and anxiety in critically ill patients nursed in ICU.

Prevention of Complications

- *Pressure ulcers*: Careful observation for breaks in skin integrity should be performed on an hourly basis. Tools like Braden Q scale may be used for monitoring pressure sores in pediatric patient.[21] Skin circulation should be improved by gentle repositioning, massage, and passive range of motion exercises of limbs. Patients who are critically ill and likely to have long stay, should be nursed on soft gel mattress or air-cushion beds to minimize the incidence of pressure ulcers.
- *Eye care*: Patients, who are sedated or paralyzed while on ventilator, are vulnerable for development of exposure keratitis. Eyes should be lubricated and taped in paralyzed patients. Lubricant gels may be used at 6-hour intervals on patients who are awake and have preserved blink reflexes while on mechanical ventilator support.
- *Prevention of malnutrition*: Enteral nutrition should be initiated early and feeds should be escalated in terms of volume and caloric intake. Actual caloric intake and weight trends should be monitored on a daily basis to identify and treat

malnutrition early so that weaning is facilitated in patients with long stay.

VENTILATORY STRATEGIES IN SPECIAL SITUATIONS (See also Specific Conditions for Guidance and Rationale in these Situations)

Pulmonary Artery Hypertension (PAH)

The ventilatory management in patients with PAH should focus on avoiding the potent triggers for pulmonary vasoconstriction[22] and avoiding hypercarbia, acidosis, hypoxemia, and excessive changes in lung volume. Children with pulmonary hypertension are generally not candidates for fast tracking. Adequate sedation and paralysis should be provided to minimize stress response. Pain control is achieved by opioid infusions like fentanyl, which maintains hemodynamic stability. In children with potential for pulmonary hypertensive crisis, postoperative pulmonary vasodilation is desirable. Usual ventilator settings aim at an arterial oxygen tension (PaO_2) between 100 and 150 mm Hg, mild respiratory alkalosis (pH 7.45–7.5), and a $PaCO_2$ between 30 and 35 mm Hg. Deepening of sedation and analgesia may be required before endotracheal suctioning or other painful procedures, to minimize triggers for increase in PVR.

Single Ventricle Physiology

Patients with single ventricle physiology (Glenn and Fontan circulation) do not have a subpulmonary pumping chamber and depend on passive pulmonary blood flow via the cavopulmonary shunts. For patients with a Glenn circulation, oxygen saturation should be kept at 80–85% and $PaCO_2$ at 45–50 mm Hg to improve cerebral blood flow and improve superior vena cava (SVC) drainage. In children with Fontan circulation the oxygen saturation should be maintained above 90%.

After a Fontan/Glenn Shunt pulmonary blood flow is passive and therefore PEEP as well as the mean airway pressure is kept at minimum physiological levels. A low-mean airway pressure promotes transpulmonary flow of blood. Any mode of ventilation with a decelerating waveform is ideal for these infants. PRVC mode will be beneficial in this setting, as the decelerating flow pattern minimizes the peak and mean airway pressures. Since spontaneous breathing improves passive pulmonary blood flow in these patients, early extubation is desirable in the postoperative period.

It is also important to remember that in children with bidirectional Glenn (BDG) circulation, the cerebral and pulmonary systems are connected in series. Pulmonary vasculature responds by vasodilatation to hyperoxemia and hypocarbia, whereas the cerebral vasculature constricts under these same circumstances resulting in systemic hypoxemia along with reduced cerebral oxygen saturation. Hypocarbia is detrimental as it decreases cerebral blood flow and consequently the SVC blood return into the pulmonary artery via the Glenn anastomosis. Bradley et al. showed that after BDG, hyperventilation resulted in a significant decrease in arterial PO_2, reduction in systemic arterial oxygen saturation and reduction in transpulmonary gradient.[23] Hence, it is advisable to maintain the $PaCO_2$ between 40 and 45 mm Hg in these infants to improve cerebral blood flow, and consequently the pulmonary blood flow and systemic oxygen saturation.

While high PEEP may be detrimental for the Fontan circulation, a very low PEEP may promote atelectasis and increase the PVR. Generally, a PEEP of 2–3 cmH_2O is advocated.[24] A negative intrathoracic pressure has hemodynamic benefits and efforts should be made to extubate patients with Glenn or Fontan at the earliest.

To summarize, short inspiratory times, longer expiratory time to allow passive pulmonary blood flow, lower mean airway pressures, minimal PEEP, and early extubation are usually adopted strategies in patients with Glenn/Fontan circulation.

Patients with Left to Right Shunts

This includes patients with ventricular septal defects, atrial septal defects, atrioventricular septal defects or a hemodynamically significant patent ductus arteriosus. These patients may sometimes be ventilated in the preoperative period, due to cardiac failure or lung complications. The ventilator settings should aim to avoid factors that decrease PVR and increase pulmonary blood flow. Hence, hyperventilation and excessive oxygen administration is not recommended in these group of patients. A low FiO_2 targeting an oxygen saturation around 90% and a slightly raised arterial PCO_2 between 45–50 mm Hg is desirable.[6] Additionally, a modest elevation of PVR with PEEP may help to further decrease pulmonary blood flow. Postoperatively, after elimination of shunt a subset of patients who are prone to reactive pulmonary hypertension (or persistant pulmonary hypertension) may require measures to lower PVR. If residual shunts complicate the hemodynamic management in the postoperative period, then decisions on ventilatory strategies should be taken based on whether the PVR or high-pulmonary blood flows are preventing patients from being extubated.

Systemic to Pulmonary Arterial Shunts

In patients with systemic to pulmonary artery (PA) shunts, a balance between systemic and pulmonary circulation has to be maintained. Increase in the SaO_2 > 90% usually implies pulmonary over circulation. Pulmonary over circulation may sometimes be accompanied by signs of inadequate systemic perfusion, such as increased serum lactate level, metabolic acidosis and reduced urine output. Ventilator strategies should aim to avoid factors that lower PVR. This is achieved by low FiO_2, higher PCO_2 (45–50 mm Hg) and mild respiratory acidosis. If there is persistent evidence of systemic hypoperfusion, systemic vasodilation with afterload reducing agents like milrinone, levosimendan, or enalapril may be considered. If the child is adequately perfused (no base deficit, normal lactate, and adequate urine output), reduction in the inspired oxygen concentration alone is required.

Duct Dependent Systemic Circulation

This includes patients with hypoplastic left heart syndrome and its variants that require careful balance between systemic and pulmonary blood flow. These patients are prone to develop systemic hypoperfusion secondary to large flow of blood to the pulmonary circulation. Ventilation should avoid factors that lower PVR such as the use of higher FiO_2 and alkalosis. A low FiO_2 and higher PCO_2 (45–50 mm Hg) will help to maintain adequate systemic perfusion and minimize steal into the pulmonary circulation.

Right Ventricular Dysfunction

Right ventricular dysfunction can complicate postoperative course of patients after congenital heart surgery in some cases (e.g., after tetralogy of Fallot repair). This may be due to the effects of ventriculotomy or excessive resection of infundibular tissue, or due to the restrictive RV physiology developing in a hypertrophied right ventricle after CPB. These patients tend to develop pleural effusions and ascites with increased intra-abdominal pressure. The right ventricle is extremely sensitive to the cardiopulmonary interactions. Mechanical ventilation settings should focus on optimizing lung volumes after drainage of pleural/peritoneal effusions and maintaining low intrathoracic pressures. This will help to optimize RV preload. Ventilatory strategy should target a low mean airway pressure (low P_{aw}) while maintaining lung volume at FRC. Lower tidal volumes and short inspiratory times may be beneficial.[25] Maintaining a low P_{aw} will also promote the transpulmonary flow of blood, which in turn is the main preload to the left heart. Effects of increased intrathoracic pressure on preload during positive pressure ventilation will be magnified by hypovolemia, so maintenance of adequate intravascular volume is important in these children. PVR is generally low in these patients, but care must be taken to avoid factors that increase the PVR (acidosis, hypercarbia, hypoxemia, large tidal volumes, or high PEEP). It is generally conceived that those patients with cardiac output predicated by RV dynamics predominantly benefit from early extubation and tetralogy of Fallot seems a well-established surgical model to study this approach.[26,27] It is, however, also worthwhile to play Devil's advocate here: in neonates although the absolute work of breathing is about 10% that of adults this is achieved at higher oxygen cost and lower mechanical efficiency. Severely compromised cardiac output including conditions such as RV restrictive physiology can unmask oxygen demand supply mismatch that could then trigger extubation failure.

Left Ventricular Dysfunction

The beneficial effect of mechanical ventilation in patients with LV dysfunction is by decreasing the LV afterload. The main determinant of LV afterload is the LV wall stress, which in turn depends on LV transmural pressure. Transmural pressure is the difference between LV systolic pressure and intrathoracic pressure. As intrathoracic pressure increases, the transmural pressure

decreases and afterload decreases. Positive intrathoracic pressure during mechanical ventilation decreases the systemic afterload and the work of breathing. Physiological levels of PEEP help to maintain alveolar patency and improve lung volumes in patients who develop secondary atelectasis, as a result of LV failure induced pulmonary edema. However, higher level of PEEP may be counterproductive in patients with low-cardiac output and hypotension, as it further decreases the ventricular preload.

WEANING FROM MECHANICAL VENTILATION

After an uncomplicated or simple procedure, when cardiorespiratory dysfunction is minimal, early extubation may be considered once child wakes up from anesthesia. Factors that contribute to delay weaning include younger age, pre-existing lung disease, long bypass time with resultant capillary leak syndromes, residual cardiac lesions, delayed sternal closure, and pulmonary hypertension.[28,29] Extubation should be attempted when sustained independent respiration seems likely and when both oxygen and ventilation requirements are sufficiently low.

The weaning practices vary from institution to institution and till date a clear-cut criteria has not been established. However, the general guidelines for weaning children after surgery for CHD include the following:

- Hemodynamic stability with minimal inotropic support.
- Reliable rhythm (sinus or paced).
- Absent or minimal drainage from chest drains.
- Absence of pulmonary hypertensive crisis.
- Appropriate neurological status to ensure airway protection.
- Chest radiograph without significant lung pathology.

- Appropriate blood gases given the underlying physiology.
- Absence of any major residual cardiac defect.

Successful extubation of most infants is most likely to occur when a low rate of SIMV/PRVC is well-tolerated. In infants being weaned from PRVC mode the decrease in RR is best accomplished by limiting the inspiratory time to around 0.5–0.6 seconds and gradually increasing expiratory time. Though steroids have proven benefits in preventing postextubation stridor in adult critically ill patients, its role in pediatric population is not clear.[30] It is worthwhile considering the use of a single dose of dexamethasone, typically administered 4-6 hours prior to extubation in high-risk patients who are prone for developing postextubation stridor.

One of the suggested criteria for extubation includes the following:

- *Minimal ventilatory settings*: FiO_2 <0.5, back up ventilatory rate <10 breaths/min, PIP ≤25 cm H_2O, spontaneous effective tidal volume ≥6 mL/kg, and pressure support <10 cm H_2O. Spontaneous breathing trials through a "T" piece were not encouraged in neonates and infants earlier, due to concerns of increased work of breathing while breathing spontaneously through a narrow ETT. However, the tubes in these patients are shorter and lower flows are generated by the infant compared to the adult. Hence, it is reasonable to allow a trial of spontaneous breathing with a "T" piece or the use of 8–10 cm H_2O PSV for up to 2 hours before attempting extubation in children.[31]

Nursing Considerations before Weaning and Extubation

- Obtain the confirmation of the intensivist or anesthesiologist to initiate weaning.
- Inform respiratory therapist about the plan to wean the infant, so they can plan the course of weaning after discussion with the intensivist/on call pediatric cardiac anesthetist.
- Decrease the rate of opioid infusion to levels required to maintain adequate pain relief.
- Stop intermittent dose of sedatives like midazolam.
- Decrease the set RR as per the physician's instruction to allow more patient initiated breaths. The ventilator settings have to be cross checked by the RT as the weaning is in progress.
- A single dose of dexamethasone 0.25 mg/kg is administered at least 4 hours before planned extubation to minimize airway edema.
- Routine reversal of skeletal muscle relaxants is not indicated if sufficient time has elapsed after the administration of these drugs and the motor power is adequate. If evidence of residual neuromuscular blockade is present administer neostigmine 50 µg/kg and glycopyrrolate 10 µg/kg intravenously as a slow injection.
- If the child is on enteral feeds, feeds are withheld 4 hours prior to extubation to minimize the risk of aspiration.
- Observe the child closely for signs of respiratory distress. Tachypnea, subcostal retractions, paradoxical breathing, nasal flaring or use of accessory muscles of respiration may indicate failure to tolerate weaning. In such situations notify the physician and analyze the probable cause of respiratory distress.
- Breathing results in oxygen expenditure and in a patient with borderline cardiac function, precious oxygen is lost to the respiratory muscles; which while on full

ventilation was used by the other vital organs. In such situations, observe the child for signs of low cardiac output such as cool extremities, feeble pedal pulses, generalized mottling, hypotension, decreased urine output, increased lactate levels and metabolic acidosis in ABG samples.

- It is beneficial to remove the mediastinal/pericardial drains before extubation as it will minimize the chance of respiratory embarrassment due to pain. This should be done after obtaining the surgeon's or intensivist's orders, if the drainage is minimal or nil.
- Obtain a blood gas sample 20 minutes after the child is on PSV or VSV before extubating the patient.

MANAGING EXTUBATION FAILURE

Weaning failure is a reality. If weaning failure occurs, a re-evaluation of the patient for both surgical and intensive care problems should be carried out. The systematic evaluation of a patient with extubation failure is provided in a separate chapter. Reintubations can be traumatic, and hence adequate interval should be allowed between reintubation and the subsequent extubation attempt.

SUMMARY

Mechanical ventilation in postoperative cardiac surgical patients requires a comprehensive understanding and expertise on the unique needs of pediatric patients and their diverse cardiorespiratory physiology. Meticulous nursing care with attention to patient safety and monitoring is of paramount importance to avoid ventilator associated complications. Extubation should be attempted at the earliest possible window to avoid complications related to mechanical ventilation.

REFERENCES

1. Polito A, Patomo E, Costello JM, Salvin JW, Emani SM, Rajagopal S, et al. Perioperative factors associated with prolonged mechanical ventilation after complex congenital heart surgery. Pediatr Crit Care Med. 2011;12:e122-6.
2. Cooper DS, Costello JM, Bronicki RA, Stock AC, Jacobs JP, Ravisankar C, et al. Current challenges in cardiac intensive care: Optimal strategies for mechanical ventilation and timing of extubation. Cardiol Young. 2008;18: 72-83.
3. Rimensberger PC, Hammer J. Mechanical ventilation in the neonatal and pediatric setting. In: Tobin MJ (Ed). Principles and Practice of Mechanical Ventilation, 3rd edition. New York: McGraw Hill Medical; 2013. pp. 573-627.
4. Cohen G, Katz-Salamon M. Development of chemoreceptor responses in infants. Respir Physiol Neurobiol. 2005;149:233-42.
5. Hassan A, Gossage J, Ingram D, Lee S, Milner AD. Volume of activation of Herring–Breuer reflex in the newborn infant. J Appl Physiol. 2001;90:763-9.
6. Shekerdemian L, Bohn D. Cardiovascular effects of mechanical ventilation. Arch Dis Child. 1999;80:470-80.
7. Balachandran R, Vadlamudi K, Krishna Kumar R. Cyanotic heart disease in a neonate. In: Rajiv PK, Lakshminrusinha S, Vidyasagar D (Eds). Essentials of Neonatal Ventilation. India: Elsevier; 2018.
8. Duke DJ. Cardiovascular effects of mechanical ventilation. Crit Care Resuscit. 1999;1:388-99.
9. Rimensberger PC, Heulitt MJ, Melines J, Pons M, Bronicki RA. Mechanical ventilation in the pediatric cardiac intensive care unit. The essentials. World J Pediatr Congenit Heart Surg. 2011;2:609-19.
10. Klingenberg C, Wheeler KI, McCallion N, Morley CJ, Davis PG, Cochrane Neonatal Group. Volume-targeted versus pressure-limited ventilation in neonates. Cochrane Database Syst Rev. 2017;10:CD00366.
11. Prella M, Feihl F, Domenighetti G. Effect of short-term pressure controlled ventilation on gas exchange, airway pressures and gas distribution in patients with acute lung injury or ARDS: comparison with volume controlled ventilation. Chest. 2002;122:1382-8.
12. Kocis CK, Dekeon MK, Rosen HK, Bandy KP, Croley DC, Bove EL, et al. Pressure regulated volume control vs volume controlled ventilation

in infants after surgery for congenital heart disease. Pediatr Cardiol. 2001;22:233-7.

13. Fan E, Sorbo LD, Goligher EC, Hodgson CL, Munshi L, Walky AJ, et al. An official American Thoracis society/European society if intensive care medicine/society of critical care medicine guideline: Mechanical ventilation in adult patients with acute respiratory distress syndrome. Am J Respir Crit Care Med. 2017;195:1253-63.

14. Rimensberger PC, Cheifetz IM, Kneyber MCJ. The top ten unknowns in paediatric mechanical ventilation. Intensive Care Med. 2018;44:366-70.

15. Zucker HA. The airway and mechanical ventilation. In: Chang AC, Hanley FL, Wernovsky G, Wessel DL (Eds). Pediatric Cardiac Intensive Care. Baltimore: Williams and Wilkins; 1998. pp. 95-105.

16. Cheifetz IM. Pediatric ARDS. Respir Care. 2017;62:718-31.

17. Al Eyadhy E. Mechanical ventilation following Glenn and Fontan surgeries: Ongoing challenge! J Saudi Heart Asso. 2009;21:153-57.

18. Couchman BA, Wetzig SM, Coyer FM, Wheeler MK. Nursing care of the mechanically ventilated patient: What does the evidence say? Part One. Intens Crit Care Nurs. 2007;23:4-14.

19. Coyer FM, Wheeler MK, Wetzig SM, Couchman BA. Nursing care of the mechanically ventilated patient: What does the evidence say? Part two. Intens Crit Care Nurs. 2007;23:71-80.

20. Rocha G, Soares P, Goncalves A, Silva AI, Almeida D, Figuerido S, et al. Respiratory care for the ventilated neonate. Can Respir J. 2018;2018:1-12.

21. Curley MAQ, Razmus IS, Roberts KE, Wypij D. Predicting pressure ulcer risk in pediatric patients: The Braden Q scale. Nurs Res. 2003;52:22-33.

22. Kulik TJ. Pulmonary hypertension. In: Chang AC, Hanley FL, Wernosvsky G, Wessel DL (Eds). Pediatric Cardiac Intensive. Baltimore: Williams and Wilkins; 1998. pp. 497-506.

23. Bradley SM, Simsic JM, Mulvihill DM. Hypoventilation improves oxygenation after bidirectional superior cavopulmonary connection. J Thorac Cardiovasc Surg. 2003;126:1033-9.

24. Williams DB, Kiernan PD, Metke MP, Marsh HM, Danielson GK. Hemodynamic response to positive end expiratory pressure following right atrium-pulmonary artery bypass (Fontan) procedure. Thorac Cardiovasc Surg. 1984;87:856-61.

25. Aronson LA, Dent CL. Post-operative respiratory function and its management. In: Lake C, Booker PD (Eds). Pediatric Cardiac Anesthesia, 4th edition. Philadelphia: Lippincott Williams and Wilkins; 2005. pp. 682-704.

26. Mahle WT, Jacobs JL, Jacobs ML, Kim S, Kirshbom PM, Pasquali SL, et al. Early extubation after repair of tetralogy of Fallot and the Fontan procedure: an analysis of the Society of Thoracic Surgeon's Congenital heart surgery database. Ann Thorac Surg. 2016;102:850-8.

27. Mahle WT, Nicolson SC, Hollenbeck-Pringle D, Gaies MC, Witte MK, Lee EK, et al. Utilising a collaborative learning model to promote early extubation after cardiac surgery. Pediatr Crit Care Med. 2016;17:939-47.

28. Mittnacht AJ, Hollinger I. Fast tracking in pediatric cardiac surgery-the current standing. Ann Card Anaesth. 2010;13:92-101.

29. Alam S, Shalini A, Hegde RG, Mazahir R, Jain A. Predictors and outcome of early extubation in infants post cardiac surgery. Ann Card Anaesth. 2018;21:402-6.

30. Jaber S, Jung B, Chanques G, Bonnet F, Marret E. Effects of steroids on reintubation and post-extubation stridor in adults. A meta-analysis of randomised controlled trials. Crit Care. 2009;13:R49.

31. Newth CJL, Venkataraman S, Willson DF, Meert KL, Harrison R, Michal Dean J, et al. Weaning and extubation readiness in pediatric patients. Pediatr Crit Care Med. 2009;10:1-11.

Extubation Protocol after Congenital Heart Surgery

Rakhi Balachandran, Suresh G Nair

Reviewed by: Aveek Jayant

■ INTRODUCTION

Extubation is considered as one of the crucial events in the postoperative recovery of the patient after pediatric cardiac surgery. Traditionally, most of the patients were mechanically ventilated for a variable period of time in the postoperative intensive care unit and considered for extubation after ensuring their cardiorespiratory stability and neurological status. However, with the refinements in surgical and anesthetic techniques, early extubation and fast tracking is feasible in many patients after congenital heart surgery.[1-3] Weaning from mechanical ventilation and extubation can be accomplished in the operating room or the postoperative intensive care unit depending on centers' experience, technical expertise and weaning protocol. Regardless of the location and timing of extubation, one has to ensure stable hemodynamics, minimal postoperative bleeding, adequate level of consciousness and reversal of neuromuscular blockade before extubation.[4] Extubation should be undertaken with extreme caution because complications in the periextubation period in critically ill children can lead to significant hemodynamic disturbances and extubation failure. Specific concerns that should be anticipated in immediate postextubation period in a pediatric cardiac surgical patient include the occurrence of postextubation stridor, pulmonary hypertensive crisis, and low cardiac output state. Extubation should always be performed by an individual who is capable of performing immediate reintubation and resuscitation should the need arise in the postoperative period. This chapter gives an overview of the practical aspects that need to be considered while performing an extubation in the pediatric cardiac intensive care unit (PCICU).

■ PREPARATION FOR EXTUBATION

Personnel

Once the decision for extubation is made by the intensive care team and weaning criteria are met, attending anesthesiologist or intensivist, bedside nurse and respiratory therapist need to be physically present at the bedside to conduct extubation process.

Equipment

Extubation after congenital heart surgery can be potentially complicated by extubation failure and need for reintubation in some patients. Hence, all equipment necessary for reintubation and emergency resuscitation should be ready at the bedside before anticipated extubation as follows:

- Endotracheal tube (ETT) of appropriate size (keep one size smaller, and one size bigger tube to be used if required). Immediate postextubation airway edema may not permit the same size of the originally placed tube

- Oral airways of appropriate sizes
- 2 working laryngoscopes with curved and straight blades
- Magill's forceps
- Ambu bag with supplemental oxygen
- Suction catheter of appropriate sizes (size of the catheter should be less than half the inner diameter of the ETT usually size 6, 8, or 10) and wall source for suction (ensure that the system is working well)
- Adhesives for securing the ETT
- 5 mL syringe for deflating endotracheal tube cuff
- Medications: Inj. Vecuronium 1 mg/mL, Inj. fentanyl 5–10 μg/mL, Inj. midazolam 0.25 mg/mL and emergency medications (adrenaline 20 μg/mL, atropine 10 μg/mL, calcium gluconate 100 mg/mL, preservative free 2% lignocaine 20 mg/mL, sodium bicarbonate 1 mEq/mL) should be preloaded and available at the bed side. Opioid receptor antagonist Naloxone should be available if required while extubating neonates on prolonged opioid infusions who exhibit respiratory depression
- Nebulizer kit with appropriate medication (salbutamol, budesonide or adrenaline)
- Oxygen mask/nasal cannula/nasal continuous positive airway pressure (CPAP) devices/high flow nasal cannula equipment
- Pacemaker with cables
- Defibrillator.

Monitoring

- Continuous SPO_2 monitoring
- Invasive arterial blood pressure monitoring
- ECG monitoring
- $ETCO_2$ (end tidal carbon dioxide) monitoring (if available).

NURSING CONSIDERATIONS AND EXTUBATION PROCESS

1. Obtain physician order for extubation.
2. Ensure that the pharmacological agents for reversal of neuromuscular blockade are administered. Reversal of neuromuscular blockade should be based on timing of last dose of muscle relaxant and motor activity.
3. Ensure that the pressure support arterial blood gas is obtained and brought to the attention of the attending anesthesiologist/physician.
4. Ensure the presence of attending anesthesiologist/intensivist at extubation.
5. Ensure the presence of a reliable arterial access and intravenous (IV) access at the time of extubation.
6. Necessary equipment and drugs should be kept ready at the bedside.
7. NPO (nil per os) hours should be confirmed. Gastric decompression should be done via the suction of nasogastric tube before extubation and should be left open.
8. Gentle ETT suction is performed using all sterile precautions. Intermittent positive pressure breaths should be given with bag valve mask device with oxygen supplementation to prevent atelectasis between each passage of suction catheter. Once the ETT is clear of secretions, the nasopharynx and oral cavity are also cleared of the secretions. If a cuffed tube is in place, ensure that the nasopharynx and oral cavity are cleared of secretions before deflating the cuff to minimize the risk of aspirating the secretions.

9. The tapes securing the ETT should be gently loosened after dabbing with normal saline or sterile water. The ETT is then gently removed while continuously applying positive pressure.

10. The appropriate supplemental oxygen delivery device is then attached. This can be an oxygen mask, nasal cannula, nasal CPAP or high flow nasal cannula system.

11. *Choosing the FiO_2 (fraction of inspired oxygen) after extubation*: FiO_2 requirement after extubation should be chosen according to the circulatory physiology that is unique to each type of congenital heart disease. Typically an oxygen saturation >90% is desirable in two ventricle physiology and >75% in single ventricle palliative procedures. In single ventricle patients who need precise balance between systemic and pulmonary circulation, FiO_2 needs to be carefully titrated with the help of air-oxygen blenders connected to wall outlets (e.g., Blalock-Taussig shunt, Norwood procedure, pulmonary artery banding, etc.). Alternatively patients can be maintained on nasal cannula with lower flow rates or on room air to maintain a saturation >75%.

SUPPLEMENTAL OXYGEN THERAPY DEVICES AFTER EXTUBATION

Oxygen Mask

Patients with normal lung compliance, minimal/no chest wall edema, adequate negative fluid balance, and breathing comfortably on pressure support/volume support mode of ventilation prior to extubation should be transitioned to oxygen mask with a flow of 3–5 L/min. The FiO_2 delivered through face masks varies depending on the patients inspiratory flow rate and the oxygen flow into the system.[5] The FiO_2 delivered by face mask typically do not exceed 0.5%. Face masks may be uncomfortable for children and can interfere with feeding. Patients should be carefully monitored for signs of increased work of breathing such as nasal flaring, subcostal retraction, or presence of stridor in the postextubation period. They should also be monitored for adequacy of peripheral circulation by noting the warmth of extremities and adequacy of peripheral pulses. A blood gas should be obtained 1 hour after extubation (or earlier if clinical situation dictates so) to assess oxygenation and ventilation. Patients can be weaned off to room air 24 hours after extubation once they are deintensified, and chest X-ray shows no evidence of lung pathology.

Nasal Cannula

Nasal cannula/prongs are designed with two short tubes that lie just inside the tip of the nostril and is available in different sizes. Standard flow rates of oxygen include 0.5 L/min for neonates, 1–2 L/min for infants and 1–4 L/min for older children.[6] Humidification is not mandatory with standard flow rates, as the natural mechanisms in the nostril are sufficient to heat and humidify oxygen at low flow rates. Typically, the FiO_2 delivered varies from 0.35 to 0.45% depending on the flow rates. Care should be taken that the nose is not occluded with mucus especially when using higher flow rates. Saline nasal drops may be used to clear and moisten the nostrils if required.

Noninvasive Ventilation Devices

Noninvasive respiratory support can be used in the treatment for respiratory failure after extubation or as a preventive measure in patients at high risk for extubation failure after pediatric cardiac surgery.[7,8] Kovacikova et al. studied 107 noninvasive positive pressure ventilations in 82 pediatric cardiac patients and found an overall success rate of 59.8% in preventing tracheal intubation. Among 73 prophylactic noninvasive positive pressure ventilation episodes postextubation, tracheal reintubation was averted in 41 (56%).[9]

Definition of Noninvasive Ventilation

Noninvasive ventilation (NIV) is defined as any mode of assisted ventilation that delivers positive pressure throughout the respiratory cycle, with additional phasic increase in airway pressure, without the presence of an endotracheal tube. These additional phasic increase in airway pressure can either be synchronized to the infant's respiratory effort or nonsynchronized depending on the delivery system used. Nonsynchronized NIV can be delivered by any of the critical care ventilators, while synchronized NIV requires specific ventilators that have triggering mechanisms. Typically, NIV is provided via the use of continuous positive airway pressure (CPAP) or bilevel positive airway pressure (BiPAP) through conventional critical care ventilators.

Physiological Benefits of Noninvasive Ventilation

- CPAP/BiPAP splints the airway throughout the respiratory cycle and provides effective chest wall stabilization.
- CPAP/BiPAP prevents alveolar collapse, promotes recruitment of alveoli and increases functional residual capacity.
- Improves lung compliance, improves ventilation perfusion matching and oxygenation.
- CPAP/BiPAP reduces the work of breathing. Synchronized NIV support leads to a reduction in respiratory rate (RR), reduces respiratory efforts and also reduces the $PaCO_2$ secondary to the larger tidal volumes generated during spontaneous breaths.
- CPAP decreases left ventricular afterload, also regulating the preload to the over-loaded ventricle(s) and can therefore offer nonpharmacologic support to the failing ventricle(s).
- CPAP, by restoring respiratory and/ or chest wall mechanics reduces the oxygen consumption of the respiratory apparatus—this could be important in whole body oxygen flux in the PCICU setting where oxygen delivery is sometimes marginal.

Indications for Nasal CPAP/BiPAP after Pediatric Cardiac Surgery

- Neonates and young infants with poor lung compliance and evidence of fluid retention as indicated by chest wall edema or radiological evidence of pulmonary congestion.
- Patients with postoperative diaphragm palsy.
- As a bridge to early extubation in fast track pediatric cardiac surgery.
- Patients with left ventricular dysfunction in the postoperative period as the increase in intrathoracic pressure will decrease the left ventricular afterload [e.g., patients undergoing repair of anomalous origin of left coronary artery from pulmonary artery (ALCAPA) with ventricular dysfunction]. It may also be beneficial in circumstances where an afterload mismatch can occur after the corrective surgery [e.g., mitral valve repair or replacement in a patient with severe mitral regurgitation (MR)].
- Patients with likelihood of a noncompliant left ventricle with a high left ventricular

end diastolic pressure (LVEDP) after corrective surgery (e.g., complex two ventricle conversions after initial single ventricle palliation, tetralogy repair with placement of a right ventricle to pulmonary artery conduit, etc.).

Techniques/Interfaces for Providing Noninvasive Ventilation

- Nasal CPAP/BiPAP
- BiPAP masks with specific BiPAP delivery systems
- Heated humidified high flow nasal cannula.

Continuous positive airway pressure may be delivered by devices that vary CPAP level by mechanisms other than flow variation (continuous flow CPAP) or by devices that vary CPAP level predominantly by altering the flow rate (variable flow devices). Continuous flow CPAP is usually delivered by infant ventilators and bubble CPAP system. In the former, the level of CPAP is altered by varying the size of the expiratory orifice in conjunction with flow control and pressure transducers. BiPAP may also be delivered with the help of standard BiPAP machines with appropriately fitting face masks for older children.

At our center nasal CPAP/BiPAP delivered by conventional ventilators, is often utilized to bridge patients after extubation following congenital heart surgery and the following section will primarily elaborate the practical aspects of delivering nasal CPAP/BiPAP using this method.

Therapeutic Targets of CPAP/BiPAP

- Stabilization of FiO_2 by reduction in the FiO_2 to <0.5 and maintenance of $PaCO_2$ between 40 and 45 mm Hg.
- Reduction in the work of breathing as indicated by a decrease of RR by 30–40% and a decrease in the severity of retractions, grunting and nasal flaring.

- Improvement in lung volumes and appearance of lung on the chest radiograph.

Practical Guidelines for the Use of CPAP/BiPAP and NIV with Conventional Ventilators

- In the current institutional practice at our center, a nasotracheal tube (a refashioned endotracheal tube) measured from the ala nasi to the tragus of the ear is introduced through one nostril and connected to the ventilator in the CPAP mode. The nostril is humidified with saline nasal drops before insertion to prevent injury due to crusting.
- *Initiation and setting up*: Start with nasal CPAP of 4–5 cm H_2O and an FiO_2 of 0.4–0.6. FIO_2 is titrated depending on the circulatory physiology and the underlying lung condition of the patient. It will be desirable to use as low FIO_2 as feasible in neonates or preterm infants to avoid the side effects of oxygen toxicity. If the primary aim is to increase the arterial oxygenation then the mean airway pressure has to be maintained at higher levels. This is achieved by slowly increasing the CPAP applied till the desired level of oxygenation is obtained. If the strategy has been initiated to augment ventilation (wash out CO_2), then BiPAP should be provided by setting a PEEP as well as a pressure support of 3–5 cm H_2O above the level of PEEP.
- Ideally, CPAP/BiPAP should be slowly increased by 1 cm H_2O every 15 minutes observing the comfort level of the patient. Typically, a PEEP of 5–7 cm H_2O and a pressure support of 3–5 cm H_2O above PEEP are used. Introduction of BiPAP or pressure support during the inspiratory phase will augment the delivered tidal volume and help washout of CO_2.

- *Humidification*: The inspired gases should always be heated and warmed to 37°C. Crust formation on the tube is common if the infant inhales dry gases for prolonged periods. On most occasions, the contralateral nostril is occupied by a nasogastric feeding tube. As obligatory nasal breathers, if the endotracheal cannula gets blocked with dry encrustations, these infants suffocate and develop cardiorespiratory events.
- It is prudent to put a nasogastric tube to prevent gastric distension while using CPAP/BiPAP. Nasogastric tube should always be left open during CPAP/BiPAP therapy except for an hour after feeds. If intermittent second hourly feeds are given, the nasogastric tube should be kept closed for at least an hour after feeding, for preventing the feeds from draining back out through the tube. Feeding may be attempted with caution if the infant appears stable on CPAP mode. Post-pyloric feeding and continuous feeds are reasonable in infants who are at risk of aspiration.
- It is reasonable to continue analgesics and mild sedatives to improve comfort levels and minimize stressors in patients on CPAP.
- Gentle suction by passage of a lubricated catheter or feeding tube can help to clear secretions periodically and maintain patency of airway.
- A chest X-ray is beneficial to support clinical findings and rule out any complication related to the use of CPAP (hyperinflation, air trapping, pneumothorax, etc.)
- Infants typically show a clinical improvement (reduction in respiratory rate, reduction in signs of respiratory distress), or improvement in ABG within an hour of CPAP/NIV. If there is deterioration or no significant changes in the clinical status, then more invasive techniques should be considered to improve the respiratory status of the infant.

CPAP/BiPAP Use in Patients on Specific Noninvasive Ventilators

CPAP/BiPAP is sometimes delivered by specific noninvasive ventilators. These ventilators differ from the conventional critical care ventilators in that they have only a single tubing that is connected to the face mask or nasal prongs. There are certain important aspects of these ventilators that merit attention.

- Single ventilator tubing passes from the ventilator to the patient. The expired gases from the patient should escape through a "swivel leak" that is placed in the tubing near the patients' end. This should always be left open. Alternatively, exit pores may be present on the mask attached to the face of the child, which should be left open for exhalation.
- A minimum CPAP of 4 cm H_2O is mandatory in these ventilators to prevent rebreathing of expired gases.
- For patients requiring BiPAP, an inspiratory positive airway pressure (IPAP) and an expiratory positive airway pressure (EPAP) need to be set.
  - Since these ventilators use only air, special ports are available for connection of oxygen source. Some specific noninvasive ventilators are available that is capable of generating an FiO_2 close to 0.8–1.

Complications Associated with the Use of CPAP

- Overdistention or atelectasis of the lungs can occur, if an inappropriate CPAP level is used. Overdistention is more common when a variable flow CPAP system is used.

- Nasal prongs can cause necrosis of the nasal septum, if the prongs are not properly placed or are used for long periods of time.
- CPAP should be cautiously used in preterm infants because of the propensity for intracranial hemorrhage due to fluctuations in CO_2 levels and increased cerebral venous pressure.
- Gaseous distension of the abdomen can sometimes occur in patients on CPAP. This can lead to feed intolerance or vomiting. In such patients it is prudent to opt for post-pyloric feeding or continuous feeds to minimize the risk of aspiration.
- Pneumothorax or other gas leaks including worsening of surgical emphysema may occur during CPAP although none have been reported in randomized studies till date.
- Blockage of the nasal cannula, in association with blockage of the other nostril (either because of a nasogastric tube or nasal congestion) can have catastrophic results in very small infants, who are obligatory nasal breathers.

Relative contraindications or when CPAP/ BiPAP should be used with caution

- Patients with abdominal distention
- Impaired neurological status
- Lobar pneumonia, pneumothorax, collapse of one lung—risk of hyperinflation of the contralateral lung with possibility of barotrauma.

MONITORING IN THE ICU AFTER EXTUBATION

- Arterial blood pressure, heart rate, SaO_2, respiratory rate and pattern of breathing should be continuously observed to identify hemodynamic instability or respiratory distress in the post-extubation period.

- Children with pulmonary hypertension should be closely monitored for development of pulmonary hypertensive crisis in the postextubation period.
- A blood gas sample should be obtained 20–30 minutes after extubation to assess the adequacy of ventilation and oxygenation. Samples can be obtained earlier if the child deteriorates or needs an emergent reintubation.
- A chest X-ray should be ordered at the bedside after extubation.

COMMON COMPLICATIONS IN THE IMMEDIATE POSTEXTUBATION PERIOD

Postextubation Stridor

This is a potential complication observed in the ICU in the postextubation period after congenital heart surgery.[10] This is most often due to airway edema, which is likely to occur after cardiac surgery under cardiopulmonary bypass.

Treatment

Administer supplemental oxygen via nasal prongs or oxygen mask. If stridor is exaggerated by crying and agitation, efforts should be made to pacify the child. Judicious use of sedatives without compromise of the airway can be attempted. Secretions obstructing the airway should be gently cleared by suctioning. Though traditionally, nebulized racemic epinephrine has been advocated for treatment of stridor, nebulized L-epinephrine 1:1,000 solution at a dose of 5 mL irrespective of the weight of the patient can be a reasonable alternative if racemic epinephrine is not available.[11-13] Nebulized epinephrine promote local vasoconstriction in the airway mediated by alpha-1-receptor stimulation and thus alleviate airway edema.

Treatment with intravenous dexamethasone at a dose of 0.2–0.5 mg/kg may be considered for a short duration to decrease airway edema contributing to stridor.[11]

Pulmonary Hypertensive Crisis

This is a probable complication, which can occur after extubation in patients with preoperative pulmonary hypertension, residual left to right shunts after surgery, or significant atrioventricular valve regurgitation.

Diagnosis

The pathognomonic features of pulmonary hypertensive crisis are a combination of high pulmonary artery (PA) pressures, systemic hypotension and desaturation. This will manifest as elevation of PA pressure to systemic levels (if PA line is present). If PA line is not available for monitoring, this is diagnosed by associated hemodynamic instability and desaturation. Management is by providing supplemental oxygen, quietening the child and clearing the airway of secretions if any. A blood gas should be obtained to rule out hypoxemia, hypercarbia or acidosis, which can aggravate pulmonary hypertension. Noninvasive ventilation may be considered in lung pathologies contributing to abnormal gas exchange and acidosis.

Extubation Failure

This is a likely complication after extubation in the postoperative period. Most common predisposing factors include young age, increased surgical complexity, residual lesions and pulmonary complications. It is important to perform a systematic evaluation in patients who have failed extubation and identify the probable causes. Extubation failure and its management in PCICU is elaborated in a separate chapter in this book.

CRITERIA FOR ELIGIBILITY FOR TRANSFER FROM THE PCICU TO STEP DOWN INTERMEDIATE CARE UNIT AFTER EXTUBATION

1. Patients should maintain normal respiratory, cardiovascular and neurological status for more than 4 hours after extubation.
2. Patients should not be on noninvasive modes of ventilator support.
3. Arterial blood gases should demonstrate acceptable $PaCO_2$ and PO_2 levels, given the cardiovascular physiology.
4. Normal serum lactate levels and absence of metabolic acidosis.
5. Patients should not require more than one inotrope for maintaining cardiac output.

SUMMARY

Extubation of a patient after congenital heart surgery is a high-risk procedure. This has to be performed after stabilization of cardiopulmonary status after the surgery. Anticipation of probable complications, careful monitoring during extubation and timely use of noninvasive respiratory support when indicated, can improve success rates after extubation.

REFERENCES

1. Neirotti RA, Jones D, Hackbarth R, Paxson FG. Early extubation in congenital heart surgery. Heart Lung Circ. 2002;11(3):157-61.
2. Mittnacht AJC, Thanjan M, Srivastava S, Joashi U, Bodian C, Hossain S, et al. Extubation in the operating room after congenital heart surgery in children. J Thorac Cardiovasc Surg. 2008;136(1):88-93.
3. Garg R, Rao S, John C, Reddy C, Hegde R, Murthy K, et al. Extubation in the operating room after cardiac surgery in children: a prospective observational study with multidisciplinary coordinated approach. J Cardiothorac Vasc Anesth. 2014;28(3):479-87.
4. Aronson LA, Dent CL. Postoperative respiratory function and its management. In: Lake C, Booker PD (Ed). Pediatric Cardiac Anesthesia,

4th edition. Philadelphia: Lippincott Williams and Wilkins: 2005. pp. 682-704.

5. Frey B, Shann A. Oxygen administration in infants. Arch Dis Child Fetal Neonatol Ed. 2003;88:F84-F88.

6. World Health Organization.(2016). Oxygen therapy for children: a manual for health workers. [online] Available from: http://www.who.int/iris/handle/10665/204584. [Last Accessed March, 2021].

7. Gandhi H, Mishra A, Thosani R, Acharya H, Shah R, Surti J, et al. Elective nasal continuous positive airway pressure to support respiration after prolonged ventilation in infants after congenital cardiac surgery. Ann Pediatr Cardiol. 2017;10(1):26-30.

8. Zhang CY, Tan LH, Shi SS, He XJ, Hu L, Zhu LX, et al. Noninvasive ventilation via bilevel positive airway pressure support in pediatric patients after cardiac surgery. World J Pediatr. 2006;2:297-2

9. Kovacikova L, Skrak P, Dobos D, Zahorec M. Noninvasive positive pressure ventilation in critically ill children with cardiac disease. Pediatr Cardiol. 2014;35:676-83.

10. Sreedharan KJ, Nair SG, Rakhi B, Rakhi KR, Vazhakkat JD, John J. Postextubation stridor in pediatric cardiac surgery patients. Ind J Resp Care. 2013;2:220-6.

11. Bjornson CL, Johnson DW. Croup in the pediatric emergency department. Pediatr Child Health. 2007;12:473-7.

12. Ortis-Alvarez O. Acute management of croup in the emergency department. Peditar Child Health. 2017;22:166-9.

13. Remington S, Meakin G. Nebulised adrenaline 1:1000 in the treatment of croup. Anaesthesia. 1986;41:923-6.

High-flow Nasal Cannula Oxygen Therapy in Pediatric Cardiac Intensive Care Unit

Suresh G Nair

Reviewed by: Rakhi Balachandran

■ INTRODUCTION

High-flow nasal cannula (HFNC) oxygen therapy is a relatively new noninvasive mode of ventilatory therapy in which heated, humidified, air-oxygen mixture is delivered to the patient at a precise fractional inspired oxygen concentration (FiO_2) at flows higher than the peak inspiratory flow of the patient. Although HFNC was first introduced in preterm infants as an alternative to continuous positive airway pressure (CPAP) therapy, its simplicity and patient comfort has resulted in widespread acceptance of the technique in both adults and children. Over the years, HFNC has been used in a variety of pediatric conditions including bronchiolitis, pneumonia, cardiomyopathy, postextubation, neonatal respiratory distress syndrome, apnea of prematurity, and obstructive sleep apnea. However, a recent Cochrane systematic meta-analysis which evaluated nine studies where HFNC was compared with conventional oxygen therapy, CPAP and bilevel positive airway pressure (BiPAP), concluded that they could not determine the safety or effectiveness of HFNC as a form of respiratory support.[1]

▌ RATIONALE FOR HFNC THERAPY IN PEDIATRIC CARDIAC PATIENTS

There is a paucity of literature regarding the use of HFNC as a postextubation therapy in cardiac surgical children. However, it seems logical to use this modality to improve respiratory failure and low cardiac output syndrome (LCOS) which are frequent complications after cardiac surgery. Common causes of respiratory failure after pediatric cardiac surgery include fluid accumulation which reduces pulmonary compliance and increase the work of breathing, increased pulmonary vascular resistance (PVR), muscle weakness, diaphragmatic fatigue, and tissue edema. Secondly, upper airway obstruction (UAO) is not uncommon after cardiac surgery and application of some form of positive pressure to the upper airway can relieve this obstruction. The UAO leads to large swings in intrapleural pressure, which in turn can affect the afterload to the left ventricle (LV) particularly when there is coexistent ventricular dysfunction. The excessive diaphragmatic movements can increase the oxygen consumption by the muscles, which could otherwise be utilized by more important organs of the body. Use of HFNC has beneficial effects in respiratory failure situations by decreasing respiratory rate, improving oxygenation and facilitating CO_2 washout. It has also been associated with improved patient comfort, decreased reintubation rates, and reduced postoperative complications.

■ HOW DOES HFNC THERAPY WORK?

High-flow nasal cannula provides heated, humidified gases at flows higher than the patient's peak inspiratory flow during the inspiratory phase. By flushing the nasopharyngeal space with fresh gas, it limits CO_2 rebreathing and thereby reduces $PaCO_2$. It also reduces the anatomical dead space by providing a nasopharyngeal source of fresh gas for the subsequent breath. During inspiration, HFNC maintains a pharyngeal positive pressure, which reduces the nasopharyngeal inspiratory resistance. HFNC also maintains a certain amount of positive end-expiratory pressure (PEEP) that helps maintain the patency of airways during the expiratory phase. The amount of PEEP generated is variable (2-7 cmH_2O) and is dependent on the cannula size, total gas flow and mouth opening. The beneficial effects of HFNC can be summarized as:

- Washout of nasopharyngeal dead space resulting in improved oxygenation and lower CO_2 in the alveoli.
- Reduced inspiratory nasopharyngeal resistance and reduced work of breathing by providing gas at flows higher than the peak inspiratory flow of the patient.
- Improved lung compliance by providing a variable amount of PEEP.
- Decreasing patient work expenditure to heat inspired gases by providing 100% humidified inspired gases.
- Improved mucociliary clearance.[2]

HFNC IN POSTCARDIAC SURGICAL PATIENTS: EFFECTS ON HEMODYNAMICS

In general, respiratory failure in the presence of LCOS is detrimental to the child who is just extubated. The large swing in intra-thoracic pressure (transpulmonary pressure) significantly alters the afterload to the LV and the excess movement of the diaphragm increases the total body oxygen consumption. HFNC by improving the oxygenation and removal of CO_2 settles the respiratory overdrive and sympathetic stimulation. The mild increase in PEEP reduces the afterload to the LV while reducing the UAO seen in some patients.

HFNC in Children with Two Ventricles

It is important to consider the variable effects of HFNC on the cardiac and respiratory physiology in children with the varying pathophysiology associated with complex congenital heart disease (CHD). In patients with normal lungs, if the PEEP exerted by HFNC leads to increase in lung volumes above the functional residual capacity (FRC), it would result in an increase in pulmonary vascular resistance (PVR). On the other hand, in patients with atelectasis, restoration of the FRC by opening up of collapsed alveoli should result in an improvement or reduction in PVR.[3] In patients with poor LV function the positive pressure (PEEP) exerted by HFNC can have beneficial effect on cardiac output due to a reduction in afterload, which outweighs the negative effects on venous return. Whereas, in patients with good LV function the reduction in venous return due to the PEEP effect of HFNC may predominate over the reduction in afterload and generate a net negative effect.[3]

HFNC in Single Ventricle Physiology

The effects of HFNC in patients with single ventricle (SV) physiology may be more complex. In patients where HFNC has restored the FRC, there may be an inadvertent increased pulmonary blood flow as compared to systemic flow, due to the reduction in the PVR. This negative effect may, however, be offset by the reduced oxygen consumption of the respiratory muscles through the effects of HFNC on cardiac output (CO) due to reduction in afterload to the LV and stabilization of sympathetic nervous system activity.[3]

After a Fontan procedure in patients with good ventricular function, the negative impact of PEEP generated by HFNC on venous return may dominate over its beneficial effect on afterload reduction to the single ventricle.[4] In patients with Fontan and poor ventricular function, the afterload reduction may be beneficial in terms of improved CO and reduced myocardial oxygen consumption, while the restoration of FRC may improve the PVR in presence of pulmonary edema or atelectasis.

HFNC IN PEDIATRIC CARDIAC SURGERY: LITERATURE EVIDENCE

There are only two studies of HFNC in postoperative pediatric cardiac surgical patients. In a study of 89 children, Testa et al. compared 89 children randomized to either conventional oxygen therapy or HFNC,[5] there was no significant difference in the $PaCO_2$, duration of therapy or intensive care unit (ICU) length of stay. However, patients in the HFNC group had significantly higher PaO_2, PaO_2/FiO_2 and lower respiratory rates during the first 48 hours of therapy. Treatment failure was significantly lower in the HFNC group. The authors concluded that the improved oxygenation was responsible for the lower respiratory rate and this resulted in overall improvement in treatment outcome. The study included both cyanotic and acyanotic children.

The second study was an observational study in very small children who developed acute respiratory failure immediately after extubation. The study was conducted in a mixed group of single ventricle and two ventricle repair patients undergoing major procedures. The authors noticed that HFNC immediately reduced the respiratory rate and systolic blood pressure of the patient while PaO_2, $PaCO_2$, lactate, and heart rate did not show any significant changes. These changes were observed in patients with

serial circulation while not appreciated in patients with single ventricles. The authors hypothesized that the improvement in respiratory distress and reduction in respiratory rate, was responsible for the drop in systolic blood pressure, a reflection of reduced sympathetic activity.[6]

HOW TO SETUP HFNC?

There is no consensus on how to use HFNC. The PEEP effect generated by HFNC is very variable as per available studies. The amount of PEEP generated is dependent on the set flow rate, weight/size of the patient and ratio of nasal cannula diameter/size of nares; with higher PEEP being generated when the mouth is kept closed.[2] In general, the PEEP generated is between 2 and 7 cmH_2O. It is also important to remember that as compared to CPAP system where a safety valve protects the airway pressure, in HFNC, it is possible that high levels of PEEP can be generated, as the only escape for the high gas flow is between the cannula and the nares and through the mouth.[2]

The flow that is generally used is about 2 L/kg/min (0.5–3 L/kg/min). A maximum of 10 L/min is normally used. Higher flows are not used, as it may be associated with complications in small children. Higher flows up to 50 L are used in older children and adults. According to Hutchings et al., the initial FiO_2 is set at 0.4 and increased to 0.5 if the SpO_2 is < 92%.[7] According to these authors who have used Paediatric Early Warning Scores (PEWS) to initiate HFNC, the noninvasive support can be initiated when the infant reaches the initial respiratory trigger of PEWS and the support can be stopped when the child maintains a SpO_2 > 92% with FiO_2 of 0.4.

Caution should be exercised when using flows greater than 1 L/kg/min or total flows greater than 10 L/min in settings outside the ICU.[2,7] At high flow rates above 4 L/min, drug delivery of nebulized medications is also debatable due to the immediate washout effect of the flow from HFNC.

IS HFNC SUPERIOR TO CPAP THERAPY?

Most studies comparing HFNC to CPAP has shown that patient comfort with HFNC is superior to CPAP.[2] This may be in terms of dryness of mouth or ability to communicate with the children. One study from Australia and New Zealand directed at senior medical and nursing staff concluded that in spite of lack of proper guidelines for use of HFNC, the noninvasive mode was easy to administer and more comfortable for infants.[8]

In the study by Testa et al., although HFNC was superior to CPAP in terms of oxygenation and reduction in respiratory rate, the former technique did not influence the duration of noninvasive ventilator therapy or the ICU stay. In a randomized controlled study comparing conventional oxygen therapy with CPAP and HFNC in children with pneumonia, CPAP therapy was significantly better than conventional oxygen therapy in terms of death, reintubation and clinical failure.[9] However, the authors could not find any significant difference between CPAP and HFNC in this study.

In a "before-after", single center study where the practice changed from nasal CPAP to HFNC in infants with bronchiolitis, the authors could not find any difference between the two noninvasive techniques in terms of respiratory rate, heart rate, FiO_2 requirements and CO_2 evolution. Failure rates were not significantly different between the two techniques.[10]

McKiernan et al. showed that the intubation rates for children with bronchiolitis decreased significantly from 23% to 9% with the introduction of HFNC.[11] Those children with greatest reduction in respiratory rate after HFNC initiation were the least likely to get intubated. Schibler et al. showed that in a subset of patients with bronchiolitis admitted to the pediatric ICU, the intubation rate dropped from 37 to 7% with the introduction of HFNC in their practice.[12]

However, till date there is no study that has shown a clear superiority of CPAP over HFNC although most studies agree that HFNC is probably noninferior to CPAP therapy.

COMPLICATIONS ASSOCIATED WITH HFNC

Most studies have shown that HFNC is a relatively safe technique to be applied in the pediatric ward, during transport or in the ICU.[2] However, it is important to remember that unlike CPAP that is delivered by systems with integrated pressure relief valves, it is neither possible to regulate or assess the pressure that is applied to the upper airway when HFNC is being used. The two studies conducted in postcardiac surgical children have shown that it is a relatively safe technique to be applied in the ICU.[5,6] Possible complications of HFNC include pneumothorax, pneumomediastinum, gastric distention and gastric aspiration.

CONCLUSION AND FUTURE

High-flow nasal cannula is a relatively safe, well-tolerated, and comfortable way of giving oxygen therapy in children following cardiac surgery. Although it is postulated that washout of the nasopharyngeal dead space is responsible for the improved oxygenation and washout of CO_2, some level of PEEP secondary to the distending effect is possibly responsible for the beneficial effect. Although most studies till date have not shown an overall superiority, the fact that reintubation rates and step up to CPAP therapy has been low is very encouraging. Overall, the ease of application and improved patient tolerance have encouraged clinicians to persist with this technique in most ICUs.

However, cost consideration of HFNC delivery systems is an important concern in limited resource environments, and might necessitate selective use of this facility only in those patients requiring prolonged noninvasive ventilator support.

In cardiac surgery, a lot of interesting possibilities exist for future evaluation. What would be the physiological response to various types of cardiac physiology; single ventricle versus two ventricle repair or high versus low pulmonary circulation, effects in patients with systemic to pulmonary shunt patients? These are areas where future research can give valuable information. Finally, what is the ideal flow rate to be maintained? It is possible that there is an ideal flow rate where the beneficial effect of HFNC can be maximized?

■ REFERENCES

1. Mayfield S, Jauncey-Cooke J, Hough JL, Schibler A, Gibbons K, Boggosian F, et al. High flow nasal cannula for respiratory support in children. Cochrane Database Syst Rev. 2014;3:CD009850.
2. Mikalsen IB, Davis P, Oymar K. High flow nasal cannula in children: a literature review. Scand J Trauma Resusc Emerg Med. 2016;24:93.
3. Inata Y, Tekeuchi M. Complex effects of high-flow nasal cannula therapy on hemodynamics in the pediatric patient after cardiac surgery. J Int Care. 2017;5:30.
4. Bronicki RA, Penny DJ, Anas NG, Furhman B. Cardiopulmonary interactions. Paed Crit Care Med. 2016;17(8 Suppl 1):S182-193.
5. Testa G, Iodice F, Ricci Z, Vitale V, DeRazza F, Haiberger R, et al. Comparative evaluation of high flow nasal cannula and conventional oxygen therapy in paediatric cardiac surgical patients: a randomized controlled trial. Interact Cardiovasc Thorac Surg. 2014;19:456-61.
6. Shioji N, Iwasaki T, Kanazawa T, Shimizu K, Suemori T, Sugimoto K, et al. Physiological impact of high flow nasal cannula therapy on post-extubation acute respiratory failure after pediatric cardiac surgery: a prospective observational study. J Int Care. 2017;5:35.
7. Hutchings FA, Hilliard TA, Davis PJ. Heated humidified high-flow nasal cannula therapy in children. Arch Dis Child. 2015;100:571-5.
8. Manley BJ, Owen L, Doyle LW, Davis PG. High-flow nasal cannula and nasal continuous positive airway pressure. J Paediatr Child Health. 2012;48:16-21.
9. Chisti M, Salam MA, Smith JH, Ahmed T, Pietroni MA, Shahunja KM, et al. Bubble continuous positive airway pressure for children with severe pneumonia and hypoxemia in Bangladesh: an open, randomized controlled trial. Lancet. 2015;386:1057-65.
10. Metge P, Grimaldi C, Hassid S, Thomachot L, Loundou A, Martin C, et al. Comparison of high flow humidified nasal cannula to nasal continuous positive airway pressure in children with acute bronchiolitis: experience in a pediatric intensive care unit. Eur J Pediatr. 2014;173:953-8.
11. McKiernan C, Chua C, Visintainer PF, Allen H. High flow nasal cannula therapy in infants with bronchiolitis. J Pediatr. 2010;156:634-8.
12. Schibler A, Pham TM, Dunster KR, Foster K, Barlow A, Gibbons K, et al. Reduced intubation rates for infants after introduction of high-flow nasal prong oxygen therapy. Int Care Med. 2011;37:847-52.

Extubation Failure after Pediatric Cardiac Surgery

Rakhi Balachandran, Amitabh C Sen

Reviewed by: Amitabh C Sen

INTRODUCTION

Recent advances in surgery, improved perfusion strategies during cardiopulmonary bypass, as well as refinements in perioperative anesthetic techniques have made successful extubation feasible after congenital heart repair with a shorter ventilation time and fewer complications. Consequent to a paradigm shift towards early extubation and fast track care in the current era, the pediatric cardiac intensivist is faced with the unique challenge of facilitating early extubation while preventing reintubation after separation from mechanical ventilation.[1] However, in spite of optimum perioperative pharmacological and hemodynamic interventions, a subset of patients continue to develop extubation failure in the postoperative period. Since extubation after surgery is a planned process, extubation failure rates also reflect intensive care and hospital practices; and as such have emerged as an important quality metric often used to compare performance between centers.[2] In low-middle-income countries (LMIC) failed extubation poses substantial challenges to resource allocation due to extended morbidity, need for intensive care and escalation of healthcare associated costs. Failed extubation after congenital heart surgery thus merits serious concern; and a comprehensive evaluation and systematic troubleshooting is imperative to ensure optimal survival with minimum morbidity. This chapter attempts to discuss the common risk factors for extubation failure and provides a systematic approach to the management of this complication in the pediatric cardiac intensive care unit (PCICU).

DEFINITION OF EXTUBATION FAILURE

Extubation failure is defined as need for reintubation within 48 hours of planned extubation.[2] Though varying time frames ranging from 24 to 72 hours have been used to define extubation failure in the postoperative period, the duration of 48 hours seems most appropriate in the current era where noninvasive ventilation techniques are often used by intensivists to bridge the periextubation period in high-risk patients.[2]

INCIDENCE OF EXTUBATION FAILURE

The overall reported incidence of extubation failure in pediatric cohorts varies from 5.8% to 15.6%.[2-5] Younger age being an established risk factor for failed extubation, current rates in neonatal population has been stated to be 11–17.5%.[1,6-8] In a study done at our center (unpublished data), we observed an incidence of 9.4% in a cohort of 1282 patients undergoing congenital heart surgery.

RISK FACTORS FOR FAILED EXTUBATION AFTER CARDIAC SURGERY

The identification of risk factors can facilitate development of preventive strategies for modifiable risk factors and improve postoperative outcomes. Efforts to reduce extubation failure rates have evolved as a potential quality improvement strategy in pediatric cardiac intensive care. Young age, genetic syndromes, surgical complexity, delayed sternal closure, postoperative infections/complications and duration of mechanical ventilation had been earlier identified as risk factors for failed extubation among pediatric patients of all ages in cardiac intensive care units.[2,9-13] A multicenter study analyzing data of 1,478 patients at eight hospitals in Pediatric Cardiac Critical Care Consortium identified 100 extubation failures (5.8%) among 1,734 ventilation episodes.[2] Interestingly, in multivariate analysis, duration of mechanical ventilation was the only factor which was significantly associated with extubation failure. Also, the failure rates were significantly lower in the cohort of patients extubated in the operating room (3%, n = 503). This data strongly justifies implementing strategies for early extubation as a quality control initiative to minimize extubation failure rates.

As an increasing number of neonates undergo early primary repair for complex CHD in the current era, the risk factors pertaining to this vulnerable population has been the focus of recent studies on extubation failure.[1,6-8] In a multicenter cohort of 899 neonates from 14 pediatric Cardiac Critical Care Consortium centers the incidence of extubation failure was 11% (unadjusted rates ranged from 5 to 22% across centers).[1] In multivariate analysis, airway anomaly was the only factor that emerged as an independent risk factor for extubation failure (OR 3.1; CI 1.4–6.7). Neonates who failed extubation had greater median postoperative length of stay (33 days vs. 23 days, p = 0.001), and higher in-hospital mortality (8% Vs 2%, p = 0.002). The variation in failure rates across centers suggests scope for improvement by instituting better periextubation care in centers with worse outcomes.

A study done at the author's center, revealed higher incidence in neonates, nutritionally challenged, associated chromosomal anomaly, and those <5th percentile of body mass index (BMI). Pulmonary artery banding, Ebstein's anomaly repair, repair of anomalous left coronary artery from pulmonary artery (ALCAPA), arterial switch operation with ventricular septal defect (VSD) closure, and aortic arch repair were more frequently associated with failed extubation. Mortality was significantly higher in failed extubation group (6.7 vs. 2.4%).

POTENTIAL CAUSES OF EXTUBATION FAILURE

- *Cardiac causes*: Low cardiac output syndrome due to ventricular dysfunction, residual cardiac defects, atrioventricular (AV) valve regurgitation, right ventricular outflow tract obstruction (RVOTO), left ventricular outflow tract obstruction (LVOTO), pulmonary artery hypertension (PAH), inadequate pulmonary blood flow, unsuspected additional lesions (e.g., ALCAPA, VSD, aortopulmonary collaterals).
- *Pulmonary causes*: Pneumonia, pulmonary congestion and pulmonary edema, lung collapse, pleural effusion, pneumothorax, pulmonary edema.
- *Airway issues*: Subglottic edema, bronchospasm, vocal cord palsy, vocal cord edema, laryngeal web, retained secretions, choanal atresia, tracheobronchomalacia, laryngomalacia, extrinsic airway

compression (by rings and slings or enlarged cardiac chambers).

- *Neuromuscular*: Diaphragm palsy, myasthenia, cerebrovascular accidents, excessive sedation or narcotic dependency/withdrawal, critical illness neuropathy.
- *Gastrointestinal complications*: Neonatal necrotizing enterocolitis (NEC), gastroesophageal reflux disease (GERD) with microaspiration.
- *Miscellaneous*: Malnutrition, sepsis, fever, fluid overload, metabolic abnormalities [hypophosphatemia, hyponatremia, hypomagnesemia, increased blood urea nitrogen (BUN), hyperammonemia], prolonged ventilation, intubation for post-operative interventions.

Analysis of data (unpublished) from a prospective cohort of patients undergoing pediatric cardiac surgery at our center revealed the following factors as the frequently observed causes for postoperative extubation failure. The major causes were divided into cardiovascular, respiratory and other causes. Cardiovascular causes (42%), included systemic ventricular dysfunction, AV valve regurgitation, pulmonary hypertension, residual lesions, arrhythmias, and pulmonary edema. Respiratory causes (43%) were upper airway obstruction, small airway obstruction, lung collapse, and ventilator associated pneumonia. Other causes (14%) observed were sepsis, seizures, apnea, diaphragm palsy, pneumothorax, pleural effusion, and re-exploration.

SYSTEMATIC EVALUATION FOR FAILED EXTUBATION

Extubation failure should be viewed as a critical event and a systematic evaluation for further management is required to facilitate successful extubation in the subsequent attempt.

TABLE 1: Checklist for failed extubation.

Step 1	Review of periextubation events
Step 2	Detailed physical examination
Step 3	Identifying specific cause by systems evaluation

Systems evaluation	Diagnostic tests
Airway evaluation	Fiberoptic laryngoscopy/bronchoscopy
Cardiac disease	• Detailed echocardiogram for anatomy and cardiac function • Contrast echocardiogram-Collaterals/intracardiac shunts • Cardiac catheterization
Lung disease	• Chest X-ray • Bronchoalveolar lavage (BAL) culture • Computed tomographic (CT) Scan
Diaphragm evaluation	• Screening echocardiogram • Fluoroscopy
Gastroesophageal reflux/swallowing dysfunction	Barium swallow, dynamic swallowing study
Laboratory tests	Serum sodium, serum potassium, serum magnesium, serum phosphorus, serum magnesium, serum calcium, blood urea nitrogen, serum ammonia *Sepsis screen*: Blood culture, blood counts, procalcitonin after 5th postoperative day
Nutritional evaluation	Anthropometric measurements, serum albumin

Checklist for Failed Extubation

A checklist of action items for systematic approach to a patient with failed extubation is provided in **Table 1**. The need for invasive diagnostic tests should be decided on a case by case basis after collective consideration of the multi-disciplinary team involved in the patient's care.

MANAGEMENT AFTER FAILED EXTUBATION[14-16]

The following measures are worth considering for all patients who require extended mechanical ventilation after an unsuccessful extubation.

General Measures

1. Inform family about the procedure and circumstances leading to it. Discuss the probable course of further stay and care plan.
2. Detailed evaluation as discussed in **Table 1**.
3. Review the need for invasive monitoring and consider re-siting monitoring catheters as appropriate.
4. Institute appropriate sedation and analgesia. Consider cycling of pharmacologic agents to minimize withdrawal, narcotic dependency and over sedation. Daily sedation interruption (DSI) as per clinical status to assess readiness for extubation. If ventilation is reinstituted for stridor, take additional precautions to keep the patient quiescent and prevent fighting the ventilator.
5. *Optimize nutrition*: Restart nasogastric feeds if not planning extubation within next 24 hours. Calorie/protein intake should be optimized. Monitor prescribed calories and actual achieved calorie intake to ensure daily achievement of caloric goals. Monitor weight trends as per feasibility in the state of critical illness. If calorie requirements are not met due to need for frequent feed interruptions, calorie dense feeds/partial parenteral nutrition may be considered to meet energy and protein targets.
6. Consider sepsis, and screen appropriately. If preliminary clinical evaluation strongly suggests infection, escalation of antibiotic therapy is reasonable after sending appropriate laboratory samples. If the screening tests are negative for sepsis, rationalize antibiotic use by appropriate de-escalation based on hospital antibiogram.
7. *Optimize fluid therapy*: Fluid management is often challenging as it requires focused efforts to strike a balance between reducing fluid overload to facilitate extubation, while allowing enough fluid intake for achieving caloric needs.

Specific System-wise Measures

This depends on the primary underlying cause of reintubation as revealed by relevant investigation. A suggested list of key interventions for pathologies related to each system is enumerated here.

Cardiovascular System

Low cardiac output state:
- Identify the cause by echocardiography/catheterization
- Residual lesions to be identified and addressed
- Optimize inotropes and afterload reducing agents
- Ventilator manipulation for optimizing the balance between systemic and pulmonary circulation in single ventricle scenarios or in patients with intracardiac shunts
- Meticulous fluid management/diuretic therapy to prevent fluid overload.

Pulmonary artery hypertension (PAH):
- Identify the cause for PAH
- Address residual lesions which might increase the pulmonary blood flow (AV valve regurgitation, VSD, aortopulmonary collaterals, pulmonary vein obstruction)
- Treat underlying lung disease which may impair gas exchange and trigger PAH—pneumonia, retained secretions, pulmonary edema, pneumothorax, pleural effusion
- *Consider pulmonary vasodilators*: Sildenafil/Bosentan.

Respiratory System

Upper airway obstruction:

- *Consider short course of steroids in the periextubation period*: Dexamethasone at a dose of 0.25–0.5 mg/kg intravenously at 8th hourly intervals for 24 hours is the preferred practice at our center.
- Ensure adequate sedation to prevent the patient from fighting the ventilator and further increasing airway edema.
- *Treatment for reflux and possible aspiration of gastroesophageal contents*: Ensure appropriate positioning with head end of bed elevation to 30–45 degrees. Prokinetic agents like domperidone and proton pump inhibitors are reasonable in established reflux based on swallowing study.
- Monitor for air leak around endotracheal tube which is suggestive of reduction in airway edema.
- Maintain a negative fluid balance as permitted by hemodynamic status to minimize overall fluid overload and laryngeal edema.
- Surgical treatment of anatomical causes if deemed significant on evaluation (e.g., subglottic stenosis/subglottic web, etc.).

Pulmonary complications:

- Institute ventilator-associated pneumonia (VAP) prevention bundle—head end of bed elevation, daily sedation vacation, assessment of readiness to extubate, prevention of deep vein thrombosis (DVT), peptic ulcer prophylaxis, age appropriate oral hygiene measures. 0.1% Chlorhexidine oral care is employed in children > 6 years[17]
- Lung protective ventilator strategies: The present strategy is to use lower tidal volumes of 6–8 mL/kg for all infants and children and the lowest feasible FiO_2 to maintain acceptable oxygen saturation in accordance with the cardiovascular physiology
- Ensure humidification of inspired gases
- Treat pneumonia, consolidation, lung collapse, effusion
- Bronchodilators if evidence of bronchospasm
- Chest physiotherapy, postural drainage and clearance of secretions
- Frequent position change to prevent atelectasis
- Prone positioning to treat refractory atelectasis/consolidation/acute respiratory distress syndrome (ARDS)
- Appropriate antibiotic therapy for infective pulmonary complications. Consider BAL to identify pathogen and target therapy
- Fluid restriction and maintaining a negative fluid balance by aggressive diuresis if increased pulmonary blood flow/pulmonary congestion is suspected.

Phrenic nerve palsy:

- Consider diaphragm plication
- Use of noninvasive ventilation or high flow nasal cannula to bridge extubation
- Ensure adequate nutrition to preserve respiratory muscle mass.

Malnutrition

- Allow appropriate fluid intake to facilitate delivery of nutrition
- Prescribe appropriate calories and fluid goals daily
- High protein diet
- Provision of micronutrients
- Daily monitoring of prescribed calories versus achieved calories
- Periodic weight measurements
- Provide a comfortable environment and minimize common stressors to ensure adequate rest and normal sleep cycles.

Neuromuscular

- Avoid continuous use of paralytic agents if long duration of ventilation is anticipated, as this can facilitate lung collapse and loss of muscle mass due to disuse atrophy.
- Ensure adequate intake of micronutrients particularly phosphorus and magnesium, the deficiency of which can contribute to respiratory muscle weakness and delay weaning from mechanical ventilation.
- Physiotherapy and range of motion exercises to the joints to prevent stiffening and development of contractures. This helps to improve skin circulation and prevent ulcer formation.

Skin

- Prevention of pressure ulcers
- Frequent monitoring for pressure ulcers and treatment if any
- Frequent position change
- Use of airbed/water bed to facilitate better skin circulation
- Application of emollients to prevent drying and flaking of skin that can lead to development of ulcers. Coconut oil is an excellent, cost effective emollient.

Eye Care

- Taping of eyes if paralyzed and ventilated
- Apply tear substitutes every 2—4 hour to prevent drying of eye
- Monitor periodically for exposure keratitis, lid edema, pressure ulcers around the eye.

Metabolic

- Monitor and treat electrolyte imbalances
- Optimize blood glucose control
- Diagnose and treat micronutrient deficiency
- Diagnosis and treatment of hyperpyrexia.

Renal/Gastrointestinal

- Daily Intake output monitoring and assessment of fluid status
- Peritoneal dialysis for established acute kidney injury (AKI)
- Monitor for cumulative toxicity of common drugs and their prolonged effects (especially sedative/paralytic agents, antibiotics) in AKI which can interfere with subsequent extubation. Appropriate drug doses depending on renal clearance should be prescribed to reduce drug toxicity
- Diagnosis and treatment of NEC
- Diagnosis and treatment of intestinal obstruction/mesenteric ischemia due to systemic steal.

PLANNING SUBSEQUENT EXTUBATION

The planning, execution and estimated time frame for the next extubation depend on the primary cause of re-intubation. Adequate time has to be allowed to optimize the patient and correct the underlying pathology before planning the subsequent extubation in order to ensure favorable outcomes.

Assessment of Extubation Readiness

- Primary condition for extubation failure should be adequately treated
- Patient should be hemodynamically stable
- Manageable respiratory secretions
- Patient should be weaned to low ventilator settings
- FiO_2 should be < 0.5
- Patient should be weaned off sedation, awake, responsive. However, analgesia should be maintained
- Adequate respiratory muscle strength and effort

- *ETT leak*: A leak test, when air is audibly leaking around ETT at low pressure <20–25 cmH$_2$O may be helpful to rule out upper airway edema
- Ensure absence of withdrawal from narcotic or benzodiazepines.

Use of Spontaneous Breathing Trial

It is rational to use a spontaneous breathing trial (SBT) of 30 minutes to 2 hours on patients deemed ready for extubation as detailed earlier.[18,19] The patient can be either allowed to breathe through an ETT connected to T piece with oxygen source or CPAP/Pressure Support Ventilation at 6–10 cm H$_2$O above PEEP. A constant vigil has to be maintained by the attending physician and the bedside nurse to detect weaning intolerance, impending respiratory failure or low cardiac output state. If not tolerating weaning, SBT should be interrupted and ventilator support intensified. In patients who fail SBT, it is justified to ventilate for another 24 hours before attempting another trial to prevent respiratory muscle fatigue. In patients who tolerate SBT, a blood gas should be obtained on pressure support before extubation. The decision to bridge through noninvasive ventilation at subsequent extubation depends on the patient status and respiratory muscle recovery. In newborns and young infants, a brief period of noninvasive ventilation is reasonable to decrease work of breathing, and increase success rates at second extubation. This can be transitioned to nasal cannula after 24–48 hours once patient status is deemed stable.

The role of corticosteroids in prevention of postextubation stridor is not clear in pediatric population. The practice of administering periextubation steroids have been extrapolated from adult literature.[20-22] A single dose of dexamethasone (0.25–0.5 mg/kg) may be administered 4-6 hours prior to planned extubation to minimize airway edema. In patients who had upper airway obstruction leading to reintubation, parenteral steroids may be given for 24 hours in the periextubation period.

■ SUMMARY

Extubation failure remains a challenging complication after congenital heart surgery. A combination of protocolized weaning, assessment of respiratory function mechanics, attention to postoperative cardiac reserve during subsequent weaning, meticulous attention to nutritional rehabilitation given the perioperative constraints such as fluid restriction and feed interruptions, and understanding of risk factors for failed extubation may help to reduce the overall duration of ventilator support and further extubation failures.

■ REFERENCES

1. Bennyworth BD, Mastropietro CW, Graham EM, Klugman D, Costello JM, Zhang W, et al. Variation in extubation failure rates after neonatal cardiac surgery across Pediatric Cardiac Critical Care Consortium hospitals. J Thorac Cardiovasc Surg. 2017;153:1519-26.
2. Gaies M, Tabbutt S, Schwartz SM, Bird GL, Alten JA, Shekerdemian LS, et al. Clinical epidemiology of extubation failure in the pediatric cardiac ICU: a report from the Pediatric Cardiac Critical Care Consortium. Pediatr Crit Care Med. 2015;16:837-45.
3. Davis S, Worley S, Mee RB, Harrison AM. Factors associated with early extubation after cardiac surgery in young children. Pediatr Crit Care Med. 2004;5;63-8.
4. Shahbah DA, Abo-Elnaga AM, El Moghazy EM. Perioperative risk factors for prolonged mechanical ventilation following cardiac surgery for congenital heart disease in pediatric patients. Egypt Soc Cardiothorac Sur. 2012; 20:13-20.8
5. Shi S, Zhao Z, Liu X, Shu Q, Tan L, Lin R, et al. Perioperative risk factors for prolonged mechanical ventilation following cardiac surgery in neonates and young infants. Chest. 2008;134(4):768-74.

6. Mastropietro CW, Cashen K, Grimaldi LM, Narayana Gowda KM, Piggott KD, Wilhelm M, et al. Extubation failure after neonatal cardiac surgery: a multicentre analysis. J Pediatr. 2017;182:190-6.

7. Miura S, Hamamoto N, Osaki M, Nakano S, Miyakoshi C. Extubation failure in neonates after cardiac surgery: prevalence, etiology and risk factors. Ann Thorac Surg. 2017;103:1293-98.

8. Laudato N, Gupta P, Walters HL3rd, Delius RE, Mastropietro CW. Risk factors for extubation failure following neonatal cardiac surgery. Pediatr Crit Care Med. 2015;16:859-67.

9. Manrique AM, Feingold B, Di Filippo S, Orr R, Kuch BA, Munoz R. Extubation after cardiothoracic surgery in neonates, children and young adults. One year of institutional experience. Pediatr Crit Care Med. 2007;8:552-5.

10. Shu Q, Shi S, Zhang XH, Piedmonte M, Drummond-Webb JJ, Mee RB. Risk factors for failed extubation after open heart surgery in infants. World J Pediatr. 2005;1:69-72.

11. Harrison AM, Cox AC, Davis S, Piedmonte M, Drummond-Webb JJ, Mee RB. Failed extubation after cardiac surgery in young children. Prevalence, pathogenesis, and risk factors. Pediatr Crit Care Med. 2002;3;148-52.

12. Polito A, Patorno E, Costello JM, Salvin JW, Emani SM, Rajagopal S, et al. Perioperative factors associated with prolonged mechanical ventilation after complex congenital heart surgery. Pediatr Crit Care Med. 2011;12:e122-6.

13. Gupta P, Wetzel RC. Risk factors for mechanical ventilation and reintubation after pediatric heart surgery. J Thorac Cardiovasc Surg. 2016;151:451-8.

14. Backer CL, Baden HP. Perioperative care. In: Mavroudis C, Backer CL (Eds). Pediatric Cardiac Surgery, 3rd edition. Philadelphia: Mosby; 2003. pp. 119-42.

15. Aronson LA, Dent CL. Postoperative respiratory function and its management. In: Lake C, Booker PD (Eds). Paediatric Cardiac Anaesthesia, 4th edition. Philadelphia: Lippincott Williams and Wilkins; 2005. pp. 682-704.

16. Roth SJ. Post-operative care. In: Chang AC, Hanley FL (Eds). Paediatric Cardiac Intensive Care. Baltimore: Williams and Wilkins; 1998. pp. 163-87.

17. Cooper VB, Haut C. Preventing ventilator associated pneumonia in children: an evidence based protocol. Crit care Nurse. 2013;33:21-30.

18. Johnston C, Lucas de silva P. Weaning and extubation in pediatrics. Curr Respir Med Rev. 2012;8:68-78.

19. Newth CJ, Venakataraman S, Wilson DF, Meert KL, Harrison R, Dean JM, et al. Weaning and extubation readiness in pediatric patients. Pediatr Crit Care Med. 2009;10:1-11.

20. Khemani RG, Randolph A, Marcowitz B. Corticosteroids for the prevention and treatment of stridor in neonates children and adults. Cochrane Database Syst Rev. 2009;8:CD001000.

21. Bjornson CL, Johnson DW. Croup in the pediatric emergency department. Paediatr Child Health. 2007;12:473-7.

22. Maloney E, Meakin GH. Acute stridor in children. Cont Educ Anaesth Crit Care Pain. 2007;7:183-7.

13

CHAPTER

Management of Undernutrition and Failure to Thrive in Children with Congenital Heart Disease in Low- and Middle-income Countries

Andrew C Argent, Rakhi Balachandran, Balu Vaidyanathan, Amina Khan, R Krishna Kumar

Reviewed by: R Krishna Kumar

■ INTRODUCTION

Many children with congenital heart disease (CHD) are underweight for age[1-11] and/or stunted (even at an early age). Being significantly underweight for age and wasted has been associated with higher perioperative morbidity and mortality in children with CHD.[12] In addition the perioperative period is frequently complicated by difficulties with enteral nutrition (EN),[10,13] and potentially with increased nutritional losses associated with problems such as chylothorax.

There is a significant burden of childhood undernutrition in low- and middle-income countries (LMICs) where some 90% of the children born with CHD across the world live.[14] The coexistence of CHD increases the likelihood and severity of undernutrition and this adds to challenges for the management of CHD including: resource constraints; late presentation and diagnosis; and perioperative infection.[15-18] The number of children, including infants and newborns being operated for CHD has recently increased in these regions.[15]

This review seeks to summarize existing evidence on prevalence of undernutrition and CHD and its impact on surgical outcomes with a focus on implications for LMICs. An effort has been made to identify specific gaps in knowledge as a basis for future multicenter studies.

■ DEFINITION OF MALNUTRITION IN CONGENITAL HEART DISEASE

In the context of CHD, it is important to reach a clear consensus on what is meant by malnutrition. Simple measurements (height, weight, skinfold thickness, etc.) and their relationships (weight for height, etc.) have been the basis of most definitions of nutritional status.[19] It is not possible to exclude malnutrition on the grounds of normal anthropometry alone, as there may be children with acute malnutrition who fall within the "normal" ranges for standard anthropometry.[20] Green Corkins has recently highlighted the importance of a full clinical evaluation (vs. simply viewing anthropometry) in the assessment of nutrition status in children.[21]

Mehta et al. defined malnutrition as: "an imbalance between nutrient requirement and intake, resulting in cumulative deficits of energy, protein, or micronutrients that may negatively affect growth, development, and other relevant outcomes"[22] (**Fig. 1**). Ideally, any assessment of nutrition and investigations on the role of nutrition in patient management should include data regarding growth over a period of time; actual dietary intake available (and provided); evidence for malabsorption; evidence of inflammatory processes and evidence of any underlying disease.[23]

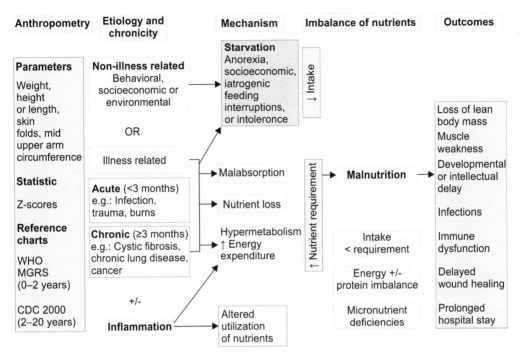

Fig. 1: Approach to malnutrition.
WHO: World Health Organization; MGRS: Multicentre Growth Reference Study, CDC: Center for Disease Control

▍FAILURE TO THRIVE IN CHILDREN WITH CONGENITAL HEART DISEASE

The basis of growth failure or underweight in CHD appears to be multifactorial and may differ in etiology from patient to patient. It includes the underlying cardiac anomaly,[24] hemodynamic factors, hypoxemia, inadequate calorie, or macronutrient intake,[1,13,25-28] increased energy expenditure relative to intake,[29-31] increased inflammation,[32] or associated comorbidities that include gut dysfunction,[25] respiratory infections, associated genetic syndromes and reduced growth potential.[7,33-37]

A study of anthropometric data in children with CHD in India showed that recorded dietary intake was not associated with the probability of being underweight.[6] Another study concluded that there was no reduction in intake in children with CHD relative to normal children, while "normal serum prealbumin and albumin in the infants with

CHD ruled out protein-calorie malnutrition".[36] The plasma amino acid profile was normal preoperatively in a group of children with CHD, regardless of anthropometric values.[38] A study from Latin America of children with CHD showed that anthropometric measures of malnutrition were present in >80% of the children; albumin and pre-albumin levels were lower than in normal controls (although transferrin levels were no different), and that failure to thrive was worse in children with pulmonary hypertension.[39]

In LMICs with resource limitations, the prevalence of abnormal preoperative anthropometry is high due to late presentation, delay in corrective intervention, and frequent hospitalizations due to respiratory infections.[6,16] In a cohort of 100 consecutive infants undergoing ventricular septal defect (VSD) closure, severe underweight (weight Z-score <−3) was observed in 46%

of patients.[33] In a prospective study of 476 consecutive patients undergoing corrective intervention for CHD, Vaidyanathan et al. reported Z-scores < −2 in 59% (weight), 26.3% (height), 55.9% (weight/height), respectively; Z-scores <−3 were observed in 27.7% (weight), 10.1% (height), and 24.2% (weight/height).[6] Congestive heart failure, older age at correction and limited growth potential as suggested by lower birth weight for gestation, lower parental anthropometry and genetic syndromes were identified as predictors of "malnutrition". The International Quality Improvement Collaborative for Congenital Heart Surgery in LMICs uses a registry to collect data from over 50 sites. An analysis of data from 15,049 patients with CHD revealed that >50% of children had weight Z-scores of −3 or less) and 12% had an emaciated appearance prior to their surgery.[15]

While anthropometric measurements in children with CHD are frequently abnormal, classical features of malnutrition such as skin changes, presence of edema, hair changes, etc., are relatively rare in children with CHD. In the setting of malnutrition in Africa, a discrepancy between clinical signs of acute malnutrition and the anthropometry[20] may be an important issue to pursue.

Finally, there is evidence that micro-nutrient deficiencies may be relatively common in children with CHD,[40] this has never been explored in LMICs where it is even more likely to be an issue.

IMPACT OF PREOPERATIVE STATE ON POSTOPERATIVE OUTCOME

Because of their lower protein and energy reserves, infants, and newborns may be particularly vulnerable to the hypercatabolic state that is expected following heart surgery[41,42] (although hypercatabolism may not follow all pediatric cardiac surgery[43]). This situation is further worsened by comorbidities such as undernutrition and major infections (see **Fig. 1**). When the acute phase of metabolic stress resolves, the anabolic phase begins, resulting in somatic growth, with decreasing concentrations of acute-phase reactants, proteins, and total urinary nitrogen values, and with increasing concentrations of visceral proteins.[44] The timing of transition to the anabolic phase is influenced by the extent of "surgical stress", associated comorbidities, quality of nutritional support, and a number of other potential factors.

Within that framework, there has been concern that cardiac surgery in underweight children with CHD would be associated with worse outcomes. However, there is very little evidence to support the notion that lower weights are associated with poorer surgical outcomes. In a study published in 1992, Hardin et al. compared two groups of patients undergoing closure of the VSD (>4 kg and <4 kg) and found no significant difference in outcomes.[45]

In a study from Southern India on 100 consecutive infants undergoing surgical closure of the VSD, 46% had weight Z-scores of −3 or lower but this did not affect post-operative mortality or morbidity [duration of mechanical ventilation, length of stay in the intensive care unit (ICU), or hospital].[16] A more recent prospective study of 1,028 infants from the same center studied the impact of preoperative factors on post-operative outcomes after congenital heart surgery,[17] weight Z-score <−3 and LBW (<2.5 kg) did not adversely affect mortality or morbidity. These results reinforce the strategy of early correction of congenital heart defects irrespective of nutritional status. Preoperative optimization of nutritional status through aggressive feeding is not necessary in most patients, but it may make sense to use this technique, if there are ongoing delays in access to surgical repair.

CORRECTION VERSUS PALLIATION

The question of correction versus palliation in a severely undernourished child with CHD is likely to be dictated by several factors that include the specific defect, the experience and expertise of the surgical and intensive care teams and associated comorbidities. Relatively simple CHD that can be corrected through a single operation, such as a VSD should be closed surgically. A study in South Africa demonstrated that when the realities of a staged approach using pulmonary artery bands (including loss to follow-up, delays in definitive procedures, the challenges of two surgical procedures in a context with limited surgical time, etc.) were taken into account, mortality after a staged approach using pulmonary artery banding was higher than primary surgical closure of the VSD.[46] There are clearly situations where pulmonary artery banding may be a useful stage en route to full correction (particularly in complex situations).

MANAGEMENT OF UNDERNUTRITION

Cardiac teams in LMICs will frequently be faced with children with CHD who are underweight, thin, and stunted. The first response should be to regard that as further evidence that the diagnosis of CHD is being delayed, and to focus on interventions to improve early diagnosis and referral.

A full preoperative assessment of nutritional status should be performed as discussed below. Evidence that the patient is severely underweight should not be used as an indication to delay surgical intervention. If anything it should be used as motivation for surgery as soon as possible. However, if there are delays, there may be opportunities to focus on improvement of nutritional status while awaiting surgery.

Preoperative Assessment of Nutritional Status

A full preoperative assessment should be obtained as it provides essential baseline information for further monitoring of progress following surgical correction. This would typically include accurate measurements of height, weight, and head circumference. The measurement of biceps or triceps skinfold thickness is a simple method for determining fat stores, which is not routinely performed during preoperative assessment[19] but might provide useful data for follow up (both for individual patients and for patient groups). Laboratory tests that include plasma levels of albumin, transferrin, prealbumin, and retinol-binding protein are seldom undertaken because they are thought to be of limited value.

Nutritional Support in Pediatric Cardiac Intensive Care Unit

Significant caloric supplementation in children with CHD could lead to improved growth,[47] and in some improved growth could be achieved using continuous enteral feeds.[48-50]

Enteral nutrition is the preferred mode of nutritional support in pediatric intensive care units (PICU).[51] EN is physiological, has a favorable effect on the intestinal mucosa and has fewer complications compared to parenteral nutrition (PN).[52,53] It has the additional benefit that it is considerably cheaper than PN and more easily available in LMIC. Intragastric feeding is the most common route, and there is insufficient data to recommend use of postpyloric feeding unless there are particular concerns such as poor tolerance of gastric feeding or evidence of gastroesophageal reflux with aspiration. In a single randomized control trial in 74 critically ill children, a higher number of patients with postpyloric feeding reached caloric goals.[54]

There are particular challenges with the feeding of neonates prior to surgery, but in most cases it is possible to start enteral feeding (even while on prostaglandins) although many of these infants may continue to require gavage feeding postoperatively.[55]

Postoperative Feeding

Postsurgery enteral feeds should be initiated as soon as possible, and PN should only be used, if absolutely essential. Recent data suggests that early PN (within 7 days of admission) in the PICU is associated with worse patient outcomes.[56]

Initiation and Advancement of Feeds

The guidelines for withholding feeds after pediatric cardiac surgery are not clearly defined and there is extremely limited data available specific to LMICs. The most common concern in early initiation of feeds is the potential for low cardiac output with gut hypoperfusion, especially in neonates with duct-dependent circulation, leading to necrotizing enterocolitis.[57,58] With careful monitoring and slow advancement of feeds, early EN is feasible in most neonates within the first 24 hours. In a retrospective review of 67 neonates, including 52 patients with duct-dependent circulation, undergoing surgical repair, postoperative enteral feeds could be initiated within 3 days in 98.5% (n = 66); 64 patients could reach full feeds at a median duration of 7.5 days following surgical correction.[55]

In neonates and young infants, feeds are typically started (within 12-24 hours of surgery) at 1 mL/kg/hr and advanced at the same rate every 4-6 hours to reach the goal volume. Though continuous feeds have not been shown to minimize aspiration or feed intolerance, it is sometimes resorted to, in infants with poor weight gain and feeding complications.[49] Feeds are withheld before extubation, around invasive procedures, in patients with hemodynamic instability, or in impending respiratory failure.

In the early postoperative phase feed volume is dictated by the maintenance fluid rate. Fluid intake is usually restricted to 50–80% of maintenance rates in neonates and infants undergoing open-heart surgery.[59] Based on studies in patients with CHD the resting energy expenditure (REE) is estimated to be 55–75 kcal/kg/day in the first 3–5 days.[60] This can guide initial feeding, which can be escalated to 120–150 kcal/kg/day on transitioning to step down care to facilitate catch up growth in infants.

Protein intake is crucial as protein catabolism could manifest as loss of respiratory muscle mass, failed weaning, poor weight gain, depressed immune function, and poor wound healing. In a small study from Brazil patients became anabolic postcardiac surgery with a calorie intake of 54 kcal/kg/day and a protein intake of 1.1 g/kg/day.[42] The decline in C-reactive protein levels, to values less than 2 mg/dL is considered an indirect marker of the onset of anabolic phase in critically ill patients; however, its relevance in postcardiac surgical patients has not been proven.[59]

For neonates and infants (in LMICs particularly), human breast milk is the preferred form of enteral feeding, although the practicalities of maintaining breast milk production in this context may be challenging.[61] Breast milk is cost effective, has immunological benefits, promotes better absorption of trace elements and may even lower the risk of necrotizing enterocolitis when used exclusively.[62] In the setting where tight fluid restriction is required, it may be necessary to increase the energy density of feeds (both formula and expressed breast milk). An energy density of approximately 1 kcal/mL is well-tolerated. Further increases should be monitored carefully as high-calorie density may precipitate osmotic diarrhea. Cost effective options to fortify formula feeds include additives such as coconut oil or medium chain triglyceride oil. An algorithm to initiate and escalate feeds is given in **Flowchart 1**.

A feeding gastrostomy or jejunostomy may be a reasonable option when long-term EN is required in children.[63,64] It may also be considered in patients with gastroesophageal

Flowchart 1: Algorithm for postoperative nutrition.

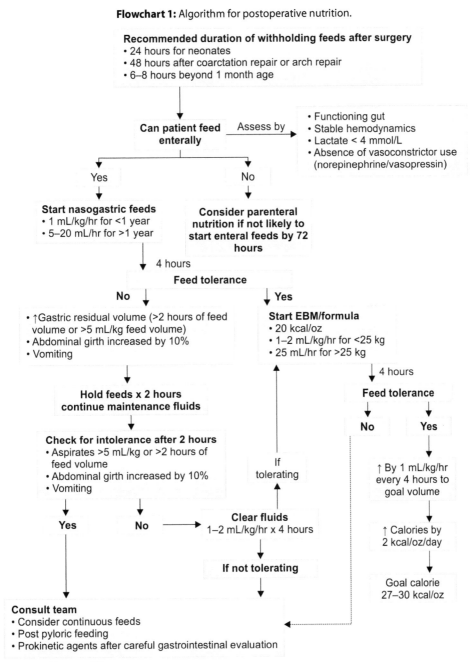

(EBM: expressed breast milk)

reflux, aspiration or severe failure to thrive. In a retrospective cohort of 54 patients who required gastrostomy (G) tube placement after surgery for single ventricle palliation, patients who underwent earlier placement of G tube had a shorter ICU stay and hospital stay.[64]

Monitoring EN

Monitoring EN should include regular audits of weight, fluid, and dietary intake, calories prescribed and calories achieved gastrointestinal function, feeding tube integrity, and feeding complications. Undue attention to gastric residual volumes is a deterrent to enteral feeding in critical care settings. Decisions to interrupt feeds should be taken considering signs of feeding intolerance such as distention, vomiting or diarrhea rather than relying on residual volumes alone.[65] The most important aspect of monitoring EN perhaps is to detect and minimize interruptions in feeding. In a recent prospective study in a PICU, implementation of a stepwise EN algorithm led to a significant decrease in the number of avoidable episodes of EN interruption (n = 3 vs. n = 51, p = 0.0001), shortened the time to reach energy goal from 4 days to 1 (p <0.0001) and also resulted in a higher proportion of patients reaching the energy goal (99% vs. 61%, p = 0.01).[66]

Underfeeding is common in critically ill pediatric patients even in most advanced units.[67-69] Algorithm led nutrition therapy and attention to energy and protein goals by dedicated nutrition support teams has translated to better postoperative outcomes in developed countries.[68,69] However, in emerging economies there is a perceived lack of dedicated nutrition support teams. A viable option is to utilize existing personnel in monitoring and supervising nutrition delivery. The initial phase should focus on education of in-house staff to bridge the knowledge gaps in feeding practices.[70] As primary caregivers, intensive care nurses should be empowered to initiate, monitor, and maintain nutrition delivery in postoperative phase. A nutrition algorithm can be formulated to serve as a clinical aid to guide the therapy (**Flowchart 1**). This can also be successfully integrated into the multidisciplinary ICU rounds as nurse led nutrition rounds.[71]

There is very limited data on recommendations for feeding children who were previously underweight and failing to thrive. We would recommend that such children be started on the nutritional program as above, together with close monitoring of progress and weight gain. Failure to gain weight should stimulate renewed focus on adequacy of the cardiac repair; presence of complications such as chylothorax (with associated nutritional deficits) and the possibility of other underlying conditions that may cause malabsorption of enteral feeds. In addition there needs to be focus on optimization of the diet available to the child, and provision of supplements of essential macro and micronutrients.

Parenteral Nutrition

The overall use of PN in critical care settings in developing countries is reported to be very low.[72] This is primarily due to prohibitive costs and lack of dedicated personnel to ensure safe prescription and delivery. Added to this are the biological complications related to PN including infection, venous thrombosis, electrolyte imbalances, and PN-induced cholestasis.[73] Notwithstanding these concerns, the use of PN may be warranted in critically ill patients after congenital heart surgery in situations where enteral feeding is contraindicated or is insufficient to promote adequate growth. Prescription of PN is a complex process with potential for errors and appropriate precautions and systems are vital.[74]

Though EN is the preferred mode of nutrition support in critically ill patients it may be intuitive to assume that initiating early PN might hasten recovery in critically ill patients, where early EN is contraindicated. However, in a recent multicenter randomized controlled trial of 1,440 patients comparing early versus late (>1 week) PN, late PN was associated with less infection [10.7% vs. 18.5% (OR:0.48, CI:0.35–0.66)], lower ICU stay (6.5 ± 0.4 days vs. 9.2 ± 0.8 days), shorter duration of ventilation and shorter length of hospital stay.[56] They concluded that withholding PN for a week in the ICU was clinically superior to providing earlier PN. Thus, withholding early PN in resource limited settings may be justified to save costs and avoid prolongation of ICU care.

Nutrient Sources in PN

Parenteral nutrition should meet energy and protein requirements as well as fluid and electrolyte needs in the postoperative period. Energy needs are ideally calculated using indirect calorimetry, double-labeled water method or standard equations to calculate REE. Schofield equation, which utilizes both height and weight, is considered appropriate as it is least likely to underestimate REE[75,76] (**Table 1**). Surgery and cardiopulmonary bypass elicit a substantially elevated metabolic response and catabolic phase. During this phase energy requirements are met by endogenous production of glucose and excess exogenous energy provision can lead to energy imbalance. In acute phase of critical illness, the energy supply is recommended to be equal to or less than measured REE intake. In the stable and recovery phase, energy intakes can be boosted by approximately 1.3 times that of REE.[76] Energy requirements as per stage of critical illness are depicted in **Table 2**.[76]

Protein supplementation in PN is primarily achieved by amino acid solutions. Typically, the amino acid requirements are

TABLE 1: Schofield equation for calculating REE (kcal/day).[76]

Age	Boys	Girls
0–3 years	59.5 × (Wt in kg) – 30	58.3 × (Wt in kg) – 31
3–10 years	22.7 × (Wt in kg) + 504	20.3 × (Wt in kg) + 486
10–18 years	17.7 × (Wt in kg) + 658	13.4 × (Wt in kg) + 692

(REE: resting energy expenditure)

TABLE 2: Energy requirements (kcal/kg/day) for PN in different phases of disease (ESPGHAN 2018).

Age	2005 (ESPGHAN)	2016 (Recovery)	2016 (Stable)	2016 (Acute)
Preterm	110–120	90–120		45–55 (day 1)
0–1 year	90–100	75–85	60–65	45–50
1–7 years	75–90	65–75	55–60	40–45
7–12 years	60–75	55–65	40–55	30–40
12–18 years	30–60	30–55	25–40	20–30

Acute phase = Resuscitation phase (sedation, ventilation, vasopressors, fluid resuscitation)
Stable phase = Patient is stable on or can be weaned from vital support
Recovery phase = Patient who is mobilizing
(PN: parenteral nutrition; ESPGHAN: European Society of Paediatric Gastroenterology, Hepatology and Nutrition)

TABLE 3: Parenteral amino acid requirements (ESPGHAN 2018).

Age	Amino acids (g/kg/day)
Preterm infants	1.5–3.5
Term neonates	1.5–3.0
1 months–3 years	1.0–2.5
3–18 years	1.0–2.0

(ESPGHAN: European Society of Paediatric Gastroenterology, Hepatology and Nutrition)

TABLE 4: Parenteral glucose infusion rates (mg/kg/min) in PN (ESPGHAN 2018).

	Acute phase	Stable phase	Recovery phase
28 days–10 kg	2–4	4–6	6–10
11–30 kg	1.5–2.5	2–4	3–6
31–45	1–1.5	1.5–3	3–4
>45 kg	0.5–1	1–2	2–3

- Newborn < 28 days of age with acute phase of illness should receive 2.5–5 mg/kg/min of parenteral glucose supply guided by blood glucose levels.

(PN: parenteral nutrition; ESPGHAN: European Society of Paediatric Gastroenterology, Hepatology and Nutrition)

lower in exclusively parentally fed infants due to decreased intestinal uptake of amino acids.[77] Adequacy of amino acid intake is reflected by anthropometry, nitrogen balance, serum albumin, prealbumin, and blood urea nitrogen (BUN) levels. The amount of amino acids needed to achieve a positive nitrogen balance is optimal and recommendations are made based on studies on individual patient age groups (**Table 3**).[77] If renal function and hydration is normal, a BUN between 10 and 20 mg/dL reflects an amino acid intake that is adequate for protein anabolism.[78] Energy needs in PN are met by carbohydrates and lipids. Dextrose in its monohydrate form (d-glucose) is the carbohydrate in PN, which form the chief source of nonprotein calories (60–75%) and adds to the osmolality of the PN solution. The safe limits of dextrose supplementation have been set, based on the rates, which match glucose production and oxidation. In critically ill patients, the glucose utilization and metabolism may be modified depending on phase of illness and the extrinsic supply of glucose, resulting in substantial risk of hyper and hypoglycemia.[79,80] Hyperglycemia will in turn promote lipogenesis and fat deposition leading to steatotic states. High carbohydrate intake induces insulin resistance to protect the liver from glucose overload resulting in a counterproductive increase in hepatic glucose production.[81] Additionally, increased carbon dioxide production with excess glucose may pose challenges during weaning patients from mechanical ventilation. Hence, glucose administration in PN should not exceed the maximum rate of glucose oxidation. The typical glucose delivery rates of approximately 5 mg/kg/min has been proposed in the first week of injury in critically ill patients based on a study in pediatric patients with burns.[82] The general guidelines for parenteral carbohydrate intake based on age and phase of illness is depicted in **Table 4**.[83] The osmolarity of solutions should be restricted to less than 1,000 mosm/L if peripheral access is utilized.

Diversification of energy supply by adding lipid emulsions and amino acids will help to ameliorate the need for excess glucose supply. Lipid emulsions in PN should provide 25–50% of nonprotein calories. Lipids are generally administered as intravenous lipid emulsion (ILE) which can be 20% ILE, (2 kcal/mL) or 10% ILE (1.1 kcal/mL). Lipids decrease the osmolality of PN solutions, provide essential fatty acids, enhance the delivery of lipid soluble vitamins A, D, E, and K and improve the net nitrogen balance.[84]

However, increased lipid infusion rates can saturate lipoprotein lipase capacity and may lead to increase in serum triglyceride levels. It may also potentiate adverse effects like reticuloendothelial system overload. Hence, continuous infusions of lipid emulsion with gradual increments in lipid intake at the rate of 0.5–1 g/kg/day and close monitoring of triglyceride levels will be ideal. The recommended maximum intake is 4 g/kg/day in preterm and term infants. In children, parenteral lipid intake should not exceed 3 g/kg/day. The upper limit of triglyceride levels should not exceed 265 mg/dL in infants and 400 mg/dL for older children.[84] The currently available lipid emulsions are soy-based preparations and omega 3 fatty acid preparations derived from fish oil. For short-term PN composite ILEs with or without fish oil should be the first choice treatment due to better provision of balanced nutrition.[84] In a recent randomized controlled trial in infants undergoing open heart surgery, fish oil-based lipid emulsions have been found to reduce tumor necrosis factor (TNF)-alpha concentrations and ameliorate inflammatory response after cardiac surgery.[85] Some of the existing concerns associated with lipid emulsions for which substantial evidence is lacking include impaired clearance in septic patients, and a risk of thrombocytopenia due to reduced platelet life span.[86] In patients with unexplained thrombocytopenia, serum triglyceride composition should be monitored and a reduction in lipid dosage may be considered. In addition to macronutrients patients on long-term PN should also receive electrolytes, trace elements and vitamins.

TABLE 5: Daily electrolyte and mineral requirements for pediatric patients.[87]

Electrolyte	Preterm neonates	Infants and children	Adolescents and children > 50 kg
Sodium	2–5 mEq/kg	2–5 mEq/kg	1–2 mEq/kg
Potassium	2–4 mEq/kg	2–4 mEq/kg	1–2 mEq/kg
Calcium	2–4 mEq/kg	0.5–4.0 mEq/kg	10–20 mEq
Phosphorus	1–2 mmol/kg	0.5–2 mmol/kg	10–40 mmol
Magnesium	0.3–0.5 mEq/kg	0.3–0.5 mEq/kg	10–30 mEq
Acetate	As per acid base balance	As per acid base balance	As per acid base balance
Chloride	As per acid base balance	As per acid base balance	As per acid base balance

Source: Mirtallo J, Canada T, Johnson D, Kumpf V, Petersen C, Sacks G, et al. Safe practices for parenteral nutrition. Task force for the revision of safe practices for parenteral nutrition. J Parent Enter Nutr. 2004;28:S39-70.

TABLE 6: Trace element daily requirements in pediatric patients.[87]

Trace elements	Preterm neonates <3 kg (µg/kg/day)	Term neonates/infants 3–10 kg (µg/kg/day)	Children 10–40 kg (µg/kg/day)	Adolescents >40 kg
Zinc	400	50–250	50–125	2–5 mg
Copper	20	20	5–20	200–500 µg
Manganese	1.0	1.0	1.0	40–100 µg
Chromium	0.05–0.2	0.2	0.14–0.2	5–15 µg
Selenium	1.5–2.0	2.0	1.0–2.0	40–60 µg

Source: Mirtallo J, Canada T, Johnson D, Kumpf V, Petersen C, Sacks G, et al. Safe practices for parenteral nutrition. Task force for the revision of safe practices for parenteral nutrition. J Parent Enter Nutr. 2004;28:S39-70.

The daily requirements of micronutrients for PN[34,87] are depicted in **Tables 5** and **6**.

A Feasible PN Strategy in LMIC

In pediatric cardiac intensive care units of LMIC, considering the existing logistics and resource limitations, PN should be prescribed only if absolutely indicated. With lack of dedicated nutrition support teams and in house total parenteral nutrition (TPN) formulating facility in LMIC the pediatrician/pediatric cardiac intensivist in conjunction with the nurse leader and the hospital clinical pharmacist should be in charge of prescribing and ensuring safe administration of PN. A combined nutrition rounds by pediatric cardiac intensivisit, nurse leader, and assigned nurse would be beneficial to evaluate the patient on a day-to-day basis and review PN prescription and delivery. A daily attempt should be made to assess the feasibility of reintroducing EN as early as clinical condition permits. Trophic feeds should be encouraged wherever feasible to prevent intestinal mucosal atrophy.[73] Strict attention to aseptic practices to minimize infectious complications is of paramount importance. Monitoring during PN should include careful biochemical monitoring for complications and maintenance of stability of nutrient solutions. The common complications include metabolic complications, infections, vascular thrombosis, and PN-related cholestasis. Periodic assessment of nutritional status is ideal to monitor growth and recovery.

NUTRITIONAL RECOVERY AFTER CORRECTIVE SURGERY

Studies from advanced nations have previously reported normalization of somatic growth typically 6–12 months after corrective congenital heart surgery.[34,88] Weintraub et al. reported that after surgical closure of VSD in infancy, growth parameters were almost comparable to the reference population by 5.7 years.[34] However, in a study from Southern India the nutritional recovery on follow-up after VSD closure in infancy was suboptimal, with weight, and height Z-scores <−2 in 42% and 27% of patients, respectively.[89] In a larger study with all forms of CHD, the same authors reported significant catch-up growth after correction, typically within 3–12 months after correction followed by plateauing of the growth curves after a year.[90] This reflects an immediate catch-up growth in short-term due to correction of the hemodynamic derangement, while other determinants of growth such as dietary and constitutional factors play a more important long-term role. Suboptimal nutritional recovery with persistent weight Z-score <−2 was observed in 27.3% of patients and this was predicted by lower weight Z-score at surgery, lower birth weight, and lower parental anthropometry.[90] It is also important to identify patients at risk of sub-optimal recovery (those with lower growth potential) before intervention so that targeted nutritional rehabilitation may be provided on follow-up.

Review Postsurgery and Surgical Recovery

Following PICU discharge close attention to nutrition is required, particularly in some subsets of patients[91] such as those with total cavopulmonary connection (TCPC) circulation following complex CHD[92] and this may be challenging to achieve in resource limited settings.

FUTURE DIRECTIONS

Ideally, nutritional support for children with CHD should be based on data that is appropriate to specific environments. Much of the current data on children with CHD is limited to a relatively small spectrum of cardiac anomalies, and as increasingly complex CHD is addressed in LMICs, the issues related to nutrition may well change and require different approaches. The maintenance of regional databases of information and outcomes would provide an ideal basis for future research in this area. Much work may also need to be done in the areas of quality control and research implementation in order to carry through what is already known into clinical practice. There may also need to be increased focus on the supporting teams and structures that are implemented around teams that work with CHD in LMICs.

■ CONCLUSION

The overall management of children with CHD may be complex, and attention to nutrition is a critical element of that care. In general, nutritional support is relatively inexpensive, but it does rely on the existence of a structured system within the cardiac care environment to ensure appropriate recognition of the particular role of nutrition in a specific child. Repeated and accurate measurement of growth parameters together with detailed attention to nutritional intake and tolerance is essential to facilitate optimal postoperative recovery.

■ ACKNOWLEDGMENT

Reproduced with permission from Argent AC, Balachandran R, Vaidyanathan B, Khan A, Krishna Kumar R. Management of undernutrition and failure to thrive in children with congenital heart disease in low- and middle-income countries. Cardiol Young. 2017;27(S6):S22-30. (DOI: 10.1017/S104795111700258X).

■ REFERENCES

1. Unger R, DeKleermaeker M, Gidding SS, Christoffel KK. Calories count. Improved weight gain with dietary intervention in congenital heart disease. Am J Dis Child. 1992;146:1078-84.
2. Arodiwe I, Chinawa J, Ujunwa F, Adiele D, Ukoha M, Obidike E. Nutritional status of congenital heart disease (CHD) patients: burden and determinant of malnutrition at university of Nigeria teaching hospital Ituku - Ozalla, Enugu. Pak J Med Sci. 2015;31:1140-5.
3. Cameron JW, Rosenthal A, Olson AD. Malnutrition in hospitalized children with congenital heart disease. Arch Pediatr Adolesc Med. 1995;149:1098-102.
4. Okoromah CA, Ekure EN, Lesi FE, Okunowo WO, Tijani BO, Okeiyi JC. Prevalence, profile and predictors of malnutrition in children with congenital heart defects: a case-control observational study. Arch Dis Child. 2011;96:354-60.
5. Toole BJ, Toole LE, Kyle UG, Cabrera AG, Orellana RA, Coss-Bu JA. Perioperative nutritional support and malnutrition in infants and children with congenital heart disease. Congenit Heart Dis. 2014;9:15-25.
6. Vaidyanathan B, Nair SB, Sundaram KR, Babu UK, Shivaprakasha K, Rao SG, et al. Malnutrition in children with congenital heart disease (CHD) determinants and short term impact of corrective intervention. Indian Pediatr. 2008;45:541-6.
7. Varan B, Tokel K, Yilmaz G. Malnutrition and growth failure in cyanotic and acyanotic congenital heart disease with and without pulmonary hypertension. Arch Dis Child. 1999;81:49-52.
8. Venugopalan P, Akinbami FO, Al-Hinai KM, Agarwal AK. Malnutrition in children with congenital heart defects. Saudi Med J. 2001;22:964-7.
9. Villasis-Keever MA, Aquiles Pineda-Cruz R, Halley-Castillo E, Alva-Espinosa C. Frequency and risk factors associated with malnutrition in children with congenital cardiopathy. Salud Publica Mex. 2001;43:313-23.
10. Leite HP, Fisberg M, Novo NF, Nogueira EB, Ueda IK. Nutritional assessment and surgical risk markers in children submitted to cardiac surgery. Sao Paulo Med J. 1995;113:706-14.
11. Ehlers KH. Growth failure in association with congenital heart disease. Pediatr Ann. 1978;7:750-9.

12. Anderson JB, Beekman RH 3rd, Border WL, Kalkwarf HJ, Khoury PR, Uzark K, et al. Lower weight-for-age z score adversely affects hospital length of stay after the bidirectional Glenn procedure in 100 infants with a single ventricle. J Thorac Cardiovasc Surg. 2009;138:397-404.e1.

13. Schwalbe-Terilli CR, Hartman DH, Nagle ML, Gallagher PR, Ittenbach RF, Burnham NB, et al. Enteral feeding and caloric intake in neonates after cardiac surgery. Am J Crit Care. 2009;18:52-7.

14. Tchervenkov CI, Jacobs JP, Bernier PL, Stellin G, Kurosawa H, Mavroudis C, et al. The improvement of care for paediatric and congenital cardiac disease across the World: a challenge for the World Society for Pediatric and Congenital Heart Surgery. Cardiol Young. 2008;18(Suppl 2):63-9.

15. Jenkins KJ, Castaneda AR, Cherian KM, Couser CA, Dale EK, Gauvreau K, et al. Reducing mortality and infections after congenital heart surgery in the developing world. Pediatrics. 2014;134: e1422-30.

16. Vaidyanathan B, Roth SJ, Rao SG, Gauvreau K, Shivaprakasha K, Kumar RK. Outcome of ventricular septal defect repair in a developing country. J Pediatr. 2002;140:736-41.

17. Reddy NS, Kappanayil M, Balachandran R, Jenkins KJ, Sudhakar A, Sunil GS, et al. Preoperative determinants of outcomes of infant heart surgery in a limited-resource setting. Sem Thorac Cardiovasc Surg. 2015;27:331-8.

18. Bernier PL, Stefanescu A, Samoukovic G, Tchervenkov CI. The challenge of congenital heart disease worldwide: epidemiologic and demographic facts. Sem Thorac Cardiovasc Surg Pediatr Cardiac Surg Ann. 2010;13:26-34.

19. WHO. (2017). Global Database on Child Growth and Malnutrition. [online] Available from: https://www.who.int/nutgrowthdb/en/. [Last accessed February, 2021].

20. Van den Broeck J, Meulemans W, Eeckels R. Nutritional assessment: the problem of clinical-anthropometrical mismatch. Eur J Clin Nutr. 1994;48:60-5.

21. Green Corkins K. Nutrition-focused physical examination in pediatric patients. Nutr Clin. Prac. 2015;30:203-9.

22. Mehta NM, Corkins MR, Lyman B, Malone A, Goday PS, Carney LN, et al. Defining pediatric malnutrition: a paradigm shift toward etiology-related definitions. JPEN. 2013;37:460-81.

23. Becker P, Carney LN, Corkins MR, Monczka J, Smith E, Smith SE, et al. Consensus statement of the Academy of Nutrition and Dietetics/American Society for Parenteral and Enteral Nutrition: indicators recommended for the identification and documentation of pediatric malnutrition (undernutrition). Nutr Clin Prac. 2015;30:147-61.

24. Blasquez A, Clouzeau H, Fayon M, Mouton JB, Thambo JB, Enaud R, et al. Evaluation of nutritional status and support in children with congenital heart disease. Eur J Clin Nutr. 2016;70:528-31.

25. Yahav J, Avigad S, Frand M, Shem-Tov A, Barzilay Z, Linn S, et al. Assessment of intestinal and cardiorespiratory function in children with congenital heart disease on high-caloric formulas. J Pediatr Gastroenterol Nutr. 1985;4:778-85.

26. Thommessen M, Heiberg A, Kase BF. Feeding problems in children with congenital heart disease: the impact on energy intake and growth outcome. Eur J Clin Nutr. 1992;46:457-64.

27. Hansen SR, Dorup I. Energy and nutrient intakes in congenital heart disease. Acta Paediatr. 1993;82:166-72.

28. Nicholson GT, Clabby ML, Kanter KR, Mahle WT. Caloric intake during the perioperative period and growth failure in infants with congenital heart disease. Pediatr Cardiol. 2013;34:316-21.

29. Menon G, Poskitt EM. Why does congenital heart disease cause failure to thrive? Arch Dis Child. 1985;60:1134-9.

30. Barton JS, Hindmarsh PC, Scrimgeour CM, Rennie MJ, Preece MA. Energy expenditure in congenital heart disease. Arch Dis Child. 1994;70:5-9.

31. Mitchell IM, Davies PS, Day JM, Pollock JC, Jamieson MP. Energy expenditure in children with congenital heart disease, before and after cardiac surgery. J Thorac Cardiovasc Surg. 1994;107:374-80.

32. Goulart MR, Schuh DS, Moraes DW, Barbiero SM, Pellanda LC. Serum C-reactive protein levels and body mass index in children and adolescents with CHD. Cardiol Young. 2016:1-7.

33. Mehrizi A, Drash A. Growth disturbance in congenital heart disease. J Pediatr. 1962;61:418-29.

34. Weintraub RG, Menahem S. Growth and congenital heart disease. J Paediatr Child Health. 1993;29:95-8.

35. Ackerman IL, Karn CA, Denne SC, Ensing GJ, Leitch CA. Total but not resting energy expenditure is increased in infants with ventricular septal defects. Pediatrics. 1998;102:1172-7.

36. Salzer HR, Haschke F, Wimmer M, Heil M, Schilling R. Growth and nutritional intake of infants with congenital heart disease. Pediatr Cardiol. 1989;10:17-23.

37. Matthiesen NB, Henriksen TB, Gaynor JW, Agergaard P, Bach CC, Hjortdal VE, et al. Congenital heart defects and indices of fetal cerebral growth in a nationwide cohort of 924,422 live born infants. Circulation. 2016;133:566-75.

38. Villares JM, Leal LO, Diaz IS, Gonzalez PG. [Plasma aminogram in infants operated on complex congenital heart disease]. Nutr Hospital. 2008;23:283-7.

39. Leite HP, de Camargo Carvalho AC, Fisberg M. [Nutritional status of children with congenital heart disease and left-to-right shunt. The importance of the presence of pulmonary hypertension]. Arq Bras Cardiol. 1995;65: 403-7.

40. Steier M, Lopez R, Cooperman JM. Riboflavin deficiency in infants and children with heart disease. Am Heart J. 1976;92:139-43.

41. Finnerty CC, Mabvuure NT, Ali A, Kozar RA, Herndon DN. The surgically induced stress response. JPEN. 2013;37:21s-9s.

42. Teixeira-Cintra MA, Monteiro JP, Tremeschin M, Trevilato TM, Halperin ML, Carlotti AP. Monitoring of protein catabolism in neonates and young infants post-cardiac surgery. Acta Paediatr. 2011;100:977-82.

43. Mehta NM, Costello JM, Bechard LJ, Johnson VM, Zurakowski D, McGowan FX, et al. Resting energy expenditure after Fontan surgery in children with single-ventricle heart defects. JPEN. 2012;36:685-92.

44. Jones MO, Pierro A, Hammond P, Lloyd DA. The effect of major operations on heart rate, respiratory rate, physical activity, temperature and respiratory gas exchange in infants. Eur J Pediatr Surg. 1995;5:9-12.

45. Hardin JT, Muskett AD, Canter CE, Martin TC, Spray TL. Primary surgical closure of large ventricular septal defects in small infants. Ann Thorac Surg. 1992;53:397-401.

46. Brooks A, Geldenhuys A, Zuhlke L, Human P, Zilla P. Pulmonary artery banding: still a valuable option in developing countries? Eur J Cardiothorac Surg. 2012;41:272-6.

47. Jackson M, Poskitt EM. The effects of high-energy feeding on energy balance and growth in infants with congenital heart disease and failure to thrive. Brit J Nutr. 1991;65:131-43.

48. Bougle D, Iselin M, Kahyat A, Duhamel JF. Nutritional treatment of congenital heart disease. Arch Dis Child. 1986;61:799-801.

49. Vanderhoof JA, Hofschire PJ, Baluff MA, Guest JE, Murray ND, Pinsky WW, et al. Continuous enteral feedings. An important adjunct to the management of complex congenital heart disease. Am J Dis Child. 1982;136:825-7.

50. Schwarz SM, Gewitz MH, See CC, Berezin S, Glassman MS, Medow CM, et al. Enteral nutrition in infants with congenital heart disease and growth failure. Pediatrics. 1990;86: 368-73.

51. Skillman HE, Mehta NM. Nutrition therapy in the critically ill child. Curr Opin Crit Care. 2012;18:192-8.

52. Zamberlan P, Delgado AF, Leone C, Feferbaum R, Okay TS. Nutrition therapy in a pediatric intensive care unit: Indications, monitoring, and complications. JPEN. 2011;35:523-9.

53. Mehta NM. Approach to enteral feeding in the PICU. Nutr Clin Prac. 2009;24:377-87.

54. Meert KL, Daphtary KM, Metheny NA. Gastric vs small-bowel feeding in critically ill children receiving mechanical ventilation: a randomized controlled trial. Chest. 2004;126:872-8.

55. Natarajan G, Reddy Anne S, Aggarwal S. Enteral feeding of neonates with congenital heart disease. Neonatology. 2010;98:330-6.

56. Fivez T, Kerklaan D, Mesotten D, Verbruggen S, Wouters PJ, Vanhorebeek I, et al. Early versus late parenteral nutrition in critically ill children. N Engl J Med. 2016;374:1111-22.

57. Jeffries HE, Wells WJ, Starnes VA, Wetzel RC, Moromisato DY. Gastrointestinal morbidity after Norwood palliation for hypoplastic left heart syndrome. Ann Thorac Surg. 2006;81:982-7.

58. Giannone PJ, Luce WA, Nankervis CA, Hoffman TM, Wold LE. Necrotizing enterocolitis in neonates with congenital heart disease. Life Sci. 2008;82:341-7.

59. Owens JL, Musa N. Nutrition support after neonatal cardiac surgery. Nutr Clin Prac. 2009; 24:242-9.

60. De Wit B, Meyer R, Desai A, Macrae D, Pathan N. Challenge of predicting resting energy expenditure in children undergoing surgery for congenital heart disease. Pediatr Crit Care Med. 2010;11:496-501.

61. Torowicz DL, Seelhorst A, Froh EB, Spatz DL. Human milk and breastfeeding outcomes in infants with congenital heart disease. Breastfeed Med. 2015;10:31-7.

62. Sullivan S, Schanler RJ, Kim JH, Patel AL, Trawöger R, Kiechl-Kohlendorfer U, et al. An exclusively human milk-based diet is associated with a lower rate of necrotizing enterocolitis than a diet of human milk and bovine milk-based products. J Pediatr. 2010;156:562-7.e1.

63. Hofner G, Behrens R, Koch A, Singer H, Hofbeck M. Enteral nutritional support by percutaneous endoscopic gastrostomy in children with congenital heart disease. Pediatr Cardiol. 2000;21:341-6.

64. El-Sayed Ahmed MM, Alfares FA, Hynes CF, Ramakrishnan K, Louis C, Dou C, et al. Timing of gastrostomy tube feeding in three-stage palliation of single-ventricle physiology. Congenit Heart Dis. 2016;11:34-8.

65. Lee JH, Rogers E, Chor YK, Samransamruajkit R, Koh PL, Miqdady M, et al. Optimal nutrition therapy in paediatric critical care in the Asia-Pacific and Middle East: a consensus. Asia Pacific J Clin Nutr. 2016;25:676-96.

66. Hamilton S, McAleer DM, Ariagno K, Barrett M, Stenquist N, Duggan CP, et al. A stepwise enteral nutrition algorithm for critically ill children helps achieve nutrient delivery goals. Pediatr Crit Care Med. 2014;15:583-9.

67. Martinez EE, Smallwood CD, Bechard LJ, Graham RJ, Mehta NM. Metabolic assessment and individualized nutrition in children dependent on mechanical ventilation at home. J Pediatr. 2015;166:350-7.

68. Mehta NM, Bechard LJ, Cahill N, Wang M, Day A, Duggan CP, et al. Nutritional practices and their relationship to clinical outcomes in critically ill children—an international multicenter cohort study. Crit Care Med. 2012;40:2204-11.

69. Mehta NM, Bechard LJ, Zurakowski D, Duggan CP, Heyland DK. Adequate enteral protein intake is inversely associated with 60-d mortality in critically ill children: A multicenter, prospective, cohort study. Am J Clin Nutr. 2015;102:199-206.

70. Martinez EE, Bechard LJ, Mehta NM. Nutrition algorithms and bedside nutrient delivery practices in pediatric intensive care units: an international multicenter cohort study. Nutr Clin Prac. 2014;29:360-7.

71. Balachandran R, Nair SG, Gopalraj SS, Vaidyanathan B, Kumar RK. Dedicated pediatric cardiac intensive care unit in a developing country: Does it improve the outcome? Ann Pediatr Cardiol. 2011;4:122-6.

72. Ramakrishnan N, Shankar B, Ranganathan L, Daphnee DK, Bharadwaj A, Venkataraman R. Parenteral nutrition support: Beyond gut feeling? Quality control study of parenteral nutrition practices in a Tertiary Care Hospital. Indian J Crit Care Med. 2016;20:36-9.

73. Heine RG, Bines JE. New approaches to parenteral nutrition in infants and children. J Paediatr Child Health. 2002;38:433-7.

74. Boullata JI, Gilbert K, Sacks G, Labossiere RJ, Crill C, Goday P, et al. A.S.P.E.N. clinical guidelines: parenteral nutrition ordering, order review, compounding, labeling, and dispensing. JPEN. 2014;38:334-77.

75. Sentongo TA, Tershakovec AM, Mascarenhas MR, Watson MH, Stallings VA. Resting energy expenditure and prediction equations in young children with failure to thrive. J Pediatr. 2000;136:345-50.

76. Joosten K, Embleton E, Yan W, Senterre T. ESPGHAN/ESPEN/ESPR guidelines on pediatric parenteral nutrition: Energy. Clin Nutr. 2018;37:1-6.

77. van Goudoever JB, Carnielli V, Darmaun D, Sainz de Pipaon M. ESPGHAN/ESPEN/ESPR/CSPEN guidelines on pediatric parenteral nutrition: Aminoacids. Clin Nutr. 2018;37:2315-23.

78. Schulman RJ, Phillips S. Parenteral nutrition in infants and children. J Pediatr Gastroenterol Nutr. 2003;36:587-607.

79. Robin AP, Carpentier YA, Askanazi J, Nordenström J, Kinney JM. Metabolic consequences of hypercaloric glucose infusions. Acta Chir Belg. 1981;80:133-40.

80. Geukers VG, Li Z, Ackermans MT, Travers S, Weber ML, Wentz AE, et al. High carbohydrate/low protein-induced hyperinsulinemia does not improve protein balance in children after cardiac surgery. Nutrition. 2012;28:644-50.

81. Agius L. High carbohydrate diets induce hepatic insulin resistance to protect liver from substrate overload. Biochem Pharmacol. 2013;85:306-12.

82. Dylewski ML, Baker M, Prelack K, Weber JM, Hursey D, Lydon M, et al. The safety and efficacy of parenteral nutrition among pediatric patients with burn injuries. Pediatr Crit Care Med. 2013;14:e120-5.

83. Mesotten D, Joosten K, van Kempen A, Verbruggen S. ESPGHAN/ESPEN/CSPEN guidelines on pediatric parenteral nutrition: Carbohydrates. Clin Nutr. 2018;37:2337-43.

84. Lapillonne A, Mis NF, Goulet O, van den Akker CHP, Wu J, Koletzko B. ESPGHAN/ESPEN/ESPR/CSPEN guidelines on pediatric parenteral nutrition: Lipids . Clin Nutr. 2018;37:2324-36.

85. Larsen BM, Goonewardene LA, Joffe AR, Van Aerde JE, Field CJ, et al. Pretreatment with an intravenous lipidemulsion containing fish oil (Eicosapentaenoic acid and Docosahexaenoic Acid) decreases inflammatory markers after open heart surgery in infants, a randomized controlled trial. Clin Nutr. 2012;31:322-9.

86. Koletzko B, Goulet O, Hunt J, Krohn K, Shamir R. Guidelines on Paediatric Parenteral Nutrition of the European Society of Paediatric Gastroenterology, Hepatology and Nutrition (ESPGHAN) and the European Society for Clinical Nutrition and Metabolism (ESPEN), Supported by the European Society of Paediatric Research (ESPR). J Pediatr Gastroenterol Nutr. 2005;41(Suppl 2):S1-87.

87. Mirtallo J, Canada T, Johnson D, Kumpf V, Petersen C, Sacks G, et al. Safe practices for parenteral nutrition. Task force for the revision of safe practices for parenteral nutrition. J Parent Enter Nutr. 2004;28:S39-70.

88. Cheung MM, Davis AM, Wilkinson JL, Weintraub RG. Long term somatic growth after repair of tetralogy of Fallot: evidence for restoration of genetic growth potential. Heart. 2003;89:1340-3.

89. Vaidyanathan B, Roth SJ, Gauvreau K, Shivaprakasha K, Rao SG, Kumar RK. Somatic growth after ventricular septal defect in malnourished infants. J Pediatr. 2006;149:205-9.

90. Vaidyanathan B, Radhakrishnan R, Sarala DA, Sundaram KR, Kumar RK. What determines nutritional recovery in malnourished children after correction of congenital heart defects? Pediatrics. 2009;124:e294-9.

91. Medoff-Cooper B, Ravishankar C. Nutrition and growth in congenital heart disease: a challenge in children. Curr. Opin Cardiol. 2013;28:122-9.

92. Glockler M, Severin T, Arnold R, Greiner P, Schwab KO, Uhl M, et al. First description of three patients with multifocal lymphangiomatosis and protein-losing enteropathy following palliation of complex congenital heart disease with total cavo-pulmonary connection. Pediatr. Cardiol. 2008;29:771-4.

14

CHAPTER

Management of Patients with Open Sternum after Pediatric Cardiac Surgery

Rakhi Balachandran, Brijesh P Kottayil

Illustration: Balaji Srimurugan

Reviewed by: Brijesh P Kottayil

■ INTRODUCTION

Delayed sternal closure refers to leaving the sternum open for a variable period of time after open cardiac surgery. Typically the decision to leave the sternum open is electively taken at the end of the primary cardiac surgical procedure depending on the clinical and hemodynamic status of the patient. Rarely a patient who had a primary sternal closure might require reopening of the sternum in the postoperative period following any adverse hemodynamic event. Sternal closure after open cardiac surgery can sometimes cause cardiac compression, an elevation in right and left ventricular end diastolic pressures, decreased ventricular filling and subsequently a reduction in cardiac output.[1] This is likely to be due to a disproportion between the available retrosternal space and an edematous heart resulting in a clinical picture indistinguishable from cardiac tamponade.[1,2] Chest closure can also fix the volume of thoracic cage and decrease overall chest wall compliance affecting ventilatory mechanics. Leaving the sternum open can mitigate the diastolic filling restriction and impairment of myocardial function that occurs due to increased pericardial pressure following chest closure.[3-5] Concomitantly, it also helps to avoid the worsening of pulmonary mechanics and gas exchange which are likely to occur at the time of

sternal approximation. The reported frequency of delayed sternal closure in pediatric cardiac surgery ranges from 3.45 to 11%.[2,6-8] Some of the established risk factors that predict delayed sternal closure include age less than 7 days, diagnosis of interrupted aortic arch or total anomalous pulmonary venous connection, cardiopulmonary bypass time >185 minutes, aortic cross clamp time >98 min and post bypass central venous oxygen saturation <51%.[8] In the current era, open sternum strategy becomes more relevant in the context of early primary repair of complex congenital heart disease in neonates and infants requiring longer surgical support times. Intuitively, the benefit of open sternum is greater in neonates and infants due to the larger cardiac size relative to thoracic cavity. Despite the purported favorable cardiopulmonary benefits in selected subset of pediatric cardiac surgical patients, delayed sternal closure is often accompanied by a need for prolongation of intensive care and increased propensity for postoperative infections.[7,9] The care of postoperative patients with open sternum in the intensive care unit is challenging and necessitates intense hemodynamic monitoring with diligent nursing care. This chapter provides an overview of management of patients with open sternum in the pediatric cardiac intensive care unit (PCICU).

INDICATIONS FOR DELAYED STERNAL CLOSURE[10]

- Significant myocardial edema
- Hemodynamic instability with depressed myocardial function
- Refractory arrhythmias
- Inadequate intraoperative hemostasis
- Pulmonary edema and poor lung compliance
- To provide access for external cardiac support systems.

BENEFITS OF LEAVING STERNUM OPEN

- Easy access for the surgeon, in terms of controlling a bleed and clot evacuation.
- Facilitates internal cardiac massage in the event of resuscitation.
- Improves hemodynamic stability by improving ventricular compliance, which in turn improves ventricular filling and cardiac output.
- Improves thoracic cage compliance that augments pulmonary mechanics and gas exchange.

DEMERITS OF DELAYED STERNAL CLOSURE

- *High risk of nosocomial infections*: Data from a large multicenter study of 6,127 index operations with open sternum in infant population reported an incidence of at least one infection in 18.7%.[9] Prolonged duration of open sternum was associated with increased rate of infectious complications.[9]
- Frequent dressing changes and irrigation of the wound which might injure the skin.
- Lack of thoracic cage stability necessitates continued mechanical ventilatory support.
- Risk of injury to right ventricle by the sternal edges when the patient is moved.
- Nursing care and physiotherapy is limited.

- Prolonged duration of mechanical ventilation.
- Prolonged intensive care unit stay.

SURGICAL TECHNIQUE OF MAINTAINING AN OPEN STERNUM

Several techniques are employed to maintain an open sternum in the postoperative period. Typically a rigid plastic tube cut to the desired size can be used as a sternal separator, keeping the sternal edges stented .This tube is transfixed to the sternal edges with a steel wire. An Esmark/transparent serum bag membrane cut into an elliptical shape is sutured to the skin edges with a continuous suture. Alternatively a transparent iodine impregnated dressing is applied on the skin edges ensuring an airtight compartment below the dressing **(Fig. 1)**. This strategy facilitates maintenance of skin integrity by avoiding suturing of the membrane to the edges. If a sutured membrane is used, bactericidal ointment (Povidone iodine) is applied liberally to the skin- patch interface to help seal off the suture holes that might admit air into the mediastinum. The wound is dressed airtight with iodine impregnated incision drape (Ioban™ 2, 3M™, USA).

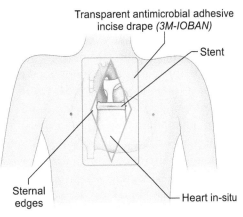

Fig. 1: Open sternum following pediatric cardiac surgery. Sternal edges are stented using a rigid plastic tube. Iodine impregnated transparent adhesive drape is used to give an airtight seal.

Use of transparent membrane allows visibility to detect pericardial collection and cardiac contractility.

■ NURSING CONSIDERATIONS[11]

Patients with open sternum are vulnerable to hemodynamic instability, postoperative bleeding and nosocomial infection. Hence, they have to be handled with extra vigil in the postoperative intensive care unit. The important nursing considerations are given here.

1. Maintain a high degree of asepsis, while handling these infants, as there is a high risk of infection.
2. Limit the number of personnel touching the infant.
3. Ensure strict hand hygiene and use of sterile gloves for sterile techniques such as endotracheal suctioning, wound dressing manipulations, and for routine body care.
4. Dressing changes are provided if there is soiling with blood or fluid. This should only be done with the concurrence of the surgical team member.
5. The Esmark/transparent dressing should be observed continuously for evidence of bulging or leaking, which indicates ongoing bleeding or tamponade. In such situations, the surgeon should be alerted immediately for partial removal of the patch and to perform mediastinal suction/exploration.
6. Ventilator tubing should not be allowed to rest directly on the sternal wound. A sterile surgical pad is used to support the ventilator tubing.
7. Sterile towel/surgical pad/Steri-Drape™ should be used to cover the Esmark while endotracheal suction is in progress.
8. Continuous invasive hemodynamic monitoring is mandatory for all patients with open sternum.
9. As there is thoracic cage instability movement of the infant should be minimized and done very carefully, especially while giving body care to the patient.
10. Physiotherapy should be restricted and should not involve percussion or vibration. Passive range of motion exercises should be performed gently, to improve circulation to the extremities as the patients are often on neuromuscular blockade.
11. As these patients with hemodynamic instability are likely to have compromised peripheral circulation or venous stasis they are vulnerable to develop pressure ulcers. They should be nursed on soft beds (water cushion beds/air beds). Periodic evaluation for development of pressure sores and gentle repositioning of extremities/body tilts can be done every 4 hours.
12. Re-exploration in the PCICU should be carried out in a sterile surgical environment. The involved personnel should wear mask, cap, sterile gown and gloves after adequate hand hygiene. Typically, a single dose of intravenous vancomycin is administered as prophylaxis against gram positive organisms. Some surgeons prefer a sternal wound irrigation with diluted vancomycin preparation instead of intravenous administration. Blood products should be kept ready by the bedside for any bleeding complications.

■ ANTIBIOTIC PROPHYLAXIS

There are no clear guidelines for antibiotic prophylaxis for open chest patients after cardiothoracic operation. Though surgical site infections are typically caused by gram positive organisms, postoperative gram negative infections have also been reported in open sternum patients. Based on this, some centers have adopted the practice of escalating antibiotic therapy in patients with open sternum. A retrospective single center study which compared three different antibiotic regimens namely cefazolin, cefazolin + vancomycin or vancomycin + meropenem observed a lower rate of blood stream infection and surgical site infection in the broad spectrum antibiotic group in open sternum patients.[12] However, in the absence of robust evidence, routine use of broad spectrum antibiotics cannot be recommended in patients with open sternum after pediatric cardiac surgery due to concerns of antimicrobial resistance. The common practice is to administer the standard surgical prophylaxis antibiotic (cefuroxime or cefazolin) for the duration for which sternum remains open and for 24 hours after sternal closure. However, in the event of sternum remaining open for longer than 48 hours, need for escalation of the antibiotics is considered based on clinical/laboratory evidence of a nosocomial infection. Appropriate specimens including blood culture, mediastinal wound swab or a mini bronchoalveolar lavage (BAL) culture should be sent before starting the second-line antibiotic.

■ HEMODYNAMIC MANAGEMENT

Invasive hemodynamic monitoring is mandatory in children with open sternum. Standard monitoring includes invasive arterial blood pressure, central venous pressure monitoring, continuous ECG monitoring, and pulse oximetry. Additionally some patients are likely to have transthoracic lines for left atrial (LA) or Pulmonary artery (PA) pressure monitoring. These lines should be properly secured and monitored continuously for waveform and pressures.

Infants with open sternum most often have moderate inotropic supports. These are usually maintained till the sternum is approximated. However, if hemodynamic stability was not the major concern for keeping the sternum open these may be judiciously tapered to acceptable levels.

■ VENTILATION

Children with open sternum need mechanical ventilator support due to thoracic cage instability. Pressure preset modes such as pressure controlled ventilation are likely to be beneficial because of the poorly compliant lungs often encountered in these group of patients. Ventilatory settings, particularly peak and plateau airway pressures as well as gas exchange should be vigilantly monitored in these patients. Arterial blood gases need to be evaluated at least 4th hourly or more frequently in critically ill patients. Hourly respiratory assessment should be made to understand the quality of breath sounds, patency of airway, adequate bilateral chest expansion and the stability of endotracheal tube. Secretions should be promptly removed by suctioning, as this facilitates expansion of atelectatic areas and improves lung compliance.

Chest X-ray is taken to assess the pulmonary and cardiac status. Moving the baby for chest X-ray should be done with extreme caution and should be carried out only in the presence of physician or a member of the surgical team.

■ PAIN AND SEDATION MANAGEMENT

Infants and neonates who undergo delayed sternal closure for hemodynamic instability or refractory bleeding should be kept quiescent by adequate neuromuscular blockade, and sedation. Adequate analgesia is mandatory to avoid increased sympathetic response in these critically ill infants. The drugs typically used are either fentanyl or morphine infusions with intermittent doses of paralytic agents. Administration of PRN doses of midazolam should be done with extreme caution as this drug can precipitate sudden hypotension in patients with depressed myocardial function.

The plane of sedation should be deepened before performing painful procedures such as endotracheal suctioning, wound exploration and sternal closure.

■ FLUID MANAGEMENT

Fluid management is in accordance with the standard body surface area method, as followed for cardiac surgery under bypass. However, fluid restriction may be critical in children with fluid overload and those with significant capillary leak. This is usually coupled with aggressive diuresis using furosemide infusion or peritoneal dialysis to accomplish adequate negative fluid balance and facilitate early sternal closure.[6,10] Fluid restriction with diuresis can also aid in decreasing extravascular lung water, improving lung compliance and gas exchange thereby facilitating early closure of the sternum. In patients with acute kidney injury in the postoperative period, fluid restriction and renal replacement therapy should be instituted till the renal function recovers.

■ NUTRITIONAL SUPPORT

Nasogastric feeds can be initiated 12–24 hours after surgery if patient is not requiring high dose vasoconstrictors (noradrenaline, high dose epinephrine or vasopressin) and the serum lactate levels remain below 4 mmol/liter. Volume of feeds should be adjusted as permitted by maintenance fluid intake allowance. If the patient cannot be initiated on enteral feeds by 72 hours, it is worth considering parenteral nutrition to meet energy and protein requirements.

▌ TIMING OF DELAYED STERNAL CLOSURE

The optimal duration for which the sternum has to be kept open is not defined. This depends on the primary indication for leaving the sternum open and the cardiorespiratory status of the patient. In a retrospective analysis by Riphagen et al. early sternal closure was feasible at a median duration of 21 hours after cardiac surgery.[2] It is clear from retrospective reviews that the morbidity related to an open sternum is worsened by the duration for which the sternum is kept open.[7,9] Open sternum increases the risk of postoperative infections, duration of ventilation and need for intensive care unit stay. Hence, it is imperative that the entire team should have a focused approach for optimizing the patient toward the primary goal of facilitating sternal closure at the earliest possible window. A reasonable strategy would be the resolution of the primary condition responsible for delaying closure, a reduction in fluid overload (measured by a total negative fluid balance) and clinical judgment.

Management of Sternum Closure in PCICU

1. Decision to close the sternum is made on the basis of hemodynamic improvement, cessation of bleeding and adequate negative fluid balance. The optimal time to sternal closure remains unclear. Resolution of the primary indication and clinical judgment may be the best guide.
2. Confirmation from the surgical team is required before preparing for sternal closure.
3. *Location*: Sternal closure can be performed in the PCICU or the operating room (OR) depending on the decision of the surgical team. Potential advantages of sternal closure in ICU include avoiding the need for transfer of a critically ill patient with open sternum to and from the OR and avoiding the anticipated hemodynamic instability resulting from the transfer itself. In the study by Nelson-McMillan et al.[9] of 6127 patients with delayed sternal closure 67% of sternal closures were performed in

ICU, 16% in OR and 17% in other locations including cathlab/hybrid suite. The location of sternal closure did not have an impact on infectious complications.

4. An additional dose of prophylactic antibiotic is administered before the anticipated closure.

5. Packed red cells and/or other blood components as required should be available at the bedside before closure.

6. Paralysis and analgesia should be supplemented before starting the procedure.

7. Ensure that all the inotrope infusions are on flow.

8. Ensure safe transfer of infants to and from the OR according to the standard practice, if the sternal closure is performed in the OR.

9. Accessibility to the pacer wires and availability of a pacemaker should be ensured before the infant is draped for the procedure.

10. Intravascular access lines should be secured and be accessible to the anesthesiologist before the surgical drapes are in place. Additional extension lines for volume infusion or inotropes should be secured at an accessible location before the patient is draped.

11. The stability and position of the endotracheal tube should be checked before the drapes are placed. If required, an endotracheal suction can be performed, to clear any secretions. The breathing circuit is positioned away from the surgical field. FiO_2 may be increased 10–20% above the baseline setting before closure.

12. Continuous hemodynamic monitoring is mandatory. Ensure that optimal tracing of ECG is available on the monitor. A reliable pulse oximetry signal should be displayed on the monitor.

13. An arterial blood gas sampling should be done before the start of the procedure.

14. Mediastinum is inspected and bacterial culture swabs should be taken from two locations before closure.

15. Gauze pieces kept inside the mediastinum for achieving hemostasis are removed and counts verified.

16. The proper placement of pacer wires and transthoracic pressure monitoring lines should be confirmed before closure.

17. Some surgeons prefer to perform antibiotic irrigation before approximating the sternal wound.

18. Close monitoring of the hemodynamics during closure is mandatory. Increase in filling pressures (CVP/LAP) with sternal approximation indicates poor ventricular compliance and may require optimization of inotropes/dilators or reconsideration of the decision for closure. Sternal approximation may also necessitate changes in the ventilator settings. Chest closure decreases the chest wall compliance often manifesting as increase in peak and plateau pressures with worsening of arterial blood gas.[10,13] This may warrant increase in mechanical ventilation settings including minute ventilation and FiO_2.[6,10] The use of pressure preset modes will help to tide over the initial period of pulmonary dysfunction as it limits harmful peak airway pressures and risk of barotrauma.

19. An arterial blood gas sample should be obtained 15 min after sternal wire approximation to assess the gas exchange, serum lactate level and acid base status.

POSTOPERATIVE CARE AFTER DELAYED STERNAL CLOSURE

The immediate period after sternal closure is very critical as substantial cardiorespiratory compromise can happen in poorly optimized patients. Close monitoring of hemodynamic status and pulmonary function is mandatory.

Hypertension can be detrimental as it increases left ventricular afterload and can precipitate ventricular failure. Hence, the cause should be evaluated and treated promptly. The FiO_2 should gradually be brought down to baseline levels, after evaluating arterial blood gases. Inotropes are continued for 24 hours after closure, to avoid sudden deterioration in myocardial function after sternal approximation. Nasogastric feeds are restarted after sternal closure if there is no evidence of low cardiac output and lactate levels remain within normal limits. Typically patients are ventilated 24 hours before attempting extubation. Diuresis and fluid restriction is continued to facilitate extubation within 24 hours of sternal closure. Surveillance should be continued for identifying nosocomial infection during further course in hospital.

■ SUMMARY

Delayed sternal closure is a useful strategy after congenital heart surgery to facilitate recovery of cardiopulmonary function. The optimal duration for which the sternum has to be kept open is dictated by the primary condition that delayed the closure. Patients with open sternum are vulnerable to postoperative infections and often need extended intensive care. A focused approach to facilitating sternal closure at the earliest window is ideal. Meticulous care by the PCICU team is mandatory to prevent complications resulting from open sternum.

■ REFERENCES

1. Gielchinsky I, Parsonnet V, Krishnan B, Silidker M, Abel RM. Delayed sternal closure following open heart operation. Ann Thorac Surg. 1981;32:273-7.
2. Riphagen S, McDougall M, Tibby SM, Alphonso N, Anderson D, Austin C, et al. Early delayed sternal closure following pediatric cardiac surgery. Ann Thorac Surg. 2005;80:678-85.
3. Kay PH, Brass T, Lincoln C. The pathophysiology of atypical tamponade in infants undergoing cardiac surgery. Eur J Cardiothorac Surg. 1989;3:255-61
4. Ott DA, Cooley DA, Norman JC, Sandiford FM. Delayed sternal closure: a useful technique to prevent tamponade or compression of heart. Cardiovasc Dis. 1978;5:15-8.
5. Riahi M, Tomatis LA, Schlosser RJ, Bertolozzi E, Johnston DW. Cardiac compression due to closure of the median sternotomy in open heart surgery. Chest. 1975;67:113-4.
6. Tabbutt S, Duncan BW, McLaughlin D, Wessel DL, Jonas RA, Laussen PC. Delayed sternal closure after cardiac operations in a pediatric population. J Thorac Cardiovasc Surg. 1997;113:886-93.
7. Ozker E, Saritas B, Vuran C, Yoruker U, Ulugol H, Turkoz R. Delayed sternal closure after pediatric cardiac operations; single centre experience: a retrospective study. J Cardiothorac Surg. 2012;7:102.
8. Samir K, Riberi A, Ghez O, Ali M, Metras D, Kreitman B. Delayed sternal closure: a life saving measure in neonatal open heart surgery: could it be predictable? Eur J Cardiothorac Surg. 2002;21:787-93.
9. Nelson-McMillan K, Hornik CP, He X, Vricella LA, Jacobs JP, Hill KD, et al. Delayed sternal closure in infant heart surgery-the importance of where and when: an analysis of the STS congenital heart surgery database. Ann Thorac Surg. 2016;102:1565-72.
10. McElhinney DB, Reddy VM, Parry AJ, Johnson L, Fineman JR, Hanley FL. Management and outcomes of delayed sternal closure after cardiac surgery in neonates and infants. Crit Care Med. 2000;28:1180-4.
11. Pye S, McDonnell M. Nursing considerations for children undergoing delayed sternal closure after surgery for congenital heart disease. Crit Care Nurse. 2010;30:50-61.
12. Hatachi T, Sofue T, Ito Y, Inata Y, Shimizu Y, Hazegawa M, et al. Antibiotic prophylaxis for open chest management after pediatric cardiac surgery. Pediatr Crit Care Med. 2019;20:801-8.
13. Main E, Elliot MJ, Stocks J, Schindler M. Effect of delayed sternal closure after cardiac surgery on respiratory function in ventilated infants. Critical Care Med. 2001;29;1798-802.

15

CHAPTER

Antibiotic Guidelines after Pediatric Cardiac Surgery

Pragnatha Komaravolu
Reviewed by: R Krishna Kumar

■ INTRODUCTION

Pediatric patients undergoing elective and emergency heart surgery are vulnerable to invasive postoperative infections. The use of extracorporeal circulation during surgery, immature immune system, hypothermia, greater surgical complexity, longer duration of surgery, use of prosthetic material for repair and presence of invasive lines and tubes predispose to increased risk of infection after pediatric cardiac surgery.[1] The common healthcare-associated infections encountered in the postoperative setting after pediatric cardiac surgery include blood stream infection, surgical site infection, ventilator-associated pneumonia and urinary tract infection (UTI). In a large cohort of 14,000 patients undergoing congenital heart surgery from the developing world, the incidence of major infection in the postoperative period was 6.9%.[2] Younger age at surgery, higher surgical complexity, lower oxygen saturation, and major medical illness were independent predictors of infection. Postoperative infections merit serious concern as they predispose to increased mortality and morbidity, necessitate broad spectrum antibiotic use, increase resource utilization, and escalate healthcare-associated costs.[2,3] Prevention of infection is an important quality improvement metric in congenital heart surgery programs and appropriate use of perioperative antibiotics is a key intervention to facilitate good

outcomes. On the contrary, inappropriate use of antibiotics often contributes to additional healthcare hazards like emergence of antibiotic resistance, development of other major infections, and the problem of *Clostridium difficile* infections.[4,5] Implementation of quality control check lists, adherence to infection control policies, and antibiotic stewardship recommendations are therefore, required to provide cost-effective care and improve surgical outcomes.[6,7] In this chapter, we have provided a brief overview of antibiotic strategies in various clinical settings encountered in the pediatric cardiac surgical patients. We would also like to reiterate that the antibiotic practices in each scenario is based on institutional practice that has evolved over years after analyzing the unit's common pattern of nosocomial infections and antibiogram.

PERIOPERATIVE ANTIBIOTIC PROPHYLAXIS IN PEDIATRIC CARDIAC SURGICAL PATIENTS

Incidence of surgical site infections (SSI) in pediatric cardiac patients varies from 2.1 to 6.3% and is known to be associated with adverse postoperative outcomes.[2,8] Perioperative antibiotic prophylaxis has become the standard of care in pediatric cardiac surgery for prevention of SSI.[9] However, there is a wide heterogeneity in practice with respect to the choice of antibiotic, dosing patterns, and duration of prophylaxis after surgery. Antimicrobial prophylaxis in cardiothoracic procedures reduces the incidence of SSI by fivefold.[10] For clean contaminated procedures, including cardiovascular surgeries, predominant pathogens causing SSI include gram-negative rods, and enterococci in addition to skin flora (*Staphylococcus aureus*, and coagulase negative staphylococci).[11]

Choice of Antibiotic for Prophylaxis

All the four generations of cephalosporins (Beta-lactam antibiotics) are effective in reducing SSI and they differ in half lives, pharmacodynamics, and pharmacokinetic properties. The later generations of cephalosporins provide better coverage for gram-negative organisms. Since *S. aureus* is the predominant microorganism causing SSI in children, most antibiotic regimes employ a first generation or second generation cephalosporin for perioperative prophylaxis. There is no convincing evidence of superiority of second generation cephalosporins over first generation agents in perioperative prophylaxis. Since, SSIs with gram-negative organisms are frequently encountered in developing countries, it is reasonable to use a second-generation cephalosporin (e.g., Cefuroxime), which can cover both gram-positive and gram-negative infections. A suggested perioperative antibiotic regime is depicted in **Table 1**.

Special Guideline in Methicillin-resistant Staphylococcus aureus (MRSA) Outbreak

Based on available evidence, the routine use of vancomycin for perioperative prophylaxis is not recommended.[1] However, specific institutions or selected group of patients, with high incidence of methicillin resistance, may benefit from receiving vancomycin as an adjuvant to primary prophylaxis, although it is unclear as to what constitutes a high incidence.

TABLE 1: Suggested perioperative antibiotic prophylaxis.

Antibiotic	Dose	Duration of prophylaxis
Cefuroxime (half life 1–2 hours)	50 mg/kg IV 8th hourly	24–48 hours
Vancomycin (In case of allergy to cephalosporins)	15 mg/kg IV 12th hourly	24–48 hours (*If administered as adjuvant prophylaxis for MRSA outbreak a single intraoperative dose will suffice*)

(MRSA: methicillin-resistant *Staphylococcus aureus*)

Sometimes vancomycin is temporarily instituted into the perioperative antibiotic regime following an outbreak of MRSA infections in the unit or hospital. Overall, vancomycin has a narrower antimicrobial spectrum, inferior tissue and bone penetration, less desirable pharmacokinetics, and slower bactericidal action compared with cephalosporins.[9] Emergence of vancomycin-resistant strains of Staphylococcus and Enterococcus is also a cause of concern with routine use. Therefore, it is rational to review the policy of vancomycin prophylaxis every 4 months, when instituted following an outbreak.[1,11]

Timing of Antibiotic Administration with Respect to Surgical Incision

The timing of antibiotic administration with respect to surgical incision is crucial in order to achieve adequate plasma concentration of the drug for effective prophylaxis. The first dose of antibiotic (Cefuroxime) should be administered beginning within 60 minutes before skin incision, to achieve adequate minimum inhibitory concentration of the drug for *Staphylococcus* spp.[9]

In patients for whom vancomycin is an appropriate prophylactic antibiotic for cardiac surgery, a dose of 1–1.5 g or a weight-adjusted dose of 15 mg/kg administered intravenously slowly over 1 hour, with completion within 1 hour of the skin incision, is recommended. A second dose of vancomycin of 7.5 mg/kg may be considered during cardiopulmonary bypass (CPB), although its usefulness is not well-established.[9]

Redosing Antibiotics during Surgery

Institution of CPB and resultant hemodilution can impact the pharmacokinetics and pharmacodynamics of antibiotics during surgery. Important alterations in plasma drug concentration can occur due to increased volume of distribution, variations in drug clearance, or sequestration into the extracorporeal circuit.[12] Most cephalosporins have a half life of 1–2 hours and hemodilution during CPB further reduces the circulating drug levels. Repeat administration of a prophylactic antibiotic during surgery should be ideally within two half-lives of the antibiotic exclusive of any influence of the effects of CPB.[9] Hence, it is rational that there should be additional dosing during surgery every 4 hours, when an operation is proceeding with an open wound beyond that period. Typically, the antibiotic dose is timed after weaning off CPB, if this happens within the four-hour time interval after the initial dose of antibiotic. However, in complex congenital heart surgery or redo surgery, which is likely to result in longer duration of CPB, the antibiotic is administered in the CPB circuit after 4 hours.

Duration of Antibiotic Prophylaxis

There is no standardization of the optimal duration of postoperative antibiotic prophylaxis. Most centers administer the prophylactic antibiotic for 24–48 hours in the postoperative period. There is no evidence of incremental benefit for prophylaxis administered longer than 48 hours.[9] On the contrary, prolonged duration of prophylaxis accounts to increasing rate of fungal infections and emergence of resistant organisms. Two large meta-analyses in adult patients undergoing open cardiac surgery comparing different antibiotic regimens for different durations have shown higher rates of sternal SSI and deep sternal wound infections in antibiotic regimes with duration less than 24 hours.[13,14] Hence, it appears most reasonable to employ a cephalosporin as the primary prophylactic agent for the first 24–48 hours, and only to use vancomycin selectively as an adjuvant agent, typically a single dose preoperatively (together with the first dose of cephalosporin) with at most one additional dose in patients of selected environments.[1] The duration of antibiotic prophylaxis should not be dependent on indwelling catheters, lines, nor drains of any type.

Duration of Antibiotic Prophylaxis in Patients with Delayed Sternal Closure

There are no clear guidelines for antibiotic prophylaxis for patients undergoing delayed sternal closure after cardiothoracic operation. Though SSIs are typically caused by gram-positive organisms, postoperative gram-negative sternal wound infections have also been reported in open sternum patients.[15] Based on this, some centers have adopted the practice of escalating antibiotic therapy in patients with open sternum. A retrospective single center study, which compared three different antibiotic regimens namely cefazolin, cefazolin + vancomycin, or vancomycin + meropenem observed a lower rate of blood stream infection and surgical site infection in the broad spectrum antibiotic group in open sternum patients.[16] However in the absence of robust evidence, routine use of broad spectrum antibiotics cannot be recommended in patients with open sternum after pediatric cardiac surgery due to concerns of antimicrobial resistance. The common practice is to administer the standard surgical prophylaxis antibiotic (cefuroxime) for the duration for which sternum remains open and for 24 hours after sternal closure. However, in the event of sternum remaining open for longer than 48 hours, need for escalation of the antibiotics may be considered based on clinical or laboratory evidence of a secondary nosocomial infection. Appropriate investigations including blood culture, mediastinal wound swab or a mini bronchoalveolar lavage (BAL) culture is then indicated to identify the likely source of infection in such cases before starting the second-line antibiotic.

ANTIBIOTIC POLICY IN SUSPECTED POSTOPERATIVE SEPSIS

Sepsis is a likely differential diagnosis for most clinical deterioration and antibiotics may be initiated, but a careful approach to the cause of deterioration often helps in de-escalating antibiotics wherever possible. Appropriate first or second-line antibiotic should be administered at the earliest, ideally within one hour of suspicion of sepsis after collecting the appropriate specimen for the culture, to identify pathogen and target therapy.

Patients with underlying immunodeficiency (e.g., DiGeorge syndrome), neonates, and patients on steroid therapy are the most vulnerable subsets. They are less likely to produce inflammatory response in sepsis and subtle clinical clues (such as unexplained hypoglycemia, persistent low-output state) merit consideration of sepsis as a possibility.

Indications and Screening Tests before Initiating Second-line Antibiotic Therapy

Postoperatively, clinical deterioration is picked up at the earliest. In children being monitored in the ICU, the key challenge in identifying sepsis in postoperative phase after cardiac surgery is the considerable overlap of signs and symptoms of inflammation, with that of sepsis. Fever is a common presenting

sign of sepsis in the pediatric populations but is not specific to sepsis. CPB triggers a systemic inflammatory response, which often presents as fever within the first 24 hours of surgery. Younger children and infants can sometimes present with hypothermia as a manifestation of sepsis. Though not very specific, some of the clinical signs, which have been associated with postoperative infection in clinical practice include, fever >38°C beyond 24 hours, persistent hypoglycemia and catecholamine-resistant hypotension. Commonly used laboratory tests for sepsis screening like total leucocyte counts, neutrophil count and platelet counts usually have limited predictive value in patients undergoing open-heart surgery as these are influenced by the systemic inflammatory response subsequent to cardiac surgery and bypass. The role of biomarkers like C-reactive protein (CRP) and procalcitonin (PCT) is also questionable in their efficacy in differentiating infection from inflammation in the early postoperative period. Both CRP and PCT increase significantly from baseline after cardiac surgery and bypass. While PCT concentrations peak at 24 hours after surgery and begin to decrease at 48 hours, CRP values continue to increase till 3rd postoperative day (POD).[17] In a single-center cohort of 275 infants undergoing cardiac surgery, postoperative CRP levels showed a linear correlation with the duration of CPB.[18] The highest mean CRP values were observed on 2nd POD and CRP trends continued to remain high in 3rd and 4th POD even in noninfected patients who had a CPB time more than 150 minutes.[18] Compared to CRP, PCT values show an earlier peak and faster decline and hence it may be more suited to differentiate sepsis from inflammation in the later postoperative period.[19] Evaluating PCT trends have also been proved to be beneficial in de-escalating or stopping antibiotic therapy in pediatric cardiac patients without adverse

TABLE 2: Suggested tests for sepsis screening.

Clinical suspicion	Investigations
Aspiration VAP LRTI (if intubated)	CXR/BAL/WCC/neutrophils/lactate (Respiratory virus panel in subset)
CLABSI	Two cultures one from catheter, and one peripheral blood culture/CRP/WCC/ neutrophil/procalcitonin/platelet/lactate
UTI	Urine microscopy and culture/CRP/WCC/neutrophil
Sepsis	2 × peripheral blood culture/procalcitonin trend/WCC/neutrophil/platelet/lactate/ blood film/glucose/PCR for sepsis panel
Meningitis	WCC/neutrophil/platelet/glucose/lactate CSF–Glucose/WCC/protein/culture/PCR MRI
SSI	Pus swab/blood culture/CRP/WCC/neutrophil
Endocarditis	3 × peripheral blood culture/ECHO for vegetation
Others (e.g., malaria/dengue)	Based on local incidence, appropriate specimens as per to the local policy

(CLABSI: central line associated blood stream infection; CRP: C-reactive protein; CSF: cerebrospinal fluid; LRTI: lower respiratory tract infection; MRI: magnetic resonance imaging; PCR: polymerase chain reaction; SSI: surgical site infection; UTI: urinary tract infection; VAP: ventilator associated pneumonia; WCC: white cell count)

outcomes.[20] Thus, while identifying sepsis remains a challenge in post-cardiac surgical patients, meticulous attention to clinical clues and initiating definitive treatment before the development of hemodynamic instability, and de-escalating antibiotics at the earliest possible window is probably a reasonable strategy in decreasing mortality associated with pediatric sepsis. However, if the patient suspected of sepsis continues to remain stable and well on assessment, it is appropriate to wait for preliminary investigations before initiating antibiotic therapy. Suggested tests useful for sepsis screening in postoperative patients are enumerated in **Table 2**.

Choice of Antibiotic

The choice of antibiotic should be based on the nature of the pathogen and sensitivity. Hospital and ICU-specific antibiograms are recommended to understand common nosocomial infections and the resistance patterns before formulating appropriate antibiotic policy. Pathogens can be bacterial,

viral, or fungal. A suggested antimicrobial strategy, which has been evolved based on experience at our center is depicted in **Table 3**.

Duration of First/Second-line Antibiotic Therapy (In Culture Proven Sepsis versus Clinical Sepsis)[21]

There are no standard guidelines specific to treatment of postoperative sepsis after pediatric cardiac surgery. However, based on available evidence on the treatment of healthcare associated infections, we propose the following optimal duration of antibiotic therapy for the commonly encountered post-operative infections in PCICU **(Table 4)**. We would also like to reiterate that the antibiotics for treatment of culture proven/clinical sepsis should be chosen based on the common microbial isolates specific to each hospital environment. In addition to appropriate antibiotic therapy, adequate source control and isolation/barrier nursing are also crucial elements to facilitate good outcomes in patients with postoperative sepsis.

TABLE 3: Common pathogens and suggested antimicrobial therapy.

Patients	Organism	Antimicrobial agent
Postoperative patient in cardiac ICU	Gram-negative bacteria (*Klebsiella, Acinetobacter, Escherichia coli*)	Extended spectrum Penicillin or third or fourth generation cephalosporin ± aminoglycoside
	Burkholderia, and Pseudomonas group	Ceftazidime monotherapy (occasionally require dual therapy for recurrent or resistant infections)
Aspiration Pneumonia	*Staphylococcus aureus* *Haemophilus influenzae* *Enterobacter* spp. *Viridans streptococci* *Peptostreptococcus* spp. *Prevotella* spp. *Porphyromonas melaninogenicus* *Fusobacterium* spp.	Cefuroxime + (metronidazole or clindamycin)
UTI	*Escherichia coli,* *Klebsiella* spp. *Proteus* spp. *Enterobacter* spp. *Enterococcus* spp.	Ampicillin ± Gentamicin
Asplenia	Encapsulated organisms (*Streptococcus, Haemophilus infleunza, Neisseria meningitides*)	Extended spectrum Penicillin or third or fourth generation cephalosporin ± aminoglycoside ± Vancomycin
Immune deficiencies / neutropenia	All pathogens including opportunistic	Extended spectrum Penicillin or third or fourth generation cephalosporin ± Aminoglycoside ± Vancomycin plus antifungals
SSI (*Staphylococcus aureus,* Group A Streptococcus)	Mild	Cephalexin or trimethoprim-sulfamethoxazole
	Severe	Cefazolin ± Clindamycin
	Necrotizing fasciitis (also consider aerobic/anaerobic) may be polymicrobial	Extended spectrum Penicillin + Vancomycin + Clindamycin
	MRSA	Vancomycin

(MRSA: methicillin- resistant *Staphylococcus aureus*; UTI: urinary tract infection; SSI: surgical site infection)

Note: Avoid beta lactams (Penicillin, cephalosporins, carbapenems) if allergic to Penicillin; consult ID/Microbiology and consider allergy testing.

TABLE 4: Suggested duration of antimicrobial therapy in sepsis.

UTI	5 days
SSI (uncomplicated)	5 days
VAP	7 days
Gram-negative bloodstream sepsis (Culture proven)	14 days
Suspected bloodstream sepsis (Culture negative)	Review antibiotic at 48 hours to stop or de-escalate. Clinical assessment and multidisciplinary discussion can help in decision making process regarding duration
Meningitis (uncomplicated)	Depends on organism isolated • *S. pneumoniae*:10–14 days • *S. aureus*: 2 weeks • Gram-negative bacilli: 3 weeks or a minimum of 2 weeks beyond the first sterile CSF culture whichever is longer.

(UTI: urinary tract infection; SSI: surgical site infection; VAP: ventilator associated pneumonia; CSF: cerebrospinal fluid)

SPECIAL CONSIDERATIONS IN PEDIATRIC CARDIAC INTENSIVE CARE UNIT

Patients on Preoperative Antibiotic Therapy

It is not uncommon for children to be treated with antibiotics prior to transfer to the surgical center. Therefore, a detailed documented, antibiotic history and review of cultures is mandatory at admission. Occasionally, one may even have to contact the referring center for culture results pending at the time of transfer. It is important to draw appropriate specimens for identifying any likely source of infection in such patients after a detailed clinical evaluation. Empiric broad spectrum antibiotics appropriate to the unit's antibiogram are then recommended in such a situation after discussion with the treating team, and subsequently changed to target therapy based on cultures.

Patients with Preoperative ICU Stay/Indwelling Invasive Lines/Mechanical Ventilation

Generally, presence of indwelling catheters or mechanical ventilation is not a routine indication to initiate antibiotic therapy. However, it is important to understand the severity of illness if a patient requires invasive monitoring and intensive support. Nosocomial infections are a likely complication in patients with invasive lines or need for ventilation and hence it is important to diagnose and treat any underlying infection prior to the surgery. In a large single center study from the developing world, which evaluated the preoperative determinants of adverse postoperative outcomes in 1,028 infants undergoing open heart surgery, preoperative intensive care unit stay, mechanical ventilation, and bloodstream infection were significantly associated with postoperative sepsis.[22] So in patients with preoperative risk factors who are presenting

for surgery, it is reasonable to send a blood culture, complete blood count (CBC), and CRP before skin incision in the operating room, and resite existing indwelling catheters as appropriate. Appropriate antibiotic prescription based on the hospital/ICU-specific antibiogram is then initiated with consideration of de-escalation if feasible in the postoperative period after evaluation of laboratory tests and clinical status.

Patients with Preoperative Sepsis (Culture Proven)

In a patient with culture positive sepsis, appropriate antibiotic therapy is mandatory prior to the surgery. A repeat negative culture along with improvement in clinical condition is recommended for best outcomes after surgery and for facilitating early postoperative recovery. In patients on preoperative antibiotic therapy for sepsis, the specific antibiotic targeting the pathogen is continued in the perioperative period for the required duration of therapy. In patients requiring valve transplants, conduits, other prosthetic material, or intraoperative pacemaker insertion, documentation of clearance of pathogen is necessary before proceeding with the planned surgery.

Patients Having Fever on Operating Table at Induction of Anesthesia

Fever can be a sign of many clinical conditions. Appropriate preanesthesia evaluation and basic infection screening should be done as standard practice, prior to all surgical procedures. However, when a patient presents with fever at induction of anesthesia, a thorough assessment should be done to rule out possibility of infection. If infection is unlikely, review of drugs/allergy, infusion rate of blood/blood components, severe dehydration, low cardiac output state, etc. should be considered. If the surgery is of an emergent nature, the surgery may proceed after drawing appropriate blood samples. The need for escalation of antibiotic is considered before commencement of surgery, after a multidisciplinary discussion of the patients' clinical profile (Immunodeficiency, neonatal age group, preoperative invasion, etc.)

Postoperative Neonates/Infants with Features of Severe Sepsis

Some of the commonly encountered clinical signs that may arouse the suspicion of severe sepsis in neonates/infants in the post-operative period include total leukocyte count <4,000/mm³, severe thrombocytopenia, hypoglycemia (blood glucose <40 mg/dL), cate-cholamine resistant shock or a persistently elevated serum lactate >4 mmol/L in the absence of myocardial dysfunction. An infant with features suggestive of sepsis should be screened for sepsis and appropriate speci-mens need to be collected before initiating antibiotic therapy. Urine, blood, and cerebro-spinal fluid (CSF) specimens are all useful to trace the source of infection and to predict the duration of therapy. Broad-spectrum antibiotics should be administered as soon as possible based on the unit's antibiogram and avoid any potential delays in an unstable patient. Whenever culture samples are not drawn prior to antibiotic administration, the reasons should be clearly documented in the clinical notes. Administration of antibiotics, should be simultaneously combined with the management of other aspects such as correction of blood glucose levels, correction of electrolyte imbalances, fluid resuscitation, and vasoactive drug therapy.

Neonates with Soft Signs of Sepsis (High White Cell Counts, Labile Blood Pressure and Borderline Blood Sugar Levels)

Typically in the postoperative period, most patients are on a restricted fluid management strategy and large negative fluid balances are to be achieved, while maintaining cardiac output. In evaluating a patient with hypoten-sion important hypovolemia has to be ruled out before considering it as a sign of sepsis. If the child is stable clinically but shows abnormal white cell/platelet counts in the immediate postoperative sample, it is rational to send blood cultures and repeat white cell/platelet counts after 6–8 hours of surgery. This is important to rule out spurious values caused by the dilutional effects of CPB on the cell counts. Although, CRP levels in the early postoperative period have limited diagnostic value, PCT kinetics may be useful in predicting outcome of invasive bacterial infection and rationalize antibiotic therapy in this patients.[23]

Neonates with Clinical Signs of Necrotizing Enterocolitis

Necrotizing enterocolitis (NEC) is a serious complication in neonates with compromised splanchnic circulation particularly in low cardiac output states or secondary to a duct-dependent systemic circulation. This condition is characterized by loss of gut mucosal integrity and bacterial translocation and if untreated can lead to extensive bowel necrosis, sepsis, and death.[24] Clinical diagnosis is generally based on abdominal signs, Bell's criteria, abdominal X-ray evaluation, and laboratory tests like total leucocyte counts/platelet counts. Multidisciplinary collaboration with involvement of the pediatric surgery team is sought in the management of these patients. Children with suspected NEC, are often managed conservatively by keeping nil per orally and with continuous nasogastric tube aspiration. Broad spectrum antibiotics with an anaerobic cover are generally recommended for treating NEC. In neonates with bowel gangrene, surgical resection, and anastomosis is necessary along with aggressive antibiotic therapy for improved survival.

Pediatric Patients with Lung Infiltrates and/or Purulent Endotracheal Secretions and/or Fever > 24 Hours

Pediatric cardiac patients are vulnerable to postoperative pulmonary dysfunction secondary to inflammatory response to CPB, fluid overload with pulmonary congestion, pulmonary venous obstruction, or increased pulmonary blood flow conditions. These patients can present a clinical and radiological picture, which is often indistinguishable from pulmonary conditions developing from an infective etiology. A postoperative patient with lung infiltrates thus merits evaluation to rule out cardiac causes as well as likely pulmonary conditions of infective etiology. Potential causes of pulmonary morbidity after pediatric cardiac surgery are listed in **Table 5**.

In a stable child with purulent respiratory secretions and fever, it is reasonable to rule out pulmonary conditions of infective origin by gram staining and culture of BAL specimen or a mini BAL specimen. If a pathogen is identified, appropriate antibiotic therapy based on sensitivity profile is indicated.

Unexplained Hyperpyrexia

Fever in the first 24 hours after surgery under CPB, without evidence of an underlying infection, is most frequently due to the systemic inflammatory response. Symptomatic treatment for temperature control alone would suffice in such situations. In an otherwise stable patient with negative cultures and persistent fever (>24 hours), postoperatively, other causes of fever have to be evaluated. While it is difficult to ascertain the diagnosis in all cases of hyperpyrexia, a multidisciplinary approach to postoperative care and early deintensification will reduce the chance of secondary bacterial infection.

Patients on Extracorporeal Membrane Oxygenation

There are no specific guidelines for antibiotic therapy in patients on extracorporeal membrane oxygenation (ECMO). In ECMO with delayed sternal closure, the general practice is to continue the prophylactic antibiotics for the duration of ECMO and for 24 hours after closure of sternum. If suspicion of postoperative infection arises, empirical antibiotic therapy based on hospital antibiogram and discontinuation of the prophylactic antibiotics is reasonable.[25] Extracorporeal circulation alters both the volume of distribution and elimination of commonly administered prophylactic antibiotics and hence appropriate dosing has to be ensured while prescribing antibiotics in these patients. Antifungal prophylaxis is commonly administered to patients on ECMO. These patients require a higher fluconazole loading dose for prophylaxis (12 mg/kg) as well as treatment (35 mg/kg).[26]

Emergent Resternotomy in ICU Following Cardiac Arrest

Significant hemodynamic instability or cardiac arrest may sometimes necessitate emergent resternotomy in ICU for resuscitation. Even though the incidence of subsequent infection is low in the cardiac arrest situation,

TABLE 5: Potential causes of pulmonary complications in pediatric cardiac patients.

Cardiac-related	Residual VSD, LV dysfunction, collateral circulation
Ventilation-related	Frequent suctioning, mechanical and barotrauma
Gastrointestinal tract-related	Reflux causing aspiration (specially in patients on sedation and muscle relaxants)
Chylothorax	Leak of Chyle
Chest drain	Inadequate drainage

(VSD: ventricular septal defect; LV: left ventricular)

full aseptic technique including gown and gloves might be regarded as best practice. However, if there is suspicion of breach in sterility during resternotomy in ICU, it is rational to escalate antibiotic therapy and send appropriate cultures. De-escalation should be then considered based on laboratory tests once the patient is stabilized. The evidence available in support of this is limited other than uncontrolled cohort studies.[27]

Patients Developing Urinary Tract Infection

Apart from iatrogenic causes of UTI due to urinary catheterization, and need for ICU observation, children, particularly neonates, can present with congenital anomalies of urinary tract. Careful history and evaluation are important preoperatively. Clues such as dilated renal pelvic diameter from antenatal scans, hypospadias, ambiguous genitalia, previous recurrent UTI requiring multiple antibiotics, chronic constipation need to be considered while evaluating for causes relating to UTI. It is important to follow aseptic technique while inserting urinary catheters. Occasionally, feeding tubes are often used as urinary catheters in infants and in such cases the length of the tube residing inside the patient's urethra has to be estimated and documented in the notes following the procedure.

Decision to remove urinary catheter should be discussed on ward rounds every day. Prolonged catherization is a common cause of iatrogenic infections. When a UTI is suspected, it is recommended to remove catheter as appropriate and send a sample for microscopy and culture prior to starting antibiotics.

■ ANTIFUNGAL THERAPY

Postoperative fungal infections are rare in pediatric cardiac surgery. The reported incidence is 0.4%.[27] Children with immuno-

deficiency and those requiring prolonged ventilation are the most vulnerable patients. Additionally, patients receiving multiple broad spectrum antibiotics for long duration are also at risk.

Screening Tests

There are no recommendations on when to initiate screening tests for fungal infection in postoperative period. However, if there is suspicion of an underlying fungal infection, blood culture (with specific medium for detection of fungi and prolonged observation of the specimen for fungal growth) may be considered.

Prophylaxis for Fungal Infections

Prophylaxis in specific group of patients such as those on ECMO, may reduce morbidity and mortality.[28] There are no recommended guidelines for routine fungal prophylaxis in patients undergoing cardiac surgery. Fluconazole prophylaxis does not provide total protection from Candida infection. It is also hypothesized that frequent fungal infections are due to under-dosing of fluconazole when used at 3–6 mg/kg and hence higher doses are recommended for postcardiac surgery patients (8–12 mg/kg).[29] An invasive fungal infection and persistent fungemia in pediatric patient is mostly likely due to prolonged antibiotic usage, prolonged indwelling catheters, or due to an underlying primary immunodeficiency.

Duration of Antifungal Therapy

The choice of antifungal agents should be based on culture and sensitivity profile. The most common isolates include *Candida albicans, Candida parapsilosis, Candida glabrata,* and *Candida krusei.* Invasive candidiasis is associated with poor survival and hence need to be aggressively treated. Recommended drugs for empirical treatment of systemic candidiasis are liposomal amphotericin B or caspofungin.[27] For proven fungal sepsis, treatment should be continued till 14 days from the last negative culture. Examination of fundus by ophthalmology and echocardiographic evaluation to rule out vegetations for all patients with fungal sepsis to monitor sequalae is reasonable. It is also ideal to follow the antifungal policy bundle checklist.

◼ COMMON ANTIBIOTIC DOSAGES/SPECIAL PRECAUTION IN ADMINISTRATION (TABLE 6)

TABLE 6: Common antibiotics, dosing and special precautions.

Antibiotic	Dosage	Precaution
Cefuroxime	50 mg/kg IV 8th hourly	
Vancomycin	15–20 mg/kg IV 8–12th hourly	Narrow therapeutic index (Follow TDM policy) Monitor renal function
Amikacin	15 mg/kg/day IV OD	Monitor renal function Auditory assessment if duration prolonged >7 days (Follow TDM policy)
Ceftazidime	25–50 mg/kg IV 8th hourly	
Cefoperazone-Sulbactum	50 mg/kg IV 8th hourly	
Piperazilline-Tazobactam	100 mg/kg IV 6–8th hourly (max 4.5 g per dose)	
Meropenem	20–40 mg/kg IV 8th hourly	
Colistin	40,000 units/kg IV 8th hourly or 1.25–2.5 mg/kg of colistin base 12th hourly (1 mg colistin base = 30,000 units)	Monitor renal function; Caution while administering in combination with other nephrotoxic drugs

(TDM: therapeutic drug monitoring; OD: once daily)

◼ REFERENCES

1. Alfonso N, Anagnostopoulos PV, Scarpace S, Weintrub P, Azakie A, Raff G, et al. Perioperative antibiotic prophylaxis in pediatric cardiac surgery. Cardiol Young. 2007;17:12-25.
2. Sen AC, Morrow DF, Balachandran R, Du X, Gauvreau K, Jagannath BR, et al. Postoperative infection in developing world congenital heart surgery programs, Data from the International Quality Improvement Collaborative. Circ Cardiovasc Qual Outcomes. 2017;10:e002935.
3. Sochet AA, Cartron AM, Nyhan A, Spaeder MC, Song X, Brown AT, et al. Surgical site infection after pediatric cardiac surgery: Impact on hospital cost and length of stay. World J Pediatr Cong Heart Surg. 2017;8:7-12.
4. Poeran J, Mazumdar M, Rasul R, Meyer J, Sacks HS, Koll BS, et al. Antibiotic prophylaxis and risk of *Clostridum difficele* infection after coronary artery bypass graft surgery. J Thorac Cardiovasc Surg. 2016;151:589-97.e1-3.
5. Gelijns AC, Moskowitz AJ, Acker MA, Argenziano M, Geller NL, Puskas JD, et al. Management practices and major infections after cardiac surgery. J Am Coll Cardiol. 2014;64:372-81.
6. Doron S, Davidson LE. Mayo Clin Proc 2011;86: 1113-23.
7. UpToDate. (2019). Antimicrobial stewardship in hospital settings. [online] Available from: https://www.uptodate.com/contents/antimicrobial-stewardship-in-hospital-settings?search=antibiotic%20duration&source=search_result&selectedTitle=1~150&usage_type=default&display_rank=1. [Last Accessed February, 2021].
8. Sohn AH, Scwartz JM, Yang KY, Jarvis WR, Guglielmo BJ, Weintrub PS. Risk factors and risk adjustment for surgical site infections in pediatric cardiothoracic surgery patients. Am J Infect Control. 2010;38:706-10.
9. Engelman R, Shahian D, Shemin R, Guy TS, Bratzler D, Edwards F, et al. The Society of Thoracic Surgeons Practice Guideline Series: Antibiotic prophylaxis in cardiac surgery. Part II: Antibiotic Choice. Ann Thorac Surg. 2007;83:1569-76.
10. Kreter B, Woods M. Antibiotic prophylaxis for cardiothoracic operations. Meta-analysis of

thirty years of clinical trials. J Thorac Cardiovasc Surg. 1992;104(3):590-9.

11. Bratzler DW, Dellinger EP, Olsen KM, Perl TM, Auwaerter PG, Bolon MK, et al. Clinical practice guidelines for antimicrobial prophylaxis in surgery. Am J Health Syst Pharm. 2013;70(3):195-283.

12. Paruk F, Sime FB, Lipman J, Roberts JA. Dosing antibiotic prophylaxis during cardiopulmonary bypass—a higher level of complexity? A structured review. Int J Antimicrob Agent. 2017; 49:395-402.

13. Lador A, Nasir H, Mansur N, Sharoni E, Biderman P, Leibovici L, et al. Antibiotic prophylaxis in cardiac surgery: systematic review and meta-analysis. J Antimicrob Chemother. 2012;67:541-50.

14. Mertz D, Johnstone J, Loeb M. Does duration of perioperative antibiotic prophylaxis matter in cardiac surgery? A systematic review and meta analysis. Ann Surg. 2011;254:48-54.

15. Ozker E, Saritas B, Vuran C, Yoruker U, Ulugol H, Turkoz R. Dealyed sternal closure after pediatric cardiac operations; single centre experience: a retrospective study. J Cardiothorac Surg. 2012;7:102.

16. Hatachi T, Sofue T, Ito Y, Inata Y, Shimizu Y, Hazegawa M, et al. Antibiotic prophylaxis for open chest management after pediatric cardiac surgery. Pediatr Crit Care Med. 2019;20:801-8.

17. Arkader R, Troster EJ, Abellan DM, Lopes MR, Junior RR, Carcillo JA, et al. Procalcitonin and C reactive protein kinetics in postoperative pediatric cardiac surgical patients. J Cardiovasc Thorac Anaesth. 2004;18:160-65.

18. Abqari S, Kappanayil M, Sudhakar A, Balachandran R, Nair SG, Kumar RK. Common inflammatory markers after cardiac surgery in infants and their relation to blood stream sepsis. Heliyon. 2019;5:e02841.

19. Davidson J, Tong S, Hauck A, Lawson S, da Cruz E, Kaufman J. Kinetics of procalcitonin and C-reactive protein and the relationship to post operative infection in young infants undergoing cardiovascular surgery. Pediatr Res. 2013;74:413-9.

20. Bobillo-Perez S, Sole-Ribalta A, Balaguer M, Esteban E, Girona-Alarcon M, Hernandez-Platero L, et al. Procalcitonin to stop antibiotics after cardiovascular surgery in a pediatric intensive care unit—The PROSACAB study. Plos One. 2019;14:e220686.

21. ICMR. (2019). Antimicrobial Stewardship Program Guideline. [online] Available from: https://www.icmr.nic.in/sites/default/files/guidelines/AMSP.pdf. [Last Accessed February, 2021].

22. Reddy NS, Kappanayil M, Balachandran R, Jenkins KJ, Sudhakar A, Sunil GS, et al. Pre-operative determinants of outcomes of infant heart surgery in a limited resource setting. Semin Thorac Cardiovasc Surg Autumn. 2015;27:331-8.

23. D'Souza S, Guhadasan R, Jennings R, Siner S, Paulus S, Thorburn K, et al. Procalcitonin and other common biomarkers do not reliably identify patients at risk for bacterial infection after congenital heart surgery. Pediatr Crit Care Med. 2019;20(3):243-51

24. Spinner JA, Morris SA, Nandi D, Costarino AT, Marino BS, Rossano JW, et al. Necrotising enterocolitis and associated mortality in neonates with congenital heart disease: a multi-institutional study. Pediatr Crit Care Med. 2020;21:228-34.

25. Jaworski R, Kansy A, Fangrat KD, Maruszewski B. Antibiotic prophylaxis in pediatric cardiac surgery: Where are we and where do we go? A systematic review. Surg Infect. 2019;20:253-60.

26. Jaworski R, Haponiuk I, Irga-Jaworska N, Chojnicki M, Steffens M, Paczkowski K, et al. Fungal infections in children in early postoperative period after cardiac surgery for congenital heart disease: A single centre experience. Interact Cardiovasc Thorac Surg. 2016;23:431-7.

27. Yap EYL. Levine A, Strang T, Dunning J. Should additional antibiotic or an iodine washout be given to all patients who suffer an emergency resternotomy on the cardiothorac intensive care unit? Interact Cardio Vasc Thorac. 2008;7:464-9.

28. Gardner AH, Prodhan P, Stovall SH, Gossett JM, Stern JE, Wilson CD, et al. Fungal infections and antifungal prophylaxis in pediatric cardiac extracorporeal life support. J Thorac Cardiovasc Surg. 2012;143(3):689-95.

29. Hope WW, Castagnola E, Groll AH, Roilides E, Akova M, Arendrup MC, et al. ESCMID (European Society of Clincal Microbiology and Infectious Diseases) for the diagnosis and management of Candida diseases 2012: Prevention and management of invasive infections in neonates and children caused by Candida spp. Clin Microbiol Infect. 2012;18 (suppl 7):38-52.

SECTION

2

Cardiac Lesion Specific
Postoperative Management

Atrial Septal Defect Repair

Rakhi Balachandran

Illustrations: Praveen Reddy Bayya, Balaji Srimurugan
Reviewed by: R Krishna Kumar

◼ INTRODUCTION

Atrial septal defect (ASD) is one of most common congenital heart diseases (CHD) with a prevalence of 1.64/1,000 live births.[1] ASD is characterized by a defect in the interatrial septum which can occur as an isolated lesion or along with other congenital heart defects. Associated lesions which can occur along with ASD include partial anomalous pulmonary venous connection, pulmonary stenosis or mitral valve abnormalities. Anatomical subtypes include ostium secundum or fossa ovalis defect, ostium primum defect, sinus venosus (SV) defect, coronary sinus defect and posterior defect. Ostium secundum ASD is the most common type that occurs in the center of the interatrial septum at the region of fossa ovalis (**Fig. 1**). Primum ASD is located at the inferior portion of the interatrial septum and is often a part of atrioventricular septal defect. SV defect is located in the superior part of the interatrial septum at the superior vena cava (SVC)-right atrium (RA) junction and is usually associated with partial anomalous pulmonary venous drainage of the right upper and middle pulmonary veins (**Fig. 2**). Surgical repair of ASD involves closure of the defect with a pericardial patch on cardiopulmonary bypass. Though standard surgical approach is through a median sternotomy, cosmetically appealing incisions such as ministernotomy, limited posterior thoracotomy, and axillary approaches are being increasingly utilized[2,3] (**Figs. 3A to C**). Catheter based closure of secundum type

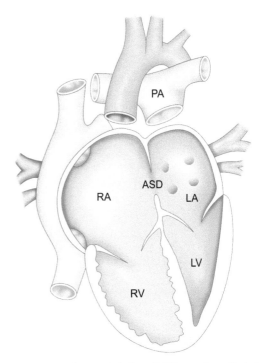

Fig. 1: Atrial septal defect (ASD) causing dilated right atrium (RA), right ventricle (RV) and pulmonary artery (PA).

(LA: left atrium; LV: left ventricle)

defects is feasible for anatomically suitable lesions. Although considered the simplest of all CHDs the following specific considerations are worth stating:

- Most centers and databases report a mortality close to zero. Therefore, no mortality or morbidity is acceptable for ASD.

- There is growing emphasis on minimally invasive cosmetic approaches (axillary/limited posterior thoracotomy); these approaches bring in some unique challenges that need to be addressed.

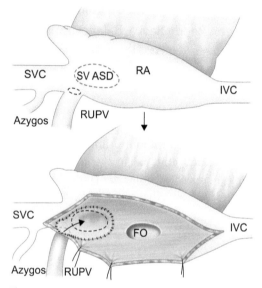

Fig. 2: Sinus venosus atrial septal defect (SV-ASD) located close to superior vena cava (SVC)-right atrium (RA) junction along with anomalous drainage of right upper pulmonary vein (RUPV). These images show patch closure of ASD with routing of RUPV to left atrium (Surgeons' view).

(FO: fossa ovalis; IVC: inferior vena cava)

■ MONITORING

Patients after ASD closure require invasive monitoring of arterial blood pressure, central venous pressure (CVP), continuous ECG monitoring, pulse oximetry and capnography.

■ MANAGEMENT

Hemodynamic and Inotrope Management

Patients undergoing ASD closure often do not require any inotropic support. However, an important subset of patients who requires close attention includes adult patients with chronic right ventricular (RV) volume over-load and subsequent poor left ventricular (LV) compliance. The removal of left to right shunt with a sudden increase in preload coupled with diminished distensibility of the left ventricle can result in acute elevation in LV filling pressures and pulmonary edema in these patients.[4] Inotropic support with

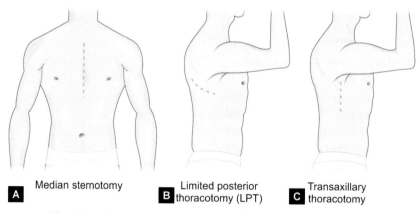

Figs. 3A to C: Various surgical approaches for atrial septal defect closure.

afterload reduction may be beneficial in these patients.[5] Usually dopamine/dobutamine at 5 µg/kg/min will suffice. Careful monitoring for postoperative arrhythmias is essential after ASD closure. CVP often remains very low after ASD closure due to highly compliant right ventricle and relative hypovolemia. Adequate filling to maintain preload is usually required to optimize cardiac output.

Fluid Management

Standard fluid management protocol for cardiac surgery under cardiopulmonary bypass is followed. Additional volume for replacing postoperative losses or for maintaining preload is administered in the form of colloids such as 6% hydroxyethyl starch in a balanced electrolyte solution (e.g., volulyte®) or crystalloids such as ringer lactate solution.

Diuretic Therapy

Diuretic therapy is usually not required as the surgical support times are very short with minimal fluid overload. However, older patients with chronic RV volume overload and heart failure may require a short course of diuretic therapy in the postoperative period.

Pain and Sedation Management

Since these patients are typically candidates for fast tracking and early recovery, analgesia and sedation protocols should focus on avoiding excessive sedation while providing maximum analgesic effects. Regional analgesia with single shot caudal epidural block or an intercostal nerve block administered by the surgeon through the thoracotomy incision at completion of surgery will facilitate reduction in perioperative dose of opioids and enable early awakening from anesthesia. Dexmedetomidine infusion is a suitable alternative to opioid infusion in patients undergoing fast tracking to provide adequate pain relief with minimal sedation.[6]

Ventilation Management and Extubation

Atrial septal defect repair is a low risk operation and patients typically tolerate extubation in the operating room or early in the postoperative period. Once patient is normothermic, neuromuscular blockade is reversed, and ventilator settings quickly scaled down for extubation.

Feeding and Nutrition

These patients usually have an uncomplicated postoperative period and oral feeds can be initiated if deemed stable after extubation.

COMMON POSTOPERATIVE COMPLICATIONS

Postoperative Arrhythmias

Postoperative arrhythmias such as atrial flutter, atrial fibrillation (AF), sinus tachycardia and nodal rhythm are all described after ASD repair.[7-9] Sinus node dysfunction is reported to be the most common bradyarrhythmia and is more frequently associated with SV type of ASD.[10] The use of Warden's technique for SV ASD closure preserves sinus node and its blood supply and has been reported to be superior in preventing this complication.[11,12] Atrial flutter and AF are most often encountered in adult patients and has been attributed to geometric remodeling resulting from the large intracardiac shunt which creates an arrhythmogenic substrate.[8] At microscopic level, changes in atrial tissue properties along with interstitial fibrosis, increase in myocyte size and alterations in ultracellular structure have been implicated in the pathogenesis of AF in patients with ASD.[8]

Postpericardiotomy Syndrome

This refers to an inflammatory condition that can occur after cardiothoracic surgery and incidence after surgical ASD closure appears particularly higher than other congenital heart operations.[13] It typically manifests 48–72 hours after surgery and presents with fever, chest pain and a pericardial friction rub. Pericardial effusion on echocardiography is a frequently associated finding. Interestingly, ASD repair had been identified as an independent risk factor that predisposes to pericardial effusions requiring readmissions after pediatric cardiac surgery.[14] Treatment includes use of anti-inflammatory agents such as aspirin or nonsteroidal anti-inflammatory drugs (NSAIDs) such as ibuprofen. Other drugs which had been explored as prevention strategies for postpericardiotomy syndrome after cardiac surgery include colchicine and steroids, however, conclusive evidence is limited.[15] Pericardiocentesis may be required in persistent effusions causing hemodynamic compromise.

SPECIAL CONSIDERATIONS FOR PATIENTS UNDERGOING ASD REPAIR THROUGH THORACOTOMY INCISIONS

Patients who undergo ASD closure through a limited posterior thoracotomy or axillary approach need meticulous attention to postoperative pain management. Thoracotomy incisions are particularly painful and can limit respiratory muscle excursions leading to atelectasis. Intraoperatively these patients will benefit from caudal epidural block or intercostal block administered via the thoracotomy incision. Postoperatively fentanyl or dexmedetomidine infusion is preferred in the early phase and adjuvant analgesics such as ibuprofen or ketorolac are often added after extubation for synergistic effect.

There is likelihood of lung compression and retraction during thoracotomy and hence these patients have to be carefully monitored for development of postoperative air leaks, pneumothorax or atelectasis. Adequate lung expansion has to be ascertained through chest X-ray and clinical evaluation at the time of extubation. The drainage tubes are sometimes left longer than usual if air leaks are detected or pneumothorax is evident in chest X-rays obtained after clamping the intercostal drains.

Though ASD closure is deemed to be a low risk surgery, in the unlikely event of a postoperative cardiorespiratory collapse, open resuscitation attempts can be technically difficult due to suboptimal access through a thoracotomy incision.

■ DEINTENSIFICATION

Most patients after ASD closure can be rapidly deintensified after extubation. Invasive lines are usually removed once inotropic supports are weaned off. Transfer to ward care can be achieved on postoperative day 1 after removal of intercostal drains and ruling out postoperative pleural or pericardial effusions.

■ DISCHARGE MEDICATIONS

These are often limited to pain relief medications. Rarely, in adults with persistent pulmonary edema, extended diuretic usage is needed for 1–2 weeks.

■ REFERENCES

1. Van der Linde D, Konings EM, Slager MA, Witzenberg M, Helbing W, Takkenberg JM, et al. Birth prevalence of congenital heart disease worldwide. A systematic review and meta-analysis. J Am Coll Cardiol. 2011;58:2241-7.
2. Hopkins RA, Bert AA, Buchholz B, Guarino K, Meyers M. Surgical patch closure of atrial septal defects. Ann Thorac Surg. 2004;77:2144-50.
3. Dodge Khatami A, Salazar JD. Right axillary thoracotomy for transatrial repair of congenital heart defects: VSD, Partial AV canal with mitral cleft, PAPVR/Warden, Cor triatriatum and ASD. Oper Techn Thorac Cardiovasc Surg. 2016;20:384-401.
4. Beyer J. Atrial Septal Defect. Acute left heart failure after surgical closure. Ann Thorac Surg. 1978;25:36-43.

5. Chang AC, Jacobs J. Atrial Septal defect. In Chang AC, Hanley FL, Wernovsky G, Wessel DL (Eds). Pediatric Cardiac Intensive Care. Pennsylvania: Lippincott Williams and Wilkins; 1998. pp. 207-12.

6. Mittnacht AJ, Hollinger I. Fast tracking in pediatric cardiac surgery—the current standing. Ann Card Anaesth. 2010;13:92-101.

7. Gatzoulis MA, Freeman MA, Siu SC, Webb GD, Harris L. Atrial arrhythmia after surgical closure of atrial septal defects in adults. N Engl J Med. 1999;340:839-46.

8. Chubb H, Whitaker J, Williams SE, Head CE, Chung NA, Wright MJ, et al. Pathophysiology and management of arrhythmias associated with atrial septal defect and patent foramen ovale. Arrhythm Electrophysiol Rev. 2014;3:168-72.

9. Williams MR, Perry JC. Arrhythmias and conduction disorders associated with atrial septal defects. J Thorac Dis. 2018;10:2940-4.

10. Bricker JT, Gillete PC, Cooley DA, McNamara DG. Dysrhythmias after repair of atrial septal defect. Tex Heart Inst J. 1986;13:203-8.

11. Okonta KE, Sanusi M. Superior sinus venosus atrial septal defect: overview of surgical options. Open J Thorac Surg. 2013;3:114-22.

12. Okonta KE, Aggarwal V. Does Wardens Procedure reduce sinus node dysfunction after surgery for partial anomalous pulmonary venous connection? Interact Cardiovasc Thorac Surg. 2012;14(6):839-42.

13. Heching HJ, Bacha EA, Liberman L. Postpericardiotomy syndrome in pediatric patients following surgical closure of secundum atrial septal defects: incidence and risk factors. Pediatr cardiol. 2015;36:498-502.

14. Elias MD, Glatz AC, O'Connor MJ, Schachtner S, Ravishankar C, Mascio CE, et al. Prevalence and risk factors for pericardial effusions requiring readmission after pediatric cardiac surgery. Pediatr Cardiol. 2017;38:484-94.

15. Imazio M, Brucato A, Ferrazi P, Pullara A, Adler Y, Barosi A, et al. Colchicine for prevention of post pericardiotomy syndrome and atrial fibrillation. The COPPS-2 randomized clinical trial. JAMA. 2014;312:1016-23.

Ventricular Septal Defect Repair

Rakhi Balachandran

Illustrations: Praveen Reddy Bayya, Balaji Srimurugan

Reviewed by: R Krishna Kumar

■ INTRODUCTION

Ventricular septal defect (VSD) is the most common congenital heart disease (CHD) in children with a prevalence of 2.62 per 1,000 live births.[1] VSD is characterized by a defect in the interventricular septum **(Fig. 1)**. The location of the defect in the interventricular septum identifies the different anatomical subsets namely perimembranous (80%), doubly committed subarterial (5–10%), muscular (5%),

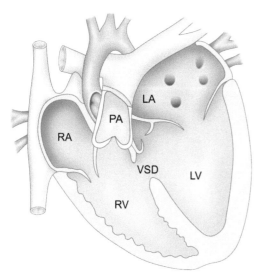

Fig. 1: Ventricular septal defect (VSD) causing dilatation of left atrium (LA) and left ventricle (LV). Increased pulmonary blood flow causes dilatation of pulmonary arteries (PA) and, over a period of time, pulmonary vascular disease.

(RA: right atrium; RV: right ventricle)

and inlet septal (5%) defects.[2] VSD may occur as an isolated defect, or in association with simple cardiac lesions such as atrial septal defect, patent ductus arteriosus, coarctation of aorta or with complex congenital lesions such as transposition of great arteries, tetralogy of Fallot and atrioventricular septal defects. Surgical closure in early infancy is the standard treatment in most established pediatric cardiac programs, as it prevents hemodynamic consequences of heart failure and pulmonary hypertension, thereby restoring normal growth and development of the infant. Nevertheless, many children present late in low middle-income countries with a poor preoperative status. The postoperative course after VSD closure is influenced by the preoperative condition, presence of pulmonary vascular disease, need for ventriculotomy during surgery, the success of concomitant valve repair if any, and the presence of residual lesions. Though isolated VSD closure is regarded as a low risk operation in the current era due to early repair and advanced perioperative care, some patients might still pose substantial postoperative challenges. Previously identified risk factors for a longer postoperative course include presence of a genetic syndrome, lower patient weight, and longer surgical support times.[3] Experience from our center suggests that low weight and preoperative undernutrition is no longer a significant risk factor for long postoperative stay.[4]

MONITORING

Standard hemodynamic monitoring includes continuous ECG monitoring, invasive arterial blood pressure monitoring, central venous pressure monitoring, pulse oximetry and capnography. Arterial blood gas analysis is usually performed every 4 hours till extubation and thereafter optimized to patient status. Pulmonary artery pressure monitoring via an intraoperatively placed pulmonary artery (PA) line was sometimes employed in patients with pulmonary hypertension in the early era to guide postoperative management. However, with the current trends of early primary repair and shorter cardiopulmonary bypass time this is no longer a routine practice.

HEMODYNAMIC AND INOTROPE MANAGEMENT

Isolated VSD closure is usually an uncomplicated procedure and patients with small/moderate VSD require only minimal inotropic support with dopamine or dobutamine at 5 µg/kg/min. Though an increased left atrial and left ventricular volume overload is preoperatively seen in patients with VSD, the left ventricular end diastolic volume (LVEDV) and left ventricular stroke output usually normalizes after surgery particularly in young infants.[5] A favorable hemodynamic response after successful closure of a left to right shunt in a patient with VSD include reflex hypertension and a low heart rate with minimal requirement of inotropes. However, presence of tachycardia and blood pressure at the lower limit of normal merits concern, and the possibility of a previously undetected ventricular dysfunction after bypass should be explored by a screening echocardiogram. Patients who are likely to have ventricular

dysfunction include those with a large VSD, need for ventriculotomy during repair or those who undergo closure of multiple VSDs where a substantial proportion of the interventricular septum is constituted by the noncontractile patch postoperatively.[6] In such patients, afterload reduction with levosimendan or milrinone is reasonable along with a low dose of epinephrine at 0.02–0.04 µg/kg/min. Though reflex bradycardia is a common phenomenon after VSD closure, careful evaluation of postoperative rhythm is important to identify atrioventricular conduction block.

It is important to monitor heart rate and rhythm continuously in the postoperative intensive care unit (ICU). Heart block is a potential complication after VSD closure due to the inherent proximity of the defect to the conduction system and likelihood of injury. Therefore, two ventricular wires and two atrial wires are desirable while separating from cardiopulmonary bypass (CPB).

There is a significant hemodynamic concern of postoperative pulmonary artery hypertension (PAH) in patients undergoing closure of large VSDs or patients presenting late for repair. Though reactive PAH consequent to a large shunt is expected to regress soon after surgery, patients with pulmonary vascular changes may have persistent PAH in the postoperative period. Such patients might require extended treatment with pulmonary vasodilators and mechanical ventilator support.

FLUID MANAGEMENT

Maintenance fluid requirements are calculated as per standard body surface area method for patients undergoing surgery under CPB. Patients with small VSDs usually do not require fluid restriction. Patients with large/moderate shunts with high pulmonary blood flow preoperatively might have postoperative pulmonary congestion after cardiopulmonary bypass. A negative fluid balance with fluid restriction and diuretic therapy is desirable in the early postoperative period after closure of large shunts in young infants. This will facilitate elimination of extravascular lung water and enable early extubation in these patients. A fluid bolus of 5 mL/kg is usually effective to treat hypotension resulting from hypovolemia in the postoperative period. An improvement in systolic blood pressure on compression of the liver margin may be used as a simple bedside test to elicit fluid responsiveness in the postoperative period.

■ DIURETIC THERAPY

Restrictive fluid strategy with aggressive diuretic therapy is the usual policy in young infants undergoing closure of large defects. Most patients benefit from a furosemide infusion at 1–2 mg/kg/day soon after arrival in ICU and a negative fluid balance of 30–50 mL/kg is usually targeted at the time of extubation in infants.

■ PAIN AND SEDATION MANAGEMENT

Most patients are started on fentanyl or morphine infusion for postoperative analgesia and sedation. Dexmedetomidine is frequently used in patients targeted for early extubation due to its analgesic and sedative properties without producing respiratory depression or chest wall rigidity typically associated with opioid use. Adjuvant agents such as paracetamol or ibuprofen may be useful for supplemental analgesia.

■ VENTILATION MANAGEMENT

- Children with small-moderate VSD with no/mild PAH, and requiring only minimal inotropic support are usually considered for early extubation on the day of surgery. Once the child is normothermic and awake, neuromuscular blockade should be reversed and ventilator settings scaled down to pressure support.
- Infants with large VSD, multiple VSDs, preoperative pneumonia or ventricular dysfunction, will usually require elective ventilation on the day of surgery. A screening echo is reasonable for assessment of ventricular function and to diagnose residual defects before planning extubation. Extubation is usually performed on postoperative day 1 after confirming a stable cardiopulmonary status.
- Children with preoperative evidence of pulmonary vascular disease, and PA systolic pressure more than two-thirds systemic pressure in the postbypass period merit sedation and ventilation on the day of surgery. All precautions to prevent pulmonary hypertensive crisis should be undertaken. It is reasonable to titrate ventilator settings to maintain a mild respiratory alkalosis (pH 7.45–7.5), partial pressure of carbon dioxide ($PaCO_2$) between 30 and 35 mm Hg and partial pressure of oxygen (PaO_2) of 100–150 mm Hg in order to avoid increase in pulmonary vascular resistance (PVR). Pulmonary vasodilator therapy should be used in conjunction with ventilator maneuvers after excluding significant residual VSD.
- Most children can be extubated to oxygen mask or nasal cannula. However, young infants with evidence of pulmonary congestion, or those who underwent prolonged preoperative ventilation might benefit from a short period of noninvasive ventilation using nasal continuous positive airway pressure (CPAP) or high flow nasal cannula oxygen therapy after extubation.

- Trisomy 21, multiple VSD, low cardiac output syndrome and a high vasoactive inotropic score have been identified as risk factors for delayed extubation after VSD closure in a single center study in Indian population.[7]

FEEDING AND NUTRITION

Patients who undergo early extubation are typically initiated on nasogastric/oral feeds 3–4 hours after extubation if remaining stable without any airway complications. Feeding is initiated with clear fluids and later transitioned to expressed breast milk/infant formula depending on the age of the infant. Infants with severe growth failure will require meticulous attention to nutritional rehabilitation once they recover from the initial catabolic phase of surgery and fluid intake is liberalized to meet calorie requirements.

COMMON COMPLICATIONS IN THE POSTOPERATIVE PERIOD

Pulmonary Hypertension

Older patients with large left to right shunts have the inherent risk of pulmonary hypertension. Early surgery is the most optimal prophylactic strategy for preventing subsequent pulmonary vascular disease.[8] Reactive pulmonary hypertension due to increased pulmonary blood flow typically resolves spontaneously in the early postoperative period after surgical correction. However, persistent pulmonary hypertension complicating the postoperative period should raise the suspicion of significant pulmonary vascular disease, residual shunts increasing pulmonary blood flow, previously undiagnosed pulmonary vein stenosis or a significant AV atrioventricular (AV) valve regurgitation.

Diagnosis

Pulmonary hypertension can be easily recognized if pulmonary artery pressure monitoring is available via an intraoperatively placed PA line. This may manifest as episodic pulmonary hypertensive crisis, or high pulmonary artery pressures more than two-thirds systemic arterial pressure, or as a low cardiac output state. Rarely this might be identified during cardiac evaluation for the cause of a failed extubation. Diagnosis is confirmed by echocardiography.

Therapeutic Measures

- Continue mechanical ventilation with appropriate ventilatory strategies for decreasing PVR
- Provide adequate sedation and pain relief
- Find out the cause of pulmonary hypertension—echocardiography, chest X-ray
- Address residual defects by surgery/intervention
- AV valve regurgitation if any, must be addressed with after load reducing measures
- Optimize inotropic supports to maintain hemodynamic stability
- Pre-existing lung infections triggering increased PVR have to be treated with appropriate antibiotics
- Correct hypoxia, hypercarbia and acidosis which can trigger pulmonary hypertensive crisis by increasing PVR
- *Specific treatment*: Pulmonary vasodilators, e.g., nitric oxide, sildenafil, bosentan.

Complete Heart Block

Heart block is a serious problem which can complicate the postoperative course in 1.3–3.5% patients.[9,10] The precise understanding of anatomy of the conduction system in relation to the VSD and the refinement of surgical techniques have substantially reduced the incidence of permanent heart block in the current era. The bundle of His traverses close to the posteroinferior margin of the VSD and the proximity is maximal in perimembranous and inlet septal type of VSD. Choosing a larger size of the patch, suturing to the right ventricular surface at least 2 mm away from the posteroinferior rim of the VSD and placement of superficial/interrupted sutures in this area are some of the described strategies to avoid injury to the conduction system.[9] The relationship of conduction system to the perimembranous VSD is depicted in **Figure 2**.

In patients who have heart block on weaning off CPB in the operating room, temporary epicardial pacing wires are placed and temporary pacing is initiated till intrinsic rhythm recovers. Though there is no published data, it is common practice at our center to administer a short course (1–2 days) of dexamethasone 0.2–0.5 mg/kg empirically to reduce edema in the conduction system near the AV node. Transient complete heart block generally reverts to sinus rhythm within a week and hence it is prudent to wait for 7–10 days after surgery before planning a permanent pacemaker. In patients whom sinus rhythm is restored, a 24-hour Holter should be obtained to exclude any likelihood of intermittent blocks in AV conduction and to document sinus rhythm. If the heart block persists beyond 10 days a permanent pacemaker is indicated.

Tachyarrhythmias

Tachyarrhythmias such as supraventricular tachycardia and junctional ectopic tachycardia may be seen in some children after VSD repair. Precipitating factors such as electrolyte imbalances, hyperthermia and high doses of catecholamines should be addressed. Specific pharmacological treatment should follow depending on the type of arrhythmia.

Ventricular Dysfunction

Ventricular dysfunction occuring in the first few days after surgical closure of VSD is most often due to afterload mismatch. Essentially, this refers to a hemodynamic adaptation after elimination of the left to right shunt that required the left ventricle to eject a large volume preoperatively. After closure of VSD the left ventricle is no longer expected to generate the same output and one of the following hemodynamic responses result. The more common response is bradycardia with relative hypertension. The echocardiogram

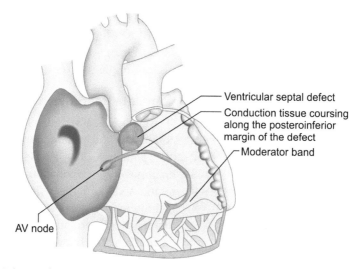

Ventricular septal defect

Conduction tissue coursing along the posteroinferior margin of the defect

Moderator band

AV node

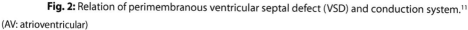

Fig. 2: Relation of perimembranous ventricular septal defect (VSD) and conduction system.[11]
(AV: atrioventricular)

in these patients reveals a preserved ejection fraction. A less common form of compensation is persistent tachycardia with reduced systolic function on the echocardiogram. This is usually a transient phenomenon that resolves in a few days. It may be prudent to avoid extubation for a day or two and use vasodilators such as milrinone.

Ventricular dysfunction may also be anticipated in patients with large VSD, need for ventriculotomy to facilitate adequate exposure during repair and in infants with multiple VSDs. Functional depression after VSD closure has been described to be usually asymmetric, mostly affecting the septal and lateral wall segments.[12] Postoperative ventricular dysfunction will clinically manifest as hemodynamic instability or low cardiac output state (cool extremities, low urine output, weak peripheral pulses). Ventricular dysfunction should also be suspected in infants who have an unexpected failed extubation in the early postoperative period.

Management

- Continue mechanical ventilatory support if indicated to decrease left ventricular (LV) afterload
- *Optimize inotrope use*: Afterload reduction with milrinone or levosimendan
- Transition through noninvasive ventilation at subsequent extubation to decrease work of breathing and reduce LV afterload.

Residual Ventricular Septal Defect

Residual VSD should be suspected by the presence of a systolic murmur in the postoperative period. Diagnosis is confirmed by echocardiography. Intraoperatively an absolute PA saturation of ≥ 80% at a fraction of inspired oxygen (FiO_2) ≤ 0.5 is suggestive of residual left to right shunt. A previously undiagnosed residual/additional VSD in the postoperative period can present as elevated

pulmonary artery pressures, low cardiac output state or failure to wean off ventilator. Large residual defects should be addressed surgically or through device closure. Inotropic support with afterload reducing agents such as Milrinone/Levosimendan is reasonable. Adoption of ventilatory strategies to mildly increase PVR and decrease the magnitude of left to right shunt is often beneficial. This typically includes choosing the lowest inspired oxygen concentration feasible to maintain a PaO_2 of >60 mm Hg and titrating the ventilator settings to target a $PaCO_2$ of 45–50 mm Hg.

Low Cardiac Output State

This may be due to residual defect, pulmonary hypertension or ventricular dysfunction. The causes for ventricular dysfunction in the postoperative period after VSD closure had been elucidated earlier. Treatment should be directed at the cause. Ventricular dysfunction should be treated with inotropic supports and afterload reducing agents such as milrinone or enalapril. Ventilatory support may need to be extended till ventricular function recovers.

Extubation Failure

Possibilities:
- Residual VSD
- Low cardiac output state-often a sequelae of large VSD requiring a large patch or afterload mismatch after VSD closure
- Preoperative pneumonia
- Fluid overload after CPB
- Persistent pulmonary hypertension.

Management is directed at the cause.

■ SPECIAL SITUATIONS

Ventricular Septal Defect with Pneumonia and Preoperative Mechanical Ventilation

A significant proportion of infants with large VSD in low middle-income countries may present to tertiary care centers with lower respiratory tract infection, cardiorespiratory failure and severe growth failure. Delayed presentation adds to the preoperative morbidity. Most often, these infants require preoperative ventilation for initial stabilization. Though the initial standard practice was an attempt to optimize with medical management, many of these infants typically fail extubation due to the presence of large left to right shunt with increased pulmonary blood flow. With growing experience many centers have acknowledged the fact that corrective surgery at the earliest window available might provide the best chance for a favorable postoperative outcome.[4,13,14] The timing of the optimal window for surgery in these critically ill infants should be judiciously based on clinical assessment with partial resolution of pneumonia, improvement in laboratory parameters suggestive of infection and evidence of reduced pulmonary artery pressures on echocardiographic assessment.[13] When compared to infants who undergo elective VSD closure, preoperatively ventilated patients are likely to have longer duration of mechanical ventilation, need for prolonged intensive care and delayed hospital discharge.[13]

■ DEINTENSIFICATION

Despite the afore-mentioned postoperative complications, VSD closure is a low risk congenital heart repair. Patients who have an uncomplicated course can be quickly deintensified with early extubation, weaning of inotropes and removal of invasive lines. Oral/nasogastric feeds can be initiated if deemed stable after extubation and transitioned to direct breastfeeds in young infants. A focused approach to nutritional rehabilitation is important in severely malnourished infants. Fortification of infant formula with indigenously available cost-effective agents

such as medium chain triglyceride (MCT) oil or institution of high calorie infant formula may be required for meeting energy goals in such patients. Appropriate parent education on nutrition care is important to ensure adequate calorie intake at home after discharge.

■ DISCHARGE MEDICATION AND NUTRITION

Most patients after VSD closure need no medications at the time of discharge. Diuretics can be stopped altogether while the child is recovering in hospital. Patients who have preoperative failure to thrive require supplementation of multivitamins and minerals in addition to nutritional rehabilitation. Catch up growth is impressive and during the first follow-up visit, most infants show remarkable weight gain.[15] An improved appetite and hunger are often noted by the parent and the advice should be to feed as demanded by the baby.

■ REFERENCES

1. Menting ME, Cuypers JA, Opic P, Utens E, Witzenberg M, van den Bosch AE, et al. The unnatural history of ventricular septal defect. J Am Coll Cardiol. 2015;65:1941-51.
2. Kouchukos NT, Blackstone EH, Hanley FL, Kirklin JK. Ventricular septal defect. In: Kirklin Barratt-Boyes Cardiac Surgery. Philadelphia: Elsevier Saunders; 2013. pp. 190-250.
3. Schipper M, Slieker MG, Schoof PH, Breur Johannes MPJ. Surgical repair of ventricular septal defect: contemporary results and risk factors for a complicated course. Pediatr Cardiol. 2017;38:264-70.
4. Reddy SN, Kappanayil M, Balachandran R, Sudhakar A, Sunil GS, Raj BR, Kumar RK. Preoperative determinants of outcomes of infant heart surgery in a limited-resource setting. Semin Thorac Cardiovasc Surg. 2015;27:331-8.
5. Cordell D, Graham TP, Atwood GF, Boerth RC, Boucek RJ, Bender HW. Left ventricular volume characteristics following ventricular septal defect closure in infancy. Circulation. 1976;54:294-8.

6. Matsuhisa H, Yoshimura N, Higuma T, Misaki T, Onuma Y, Ichida F, et al. Ventricular septal dysfunction after surgical closure of multiple ventricular septal defects. Ann Thorac Surg. 2013;96:891-7.

7. Parmar D, Lakhia K, Garg P, Patel K, Shah R, Surti J, et al. Risk factors for delayed extubation after ventricular septal defect closure: a prospective observational study. Braz J Cardiovasc Surg. 2017;32:276-82.

8. Zhu WH, Zhu XK, Shu Q. Postoperative hemodynamics of severe pulmonary hypertension caused by congenital heart disease. World J Pediatr. 2006;1:45-8.

9. Azab S, El-Shahawy H, Samy A, Mahdy W. Permanent heart block following surgical closure of isolated ventricular septal defect. Egyptian J Chest Dis Tubercul. 2013;62:529-33.

10. Edwin F, Aniteye M, Tettey M, Sereboe L, Kotei D, Tamatey M, et al. Permanent complete heart block following surgical correction of congenital heart disease. Ghana Med J. 2010;44:109-14.

11. Altaweel H, Kabbani MS, Hijazi O, Hammadah HM, Al Ghamdi S. Late presenting complete heart block after the surgical repair of ventricular septal defect. Egyptian Heart J. 2018;70:455-9.

12. Quinn TA, Cabreriza SE, Blumenthal BF, Printz BF, Altmann K, Glickstein JS, et al. Regional functional depression immediately after ventricular septal defect closure. J Am Soc Echocardiogr. 2004;17:1066-72.

13. Bhatt M, Roth SJ, Kumar RK, Gauvreau K, Nair SG, Chengode S, et al. Management of infants with large unrepaired ventricular septal defects and respiratory infection requiring mechanical ventilation. J Thorac Cardiovasc Surg. 2004;127:1466-73.

14. Vaidyanathan B, Roth SJ, Rao SG, Gauvreau K, Shivaprakasha K, Krishna Kumar R. Outcome of ventricular septal defect repair in a developing country. J Pediatr. 2002;140:736-41.

15. Banerji N, Sudhakar A, Balachandran R, Sunil GS, Kottayil B, Krishna KR. Early weight trends after congenital heart surgery and their determinants. Cardiol Young. 2020;30(1):89-94.

Surgical Closure of a Hemodynamically Significant Patent Ductus Arteriosus

Jessin P Jayashankar, Aveek Jayant
Illustration: Praveen Reddy Bayya
Reviewed by: Aveek Jayant

■ INTRODUCTION

The ductus arteriosus (DA) is a muscular artery connecting two elastic arteries with different resistances viz., the descending thoracic aorta and the pulmonary artery **(Fig. 1)**. It is a normal fetal structure that only becomes pathological if it remains patent after a predefined period postnatally.[1]

The DA is normally functionally closed by about 10-15 hours postnatally. The physio-

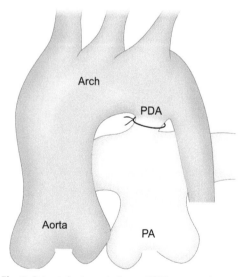

Fig. 1: Patent ductus arteriosus (PDA) connecting descending thoracic aorta and the pulmonary artery (PA).

logical impact and clinical significance of the patent ductus arteriosus (PDA) depend largely on its size, the underlying cardiac and pulmonary status of the neonate or older infant, and, when applicable premature status of birth. In utero, the drivers of ductal patency-a low oxygen tension and high doses of circulating prostaglandin from the placenta coupled with low lung metabolism predominate. At birth of the term fetus, these factors diminish and the duct closes, functionally first, and later, anatomically. When a neonate is born prematurely the functional milieu of the postnatal status is closer to that of the in utero period (although here the primary incriminating factor might often be the pulmonary insufficiency that results from prematurity) and the duct remains patent, sometimes contributing to the morbidity of preterm birth. In term infants, the PDA is essentially a left to right shunt and its pathophysiologic correlates are matched to size of the duct, and by extension, the magnitude of the shunt.[2] PDA can exist as an isolated anomaly or it can persist in association with other defects. In some of these defects the DA critically supports the systemic or pulmonary circulations and its patency is therefore linked to survival. In the preterm neonate the duct can persist and, in return, contribute to other morbid conditions such as necrotizing enterocolitis, intraventricular hemorrhage (IVH), bronchopulmonary dysplasia (BPD), and retinopathy of prematurity.[3] This arises from the preemie's inability to maintain active pulmonary vasoconstriction. A relatively less distensible left ventricle also means there are limits to increasing cardiac output without increases in left ventricular end diastolic pressures, and, by extension in left atrial and pulmonary venous pressures. When shunt sizes exceed 50% a double jeopardy sets in: (1) of low systemic blood flow compromising the gut and the cerebral circulation, and (2) alteration in pulmonary compliance disadvantageously (hampering management of lung disease that is naturally present in proportion to prematurity).

Ductal patency is a direct correlate to the extent of preterm birth. When term neonates are surveyed at 72 hours most will have a nonpatent duct. This figure drops to 98% when children are born beyond 30 weeks but before term and even further to about 54% when birth occurs at 24–25 weeks of gestation. However, even when born preterm although the duct might be patent during early infancy about 86% will achieve closure by the age of 1 year. Of note, patency also seems to be grossly disproportionate in neonates born small for gestational age (SGA). When functionally insignificant in terms of shunt potential, the duct can rarely become aneurysmal or the focus of infective endocarditis, usually not compelling enough reasons to address a restrictive duct in these times. This account of a patent duct is primarily directed toward management of the duct in the typically symptomatic term neonate or infant, sometimes in the older child. Management of the duct in the preterm neonate deserves separate treatment altogether; it is not the focus here as such children are cared for in the specialized neonatal care unit. Occasionally, we do manage an ex-preemie with a patent and symptomatic duct and a brief topical review is included.

In situations of persistent ductal patency, there occurs a reversal of ductal flow due to the normal decline in pulmonary vascular resistance (PVR) that occurs after birth with aeration and ventilation of lungs. This results in a left to right shunt from the aorta to pulmonary artery. Fully saturated aortic blood passes from the descending thoracic aorta to the pulmonary artery via the ductus, and eventually goes through the lungs into the left atrium, into the left ventricle and back to the aorta. This results in volume overload of the left heart. Ultimately, left atrial dilatation occurs along with left ventricular dilatation and hypertrophy.[2]

Increased pulmonary flow from the ductal shunting leads to increased pulmonary fluid volume, and in patients with moderate or large shunts, this causes decreased lung compliance, which may result in increased work of breathing. Increased flow returning to the left heart results in increased left atrial and left ventricular end-diastolic pressures. The left ventricle compensates by increasing stroke volume and eventually may hypertrophy to normalize wall stress. Neuroendocrine adaptations also occur, with increased sympathetic activity and circulating catecholamines that result in increased contractility and heart rate.[4,5] When the duct is large enough for all these latter effects it could also be a source of "hyperkinetic" pulmonary artery hypertension, but this is not common.[6] Duct flow is governed by the Poiseuille equation which deems this to be a function of the duct diameter, blood viscosity and the relative pressure difference between the systemic and pulmonary circulations. It follows that a high volume shunt typically accompanies relatively *low* pulmonary artery pressure (PAP).

Very rarely, a duct may be addressed surgically under cardiopulmonary bypass: this is in the adult when it is potentially calcified or if there is a ductal aneurysm in the background of previous closure or de novo. This is rare to such an extent that no special description is warranted here. A patent duct can rarely also present as grown up congenital heart disease (GUCH) with pulmonary vascular disease; this too is not the focus of this chapter.

■ MONITORING

Isolated ducti are ligated using a left posterolateral thoracotomy. At our center, it is usual to place an invasive arterial line. Most practitioners also place a central venous catheter but it can be argued from a risk benefit perspective that large bore peripheral venous access should suffice. Consideration may be given to monitor for a pulse in the lower extremity either via a pulse oximeter or the invasive arterial line in the lower limb.[6] Although very uncommon, a large duct can occasionally cause anatomic confusion with the descending thoracic aorta for noviciate surgeons. Caudal opiates in addition to an intercostal nerve block under surgical vision are usual.

Most children with isolated PDA will be weaned from mechanical ventilation within the first few hours of surgery but after an echocardiogram to assess ventricular function in the ICU in our unit. Some children with a PDA are also either SGA or suffer from low nutritional status: they would need special care in matching the postoperative plan to their preoperative status as such, beyond the PDA itself.[7-9]

■ HEMODYNAMIC MANAGEMENT

Preoperatively, and intraoperatively focus is on limiting the magnitude of the shunt itself, typically by respiratory management of oxygen and carbon dioxide tensions in a manner to increase the pulmonary vascular resistance (see later). A proportion of children with a PDA will develop an entity known as the postligation syndrome.[10,11]

For all hemodynamically significant PDA, postligation there can be a maladaptive response to a sudden increase in left ventricular (LV) afterload as the duct previously allowing decompression into the lower pressure pulmonary artery (PA) becomes extinct. The stiffer LV pressure volume relationship in this age group, occult coronary ischemia (which can increase diastolic dysfunction) and withdrawal of LV preload can produce various combinations of systolic, diastolic and combined LV functional impairment. The classical clinical manifestation is low systolic blood pressure (less than the 3rd centile) and respiratory impairment in lung mechanics and oxygenation occurring 6–12 hours after ligation. Officiously called the *postligation cardiac syndrome*,[12] this can happen in 28–45% of cases. Younger age at intervention (<28 days postnatal age), weights <1 kg,[12] lower gestational ages, and, higher ventilatory support preoperatively have been identified as risk factors.[10-13] This has also been described in older infants undergoing transcatheter or surgical closure but the severity was likely lower and may not be of clinical significance.[14,15] However, the standard echocardiographic indices used in these studies have previously shown to be not useful as assessors of this entity.[12] Outside of traditional cardiac and demographic risk factors low cortisol levels linked to a paucity of adrenal stimulation has also been documented.[16] Among the younger and smaller neonates at risk the syndrome is not innocuous and can lead to sequelae such as bronchopulmonary dysplasia and need for home oxygen.[17] Given this predilection for consequences beyond the immediate short-term, groups have advocated targeted echocardiography 1 hour after ligation to assess the left ventricular output (LVO). This is calculated as:[18,19]

$$LVO = \frac{\text{(Instantaneous ascending aortic output)} \times \text{(aortic cross sectional area)} \times 60}{\text{Weight in kg}}$$

Anticipatory use of milrinone based on this metric has reduced the incidence of this syndrome[20] in the vulnerable group. However, respiratory insufficiency still supervenes (in about 50%) in preterm neonates receiving anticipatory milrinone therapy: this is probably due to diastolic dysfunction.[13] It should specifically be stated that the use of standard echocardiographic measures of LV performance such as fractional shortening do not have adequate predictive power and there is evidence that the best metric is the LVO.[18-20]

Fluid Management

This is an individualized decision process based essentially on preoperative status (including assessing for factors causing depleted volume such as diuretic use, deliberate restriction and phototherapy) and clinical judgment. Typically most patients will receive 750–100 mL/m²/day for the first 1–2 days and thereafter appropriate for age and clinical status.

■ VENTILATORY MANAGEMENT

As adverted to above, ventilatory management is initially tweaked to increase the PVR so as to limit magnitude of shunt but there can be no universal formulation. A major practical consideration is the gas exchange impairment that follows anatomic compression of the left lung parenchyma that is a result of obtaining surgical access to the PDA. This limits the extent of permissive respiratory management intraprocedurally. In addition, limited autoregulation in preterm neonates means respiratory maneuvers cannot be drastic so as to prevent sudden fluctuations in cerebral blood flow, in turn a risk for IVH. A small subset of ex-preemies could present for hemodynamically significant ductus arteriosus (hsDA) closure at a later gestational age: some of these children may already have BPD closely linked to their actual gestational age at birth, or more subtle dysfunction that shows lung function to be intermediate between normal term infants and infants born early preterm.

Although not common at our institution some centers aspire to achieve extubation of the trachea in the operating room itself. At our institution this is typically achieved in the first few hours after surgery.

■ COMPLICATIONS

The most dramatic complication is the post-ligation cardiac syndrome. More common are residual lung dysfunction or overt collapse from surgical compression of the lung acting on the background of heart failure due to the PDA itself. The left recurrent laryngeal nerve is in anatomic jeopardy and due regard should be present to suspect and prove vocal cord dysfunction: such infants, doubtless need follow-up and caution with feeding. Sometimes there maybe a pneumothorax or more rarely a hemothorax due to intercostal drain malfunction. A chylothorax is considered rare but is by no means impossible: it calls for a paradigm of diagnosis and treatment which is troublesome.

■ REFERENCES

1. Vettukattil J. Pathophysiology of patent ductus arteriosus in the preterm infant. Curr Pediatr Rev. 2016;12:120-2.

2. Nichols DG, Ungerleider RM, Spevak PJ, Greeley WJ, Cameron DE, Lappe DG, et al. Critical Heart Disease in Infants and Children, 2nd edition. St. Louis: Mosby; 2006.

3. Clyman RI. Patent ductus arteriosus in the preterm infant. In: Gleason CA, Juul SE (Eds). Avery's Diseases of the Newborn, 10th edition. Philadelphia: Elsevier; 2018. pp. 790-800.

4. Hermes-Desantis E, Clyman R. Patent ductus arteriosus: pathophysiology and management. J Perinatol. 2006;26:S14-S18.

5. Schneider DJ, Moore JW. Patent ductus arteriosus. Circulation. 2006;114:1873-82.

6. Chang AC, Wells W. Patent ductus arteriosus. In: Chang AC, Hanley FL, Wernovsky G, Wessel DL (Eds). Pediatric Cardiac Intensive Care. Baltimore: Lippincott Williams & Wilkin; 1998. pp. 204-6.

7. Rosen DA, Rosen KR. Anomalies of the aortic arch and valve. In: Lake CL, Booker PD (Eds). Pediatric Cardiac Anaesthesia, 4th edition. Philadelphia: Lippincott Williams and Wilkins; 2005. pp. 412-7.

8. Jonas RA, Dinardo J, Laussen PC, Howe R, LaPierre R, Matte G. Patent ductus arteriosus, aortopulmonary window, sinus of Valsalva fistula, aortoventricular tunnel. Comprehensive surgical management of congenital heart disease, 2nd edition. Florida: CRC Press; 2014. pp. 267-87.

9. PDA Management following surgical closure. Neonatal Clinical Care Guidelines. Perth, Australia: King Edward memorial hospital; 2013.

10. Moin F, Kennedy KA, Moya FR. Risk factors predicting vasopressor use after patent ductus arteriosus ligation. Am J Perinatol. 2003;20(6):313-20.

11. Sehgal A, McNamara PJ. Coronary artery perfusion and myocardial performance after patent ductus arteriosus ligation. J Thorac Cardiovasc Surg. 2012;143(6):1271-8.

12. Giesinger RE, Bischoff AR, McNamara PJ. Anticipatory perioperative management for patent ductus arteriosus surgery: understanding postligation cardiac syndrome. Congenit Heart Dis. 2019;14(2):311-6.

13. Ting JY, Resende M, More K, Nicholls D, Weisz DE, El-Khuffash A, et al. Predictors of respiratory instability in neonates undergoing patient ductus arteriosus ligation after the introduction of targeted milrinone treatment. J Thorac Cardiovasc Surg. 2016;152(2):498-504.

14. Gupta S, Tharakan J, Sanjay G, Anees T, Krishnamoorthy K, Sivasankaran S, et al. Percutaneous closure of patent ductus arteriosus in children: immediate and short-term changes in left ventricular systolic and diastolic function. Ann Pediatr Card. 2011;4(2):139.

15. Abdel-Bary M, Abdel-Baseer KA, Abdel-Latif AF, Abdel-Naser MA, Nafie M, Eisa KM. Left ventricular dysfunction postsurgical patent ductus arteriosus ligation in children: predictor factors analysis. J Cardiothorac Surg. 2019;14(1):168.

16. Clyman RI, Wickremasinghe A, Merritt TA, Solomon T, McNamara P, Jain A, et al. Hypotension following patent ductus arteriosus ligation: the role of adrenal hormones. J Pediatr. 2014;164(6):1449-55.e1.

17. Ulrich TJ, Hansen TP, Reid KJ, Bingler MA, Olsen SL. Post-ligation cardiac syndrome is associated with increased morbidity in preterm infants. J Perinatol. 2018;38(5):537-42.

18. Pladys P, Wodey E, Beuchée A, Branger B, Bétrémieux P. Left ventricle output and mean arterial blood pressure in preterm infants during the 1st day of life. Eur J Pediatr. 1999; 158(10):817-24.

19. Gill AB, Weindling AM. Echocardiographic assessment of cardiac function in shocked very low birthweight infants. Arch Dis Childhood. 1993;68(1):17-21.

20. Jain A, Sahni M, El-Khuffash A, Khadawardi E, Sehgal A, McNamara PJ. Use of targeted neonatal echocardiography to prevent post-operative cardiorespiratory instability after patent ductus arteriosus ligation. J Pediatr. 2012; 160(4):584-9.e1.

Repair of Coarctation of Aorta

Rakhi Balachandran

Illustrations: Praveen Reddy Bayya
Reviewed by: R Krishna Kumar

■ INTRODUCTION

Coarctation of aorta refers to a discrete narrowing of the upper descending thoracic aorta typically located adjacent to the insertion of ductus arteriosus (**Figs. 1A and B**). Coarctation of aorta can occur either as an isolated defect or in conjunction with cardiac anomalies such as ventricular septal defect, transposition of great arteries or double outlet right ventricle. Isolated coarctation of aorta occurs with a worldwide birth prevalence of 0.34 per 1,000 live births.[1] Obstruction to left ventricular (LV) outflow results in increased LV afterload and compromises lower body perfusion. Coarctation is more common when the aortic flow is reduced during fetal life by lesions such as aortic stenosis, aortic atresia, mitral stenosis or mitral regurgitation.[2]

A neonate with critical coarctation often presents with severe heart failure and needs emergency resuscitation besides pharmacological intervention with prostaglandin E1 infusion to open the ductus arteriosus. Surgical intervention is required following the initial stabilization for facilitating optimal survival in neonates and infants. The principle of surgical repair is to maximally reduce the afterload on the systemic ventricle by eliminating any obstruction to flow between the ascending and descending aorta. The repair necessitates a brief period of aortic cross-clamp during which the distal perfusion might be affected to varying degree depending on the duration of cross clamp and the level of application of the cross clamp. The repair is generally performed through a left posterolateral thoracotomy without the use of cardiopulmonary bypass. Mild hypothermia of 34°C is provided for spinal cord protection during the period of aortic cross clamping. Resection and end to end anastomosis is the standard technique commonly employed in infants and young children with discrete coarctation and a normal aortic arch (**Fig. 1C**). Adjuvant techniques such as subclavian flap aortoplasty or patch aortoplasty may be required if augmentation of distal arch is warranted. However, with the advent of the extended arch repair, it is seldom necessary to patch or sacrifice the subclavian artery.

The chief intraoperative considerations include the effects of aortic cross clamping, control of hypertension, bleeding, potential injury to adjacent structures such as thoracic duct, phrenic nerve and recurrent laryngeal nerve and finally sequelae of ipsilateral lung compression during the procedure. Isolated coarctation repair is considered to be a low-risk procedure despite the practical challenges to the anesthesia and surgical team. The broad principles of postoperative care

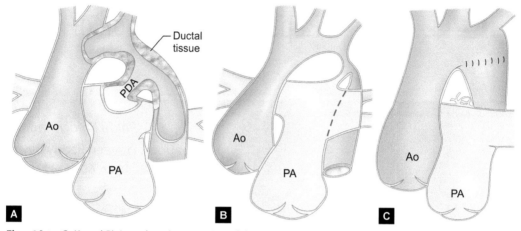

Figs. 1A to C: (A and B) Juxtaductal coarctation of the aorta (A) with patent ductus arteriosus (PDA) kept open with prostaglandin E1 infusion and (B) with absent PDA; (C) After resection and extended end to end anastomosis. (Ao: aorta; PA: pulmonary artery)

include management of sequelae of relieving the aortic obstruction, as well as monitoring for complications related to interruption of end organ perfusion during the period of aortic cross clamp. We have provided a brief overview of the postoperative management after repair of isolated coarctation of aorta in this chapter.

■ MONITORING

Standard monitoring includes invasive arterial blood pressure monitoring, central venous pressure monitoring, continuous ECG monitoring, pulse oximetry and capnography. Arterial pressure monitoring in both upper limb and lower limb is the standard practice before commencement of surgery to understand the pressure proximal and distal to the level of obstruction and also to rule out residual obstruction/gradient after repair. If axillary artery is cannulated for monitoring in the operating room, it is removed soon after arrival in intensive care unit to minimize possibility of accidental air embolism to the arch vessels. Left arm should not be used for arterial pressure monitoring if left subclavian artery is utilized for subclavian patch plasty.

■ HEMODYNAMIC MANAGEMENT

The surgery is performed without cardiopulmonary bypass and inotropes are often not necessary. However, in critically ill patients with preoperative ventricular dysfunction inotropic support may be required until ventricular function improves after surgery. Systemic hypertension is a frequent phenomenon after repair and this has been well described as paradoxical hypertension after coarctation repair. As hypertension may predispose to increased risk of bleeding from aortic suture lines, control of blood pressure may be required in early postoperative period. At our center, sodium nitroprusside or beta-blockers are usually used to control postoperative hypertension (systolic blood pressure >120 mm Hg in neonates and infants or >140 mm Hg in older children).

■ FLUID MANAGEMENT

Coarctation repair is usually performed without the use of cardiopulmonary bypass and hence, the standard fluid management policy for closed heart procedures should be followed. In critically ill patients who had preoperative renal dysfunction adequate intravascular volume has to be maintained to allow optimal renal perfusion and aggressive diuretic therapy is not generally employed. The daily fluid prescriptions range from 60 to 100 mL/kg/day during the first three postoperative days and escalated thereafter to meet the normal fluid requirements permitted for the age of the patient.

DIURETIC THERAPY

Aggressive diuresis is not indicated as most patients with preoperative renal impairment may be preload dependent, for optimal renal perfusion. However, in those patients with important ventricular dysfunction and evidence of fluid overload, it is reasonable to initiate diuretic therapy with an infusion of furosemide at 1–2 mg/kg/day.

PAIN AND SEDATION MANAGEMENT

Pain control is important to prevent postoperative hypertension and to avoid the respiratory complications secondary to a painful thoracotomy incision. A multimodal analgesia using titrated opioids, acetaminophen and nonsteroidal anti-inflammatory drugs (NSAIDs) is a reasonable postoperative strategy.[3] It is rational to minimize the dose of opioids as most of the patients who have an uncomplicated intraoperative course are candidates for early extubation. Dexmedetomidine has an opioid sparing effect and facilitates sedation without respiratory depression. Intraoperative single-shot caudal epidural blockade or intercostal blockade, are often used as adjuvants to standard analgesic therapy. In a recent retrospective review by Kynes et al., patients who received thoracic epidural analgesia for postoperative pain relief after repair of coarctation had reduced requirement for antihypertensive infusions in the postoperative period compared to patients who did not receive epidural analgesia.[4]

VENTILATION AND EXTUBATION

Patients who have an uncomplicated preoperative and intraoperative course can be considered for early extubation. Prior to extubation adequate level of awakening and absence of neurological impairment has to be ensured. Newborns with preoperative ventricular dysfunction need to be evaluated for recovery of ventricular function before planning extubation. The ipsilateral lung may be compressed during surgery for facilitating surgical access and hence residual atelectasis (lung collapse) should be ruled out on chest X-ray before extubating the patient. As recurrent laryngeal nerve courses in close proximity to aortic arch, any likely injury during dissection can contribute to postoperative vocal cord dysfunction. Patient has to be closely monitored for occurrence of postoperative stridor, dysphagia or, poor phonation after extubation.

FEEDING AND NUTRITION

In patients with duct dependent systemic circulation and compromised lower body perfusion prior to surgery, it is safe to avoid feeding for 48 hours. Postcoarctectomy syndrome is likely in some patients as the re-establishment of pulsatile blood flow after repair can trigger reflex mesenteric vasoconstriction.[5] Nasogastric decompression and intravenous fluids are often instituted in the first 48 hours to minimize this complication. After commencement of feeds, careful monitoring for signs of intolerance is important while escalating feeds.

COMMON POSTOPERATIVE COMPLICATIONS

Paradoxical Hypertension

Paradoxical hypertension is a frequent finding after repair of coarctation, attributed to elevated sympathetic nervous system activity, alterations in the renin-angiotensin-aldosterone axis and a disrupted baroreceptor response.[6-8] Hypertension needs to be treated as it increases the risk of bleeding from aortic suture lines. Paradoxical hypertension responds to beta-blockers, arterial smooth muscle relaxants, calcium channel blockers and angiotensin-converting enzyme (ACE) inhibitors.[9] The most common treatment modality in early postoperative phase is the use of vasodilators such as sodium nitroprusside or beta-blockers. Vasodilators are typically initiated if SBP >120 mm Hg in neonates or >140 mm Hg in an older patient. Orally administered beta-blockers or ACE inhibitors such as enalapril can be started for persistent hypertension once the infant is initiated on oral feeds.

Postcoarctectomy Syndrome

The early reports of postcoarctectomy syndrome describe this condition as a mesenteric arteritis characterized by symptoms such as abdominal pain and tenderness, ileus, vomiting, fever, melena and leukocytosis along with hypertension occurring about 72 hours after surgery.[10] The establishment of pulsatile blood flow after coarctation repair resulting in increased intra-arterial wall tension and intimal damage leading to mesenteric arteritis is the proposed mechanism. Coexistent arterial hypertension is a predisposing factor for the development of this complication. Control of paradoxical hypertension has been suggested to decrease the incidence of this complication.[7] Maintenance of constant vigil for abdominal signs, control of hypertension after repair and cautious feeding will help to prevent postcoarctectomy syndrome.

Paraplegia

Coarctation repair entails a brief period of aortic cross clamping during which the perfusion to spinal cord and lower body is temporarily interrupted. This leads to the potential risk of spinal cord ischemia during the period of clamping. Prolonged cross clamp times, hyperthermia, poor collateral circulation, low proximal and distal aortic blood pressures and elevated spinal fluid pressures are considered to be risk factors for spinal cord injury during coarctation repair.[3] Typically, the cross-clamp time is restricted to 20–30 minutes and a mild passive hypothermia of 34–35°C is allowed during the period of cross clamping. It is important to have a detailed assessment of the neurological status of the patient after awakening and reversal of neuromuscular blockade. Recovery of motor function of upper limbs and lower limbs has to be ensured before planning extubation.

Lung Complications

Postoperative pulmonary complications are mostly secondary to retraction and handling of the lung during the thoracotomy. Incomplete expansion of the lung after surgery can manifest as postoperative atelectasis. Recurrent laryngeal nerve injury causing stridor may complicate weaning and extubation. Unilateral vocal cord paralysis typically presents with stridor, weak cry, dysphonia, poor feeding or aspiration and is reported in pediatric cardiac surgery commonly in operations involving the aortic arch and Norwood procedure.[11] Patients with vocal cord palsy and swallowing dysfunction require appropriate nutritional rehabilitation and caregiver training before planning discharge from hopsital.

Low Cardiac Output State

In neonates and infants who have preoperative LV dysfunction secondary to coarctation, low cardiac output state can persist after coarctation repair. This may warrant a longer period of ventilation to facilitate myocardial recovery. Appropriate inotropic support with judicious use of afterload reducing agents is reasonable in this setting.

■ DEINTENSIFICATION

Inotropic supports are usually weaned off after extubation. Invasive lines can be removed once the patient is extubated and initiated on enteral feeds. Signs for feed intolerance should be aggressively sought for, while escalating feeds.

■ DISCHARGE MEDICATIONS

Typically, these patients do not need any post discharge medication other than nutritional supplements.

■ REFERENCES

1. Van der Linde D, Konings EM, Slager MA, Witzenberg M, Helbing W, Takkenberg JM, et al. Birth prevalence of congenital heart disease worldwide. A systematic review and meta-analysis. J Am Coll Cardiol. 2011;58:2241-7.
2. Kouchukos NT, Blackstone EH, Hanley FL, Kirklin JK. Coarctation of aorta and interrupted aortic arch. In: Kirklin Barrat-Boyes Cardiac Surgery, 4th edition. Philadelphia: Elsevier Saunders; 2013. pp. 1718-79.
3. Fox EB, Latham GJ, Ross FJ, Joffe D. Perioperative and anesthetic management of coarctation of aorta. Semin Cardiothorac Vasc Anesth. 2019;23:212-24.
4. Kynes JM, Shotwell MS, Walters CB, Bichell DP, Christensen JT, Hays SR. Epidurals for coarctation repair in children associated with decreased anti-hypertensive infusion requirement as measured by a novel parameter, the anti-hypertensive dosing index. Children. 2019;6:112.
5. Chang AC, Starnes VA. Coarctation of aorta. In: Chang AC, Hanley FL, Wernovsky G, Wessel DL (Eds). Pediatric Cardiac Intensive Care. Pennsylvania: Lippincott Williams and Wilkins; 1998. pp. 247-56.
6. Sealy WC. Paradoxical hypertension after repair of coarctation of aorta: a review of its causes. Ann Thorac Surg. 1990;50:323-9.
7. Fox S, Pierce WS, Waldhausen JA. Pathogenesis of paradoxical hypertension after coarctation repair. Ann Thorac Surg. 1980;29:135-41.
8. Choy M, Rocchini AP, Beekman RH, Rosenthal A, Dick M, Crowley D, et al. Paradoxical hypertension after repair of coarctation of aorta in children: balloon angioplasty versus surgical repair. Circulation. 1987;75:1186-91.
9. Roeleveld PP, Zwijsen EG. Treatment strategies for paradoxical hypertension following surgical correction of coarctation of aorta in children. World J Pediatr Congenit Heart Surg. 2017;8:321-31.
10. Ho EC, Moss AJ. The syndrome of mesenteric arteritis following repair of aortic coarctation. Pediatrics. 1972;49:40-5.
11. Pham V, Connelly D, Wei JL, Sykes KJ, O'Brien J. Vocal cord paralysis and dysphagia after aortic arch reconstruction and Norwood procedure. Otolaryngol Head Neck Surg. 2014;150:827-33.

Repair of Atrioventricular Septal Defect

Rakhi Balachandran

Illustrations: Praveen Reddy Bayya

Reviewed by: R Krishna Kumar

■ INTRODUCTION

Atrioventricular (AV) septal defects include a spectrum of malformations caused by the deficiency of AV septum or endocardial cushions. Prevalence of full spectrum of AV septal defects is estimated to be 4.1/10,000 live births while complete AV septal defects constitute 2.2/10,000 live births.[1] Anatomically, the defect is classified into partial, and complete AV septal types. Partial AV septal defects are characterized by a primum atrial septal defect (ASD) and a cleft in the anterior leaflet of the mitral valve. Complete AV septal defects consist of interatrial and interventricular communications, and a common AV valve. Complete AV septal defects are further subdivided into Rastelli Type A, B and C based on the anatomy of the left superior bridging leaflet.[2] Trisomy 21 is an important association of AV septal defect and occurs in nearly 75% of patients with complete AV septal defect.[3] AV septal defects can also occur along with other cardiac defects such as patent ductus arteriosus (10%), tetralogy of Fallot (5%), double outlet right ventricle (2%), total anomalous pulmonary venous connection and transposition of great arteries. Complete AV septal defect is repaired in early infancy to prevent the development of hypertensive pulmonary vascular disease and progression of AV valve regurgitation. Complete AV septal defects with balanced ventricles are amenable for biventricular repair whereas extreme unbalanced ventricular morphology may necessitate single ventricle palliative operations. Surgical repair typically aims at restoration of two competent AV valves, closure of ventricular septal defect (VSD) and the primum ASD. Preservation of the conduction tissue during the repair is a challenging task for the surgeon since displacement of components of the conduction system from its usual anatomical locations is likely due to the absence of AV septum. Therefore, AV block is a potential complication in the postoperative period which can increase morbidity. With early primary repair and prevention of pulmonary hypertension, the operative mortality has declined to 3.2% in the current era.[4]

■ PREOPERATIVE ASSESSMENT

The anatomy of AV septal defect is relatively complex. It is important to be aware of the specifics of the preoperative anatomy, because it has an important bearing on the quality of postoperative repair. **Figures 1A and B** illustrate the anatomy before and after surgery. A checklist of the preoperative assessment of the anatomy is depicted in **Figure 2**.

■ MONITORING

Standard hemodynamic monitoring includes arterial blood pressure, central venous

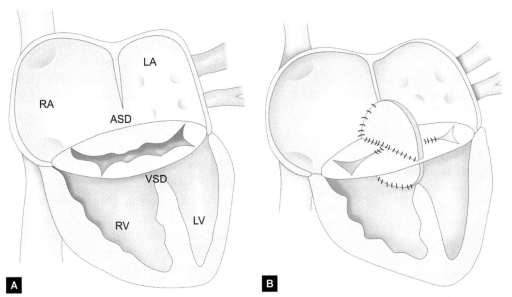

Figs. 1A and B: (A) Complete atrioventricular (AV) septal defect; (B) Anatomy after repair of complete AV septal defect.

(RA: right atrium; LA: left atrium; ASD: atrial septal defect; VSD: ventricular septal defect; RV: right ventricle; LV: left ventricle)

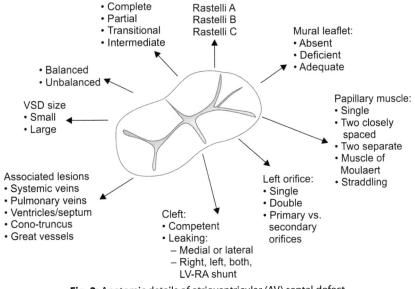

Fig. 2: Anatomic details of atrioventricular (AV) septal defect.

(VSD: ventricular septal defect; LV: left ventricle; RA: right atrium)

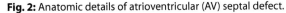

pressure (CVP), continuous ECG monitoring, pulse oximetry and capnography. With expertise in surgical repair, the practice of utilizing intracardiac lines (left atrial line/ pulmonary artery line) in the postoperative period has dramatically declined. Since heart block is an expected complication, it is worthwhile to obtain a baseline 6 lead ECG upon arrival in postoperative intensive care unit (ICU).

HEMODYNAMIC AND INOTROPE MANAGEMENT

- *Partial AV septal defect*: This repair is usually uncomplicated, and patients require mild/no inotropic support after separation from cardiopulmonary bypass (CPB). At our center, these patients usually receive dopamine or dobutamine at 5 µg/kg/min in the early postoperative period.
- *Complete AV septal defect*: This is a relatively complex repair. A postoperative screening echocardiogram is often performed to identify important residual defects such as interatrial or inter-ventricular communications or significant AV valve regurgitation/stenosis. Typically this is done in operating room (OR) itself after separation from bypass via the transesophageal probe or through epicardial screening echocardiography in small infants. The decision to reintervene can be taken immediately in the OR itself should the need arise. Pulmonary hypertension is relatively common in older patients and patients with Down syndrome. Prophylactic measures may be beneficial to prevent pulmonary hypertensive crisis in these high-risk subsets. However, it is worth mentioning that with early primary repairs and improved surgical skills this complication is becoming less frequent.[5] Most patients require only mild inotropic support and afterload reduction. Therefore, a combination of low dose epinephrine and milrinone is reasonable at separation from CPB. Aggressive volume loading

will be counterproductive as this might predispose to LV distension and AV valve regurgitation. Hypertension in the postoperative period should be vigorously treated to preserve suture lines and minimize afterload mismatch to the left ventricle. Afterload reduction with milrinone is often beneficial to avoid troublesome left AV valve regurgitation. Complete heart block is a potential complication as injury to the conduction system is possible due to the altered anatomical location. Typically, two atrial and two ventricular wires are placed before weaning from CPB. Complete heart block necessitates epicardial pacing in the early postoperative period. A dual chamber pacemaker should be available in the operating room and ICU for AV sequential pacing.

VENTILATION MANAGEMENT

- *Partial AV septal defect repair*: The repair is generally uncomplicated. These patients are candidates for early extubation.
- *Complete AV septal defect repair*: Typically, these patients are ventilated on the day of surgery due to young age, complexity of repair and longer duration of CPB. Patients who had an uncomplicated repair without any significant residual defects can be considered for extubation on postoperative day 1. A negative fluid balance is desirable during the periextubation period. Infants with pulmonary hypertension might require sedation and ventilation in the initial 24 hours to prevent pulmonary hypertensive crisis. Hypercarbia, acidosis and hypoxia should be avoided to prevent this complication. In patients who manifest pulmonary hypertension, important residual lesions should be aggressively sought for.

FLUID MANAGEMENT

- Standard fluid management protocol according to body surface area method should be followed.
- Volume boluses in infants, if required in the postoperative period, should be administered in small aliquots of 5–10 mL, carefully observing CVP and arterial blood pressure.
- Aggressive volume loading should be avoided, as sudden left ventricular distension can sometimes increase AV valve regurgitation or precipitate pulmonary edema in a patient with low ventricular compliance.

DIURETIC THERAPY

Typically, these patients are initiated on continuous infusion of furosemide at 1–2 mg/kg/day. A negative fluid balance of 25–50 mL/kg is desirable in young infants at the time of extubation to minimize fluid overload and pulmonary congestion.

PAIN AND SEDATION MANAGEMENT

Standard pain and sedation protocol are followed. Infants with Down syndrome are particularly difficult to sedate due to structural and functional alteration of opioid receptors.[5] They might require supplementation with dexmedetomidine infusion or intermittent doses of midazolam to prevent agitation during mechanical ventilation.

FEEDING AND NUTRITION

Feeding is initiated as per standard protocol. Patients are generally kept nil per oral (NPO) after surgery if planned for early extubation. Nasogastric or oral feeds are initiated 4 hours after extubation if deemed stable. In patients planned for overnight ventilation nasogastric feeds are typically started 4–6 hours after surgery and withheld thereafter in the periextubation period.

COMMON POSTOPERATIVE COMPLICATIONS

Pulmonary Hypertension[6]

This is a potential complication after AV septal defect repair especially in patients with

- Preoperative pulmonary hypertension
- Older age at the time of operation
- Patients with residual AV valve regurgitation/stenosis
- Residual VSD
- Down syndrome.

Such patients merit special attention to the following:

- Sedation and paralysis are reasonable for the first 12–24 hours in patients who are at risk for developing pulmonary hypertension in the postoperative period
- Follow the ventilator strategies to minimize factors which trigger increase in pulmonary vascular resistance.
- Deepen level of sedation before suctioning or other painful procedure in the ICU
- If pulmonary hypertension persists in the postoperative period, systematic evaluation is required to rule out important AV valve regurgitation, AV valve stenosis, or VSD.

Low Cardiac Output State

The common causes include residual AV valve regurgitation, residual VSD, ventricular dysfunction due to a large VSD patch, hemodynamically significant arrhythmia or pulmonary hypertension. It is vital to confirm the diagnosis by postoperative echocardiography.

Treatment Guidelines

Treatment should be directed at the cause.

- *Optimize afterload reduction*: It is reasonable to use afterload reducing agents such as milrinone or levosimendan in the early postoperative period. This may be switched to an orally administered agent such as enalapril after extubation.

- Inotropic support with dobutamine or epinephrine may sometimes be needed to improve contractility when there is ventricular dysfunction.
- Ensure AV synchrony by pacing if patient develops heart block.
- Aggressive volume loading should be avoided.
- Tapering of adrenergic agents is a reasonable strategy for reducing heart rate in patients with postoperative tachycardia and residual AV valve stenosis. Tachycardia impairs diastolic filling, elevates left atrial pressures and contribute to low cardiac output. Persistant tachycardia despite tapering inotropic supports may occasionally necessitate beta blocker therapy in postoperative period.
- It is reasonable to continue mechanical ventilatory support in patients with low cardiac output state till ventricular function recovers.
- If persistent hemodynamic instability exists with significant correctable residual lesion, surgical reintervention should be considered.

Arrhythmia

Postoperative period after AV septal defect repair may sometimes be complicated by arrhythmias such as AV blocks and junctional ectopic tachycardia. Arrhythmias resulting in loss of AV synchrony can adversely affect cardiac output and hence should be aggressively treated. Junctional ectopic tachycardia might require overdrive pacing, correction of electrolyte imbalances or pharmacological treatment with amiodarone or ivabradine. Heart blocks are often sequelae

of injury to an abnormally placed conduction system, during the course of surgical repair. In a large retrospective review of a spectrum of AV septal defect patients including both partial and complete types, pacemaker implantation was required in 7% patients for either AV block or sinus node dysfunction.[7] Down syndrome emerged as an independent predictor of need for pacemaker implantation.

General Guidelines

- Two atrial wires and two ventricular wires should be in place while separating from CPB
- A baseline ECG should be recorded upon arrival in ICU
- Dual chamber pacemaker with cables should be available at the bed side
- In patients who are already being paced for complete heart block, pacemaker settings and intrinsic rhythm should be reviewed on a daily basis along with clear documentation in patient records.
- If intrinsic rhythm has not recovered within 14 days, permanent pacemaker should be considered.

Facilitating LV Adaptation

In cases where an unbalanced or borderline left ventricle is considered for two ventricle repair, low cardiac output state can arise due to the smaller, less compliant left ventricle (LV) trying to adapt to the altered loading conditions. Reduction in afterload may be counterproductive in such situations. Careful titration of volume infusion while maintaining preload, optimizing heart rate to facilitate ventricular filling by preventing tachycardia, and maintenance of AV synchrony has obvious hemodynamic benefits. Selected patients may benefit from careful use of beta blockers. Non-invasive ventilatory strategies such as nasal continuous positive airway pressure (CPAP) or bilevel positive airway pressure (BiPAP) are often useful while separating these patients from mechanical ventilation since they facilitate adaptation of the systemic ventricle and reduce postextubation pulmonary edema.

■ DEINTENSIFICATION

Patients, who are extubated early, can be quickly weaned off inotropes and invasive lines. Oral feeding or breast feeding as appropriate to the age group is gradually established. In patients who have postoperative complications noninvasive ventilation and hemodynamic monitoring may be required for an extended period of time.

■ DISCHARGE MEDICATIONS

As these patients present with significant heart failure prior to surgery, diuretic therapy with furosemide is continued in postoperative period. Discharge medications are dictated by specific individual concerns. In the absence of residual lesions diuretics can be stopped at discharge.

■ REFERENCES

1. Reller MD, Strickland MJ, Riehle-Colarusso T, Mahle WT, Correa A. Prevalence of congenital heart defects in Metropolitan Atlanta, 1998-2005. J Pediatr. 2008;153:807-13.
2. Kouchukos NT, Blackstone EH, Hanley FL, Kirklin JK. Atrioventricular septal defect. In: Kirklin Barrat-Boyes Cardiac surgery, 4th edition. Philadelphia: Elsevier Saunders; 2013. pp. 1228-73.
3. Al Hay AA, MacNeill SJ, Yacoub M, Shore DF, Shinebourne EA. Complete atrioventricular septal defect, Down syndrome, and surgical outcome: risk factors. Ann Thorac Surg. 2003;75:412-21.
4. Jacobs JP, Mayer JE, Mavroudis C, O'Brien SM, Austin EH, Pasquali SK, et al. The Society of Thoracic Surgeons Congenital Heart Surgery Database 2016 Update on outcomes and quality. Ann Thorac Surg. 2016;101:850-62.
5. Pillchard J, Dadlani G, Andropoulos D. Intensive care and perioperative management of patients with complete atrioventricular septal defect. World J Pediatr Congenit Heart Surg. 2010;1:105-11.
6. Chang AC, Burke RP. Common atrioventricular canal. In: Chang AC, Hanley FL, Wernovsky G, Wessel DL (Eds). Pediatric Cardiac Intensive care. Philadelphia: Williams and Wilkins; 1998. pp. 271-287.
7. Di Mambro C, Calvieri C, Silvetti MS, Tamburri I, Giannico S, Baban A, et al. Brady arrhythmias in repaired atrioventricular septal defects: single centre experience based on 34 years of follow up of 522 patients. Pediatr Cardiol. 2018;39:1590-7.

Complete Repair of Tetralogy of Fallot with Pulmonary Stenosis

Rakhi Balachandran

Illustration: Praveen Reddy Bayya
Reviewed by: R Krishna Kumar

■ INTRODUCTION

Tetralogy of Fallot (TOF) is the most common cyanotic congenital heart defect beyond the neonatal period with a worldwide prevalence of 0.34 per 1,000 live births.[1] One of the reasons for its relative frequency is that among all the cyanotic heart defects, TOF has the best natural history often allowing survival beyond infancy. Survival is largely determined by the degree of pulmonary stenosis. Anatomically, the defect is characterized by anterior malalignment of the infundibular septum resulting in a subaortic ventricular septal defect (VSD) and varying degrees of right ventricular outflow tract obstruction (RVOTO). Aorta has a biventricular origin (overriding of Aorta). The pulmonary valve is variably dysplastic and the valve is often bicuspid with deformed leaflets. Pulmonary arterial tree may have varying degrees of hypoplasia. Right ventricular (RV) hypertrophy is the sequelae of outflow tract obstruction and unrestrictive blood flow across the large VSD. The anatomical features of TOF with pulmonary stenosis are illustrated in **Figure 1A.** Coronary artery anomalies or atrioventricular septal defects coexist in a few patients, which may pose additional surgical challenges. DiGeorge syndrome with microdeletion of q11 region of Chromosome 22 is a genetic substrate frequently associated with TOF, which can

potentially impact postoperative outcomes.[2] Other syndromes associated with TOF include, Trisomy 21, VACTERL, CHARGE, and Noonan's syndrome.[2] Associated congenital malformations such as tracheoesophageal fistula and anorectal malformations are also described in TOF. Although, the defect

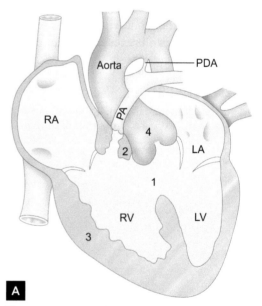

A

Fig. 1A: Tetralogy of Fallot. Note (1) the large VSD; (2) Anterior deviation of conal septum leading to a narrow RV outflow tract, small pulmonary annulus and pulmonary artery; (3) RV hypertrophy; (4) overriding of the aortic root into the RV. Aortic root is dilated and often a PDA and/or other collaterals may be found.

(RV: right ventricle; VSD: ventricular septal defect; PDA: patent ductus arteriosus ; LA: left atrium; RA: right atrium)

is typically addressed in most centers by complete repair at the age of 3–6 months[3] late presentation is common in low- and middle-income countries and corrective surgery may happen much later. Correction earlier than 3 months is reserved for selected patients with severe cyanosis or hypercyanotic spells. An earlier retrospective review had revealed longer time to extubation, longer intensive care unit (ICU) stay and hospital stay for patients operated before 3 months of age.[4]

Total correction of TOF classically includes closure of the VSD by a pericardial, dacron or polytetrafluoro ethylene (PTFE) patch and relief of RV outflow obstruction by infundibular resection, RV outflow patch or a transannular patch **(Fig. 1B)**. The evolution

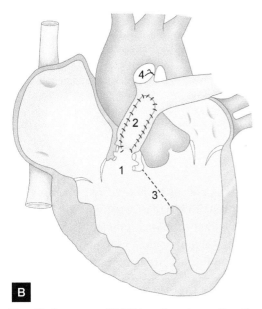

B

Fig. 1B: At surgery (1) RV bundles obstructing the outflow are either divided or excised; (2) RVOT, pulmonary annulus, and main PA are enlarged with a transannular patch; (3) VSD is closed; (4) PDA and other approachable large collaterals are occluded. The extent of intervention on the RV outflow depends on the location and severity of outflow obstruction.

(VSD: ventricular septal defect; RV: right ventricle; PDA: patent ductus arteriosus; RVOT: right ventricular outflow tract; PA: pulmonary artery)

of TOF repair to transatrial-transpulmonary approaches avoiding ventriculotomy has made a favorable impact on postoperative myocardial recovery.[5] A patent foramen ovale is often left behind to decompress the right ventricle and maintain cardiac output in some patients who are likely to develop postoperative low cardiac output state. In the last two decades, there has been a paradigm shift in the surgical techniques from complete relief of RV outflow obstruction permitting significant pulmonary regurgitation to aggressive preservation of pulmonary valve. Though valve sparing techniques are primarily directed at preventing the late complications of TOF repair such as RV dysfunction and life-threatening arrhythmias,[3,6,7] it also helps early postoperative recovery. With the expertise in pediatric cardiac surgery and intensive care, the current mortality of TOF repair in experienced centers is reported to be <1%.[8–10] In this chapter, we have given a brief overview of the postoperative management after complete repair of TOF with pulmonary stenosis.

■ PREOPERATIVE CONSIDERATIONS

It is important to be familiar with the precise anatomy of every patient who is to undergo corrective surgery. Seemingly small variations in anatomy have an important bearing on the surgical plans. **Table 1** summarizes the important anatomical variations in TOF and its relevance.

■ MONITORING

Standard hemodynamic monitoring includes continuous ECG monitoring, invasive arterial blood pressure monitoring, central venous pressure (CVP) monitoring, pulse oximetry, and capnography. Arterial blood gas analysis is performed every 4 hours till extubation and thereafter optimized to patient status.

TABLE 1: Anatomic variations in tetralogy of Fallot and their significance.

Structure	Common variation	Implications
Right ventricular outflow tract (RVOT)	Degree of stenosis at various levels: Infundibulum, valve, pulmonary annulus, main pulmonary artery (PA) bifurcation	Severe stenosis manifests early and may necessitate palliation in the newborn period; annular narrowing requires correction with a trans-annular patch with significant late sequelae; predominant stenosis of the valve may allow palliation with a balloon valvotomy in selected cases; alternatively stenting of the RVOT may need to be undertaken
Branch PAs	Stenosis of left pulmonary artery (LPA), absence of either branch PA, hypoplastic PAs	Small branch PA may not allow correction at an early age and palliation through a Blalock Taussig shunt or stenting of the RVOT may need to be undertaken, severe stenosis of LPA origin will need to be addressed at the time of surgery, absence of one branch PA may require the placement of a conduit, and ventilation perfusion considerations are important postoperatively
Pulmonary valve	Absent pulmonary valve with aneurysmal branch PAs	This results in a dramatically different manifestation. There is severe airway compression in the worst affected and the manifestations are essentially related to respiratory consequences.
Ventricular septal defect (VSD)	Extension of the VSD to the inlet or outlet septum, restrictive VSD with severe right ventricular hypertrophy and strain, additional muscular VSD	• Surgical approach needs to be tailored accordingly • Outflow extension of the VSD lowers the threshold for the placement of a trans-annular patch
Coronary arteries	Origin of left anterior descending artery from right coronary artery. This abnormal vessel may cross the RVOT	The abnormal vessel comes in the way of corrective surgery. If it is running along the pulmonary annulus and trans-annular patch is required, a conduit will need to be placed
Atrial communication	Atrial septal defects (ASD), patent foramen ovale (PFO)	While it is necessary to close an ASD, a PFO is often helpful in the early postoperative period. Many surgeons choose to leave it behind because it helps with early postoperative recovery
Aorto-pulmonary collaterals	Major aorto-pulmonary collaterals, minor bronchial collaterals	These collaterals will need to be clearly defined. They will need to be closed if their supply overlaps with the native PA supply

A baseline six lead electrocardiogram has to be recorded at admission to postoperative ICU due to the relatively high incidence of postoperative arrhythmias in this subset of patients.

HEMODYNAMIC AND INOTROPE MANAGEMENT

Key Postoperative Hemodynamic Goals

- To support RV function and to optimize the loading conditions of the RV.
- To monitor closely for postoperative arrhythmias and management.
- To diagnose and address residual/additional defects, if any.

The goal of hemodynamic management after repair of TOF is to support the RV function and to optimize preload and afterload to this chamber. Majority of patients with uncomplicated repair have a smooth postoperative recovery. These patients require minimum inotropic support. Usually, dopamine or dobutamine at 5 µg/kg/min will be adequate to support ventricular function. It is judicious to restrict the use of high doses of catecholamines to minimize the incidence of postoperative arrhythmias like junctional ectopic tachycardia (JET), which can compromise cardiac output by the loss of atrioventricular (AV) synchrony. Also, vigorous contraction of the myocardium induced by high doses of catecholamines may accentuate the dynamic component of RVOTO especially in the context of limited RV muscle resection in the current surgical era. Levosimendan or milrinone is sometimes administered in the rare patient with postoperative low cardiac output state due to left ventricular (LV) dysfunction. However, this is not absolutely essential for routine purposes. Milrinone increases the likelihood of postoperative tachyarrhythmias and should perhaps be administered with caution. Though liberal preloading of the hypertrophied RV had been the earlier strategy in the postoperative period to maintain adequate cardiac output, current valve sparing approaches and early age at corrective surgery do not mandate the need for aggressive volume loading in the postoperative period. Preload augmentation by fluid loading is guided by clinical indices of adequate cardiac output/tissue perfusion and targeting a specific "CVP cut off" is no longer the practice.

Maintenance of sinus rhythm and AV synchrony is of paramount importance in patients after TOF repair. This is to optimize the atrial contribution to ventricular filling especially in the setting of a hypertrophied RV or postoperative restrictive RV physiology with poor RV compliance. For this reason, JET needs to be managed aggressively.

Restrictive RV Physiology

A subset of patients with TOF may develop acute restrictive RV physiology in the postoperative period. This is characterized by increased RV end-diastolic pressure due to myocardial stiffness and poor compliance. Reduced compliance of the RV and poor filling results in high-systemic venous pressure predisposing to increased pleural effusions and low cardiac output. The mechanisms proposed include inadequate intraoperative myocardial protection of RV (due to its anterior location), down regulation of anti-oxidant defenses and free radical injury, severe iron loading of transferrin during cardio-pulmonary bypass (CPB) and postoperative oxidative stress.[11,12] The incidence of restrictive physiology has also been linked to duration of CPB and cross clamp times.[13] Recent studies have highlighted the use of transannular patch as an independent predictor of restrictive RV physiology.[12,13] A late diastolic antegrade pulmonary artery blood flow coincident with atrial systole on echocardiography (also known as Gatzoulis phenomenon) is an important marker of RV restrictive physiology.[14] Typically, the systolic function of RV is preserved and RV volumes are small. RV restriction can slow the postoperative recovery by contributing to low cardiac output, prolonging need for inotropes and ventilation, and predisposing to ascites and pleural effusions.[15] Measures, which can be potentially adopted to ameliorate this complication include optimizing myocardial protection during CPB, maintenance of an interatrial shunt, preservation of pulmonary valve function as much as feasible, maintenance of RV preload by optimal filling and drainage of pleural effusion and ascites.[13] Early extubation is desirable as early as feasible because spontaneous respiration improves trans-tricuspid flow and thus antegrade pulmonary blood flow by shortening the duration of pulmonary regurgitation.[15] However, in patients who need mechanical ventilation, use of shorter inspiratory times, and accepting lower tidal volumes [that allow maintenance of lowest feasible mean airway pressure (MAP)] are reasonable strategies for optimizing antegrade pulmonary blood flow.

■ FLUID MANAGEMENT

Maintenance fluid requirements are calculated as per standard body surface area method for patients undergoing surgery under CPB. Additional fluid bolus for replacement losses may be provided with crystalloids such as ringer lactate or normal saline solution. The use of fresh frozen plasma for volume expansion is no longer recommended. Fluid bolus for the treatment of hypovolemia is typically given at a dose of 5-10 mL/kg carefully monitoring the effect on CVP. An improvement in systolic blood pressure on compression of the liver margin may be used as a simple bedside test to elicit fluid responsiveness in the postoperative period.

DIURETIC THERAPY

It is important to recognize that the hypertrophied RV in patients with TOF is dependent on adequate preload. Agressive diuresis in these patients can be counterproductive as it is likely to decrease RV preload and hence cardiac output. Therefore, it is reasonable to delay the initiation of diuretic infusions for the first 8-12 hours after surgery. However, an infusion of furosemide at a lower dose of 1 mg/kg/day may be initiated afterward, if the patient has clinical signs suggestive of fluid overload.

PAIN AND SEDATION MANAGEMENT

The standard pain and sedation policy with fentanyl infusion and intermittent doses of midazolam are followed in these patients. Dexmedetomidine infusion at 0.25 µg/kg/hr is initiated in patients targeted for early extubation in the postoperative period to minimize opioid use. Beneficial effects of dexmedetomidine on prevention of postoperative tachyarrhythmias like JET have been previously described in pediatric cardiac surgical patients.[16,17]

VENTILATION MANAGEMENT

Most patients with uncomplicated intraoperative course and no residual defects are candidates for early extubation as this has obvious hemodynamic benefits including improved RV filling and cardiac output. In a recent analysis of Society of Thoracic surgeons (STS) database on early extubation after TOF repair and Fontan procedure, early extubation was performed in 31.5% of TOF repairs across 92 centers.[18] Early extubation in this analysis was associated with higher patient weight and fewer preoperative risk factors. In selected patients with important RV dysfunction and low cardiac output state, longer duration of ventilator support is sometimes required to decrease the work of breathing and support cardiac function. Spontaneous breathing increases venous return to heart by producing a combined decrease in right atrial pressure (P_{RA}) and an increase in intra-abdominal pressure due to diaphragmatic descent. The P_{RA} will remain low only if RV is compliant and its function remains normal. However, in the setting of RV dysfunction or poor RV compliance where P_{RA} remains high, the RV may not always be able to accommodate the increased preload brought about by the increased venous return during spontaneous respiration.[19] This will only bring about further increase in P_{RA} due to the inability to fill the stiff RV. Additionally, establishment of spontaneous respiration requires a substantial proportion of the cardiac output to be diverted to meet respiratory demands. In this select group of patients, it then becomes rational to continue mechanical ventilation till ventricular function and cardiac output improve. In patients on positive pressure ventilation, the ventilator strategies should aim at minimizing the MAP, decreasing inspiratory times and facilitating lower tidal volumes.[19,20] Maintaining low MAP will promote improved transpulmonary flow of blood which, in turn, is the main preload to the left heart. Pulmonary vascular resistance (PVR) is the chief determinant of RV afterload. PVR can increase at lung volumes above and below functional residual capacity (FRC). Avoiding alveolar hyperinflation by choosing lower tidal volumes of 6–8 mL/kg and minimizing atelectasis by judicious use of positive end expiratory pressure (PEEP) can prevent dramatic alterations in PVR produced by fluctuations in the lung volumes.

■ FEEDING AND NUTRITION

Patients who undergo early extubation are typically initiated on nasogastric/oral feeds 3–4 hours after extubation, if remaining stable without any airway complications. Feeding is initiated with clear fluids and later transitioned to expressed breast milk/infant formula/blend diet depending on the age of the infant.

■ COMMON COMPLICATIONS IN POSTOPERATIVE PERIOD

Although, the typical course after TOF repair is uncomplicated, it is essential to be familiar with common postoperative complications.

Postoperative Bleeding

Patients with cyanotic congenital heart disease and associated secondary erythrocytosis frequently have coagulation abnormalities due to a decrease in coagulation factor levels, thrombocytopenia and increased fibrinolytic mechanisms.[21] Hence, patients with TOF who present late with progressive cyanosis are particularly at risk for increased postoperative bleeding. Close monitoring for increased postoperative drainage and rational use of blood products guided by point of care coagulation tests like thromboelastography is beneficial.

Arrhythmias

Hemodynamically significant arrhythmias have been reported in 12% of TOF patients mostly in the first 24 hours.[22] Right bundle branch block with a change in QRS configuration is usually seen in postoperative period as a sequelae of right ventriculotomy and trauma to right bundle branch or proximal conducting system. It is necessary to obtain an ECG soon after patient is received in the ICU after surgery to document the postsurgical baseline. JET is a frequent arrhythmia, which has been reported in surgeries occurring in the vicinity of AV node and proximal conduction system such as VSD closure and RV outflow tract resection.[23] JET has been reported as frequently as 29% in patients undergoing repair of TOF in some series.[24] In a retrospective review of 322 patients undergoing correction of TOF, younger age, higher preoperative heart rate, avoidance of beta-blockers, and low serum magnesium/calcium levels were independent predictors of JET.[24] Avoidance of electrolyte imbalances, minimizing the dose of catecholamines and prevention of hyperpyrexia in the postoperative period are important measures to decrease the incidence of JET. The use of dexmedetomidine for sedation and prophylactic administration of magnesium before termination of CPB have been described for prevention of postoperative JET.[16,25,26]

Low Cardiac Output State

This refers to a reduction in cardiac output that can potentially occur in the postoperative period after corrective surgery for congenital heart disease. This is a well-recognized phenomenon that typically manifests 9–12 hours after surgery.[27] Low cardiac output state is usually diagnosed by invasive hemodynamic monitoring and clinical indicators of poor systemic perfusion like cool extremities, feeble peripheral pulses, decreased urine output, hyperlactatemia, and metabolic acidosis. CVP is usually high (up to 14–16 mm Hg) and may go up further with volume challenge especially in patients with hypertrophied RV. A low PO$_2$ in arterial blood gas is often suggestive of a right to left shunt across the interatrial communication. Patients with postoperative restrictive RV physiology or RV dysfunction are more likely to develop this complication.[15] Suboptimal myocardial protection and intraoperative myocardial injury, effects of right ventriculotomy or muscle resection and significant pulmonary regurgitation are some of the proposed etiological factors for poor RV performance after tetralogy repair.[28] As a consequence of right heart failure, hepatomegaly and third space effusions with ascites and increased pleural drainage may be evident within 48 hours. Other causes of low cardiac output state include hemodynamically significant arrhythmias with loss of AV synchrony, residual defects like RVOTO or residual VSDs, or concomitant LV dysfunction. Diagnosis of specific complications is confirmed by echocardiography.

Management

- Optimize inotropic therapy with epinephrine and milrinone/levosimendan.
- Continue mechanical ventilation to decrease stress and myocardial work.
- Maintain adequate preload to right ventricle.
- Diagnose and treat arrhythmias like JET. Maintenance of sinus rhythm and AV synchrony assumes an important part in maintaining adequate cardiac output.
- Diagnose and treat residual defects, if any.
- Drain significant third space effusions by pleural drains or peritoneal dialysis catheter, if required.
- Initiate peritoneal dialysis if oliguria persists despite optimizing preload and use of diuretic therapy.

Residual or Previously Undiagnosed Defects

Residual lesions are not uncommon after complete repair of TOF. Residual/additional VSD, RVOTO, branch pulmonary artery stenosis, severe pulmonary regurgitation, or a previously undiagnosed aortopulmonary collateral are all likely problems, which can be encountered in the postoperative period. The diagnosis is confirmed by echocardiography in most instances. However, cardiac catheterization and angiography is required when aortopulmonary collaterals are suspected. Treatment is dictated by the type and magnitude of the residual lesion. Pulmonary regurgitation and residual VSD may be poorly tolerated as the resulting volume overload will further compromise the preoperatively pressure overloaded RV. Small VSDs might be addressed with afterload reducing agents like milrinone or levosimendan to decrease the magnitude of shunt across the VSD. Significant VSD causing low cardiac output or extubation failure may necessitate a return to OR/cardiac catheterization laboratory to address the defect. RVOTO may be evident by auscultation and echocardiography. Mild obstruction is typically well-tolerated and requires maintenance of adequate preload and avoiding high dose of inotropes. Hemodynamically significant obstruction with low cardiac output state might require reintervention.

Significant aortopulmonary collaterals may sometimes manifest as pulmonary hemorrhage.[29] Postoperatively, these patients might have varying degrees of bleeding from the endotracheal tube, increased peak airway pressure, radiological evidence of lung hemorrhage, or may have an unexpected failed extubation. Increased left atrial blood return during CPB should raise the suspicion of significant aortopulmonary collateral.

Diagnosis is confirmed by cardiac catheterization and early intervention by coil embolization of the major collaterals is required to facilitate extubation and postoperative recovery.[30]

Postoperative Stridor

Postextubation stridor should be anticipated in TOF with Down syndrome or DiGeorge syndrome due to inherent airway abnormalities in these patients. This usually manifest within an hour of extubation. Mild stridor can be managed with nebulized epinephrine, inhaled steroids and keeping the patient calm and quiescent. Severe stridor may necessitate noninvasive ventilation with nasal bilevel positive airway pressure (BiPAP) or reintubation.

■ DEINTENSIFICATION

Patients who are extubated early with an uncomplicated course can be quickly weaned off inotropic supports and de-intensified. Oral/nasogastric feeds are initiated 3–4 hours after extubation. Intercostal drains may be retained longer in patients who have low cardiac output state or those with significant pulmonary regurgitation, as they can develop effusion in the later postoperative period.

■ DISCHARGE MEDICATIONS

Patients with significant pulmonary valve regurgitation or RV dysfunction post operatively might require diuretic therapy with furosemide for a variable period after discharge.

■ REFERENCES

1. Van der Linde D, Konings EM, Slager MA, Witzenberg M, Helbing W, Takkenberg JM, et al. Birth prevalence of congenital heart disease worldwide. A systematic review and meta-analysis. J Am Coll Cardiol. 2011;58:2241-7.
2. Michielon G, Marino B, Formigar R, Gargiulo G, Picchio F, Digilio MC, et al. Genetic syndromes and outcome after surgical correction of tetralogy of Fallot. Ann Thorac Surg. 2006;81:968-75.
3. Aplitz C, Webb GD, Redington AN. Tetralogy of Fallot. Lancet. 2009;374:1462-71.
4. Van Arsdell GS, Maharaj GS, Tom J, Rao VK, Coles JG, Freedom RM. What is the optimal age for repair of tetralogy of Fallot? Circulation. 2000;102:III123-9.
5. Karl TR. Tetralogy of Fallot: current surgical perspective. Ann Pediatr Cardiol. 2008;1:93-100.
6. Ito H, Ota N, Murata M, Tosaka Y, Ide Y, Tachi M, et al. Technical modification enabling pulmonary valve sparing repair of a severely hypoplastic annulus in patients with tetralogy of Fallot. Interact Cardiovasc Thorac Surg. 2013;16:802-7.
7. Bacha E. Valve sparing options in tetralogy of Fallot surgery. Semin Thorac Cardiovasc Surg Pediatr Card Surg Ann. 2012;15:24-6.
8. Karl TR, Stocker C. Tetralogy of Fallot and its variants. Pediatr Crit Care Med. 2016;17: s330-6.
9. Jacobs JP, Mayer JE, Mavroudis C, O'Brien SM, Austin EH, Pasquali SK, et al. The Society of Thoracic Surgeons Congenital Heart Surgery Database: 2016 Update on outcomes and quality. Ann Thorac Surg. 2016;101:850-62.
10. Egbe AC, Mittnacht AJ, Nguyen K, Joashi U. Risk factors for morbidity in infants undergoing tetralogy of Fallot repair. Ann Pediatr cardiol. 2014;1:13-8.
11. Chaturvedi RR, Shore DF, Lincoln C, Mumby S, Kemp M, Brierly J, et al. Acute right ventricular restrictive physiology after repair of tetralogy of Fallot: association with myocardial injury and oxidative stress. Circulation. 1999;100: 1540-7.
12. Sachdev MS, Bhagyavathy A, Varghese R, Coelho R, Kumar RS. Right ventricular dysfunction after tetralogy of Fallot. Pediatr Cardiol. 2006;27:250-5.
13. Sandeep B, Huang X, Xu F, Su P, Wang T, Sun X. Etiology of right ventricular restrictive physiology early after repair of tetralogy of Fallot in pediatric patients. J Cardiothoracic Surg. 2019;14:84-92.
14. Gatzoulis MA, Clarke AL, Cullen S, Newman CGH, Redington AN. Right ventricular diastolic dysfunction 15-35 years after repair of tetralogy of Fallot: restrictive physiology predicts superior exercise performance. Circulation. 1995;91:1775-81.
15. Cullen S, Shore D, Redington A. Characterisation of right ventricular diastolic performance

after complete repair of tetralogy of Fallot. Circulation. 1995;91:1782-9.

16. El Amrousy D, El Shmaa NS, El-Kashlan M, Hassan S, Elsanosy M, Hablas N, et al. Efficacy of prophylactic dexmedetomidine in preventing postoperative junctional ectopic tachycardia after pediatric cardiac surgery. J Am Heart Assoc. 2017;6:e004780.

17. El-Shmaa NS, El Amrousy D, El Feky W. The efficacy of pre-emptive dexmedetomidine versus amiodarone in preventing postoperative junctional ectopic tachycardia in pediatric cardiac surgery. Ann Card Anaesth. 2016;19:614-20.

18. Mahle WT, Jacobs JP, Jacobs ML, Kim S, Kirshbom PM, Pasquali SK, et al. Early extubation after repair of tetralogy of Fallot and the Fontan procedure: an analysis of The Society of Thoracic Surgeons Congenital Heart Surgery Database. Ann Thorac Surg. 2016;102:850-8.

19. Gomez H, Pinsky MR. Effect of mechanical ventilation on heart lung interactions. In: Tobin MJ (Ed). Principles and Practice of Mechanical Ventilation, 3rd edition. New York: Mc Graw–Hill Medical; 2013. pp. 821-49.

20. Aronson LA, Dent CL. Postoperative respiratory function and its management. In: Lake C, Booker PD (Eds). Pediatric Cardiac Anesthesia, 4th edition. Philadelphia: Lippincott Williams and Wilkins; 2005. pp. 682-704.

21. Tempe D, Virmani S. Coagulation abnormalities in patients with cyanotic congenital heart disease. J Cardiothorac Vasc Anaesth. 2002;16:752-65.

22. Yildirim SV, Tokel K, Saygili B, Varan B. The incidence and risk factors of arrythmias in the early period after cardiac surgery in pediatric patients. Turk J Pediatr. 2008;50:549-53.

23. Cools E, Missant C. Junctional ectopic tachycardia after congenital heart surgery Acta Anaesth Belg. 2014;65:1-8.

24. Ismail MF, Arafat AA, Hamouda TE, El Tantawy AE, Edrees A, Bogis A, et al. Junctional ectopic tachycardia following tetralogy of Fallot repair in children under 2 years. J Cardiothoracic Surg. 2018;13:60.

25. Prajapati M, Patel J, Pandya H, Patel H. Magnesium supplementation during cardiopulmonary bypass to prevent junctional ectopic tachycardia after pediatric TOF surgery-A randomised controlled study. Int J Biomed Adv Res. 2015;6:584-8.

26. He D, Sznycer-Taub N, Cheng Y, Mc Carter R, Jonas RA, Hanumanthaiah S, Moak JP. Magnesium lowers the incidence of postoperative junctional ectopic tachycardia in congenital heart surgical patients: is there a relationship to surgical procedure complexity? Pediatr Cardiol. 2015;36:1179-85.

27. Wernovsky G, Wypij D, Jonas RA. Postoperative course and hemodynamic profile after arterial switch operation in neonates and infants: a comparison of low-flow cardiopulmonary bypass and circulatory arrest. Circulation. 1995;92:2226-35.

28. Spray TL, Wernovsky G. Right ventricular outflow obstruction. In: Chang AC, Hanley FL, Wernovsky G, Wessel DL (Eds). Pediatric Cardiac Intensive Care. Baltimore: Williams and Wilkins; 1998. pp. 257-65.

29. Makhija N, Magoon R, Choudhary M, Ramakrishnan S. Bleeding in the lung complicates a routine intracardiac repair: what went wrong? Ann Card Aanesth. 2018;21:78-81.

30. Kumpf M, Schaffer J, Hofbeck M. Recurrent pulmonary haemorrhage in an infant with tetralogy of Fallot and absent pulmonary valve: interventional treatment by coil occlusion of systemic to pulmonary collateral arteries. Cardiol Young. 2013;23:443-6.

Unifocalization for Tetralogy of Fallot with Pulmonary Atresia and Major Aortopulmonary Collaterals

Aveek Jayant, Thushara Madathil
Illustrations: Praveen Reddy Bayya
Reviewed by: R Krishna Kumar

■ INTRODUCTION

Major aortopulmonary collateral arteries (MAPCA) (by definition, systemic arteries terminating in the pulmonary vascular bed) can be present in many congenital heart disease (CHD) conditions including some in which the heart is functionally single ventricle. However, by far the index condition they are often linked to is Tetralogy of Fallot with pulmonary atresia (ToF-PA). About 10% of children with a diagnosis of ToF have ToF-PA. In up to one-third of children with ToF-PA there is no ductus arteriosus, abnormal native pulmonary arteries and, intrinsically these children have a large proportion of their pulmonary vascular bed supplied by MAPCAs. Other children with ToF-PA may have relatively well formed pulmonary arteries, a ductus arteriosus, varying number of MAPCAs (some may have no significant MAPCAs as well) and are relatively spared from having distal pulmonary artery (PA) arborization abnormalities. Three distinct pulmonary artery variants are described in this condition:

1. Confluent right and left pulmonary arteries supplied by an arterial duct
2. Confluent intrapericardial pulmonary arteries coexisting with MAPCAs
3. No intrapericardial pulmonary arteries

Obviously, the most favorable situation is the first, while the most complicated management strategy is reserved for the last of the above categories. In type 2, the actual distribution of the confluent pulmonary arteries is variable, but it is generally taken for granted that if a reasonably confluent pulmonary artery is seen, about two-thirds of the lung parenchyma does have a native pulmonary artery supply. In most cases of this kind, it is also usual that most segments have a supply either from the MAPCA or the native pulmonary artery though there are many exceptions and every patient has an individualized anatomic pattern that needs to be evaluated before surgery.

It is important for intensivists to be aware of these preoperative details as these are crucial to the postoperative care of these children and often contribute in large measure to the postoperative right ventricular pressure, a clear arbiter of outcomes. The overarching principles of management for this subset of patients have been laid down by groups of surgeons from Stanford,[2] Texas[4] and Melbourne.[1] The Stanford approach involves early surgery irrespective of symptom status, incorporation of the maximum number of segments into the unifocalization pathway, relieving any obstruction in the collateral arteries till the segmental level and using native tissue in the process of pulmonary arterial repair as far as possible.[2,3]

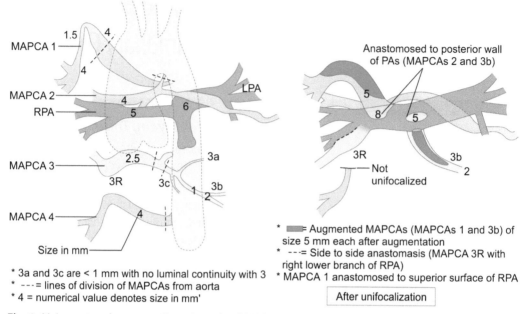

* 3a and 3c are < 1 mm with no luminal continuity with 3
* ---= lines of division of MAPCAs from aorta
* 4 = numerical value denotes size in mm'

Anastomosed to posterior wall of PAs (MAPCAs 2 and 3b)

3R — Not unifocalized

* = Augmented MAPCAs (MAPCAs 1 and 3b) of size 5 mm each after augmentation
* ---= Side to side anastomasis (MAPCA 3R with right lower branch of RPA)
* MAPCA 1 anastomosed to superior surface of RPA

After unifocalization

Fig. 1: Major aortopulmonary collateral arteries (MAPCAs) and status post unifocalization. A right ventricle-pulmonary artery conduit or systemic to pulmonary artery shunt is used to provide the pulmonary blood flow after unifocalizing the MAPCAs.

(RPA: right pulmonary artery; LPA: left pulmonary artery)

A schematic representation of the preoperative anatomy in a patient with ToF-PA with MAPCAs and the surgical repair performed is illustrated in **Figure 1**.

It should also be made clear that most of the details in the description to follow are with reference to ToF-PA and not pulmonary atresia with intact ventricular septum or other conditions with coincident presence of MAPCAs. Therefore, for functional purposes, all patients in this description also have a non-restrictive ventricular septal defect (VSD).

All patients should also be specifically assessed clinically and for the presence of 22q11 deletion syndrome by the fluorescent in-situ hybridization (FISH) test as this has important prognostic impact in postoperative course and management. A systematic airway analysis[1] using clinical symptoms and cardiac tomography is also advocated by the Stanford group. At present, unless neonates have a saturation range <75% or >90% with this condition they undergo single stage unifocalization at the age of 4–7 months; other indications for neonatal surgery are— (1) the presence of an unilateral duct to one of the pulmonary arteries, its counterpart being supplied by MAPCAs; and (2) when there is good pulmonary artery confluence and arborization to all lung segments but with dual supply additionally from MAPCAs.[5]

The major intraoperative considerations for postoperative intensive care stem from one or the other of the following technical parts of the operation:

- Long durations often mean scope for large volume fluid shifts, bleeding and need for blood products.
- Although majority of the dissection of MAPCAs is performed off pump sometimes this is not feasible and there may be an additional lengthy bypass run as well.

- Extensive dissection can often damage neural structures, including the phrenic and left recurrent laryngeal nerve—function must be assessed when indicated.
- Details of the intraoperative flow simulation study and the results with respect to the mean pulmonary artery pressure (mPAP) is relevant to determine whether the patient proceeds to complete repair, requires an open VSD or a systemic—pulmonary artery shunt. In this study while on cardiopulmonary bypass (CPB), pump flow rates are gradually raised to 3 L/min/m^2 and it is determined whether or not the mPAP < 25–30 mm Hg.
- In many cases at Stanford left atrial and pulmonary artery pressure lines are placed under direct surgical vision for postoperative monitoring.

▉ MONITORING

In addition to invasive measurements of right atrial pressure and arterial blood pressure we routinely use continuous electrocardiography, dual site temperature, pulse oximetry, and intermittently obtain arterial blood gases. The occasional patient has capnometric assessment of ventilation. The Stanford group advocates monitoring of pulmonary artery and left atrial pressures via lines placed surgically and brought out through the chest wall. Given our low volumes in this subset it should suffice to state that while we do not do this routinely we should consider using these advanced monitors (not without risk) as and when we perform the most extensive unifocalization procedures.

▉ MANAGEMENT

Hemodynamic Management and Inotropes

At our center, we predominantly use hand-made conduits designed from bovine pericardium; a small fraction of integrated valved conduits are also used. Since the mainstay of this surgery is based on recruiting the maximum volume of pulmonary vascular bed and obliterating all anatomic stenoses in this pathway, most patients are expected to separate from CPB at low right ventricular pressures ($P_{RV}/P_{LV} < 0.5$). If these pressures are higher, the entire approach to management is primarily surgical and often decided based on a flow simulation study performed on CPB; in such cases there is often a decision to either fenestrate the ventricular septal defect patch or, in some cases, the VSD is left open, and, yet in others a shunt is performed deferring primary repair. As such, it is usual to use small doses of milrinone and adrenaline at our center to assist bypass separation and in the immediate postoperative period. There is increasing use of levosimendan ostensibly because it is less arrhythmogenic though clinical evidence for this is at best, nominal. The other rationale for minimizing inotrope use is to prevent the occurrence of junctional ectopic tachycardia (JET) with its attendant adverse effects on hemodynamics. Priority is also given to readjusting the doses in use to the lowest clinically useful dose or cessation altogether in the postoperative period.

Given the nature of the incisions considerable attention should be paid to pain management, since this can contribute to sympathetic activation and predisposition to JET. Most patients receive fentanyl and dexmedetomidine to begin with in addition to paracetamol. Other units increasingly use some regional anesthesia adjuncts but these are not yet used at our center.

Blood and Fluid Management

Given the extensive nature of dissection and the length of surgery most patients receive a full component of hemostatic blood products (plasma, platelet concentrates and cryoprecipitate) in the operating room on prophylactic basis. Similar aliquots are administered in the ICU, should there be clinical bleeding or an abnormal thromboelastogram. Fluid prescriptions are usually as appropriate for age and body size, with the caveat that should there be a reperfusion lung injury, an excessive fluid balance (from hemostatic and fluid resuscitation intraprocedure and immediate postprocedure) or a congestive hepatomegaly, fluid is restricted. In the case of reperfusion lung injury fluid restriction clearly appears to shorten the time to separate from mechanical ventilation.

Ventilatory Management

Mechanical ventilation is tailored to help the stressed right ventricle, using the simple principle that the lowest pulmonary vascular resistance accrues at the functional residual capacity. Positive end-expiratory pressure (PEEP) values are tailored to the presence of lung collapse and reperfusion lung injury [the latter requires critical vigilance to lung protection so as to prevent a second insult which could result in full blown acute lung injury (ALI)/acute respiratory distress syndrome (ARDS)]. This includes judicious restriction of fluids, PEEP and titration of fractional concentration of oxygen to the lowest clinically acceptable saturation. From the clinical course quoted by the Stanford group, it seems that while subclinical reperfusion pulmonary edema is common in this group of patients it does not alter the clinical course and duration of mechanical ventilation in most patients.[6] Most patients are extubated on the first postoperative day and patients with overtly wet lungs transition through a period of continuous positive airway pressure (CPAP) therapy. Selected patients with larger areas of pulmonary edema or residual stenosis of unifocalized collaterals and resultant ventilation perfusion mismatch will require ventilation beyond 24 hours.

■ COMMON COMPLICATIONS

- Major complications arise from an inability to perform the procedure according to the preoperative plan: This may include an inability to perform the primary repair and ending up with a systemic-pulmonary artery shunt. Even with the aggressive approach from the Stanford group some children will need repeated catheter and surgical procedures for revision unifocalization. However, that particular group with its available resources is still demonstrating excellent outcomes, but low resource groups should also be aware of the practical limits on resource use. Hence, it is more essential that this surgery is only offered to such patients in whom resource use and the need for extensive procedures is assessed comprehensively in the preoperative period.
- Pulmonary reperfusion injury is a frequent occurrence and has been described in as many as 70% of patients.[6] However, in most forms it is mild and self-limiting and resolves with ventilatory support.
- Damage to adjacent neural structures, particularly the phrenic nerve can happen and should be assessed in the event of extubation failure or clinical suspicion either on ultrasound or fluoroscopy.
- Extubation failures are not uncommon and can occur due to a combination of poor lung function, airway dysfunction and sometimes even pain.
- Junctional ectopic tachycardia can occur although with preventive measures the anecdotal incidence has decreased, standard therapies such as cooling, retitration of inotropes and sometimes use of amiodarone is required. Ivabradine has recently been used with some effect.

- Catheter rehabilitation to enlarge the pulmonary bed or to gain better understanding of pulmonary hemodynamics within the first few postoperative days has rarely been required.

■ REFERENCES

1. Asija R, Ma M, Wise-Faberowski L, Presnell L, Anderson RH, McElhinney DB, et al. Tetralogy of Fallot with pulmonary atresia. In: Wernovsky G, Anderson RH, Kumar RK, Mussato KA, Redington A, Twedell JS, et al. (Eds). Anderson's Paediatric Cardiology, 4th edition. Philadelphia: Elsevier; 2019.

2. Reddy VM, Liddicoat JR, Hanley FL. Midline one stage complete unifocalisation and repair of pulmonary atresia with ventricular septal defect and major aortopulmonary collaterals. J Thorac Cardiovasc Surg. 1995;109:832-45.

3. Pawade A, Capuani A, Penny DJ, Karl TR, Mee RB. Pulmonary atresia with intact ventricular septum: surgical management based on right ventricular infundibulum. J Card Surg. 1993;8:371-83.

4. Duncan BW, Mee RB, Prieto LR, Rosenthal GL, Mesia CI, Quereshi AP, et al. Staged repair of tetralogy of Fallot with pulmonary atresia and major aortopulmonary collateral arteries. J Thorac Cardiovasc Surg. 2003;126:694-702.

5. Bauser-Heaton H, Borquez A, Han B, Ladd M, Asija R, Downey L, et al. Programmatic approach to management of Tetralogy of Fallot with major aortopulmonary collateral arteries. A 15-year experience with 458 patients. Circ Cardiovasc Interv. 2017;10:e004952.

6. Asija R, Koth AM, Velasquez N, Chan FP, Perry SB, Hanley FL, et al. Postoperative outcomes of children with tetralogy of Fallot, pulmonary atresia and major aortopulmonary collaterals undergoing reconstruction of occlude pulmonary artery branches. Ann Thorac Surg. 2016;101:2329-34.

Repair of Total Anomalous Pulmonary Venous Connection

Rakhi Balachandran

Illustrations: Praveen Reddy Bayya

Reviewed by: R Krishna Kumar

◼ INTRODUCTION

Total anomalous pulmonary venous connection (TAPVC) is a cyanotic congenital cardiac defect characterized by failure of all four pulmonary veins to connect normally to the left atrium. Instead, they drain anomalously to the right atrium via various alternative routes. Based on the site of anomalous drainage of the pulmonary veins, TAPVC exists as four different anatomical variants namely, supracardiac (45%; **Fig. 1A**), cardiac (25%; **Fig. 1C**), infracardiac (20%; **Fig. 1B**) and mixed (10%). The four pulmonary veins usually join to form a common pulmonary venous sinus, which connects via a vertical vein to the anomalous site of drainage. An atrial septal defect is essential for survival. Pulmonary venous obstruction (PVO) is often an important coexisting condition, which can lead to presentation in the early neonatal period with critical cardiopulmonary instability. The infracardiac variant is the most common type associated with PVO, and necessitates emergency surgery as a life-saving measure. Prolonged preoperative stabilization offers little benefit in these critically ill neonates as delay in surgery can aggravate pulmonary edema and pulmonary hypertension.[1] The patients with TAPVC have an inherent risk for pulmonary hypertension either due to PVO or due to increased pulmonary blood flow.

Surgical correction involves anastomosis of the common pulmonary venous chamber to the morphological left atrium under cardio-pulmonary bypass (CPB) thus redirecting the pulmonary venous blood into the left atrium. An important association of TAPVC is its occurrence as a part of heterotaxy syndromes or with a single ventricle anatomy, both of which can increase the complexity of surgical repair and adversely impact postoperative outcomes.[2,3] With advances in surgical techniques, early diagnosis and surgery, and improvement in postoperative care the overall outcomes of TAPVC in the current era have remarkably improved.[4,5] In a large retrospective review of 768 patients younger age at repair, infracardiac and mixed anatomic variants, preoperative PVO, longer CPB times and longer duration of ventilation was associated with increased mortality.[5] Post-repair PVO is a troublesome complication which challenges long-term survival. The sutureless technique for TAPVC rerouting has been reported to have reduced rates of PVO.[5,6] In this chapter, we describe the postoperative management of TAPVC without any coexistent cardiac malformation other than atrial septal defect or patent ductus arteriosus. **Figures 2A and B** depict anatomy of a supracardiac TAPVC and the anatomy after surgical repair, respectively.

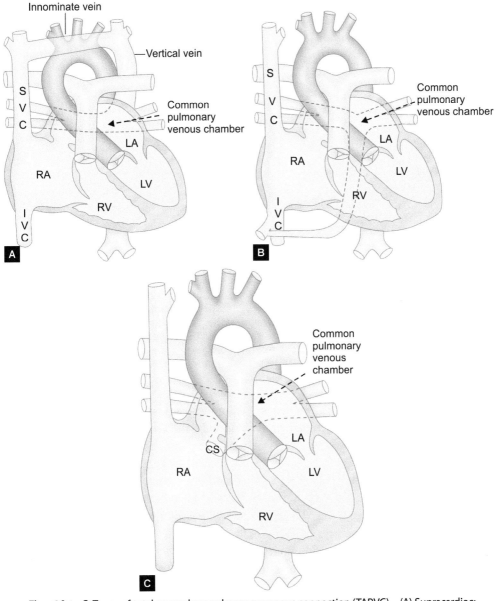

Figs. 1A to C: Types of total anomalous pulmonary venous connection (TAPVC)—(A) Supracardiac; (B) Infracardiac; (C) Cardiac.

(IVC: inferior vena cava; LA: left atrium; LV: left ventricle; RA: right atrium; RV: right ventricle; SVC: superior vena cava; CS: coronary sinus)

■ MONITORING

Standard monitoring includes invasive arterial blood pressure, central venous pressure (CVP), continuous ECG monitoring, pulse oximetry and capnography. Pulmonary arterial (PA) pressure monitoring via a catheter placed intraoperatively into the PA may be beneficial in critically ill neonates with severe

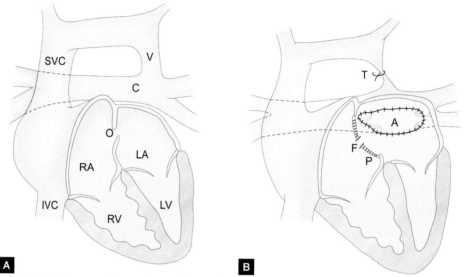

Figs. 2A and B: (A) Supracardiac total anomalous pulmonary venous connection (TAPVC): The pulmonary veins form a common chamber (C) behind the heart which drains via the vertical vein (V) into the innominate vein and hence right atrium (RA). This leads to dilated right heart, and a patent foramen ovale (O) or atrial septal defect (ASD) is essential for survival. The left atrium (LA) and left ventricle (LV) are small; (B) Postoperative anatomy after TAPVC repair: At surgery a large anastomosis (A) is created between the common chamber and posterior LA wall. The LA is enlarged by replacing the interatrial septum with a patulous pericardial patch (P) with a fenestration (F) to tide over pulmonary hypertensive crisis. Vertical vein is tied (T) after weaning off bypass

(SVC: superior vena cava; IVC: inferior vena cava; RV: right ventricle)

pulmonary hypertension,[4] but this practice is fast declining with early surgical repair and shorter bypass times in the current era.

HEMODYNAMIC AND INOTROPE MANAGEMENT

Hemodynamic status depends on the preoperative state of the patient, site of anomalous pulmonary venous drainage, pulmonary venous anatomy and presence of important PVO. Stable preoperative patients with no PVO need only minimal inotropic support. Either dopamine or dobutamine at 5 µg/kg/min will be sufficient. Critically ill patients with PVO, pulmonary hypertension, and right ventricular (RV) dysfunction may additionally require epinephrine. While there is no clear physiological basis for the use of milrinone, it continues to be used, perhaps, as a force of habit. Correction of TAPVC results in acute volume overload on the preoperatively underfilled left atrium and left ventricle. The non-compliant left atrium is poorly adapted to receive large fluid volumes, which can sometimes precipitate pulmonary edema. Hence, postoperative fluid administration should be titrated to small aliquots, or as continuous infusions in syringe pumps. The second hemodynamic concern is the high propensity for pulmonary hypertension secondary to the preoperative pulmonary hypertension, endothelial dysfunction following CPB and any coexistent substrate for PVO. Inhaled nitric oxide may be beneficial for separation from CPB in neonates with preoperative evidence of PVO.[1]

FLUID STRATEGY

Restricted fluid strategy should be followed based on preoperative status and possibility of pulmonary congestion. This is achieved by daily fluid prescriptions based on body surface area method typically followed in open heart surgery under CPB. A negative fluid balance of 30–50 mL/kg is desirable at the time of extubation.

◼ DIURETIC THERAPY

A negative fluid balance with aggressive diuresis will help to minimize pulmonary congestion, reduce extravascular lung water and thus improve lung compliance in patients with preoperative PVO. A continuous infusion of furosemide at 1–2 mg/kg/day after an initial bolus of 1 mg/kg is reasonable in the early postoperative period to prevent fluid overload. Continuous infusion should be transitioned to intermittent bolus doses after extubation and deintensification.

◼ PAIN AND SEDATION MANAGEMENT

Patients with early postoperative pulmonary hypertension are vulnerable to sympathetic stimulation and stress response. Administration of opiates, sedatives or muscle relaxants is recommended for reducing postoperative stress response and the risk of pulmonary hypertensive crisis.[7] Fentanyl infusion is typically preferred in the early postoperative period due to its potent analgesic effect and maintenance of cardiovascular stability. Additionally these patients require deeper sedation/pain control measures during endotracheal suctioning or any stressful postoperative interventions in intensive care unit (ICU).

◼ VENTILATORY MANAGEMENT AND EXTUBATION

In patients who undergo elective surgery with good pulmonary venous anatomy and no PVO, extubation can be targeted on postoperative day (POD) 1. At our center, critically ill neonates with PVO and RV dysfunction due to severe pulmonary hypertension are often electively ventilated for 24–48 hours. Typically, these are babies with very severe obstruction operated very early after birth. Preoperative PVO can result in edematous lungs with dilated lymphatic channels.[8] This may necessitate extended duration of mechanical ventilation for the recovery of pulmonary function. Maintaining adequate lung volumes and reducing pulmonary congestion are crucial to prevent postoperative pulmonary hypertension in these patients. Ventilatory settings typically target a $PaCO_2$ between 30 and 35 mm Hg, mild alkalosis (7.45–7.50) and a PaO_2 of 100–150 mm Hg. This is to avoid the potent triggers of pulmonary vasoconstriction, namely hypoxia, hypercarbia and acidosis. Positive end expiratory pressure (PEEP) may be optimized to prevent atelectasis and maintain lung volumes at Functional Residual Capacity (FRC). Endotracheal suctioning should be performed with extreme caution as the stress response can trigger a pulmonary hypertensive crisis. Additional pain relief or sedation with bolus dose of fentanyl or midazolam during endotracheal suctioning is reasonable in patients at risk for this complication.

Extubation can be a critical phase in the postoperative period of these patients and has to be planned with meticulous care. In addition to clinical evaluation for adequate systemic perfusion, recovery of pulmonary function should be ensured by arterial blood gas and chest X-ray evaluation before extubation. A postoperative screening echocardiogram for cardiac function and unobstructed pulmonary venous pathway is also desirable. Extubation should ideally be executed in the presence of intensivist as complications such as pulmonary hypertensive crisis are likely in the periextubation period. Patients should also be closely monitored for development of upper airway obstruction as this is likely to be poorly tolerated by a patient at risk for pulmonary hypertension. Neonates with decreased lung compliance and increased work of breathing after extubation may be transitioned through a short period of nasal continuous positive airway pressure or high-flow nasal cannula oxygen therapy.

■ FEEDING AND NUTRITION

Enteral feeds should be initiated 6 hours after surgery in non-neonates and stable patients undergoing elective surgery. Cautious feeding after 12–24 hours is advised in sick neonates undergoing emergency surgery, patients on high inotropic supports or if lactate levels are more than 4 mmol/L. Oral feeds should be carefully established once satisfactory cardiorespiratory status is maintained after extubation and deintensification.

■ COMMON POSTOPERATIVE COMPLICATIONS

Pulmonary Hypertension

Risk group: Pulmonary hypertension should be anticipated in patients with obstructed TAPVC, preoperatively critically ill patients requiring mechanical ventilation, infracardiac TAPVC variant and poor pulmonary venous anatomy.

Diagnosis: Pulmonary hypertensive crisis refers to an acute rise in pulmonary artery pressure and pulmonary vascular resistance (PVR) which precipitates right-sided heart failure, systemic hypotension, myocardial ischemia and sometimes bronchoconstriction.[7] In patients with indwelling PA lines, an elevation of pulmonary artery pressure more than 75% of systemic pressure along with systemic hypotension suggests pulmonary hypertensive crisis. This may be accompanied by desaturation either due to right to left shunt via an interatrial communication that is left behind during surgery to decompress

the right heart, or due to sudden pulmonary edema resulting from increased left ventricular end diastolic pressure (LVEDP) due to leftward septal shift. In the absence of a PA line, the triad of sudden onset hypotension, bradycardia and desaturation should elicit strong suspicion of this complication. Echocardiographic findings usually include a tricuspid regurgitation (TR) jet and a septal configuration suggesting pulmonary hypertension. Frequently identified triggers for pulmonary hypertensive crisis in the postoperative setting include pain, anxiety, endotracheal suctioning, hypoxia or acidosis.[7]

Management of Pulmonary Hypertensive Crisis

- Hyperventilate with 100% oxygen
- Target an arterial $PaCO_2$ of 30–35 mm Hg
- Correct acidosis if any
- Provide adequate sedation, pain relief and neuromuscular blockade
- Optimize inotropic support to support RV function
- Identify and treat any other precipitating cause
- Use specific pulmonary vasodilators such as nitric oxide or intravenous sildenafil—nitric oxide should be given at a dose of 20–40 ppm with careful monitoring of methemoglobin levels. Sildenafil can be given intravenously at a dose of 0.4 mg/kg over 3 hours followed by 1.6 mg/kg/day or by enteral route at a dose of 0.3–0.5 mg/kg Q 6–8 h
- Continue mechanical ventilation till PA pressures stabilize
- Detailed echocardiographic evaluation after stabilization to rule out pulmonary vein stenosis or narrowing of anastomotic site.

Low Cardiac Output State

This usually occurs secondary to RV dysfunction, postoperative pulmonary hypertension or hemodynamically significant arrhythmias. Treatment should be directed at the cause. Inotropic treatment with epinephrine and/or milrinone is beneficial in those with RV dysfunction. Mechanical ventilation should be electively continued. Peritoneal dialysis is instituted to support renal function if necessary. Pulmonary vasodilator therapy is often required to treat significant pulmonary hypertension.

Arrhythmias

Cardiac arrhythmias have been recognized in patients undergoing surgical correction of TAPVC.[9,10] Supraventricular arrhythmias has been reported in 15% of patients undergoing TAPVC repair and these tend to occur in supracardiac variants requiring bi-atrial incision during surgery.[10] Most of the arrhythmias are self-limiting and resolve with correction of electrolyte imbalances and reduction in catecholamine supports. Persistent tachyarrhythmias need treatment with overdrive pacing, adenosine, amiodarone or ivabradine depending on the specific type of arrhythmia.

Pulmonary Venous Obstruction

The PVO is a potential complication that occurs in 5–18% of patients undergoing TAPVC repair and can significantly affect long-term survival.[5,11] Obstruction can occur either due to individual pulmonary vein stenosis or restriction at the anastomotic site. This is usually a late complication, but sometimes may manifest in early postoperative period. Risk factors for recurrent PVO include preoperative PVO, mixed and infracardiac TAPVC variants, and longer CPB time.[5] Bando et al. had identified small pulmonary venous confluence and diffuse pulmonary venous narrowing as risk factors for postoperative PVO.[12] A sutureless technique, which includes incision into the venous confluence and extended to individual pulmonary veins followed by anastomosing insitu pericardial flaps distally to the incised veins to create a neo-left atrium, has been adopted by some centers to ameliorate this complication. The sutureless technique has been associated with a lower propensity for restenosis of pulmonary veins in patients with preoperative PVO.[5,6] Patients who develop PVO often need reinterventions and have a poor prognosis with mortality of 25%.[13] Early presentation (<6 months of surgery) and persistence of pulmonary hypertension after reintervention are risk factors for increased mortality in this subset.[13]

■ DEINTENSIFICATION

Patients who are stable preoperatively and undergoing elective surgery can be deintensified following extubation. However, patients who had PVO and pulmonary hypertension may need an extended period of postoperative stabilization, ventilation and inotropic support. In these patients, inotropes are carefully tapered after assessing cardiorespiratory stability and initiating pulmonary vasodilator therapy if required.

■ DISCHARGE MEDICATIONS

Diuretics are often necessary for about two weeks after surgery, particularly for obstructed TAPVC. Oral furosemide 1–2 mg/kg/day is often sufficient. This is because lungs tend to remain congested.

Patients who have had pulmonary hypertensive crisis in the early postoperative period often receive sildenafil for a variable number of days after discharge from the ICU. It is almost always possible to discontinue sildenafil in about a week's time with no significant risk of recurrence of this complication.

■ REFERENCES

1. Ross FJ, Joffe D, Latham GJ. Perioperative and anesthetic considerations in total anomalous

pulmonary venous connection. Semin Cardiothorac Vasc Anesth. 2016;21:138-44.

2. Khan MS, Bryant R III, Kim SH, Hill KD, Jacobs JP, Jacobs ML, et al. Contemporary outcomes of total anomalous pulmonary venous connection in patients with heterotaxy syndrome. Ann Thorac Surg. 2015;99:2136-40.

3. Hancock-Friesen CL, Zurakowski D, Thiagarajan RR, Forbess JM, del-Nido PJ, Mayer JE, et al. Total anomalous pulmonary venous connection: an analysis of current management strategies in a single institution. Ann Thorac Surg. 2005;79:596-606.

4. Warrier G, Dharan DS, Koshy S, Kumar S, Krishnanaik S, Rao SG. Repair of total anomalous pulmonary venous connection in neonates. Ind J Thorac Cardiovasc Surg. 2004;20:155-8.

5. Shi G, Zhu Z, Chen J, Ou Y, Hong H, Nie Z, et al. Total anomalous pulmonary venous connection. The Current management strategies in a pediatric cohort of 768 patients. Circulation. 2017;135:48-58.

6. Wu Y, Wu Z, Zheng J, Li Y, Zhou Y, Kuang H, et al. Sutureless technique versus conventional surgery in the primary treatment of total anomalous pulmonary venous connection: a systematic review and meta-analysis. J Cardiothorac Surg. 2018;13:69.

7. Abman SH, Hansmann G, Archer SL, Ivy D, Adatia I, Chung WK, et al. Pediatric pulmonary hypertension guidelines from American Heart Association and American Thoracic Society. Circulation. 2015; 132(21):2037-99.

8. Haworth SG, Reid L. Structural study of pulmonary circulation and of heart in total anomalous pulmonary venous return in early infancy. Br Heart J. 1977;39:80-92.

9. Saxena A, Fong LV, Lamb FK, Monro JL, Shore DF, Keeton BR. Cardiac arrhythmias after surgical correction of total anomalous pulmonary venous connection: late follow up. Pediatr Cardiol. 1991;12:89-91.

10. Zhao K, Wang H, Wang Z, Zhu H, Fang M, Zhu X, et al. Early and intermediate-term results of surgical correction in 122 patients with total anomalous pulmonary venous connection and biventricular physiology. J Cardiothorac Surg. 2015;10:172.

11. Seale AN, Uemura H, Webber SA, Partridge J, Roughton M, Ho SY, et al. Total anomalous pulmonary venous connection. Morphology and outcome from an international population-based study. Circulation. 2010;122:2718-26.

12. Bando K, Turrentine MW, Ensing GJ, Sun K, Sharp TG, Sekine Y, et al. Surgical management of total anomalous pulmonary venous connection: thirty year trends. Circulation. 1996;94: II12-II16.

13. Ricci M, Elliot M, Cohen GA, Catalan G, Stark J, de Leval MR, et al. Management of pulmonary venous obstruction after correction of TAPVC: risk factors for adverse outcome. Eur J Cardiothorac Surg. 2003;24:28-36.

24

Arterial Switch Operation

CHAPTER

Rakhi Balachandran
Illustrations: Praveen Reddy Bayya
Reviewed by: R Krishna Kumar

■ INTRODUCTION

Transposition of great arteries (TGA) accounts for 5–7% of all congenital cardiac defects with a prevalence of 0.31 per 1,000 live births.[1] TGA is described as a congenital cardiac anomaly characterized by ventriculoarterial discordance; where the aorta arises from the anatomic right ventricle (RV) and the pulmonary artery from the anatomic left ventricle (LV). The nature of atrioventricular connection differentiates the two distinct anatomic variants; D-TGA (dextro transposition of great arteries) characterized by atrioventricular concordance and CCTGA (congenitally corrected transposition of great arteries) hallmarked by atrioventricular discordance. Associated anomalies which can coexist with TGA include ventricular septal defect (VSD), coarctation of aorta, interrupted aortic arch and left ventricular outflow tract obstruction (LVOTO). For practical purposes, the term TGA in this chapter refers to D-TGA alone and does not include CCTGA or TGA associated with a functional single ventricle. Arterial switch operation anatomically "corrects" discordant ventriculoarterial connection. It involves transection of the great arteries and creation of the neo-aorta by anastomosing the ascending aorta above the level of transection to the base of original pulmonary artery (**Figs. 1A to C**). The coronary arteries need to be translocated to the neo-aorta

separately. The main pulmonary artery (MPA) with the branch pulmonary arteries above the level of transection, is brought anteriorly (LeCompte maneuver) and anastomosed to the base of original aorta with pericardial augmentation forming the future pulmonary artery. The most crucial step in the operation obviously relates to achieving a coronary transfer without any obstruction or distortion. In TGA, coronary arteries usually arise from aortic sinuses that face the pulmonary trunk irrespective of the interrelationships of the great arteries. However, several deviations from the normal pattern can potentially exist in patients with transposition which can offer technical challenges while translocating coronaries to the neo-aorta. Most of the serious postoperative adverse events after the arterial switch operation result from a compromised coronary circulation. Early arterial switch operation soon after diagnosis is being increasingly undertaken in patients with TGA due to availability of prenatal diagnosis, improving surgical expertise and increasing evidence that early operation allows improved outcomes.[2] Patients with TGA and an intact ventricular septum in whom surgery is not feasible early due to logistic reasons are transitioned through interim stabilizing measures such as prostaglandin E1 therapy or balloon atrial septostomy. Lower patient weight, intramural course of

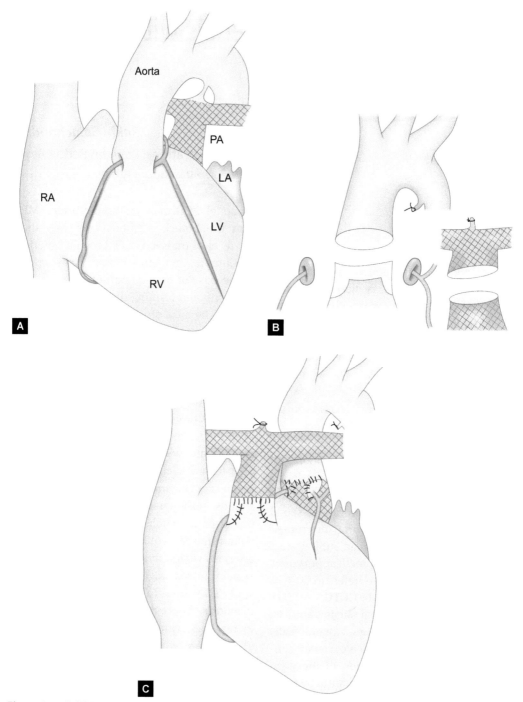

Figs. 1A to C: (A) Transposition of great arteries (TGA): Aorta arises from the anterior right ventricle (RV) and pulmonary artery from the posterior left ventricle (LV); (B) Great arteries are transected and coronary buttons explanted; (C) Great arteries switched and coronary buttons anastomosed to the pulmonary root (neo-aorta).
(RA: right atrium; LA: left atrium; PA: pulmonary artery)

coronary artery, single coronary artery, side by side great arteries, presence of LVOTO and aortic arch anomalies are factors which can pose significant surgical challenges. Some of these factors emerge as significant risk factors determining early outcomes.[3,4] With growing experience in complex neonatal surgery, most of these risk factors can be overcome to a great extent with excellent survival being reported in the current era with an operative mortality of approximately 2–3%.[5]

MONITORING AND HEMODYNAMIC MANAGEMENT

Standard monitoring should include invasive arterial blood pressure, central venous pressure, ECG, pulse oximetry and capnography. Lead II and V5 are usually monitored to diagnose arrhythmias and myocardial ischemia. It is reasonable to obtain a postoperative 6 lead ECG for comparison with preoperative baseline and to understand evolving changes in the postoperative period. New onset ST segment and T wave changes merit concern about possible coronary insufficiency. Ventricular arrhythmias may be an indirect indicator of coronary artery compromise and should be seriously investigated. Persistent tachycardia often arises in neonates with "under prepared" LV in the early postoperative period, to compensate for the low cardiac output secondary to increased afterload to the systemic ventricle.

Most neonates separate from cardiopulmonary bypass (CPB) with an inotropic support of milrinone and a low dose epinephrine (0.02–0.04 µg/kg/min). Mean arterial pressure of 35–45 mm Hg is acceptable in the post-bypass period in neonates with an intact ventricular septum. Additional systemic afterload reduction in patients who remain hypertensive can be achieved with nitroprusside or phenoxybenzamine infusion.

Hypertension should be aggressively treated as an increase in afterload can precipitate LV failure, low cardiac output and pulmonary edema. Though data on milrinone are sparse in this subset of patients, milrinone is generally preferred due to its favorable effects on maintaining a low systemic vascular resistance. At our center, nitroglycerin (NTG) is occasionally administered as an infusion in the first 24 hours in patients who had a difficult coronary transfer. However, the evidence is not strongly supportive on the use of NTG. The left ventricle in the neonate has a relatively low compliance in the postoperative period after CPB and may not tolerate sudden increases in preload. Left atrial pressure (if monitoring facility is available via an intraoperatively placed left atrial line) should be maintained below 10 mm Hg because volume infusion beyond this point may not be well-tolerated by the non-compliant ventricle after arterial switch.[6] A screening postoperative echocardiogram is rational in unstable patients to rule out important ventricular dysfunction or wall motion abnormalities.[6]

VENTILATORY MANAGEMENT

The operated neonates are usually ventilated for first 12–24 hours after surgery. A low PO_2 may be occasionally seen in the immediate postoperative period after chest closure due to reduced chest wall and lung compliance after CPB. This typically improves over 8–12 hours by the use of positive end-expiratory pressure (PEEP) and diuretic therapy. In the past, postoperative management included deep sedation, neuromuscular blockade and extended duration of ventilatory support. But with improved surgical and perfusion techniques in the current era, prolonged ventilation is seldom necessary for uncomplicated cases. In fact, early extubation minimizes postoperative complications such as pneumonia and shortens intensive care. At our center, neonates who are hemodynamically stable with good ventricular function, normal coronary anatomy, acceptable lung mechanics with adequate gas exchange on arterial blood gas evaluation and a negative fluid balance of at least 30 mL/kg are usually considered for extubation on first postoperative day. However, if there is evidence of low cardiac output, body edema, or ventricular dysfunction on echocardiography, ventilation may be continued till clinical improvement occurs. A short period of noninvasive ventilation in the form of nasal continuous positive airway pressure (CPAP) may be required in some patients to decrease work of breathing after extubation, particularly if chest wall edema or pulmonary congestion persists.

FLUID MANAGEMENT

Restricted fluid management policy for surgery under CPB is followed in the postoperative period to decrease fluid overload. In neonates with TGA and an intact ventricular septum, fluid boluses for treatment of important hypovolemia are given in aliquots of 3–5 mL/kg preferably administered as a continuous intravenous infusion to avoid sudden increases in ventricular preload.

DIURETIC THERAPY

Most neonates are initiated on a diuretic infusion of furosemide at 1–2 mg/kg/day in the postoperative period. Typically a negative fluid balance of 30–50 mL/kg is targeted in postoperative period to decrease fluid overload, reduce extravascular lung water and facilitate uneventful separation from mechanical ventilation.

PAIN AND SEDATION MANAGEMENT

Most patients are started on fentanyl infusion at 1–2 µg/kg/h in the postoperative period.

This is often combined with paracetamol for additional analgesic effect. Dexmedetomidine is an important alternative which can be used in patients who are planned for extubation on postoperative day 1 to avoid the effects of respiratory depression and chest-wall rigidity that may be associated with fentanyl.

ANTICOAGULATION

It was a common practice in the early era to initiate heparin infusion at 5–15 units/kg/h in the postoperative period to minimize the risk of coronary thrombosis. This is followed by aspirin on first postoperative day at a dose of 3–5 mg/kg via the nasogastric tube. However this policy is being abandoned in most centres. Aspirin is reserved only for patients with difficult coronary anatomy such as single coronary or that with an intramural course.

FEEDING AND NUTRITION

Enteral feeds are initiated at 12–24 hours after surgery and withheld around the period of extubation. Expressed breast milk is preferred over formula feeds whenever available. Necrotizing enterocolitis (NEC) is a likely complication in neonates who had a large ductus arteriosus preoperatively and in those who are on high inotropic supports for low cardiac output state due to mesenteric hypoperfusion. Hence, it is reasonable to delay feeding in such patients and to monitor closely for signs of feed intolerance while initiating and escalating feeds.

COMMON POSTOPERATIVE COMPLICATIONS

The results of arterial switch have improved dramatically and complications are uncommon. However, there is a list of complications that one should be familiar with, after this operation.

Increased Postoperative Bleeding

This may be due to effects of hypothermia during CPB, residual heparin effect, neonatal age group or due to bleeding from anastomotic sites. Treatment should aim at identification and correction of the cause of bleeding. Hypertension should be avoided to minimize bleeding from suture lines. In general, the need to re-explore is exceptional after the arterial switch operation.

Myocardial Ischemia

Myocardial ischemia is a potential complication of impaired coronary perfusion particularly associated with a difficult coronary transfer, as in case of single/intramural coronary artery or side by side great arterial relationship. The ICU staff should maintain a high index of suspicion for myocardial ischemia in the immediate postoperative period as mechanical obstruction to the coronary arteries due to stretching or external compression is sometimes likely after reimplantation. In addition to ECG abnormalities, unexplained ventricular dysfunction, low cardiac output state, or hemodynamically significant arrhythmias may also indicate early coronary insufficiency.[7] Coronary air emboli can also precipitate transient myocardial ischemia. Serial ECG and screening echo is usually helpful in evaluating postoperative ischemia. Traditionally, coronary vasodilators such as NTG have been used to improve myocardial perfusion after arterial switch operation although there is no evidence favoring its utility. Coronary obstruction is a serious problem and needs to be emergently addressed by revision of the anastomosis. However, in the setting of myocardial dysfunction without a demonstrable coronary obstruction, mechanical circulatory support should be considered till ventricular function recovers.

Ventricular Dysfunction

Left ventricular dysfunction often results from coronary insufficiency, inadequate myocardial protection during CPB or due to poor adaptation of the systemic ventricle to the increased afterload. Ventricular dysfunction usually manifests as low cardiac output state. Clinical signs of poor systemic perfusion should be aggressively sought for, such as poor pedal pulses, cold extremities, delayed capillary fill, increasing lactates or a fall in urine output. Mitral regurgitation secondary to papillary muscle dysfunction due to ischemia can also contribute to low cardiac output. Inotropic supports should be liberal and agents which reduce afterload such as milrinone or levosimendan are usually preferred in these circumstances. Mechanical circulatory support should be considered if pharmacotherapy is insufficient to maintain perfusion pressures. It is imperative to address any likely coronary issues along with pharmacological support for facilitating myocardial recovery.

Arrhythmias

A variety of arrhythmias have been reported in the postoperative period after arterial switch operation. Supraventricular tachycardia, junctional ectopic tachycardia and ventricular arrhythmias were identified in the early postoperative period in a retrospective review of 390 patients undergoing arterial switch operation.[8] Additionally, few instances of atrioventricular conduction defects including complete heart block (1.7%) was observed in patients who had concomitant ventricular septal defect repair with arterial switch operation. The occurrence of postoperative ventricular tachyarrhythmias after arterial switch operation should be investigated carefully since it may indicate an underlying impairment in coronary artery blood flow.

Though it may be challenging to identify coronary occlusion by echocardiography, LV dysfunction and regional wall motion abnormalities may suggest compromised coronary perfusion. Cardiac catheterization and angiography are the definitive tests for coronary artery evaluation. In the event of a confirmed coronary artery occlusion, it is usually necessary to address it through reoperation. Junctional ectopic tachycardia often responds to optimization of electrolytes, reduction in vasoactive drugs and correction of hyperthermia, but sometimes requires treatment with amiodarone or ivabradine. Persistent arrhythmias need specific anti-arrhythmic drug therapy.

DEINTENSIFICATION

Most of the neonates after an uncomplicated arterial switch are extubated within 24–48 hours. The inotropes can be weaned off 4 hours after extubation if patient is hemodynamically stable and echocardiography reveals adequate ventricular function. This is usually followed by removal of invasive lines. Nasogastric tube is removed when the baby starts accepting oral feeds and is able to maintain adequate intake.

DISCHARGE MEDICATIONS

Oral furosemide may be needed for a brief period (about a week). The role of aspirin after arterial switch is controversial. Many surgical units do not administer aspirin. In selected situations, such as intramural coronaries, where the coronary artery is opened, it may be justifiable to administer aspirin for 3 months after surgery.

REFERENCES

1. Van der Linde D, Konings EM, Slager MA, Witzenberg M, Helbing W, Takkenberg JM, et al. Birth prevalence of congenital heart disease worldwide. A systematic review and meta-analysis. J Am Coll Cardiol. 2011;58:2241-7.
2. Anderson BR, Ciarleglio AJ, Hayes DA, Quaegebeur JM, Vincent JA, Bacha EA. Earlier arterial switch operation improves outcomes and reduces costs for neonates with transposition of the great arteries. J Am Coll Cardiol. 2014;63:481-7.
3. Mekkawy A, Ghoneim A, El-Haddad O, Photiadis J, Elminshawy A. Predictors of early outcomes after arterial switch operation in patients with D-TGA. J Egypt Soc Cardiothorac Surg. 2017;25: 52-7.
4. Khairy P, Claire M, Fernandes SM, Blume ED, Powell AJ, Newburger JW, et al. Cardiovascular outcomes after the arterial switch operation for D-transposition of great arteries. Circulation. 2013;127:331-9.
5. Jacobs JP, Mayer JE, Mavroudis C, O'Brien SM, Austin EH, Pasquali SK, et al. The Society of Thoracic Surgeons Congenital Heart Surgery Database: 2016 Update on outcomes and Quality. Ann Thorac Surg. 2016;101:850-62.
6. Sarris GE, Balmer C, Bonou P, Comas JV, da Cruz E, Di Chiara L, et al. Clinical guidelines for the management of patients with transposition of great arteries with intact ventricular septum. The Task Force on Transposition of the Great arteries of the European Association for Cardio-Thoracic Surgery and The Association for European Pediatric and Congenital Cardiology. Eur J Cardiothorac Surg. 2017;51:e1-e32.
7. Vilafane J, Lantin- Hermoso R, Bhatt AB, Tweddell JS, Geva T, Nathan M, et al. Transposition of the great arteries: the current era of the arterial switch operation. J Am Coll Cardiol. 2014;64:498-511.
8. Rhodes LA, Wernovsky G, Keane JF, Mayer JE, Shuren A, Dindy C, et al. Arrhythmia and intracardiac conduction after arterial switch operation. J Thorac Cardiovasc Surg. 1995;109:303-10.

Senning/Mustard Procedure

Jessin P Jayashankar

Illustration: Praveen Reddy Bayya
Reviewed by: Aveek Jayant

■ INTRODUCTION

Following the universal acceptance and standardization of the arterial switch operation, the atrial switch operation is only performed occasionally for d-transposition of great arteries (TGA). It, however, continues to be performed as a part of the double switch operation for congenitally corrected transposition (cc-TGA). In patients with cc-TGA, this operation restores atrioventricular concordance while the ventriculoarterial concordance is corrected with one of the following options:

1. An arterial switch operation with ventricular septal defect (VSD) closure when there is no accompanying left ventricular outflow obstruction.
2. A "Rastelli" procedure with routing of anatomic left ventricle to the aorta and placement of a conduit between the anatomic right ventricle and the pulmonary arteries when there is accompanying left ventricular outflow tract obstruction.
3. Hemi-Mustard (in place of Senning), bidirectional cavopulmonary shunt and Rastelli procedures in combination; the cavopulmonary shunt is sometimes an adjunct because the Rastelli component can potentially compromise the anatomic size of the right ventricle.[1]

For those in low resource settings [with a burden of late presenting congenital heart disease (CHD) or lack of infrastructure to attempt neonatal surgery] atrial level switches could still be attempted in one of the following settings:[2]

1. Complex coronary transfer resulting from intramural coronary arteries or other variations that are considered technically very challenging.
2. D-transposition with intact ventricular septum that presents late; as technically simpler and less resource intensive alternative to the two-stage arterial switch operation.
3. In d-TGA with VSD and severe elevation of pulmonary vascular resistance. Here the Senning operation essentially serves to palliate by reducing the level of cyanosis resulting from unfavorable streaming.

Further still, care providers will need to be aware of the general surgical pathway and after care as older patients may present for conversion to anatomical repair in the face of right ventricular (systemic) failure postpalliation with an atrial switch, baffle leak or obstruction, electrophysiological abnormalities as a consequence of the operation, corrected transposition alone or in combination, and for attempts to repair the tricuspid valve.

Senning procedure is an atrial switch heart surgery performed to treat TGA. The name comes from its inventor Ake Senning, a Swedish surgeon, who first performed the surgery in 1958. This operation technically involves creation of a baffle that diverts the venous drainage into respective ventricles at the atrial level **(Fig. 1)**. This results in physiological restoration of "normal" flow of blood at the atrial level with the heart and lungs being in series; however, the left ventricle continues to remain the "subpulmonary" ventricle and right ventricle is the pump for systemic circulation (systemic ventricle).[3]

The main difference between the Senning and Mustard procedures is that in the Senning operation the baffle is created from native right atrial free-wall and atrial septum without the use of extrinsic materials. The Mustard operation, on the other hand, involves resection of the atrial septum and fashioning of a baffle with pericardium or synthetic material. These operations are performed after the neonatal period, typically between 1 month and 1 year of age. In experienced hands, the early mortality rate associated with these procedures is low (1–10%).[4] The Schumacker modification of the original Senning operation consistently enabled prevention of pulmonary pathway obstruction.[5]

■ MONITORING

Standard monitoring with invasive arterial blood pressure, central venous pressure, continuous ECG monitoring, pulse oximetry and capnography is followed in all patients. As these patients are prone for development of arrhythmias in the postoperative period, it may be worthwhile to obtain baseline ECG upon arrival in the ICU and to ensure fidelity of epicardial leads that can aid in both the treatment and diagnosis of this problem. Arrhythmias are typically a late problem of the treatment pathway and may not present in the initial perioperative period.

■ HEMODYNAMIC AND INOTROPE MANAGEMENT

When performed in the setting of late presenting d-TGA the perioperative management of this operation is usually straight forward. When performed as a component of anatomic repair of cc-TGA, due consideration has to be made toward the long duration of surgery overall and, length of cardiopulmonary bypass (CPB). There is no evidence to suggest one inotrope should be preferred over another with the caveat that inotrope use as such should be tailored to the lowest possible doses and the shortest times. The tricuspid valve can be dysmorphic and there can be some amount of tricuspid regurgitation, which needs cautious titration of fluid and ventilatory maneuvers to

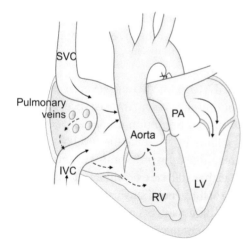

Fig. 1: Senning procedure: Atrial switch procedures baffle the superior vena cava (SVC) and inferior vena cava (IVC) drainage across the interatrial septum into the left atrium and through the mitral valve. Pulmonary veins drain into the right ventricle (RV) and enter systemic circulation.

(LV: left ventricle; PA: pulmonary artery)

aid right ventricular output. When these operations are performed in the setting of pulmonary hypertension, at our center, most patients would receive either milrinone or levosimendan as part of their inotrope prescription. A subset of patients may have reductions in right ventricular volume secondary to root translocation: these patients might receive a bidirectional Glenn shunt as a part of their surgical strategy and will be candidates for expedited separation from mechanical ventilation. If present, obstructions or leaks in the baffle or inflow tracts might require reintervention, these are typically rare. Those patients receiving a double switch need to have their ventricular function assessed periodically and their fluid and inotrope managed according to the situation.[6]

■ FLUID MANAGEMENT

Standard fluid management protocol for pediatric cardiac surgery under CPB is followed. Additional volume for replacing postoperative losses can be administered. It is advised to restrict fluid boluses in post-procedure period as these patients may already have right ventricular (systemic ventricle) dysfunction and elevated pulmonary artery pressures. Central venous pressure monitoring is reasonable to guide volume administration.

Diuretics are generally recommended in postoperative period after Senning procedure to avoid fluid overload and to facilitate extubation. Diuretics may also benefit those who are vulnerable to develop right ventricular dysfunction and elevated pulmonary artery pressures.

A continuous infusion of furosemide is generally preferred. For patients < 20 kg: 1–2 mg/kg/per day as infusion may be a sufficient dose, and for patients > 20 kg: 1–2

mg/hour infusion is a sufficient dose. Vigilant monitoring for electrolyte imbalances such as hypokalemia and hypomagnesemia is important in patients on diuretic therapy to prevent the development of arrhythmias.

■ PAIN AND SEDATION MANAGEMENT

Patients generally require good analgesia and adequate sedation after a sternotomy procedure. Patients with suboptimal analgesia may develop lung related problems such as atelectasis and lung collapse due to inadequate depth of respiration due to pain. After extubation, this can cause increased morbidity particularly in patients with high PA pressures. The combined use of opioids and nonsteroidal anti-inflammatory drugs (NSAIDs) enables pain control. Dexmedetomidine infusion at the dose of 0.5 µg/kg/hour is a good alternative, which can help to reduce the dose requirement of opioid agents.

■ VENTILATION MANAGEMENT

Early extubation can be undertaken in the intensive care unit after an echocardiogram and chest X-ray assessment.

■ COMMON POSTOPERATIVE COMPLICATIONS

Arrhythmias and Sudden Cardiac Death

Patients who have undergone the Mustard or Senning procedure are at risk of both brady- and tachyarrhythmias. The most common tachyarrhythmia is an incisional re-entrant tachycardia, sometimes described as atypical atrial flutter. Bradyarrhythmias result from sinus node dysfunction; and sinus bradycardias, sinus pauses with junctional escape rhythm as well as intermittent sino-atrial exit block are common. Sinus node dysfunction in this group appears to be more likely with increasing time from operation.

Atrial reentrant tachycardia occurs in up to 2–10% of patients after atrial baffle repair of TGA.[7] There does appear to be a small risk of high-grade atrioventricular (AV) block as a result of this procedure perhaps from injury to the AV node while creating the atrial baffle.

Baffle Obstruction and Baffle Leaks

Baffle obstruction is an infrequent but significant complication after the Mustard and Senning operations. Systemic venous baffle obstruction occurs in ~5%, whereas pulmonary venous baffle obstruction is less common (~2%).[6]

Baffle leaks are somewhat more common than obstruction. The most common site is at the suture line of the superior limb of the systemic venous baffle. Shunting may be either left-to-right or right-to-left. In patients with a large left-to-right shunt, the consequent volume loading of the systemic right ventricle may necessitate closure of the defect either surgically or by transcatheter means. In patients with important right-to-left shunts, systemic arterial desaturation ensues, likewise necessitating closure.[8]

Pulmonary Hypertension

Pulmonary vascular obstructive disease may develop in a small proportion (5–6%) of patients after Senning/Mustard procedure.[9] This complication is more common after late repair and in patients with an associated VSD.

Systemic Ventricular Dysfunction

The main focus of concern regarding the long-term future for patients with Senning or the Mustard procedure has been the function of the systemic right ventricle. Although right ventricle can tolerate functioning at systemic pressures in the short-term without difficulty, it may fail when required to do this in the long-term.[10] After 20–30 years, systemic arterial dysfunction is nearly universal and quite difficult to manage.

Tricuspid Valve Function[10,11]

Mild-to-moderate tricuspid regurgitation is relatively common in patients after Senning or Mustard procedure. The reversal of the right and left ventricular pressure relationship alters the geometry of the ventricular septum as a result of which the tricuspid valve takes on a more rounded shape. This alteration together with the displaced septal chordal attachments of the valve results in an increased tendency for tricuspid regurgitation.

■ REFERENCES

1. Zhang S, Kai Ma SL, Zhongdong H, Hao Z, Jun Y, Keming Y, et al. The hemi-Mustard, bidirectional Glenn and Rastelli procedures for anatomical repair of congenitally corrected transposition of the great arteries/left ventricular outflow tract obstruction with positional heart anomalies. Eur J Cardiothorac Surg. 2017;51(6):1058-62.
2. Sarris GE, Balmer C, Bonou P, Comas JV, da Cruz E, Di Chiara L, et al. Clinical guidelines for the management of patients with transposition of the great arteries with intact ventricular septum. Eur J Cardiothorac Surg. 2017;51(1): e1-32.
3. Horning T, O'Donnel C. Transposition of great arteries. In: Gatzoulis MA, Webb GD, Daubeney PEF (Eds). Diagnosis and Management of Adult Congenital Heart Disease, 2nd edition. Gurugram: Elsevier; 2011. pp. 513-27.
4. Ferro G, Murthy R, Sebastian VA Guleserian KJ, Forbess JM. Single centre experience with the Senning procedure in the current era. Semin Thorac Cardiovasc Surg. 2016;28: 514-20.
5. Brizard CP, Lee A, Zannino D, Davis AM, Fricke TA, d'Udekem Y, et al. Cheung. Long-term results of anatomic correction for congenitally corrected transposition of the

great arteries: a 19-year experience. J Thoracic Cardiovasc Surg. 2017;154(1):256-265.e4.

6. Dinardo JA. Transposition of great vessels. In: Lake CL, Booker PD (Eds). Pediatric Cardiac Anaesthesia, 4th edition. Philadelphia: Lippincott Williams and Wilkins; 2005. pp. 357-76.

7. Kanter RJ, Papagiannis J, Carboni MP, Ungerleider RM, Sanders WE, Wharton JM. Radiofrequency catheter ablation of supra-ventricular tachycardia after Mustard and Senning operation for d-transposition of the great arteries. J Am Coll Cardiol. 2000;35: 428-41.

8. Barron DJ, Jones TJ, Brawn DJ. The Senning procedure as part of the double switch operation for transposition of great arteries.

Semin Thorac Cardiovasc Surg Pediatr Card Surg Ann. 2011;14:109-15.

9. Yehya A, Lyle T, Pernetz MA, McConnell ME, Book WM. Pulmonary hypertension in patients with prior atrial switch procedure for D-transposition of great arteries. Int J Cardiol. 2010;143:271-5.

10. Dodge Khatami A, Kadner A, Berger F, Dave H, Turina MI, Pretre R. In the footsteps of Senning: lessons learnt from atrial repair of transposition of the great arteries. Ann Thorac Surg. 2005;79:1433-44.

11. Wernovsky G, Jonas RA. Other conotruncal lesions. In: Chang AC, Hanley FL (Eds). Pediatric Cardiac Intensive Care. Philadelphia: Lippincott Williams and Wilkins; 1998. pp. 289-301.

26

CHAPTER

Blalock-Taussig Shunt

Rakhi Balachandran

Illustration: Balaji Srimurugan

Reviewed by: R Krishna Kumar

◼ INTRODUCTION

Blalock-Taussig (BT) shunt was historically performed as the initial palliative procedure for patients with tetralogy of Fallot (TOF). Since early primary repair is advocated for TOF in the present era, the use of this procedure has been largely restricted to first stage palliation of complex single ventricle lesions with reduced pulmonary blood flow (PBF). It is also sometimes performed as the initial palliative procedure for patients with TOF with pulmonary atresia, or TOF with small branch pulmonary arteries to facilitate growth of pulmonary arteries. With the advent of stenting of the arterial duct, this operation

is performed at a much lower frequency in the recent years.

Modified BT shunt involves placement of a graft composed of expanded polytetra-fluoroethylene (PTFE) between subclavian artery and the ipsilateral branch pulmonary artery **(Fig. 1)**. It is much more commonly performed on the right side between the right subclavian and the right pulmonary artery. The flow through the shunt is regulated by the diameter and length of the graft, the site of placement of the graft (central artery or a more peripheral location) and the balance between systemic and pulmonary vascular resistance. Traditionally, BT shunt is done without the

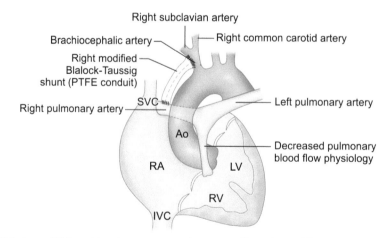

Fig. 1: Tetralogy of Fallot with pulmonary stenosis managed by right modified Blalock-Taussig shunt.
(Ao: aorta; IVC: inferior vena cava; LV: left ventricle; RA: right atrium; RV: right ventricle; SVC: superior vena cava; PTFE: polytetrafluoro ethylene)

use of cardiopulmonary bypass (CPB) through a thoracotomy incision. However, a median sternotomy approach is being increasingly favored especially in neonates, to facilitate the use of emergent CPB if necessary, for safety during resuscitation, and also due to ease of take down at a subsequent staged operation. In a recent best evidence review, sternotomy approach was also associated with less pulmonary artery distortion, ease of technical performance, ease of concomitant patent ductus arteriosus (PDA) ligation, less collateral formation in chest wall adhesions and reduction in scoliosis.[1] This procedure though simple in execution, is often complicated by relatively high postoperative mortality even in most specialized centers due to the inherent difficulty in achieving the optimum balance between systemic and pulmonary circulation and prevention of shunt failure early during postoperative recovery. Postoperative shunt occlusion and shunt over-circulation are the most important complications and account for much of the mortality and morbidity. In a large multicenter cohort of patients undergoing systemic to pulmonary artery shunts, there was a temporal increase of early mortality from 5.1 to 9.8% from first to second half of the decade which also reflected a shift in the indication for surgery from TOF toward single ventricle and pulmonary atresia in the latter decade, a group which obviously includes sicker patients.[2] Low bodyweight, small shunt size, central shunt, pulmonary over-circulation, univentricular hearts—particularly pulmonary atresia with intact ventricular septum are some of the identified risk factors for poor outcomes.[2-4] Due to the increased mortality and morbidity associated with systemic to pulmonary artery shunts a growing number of neonates and infants are alternatively being palliated in cardiac catheterization laboratory through ductal stenting, stenting of the right ventricular outflow tract or balloon pulmonary valvotomy for various congenital heart defects. Contemporary evidence shows no difference in mortality or unplanned intervention to treat cyanosis in patients who receive either palliative PDA stent or BT shunt for lesions with duct dependent pulmonary circulation. However, PDA stent patients seemed to have an advantage in terms of lower intensive care unit (ICU) stay, fewer procedural complications, and larger and more symmetrical pulmonary arteries at subsequent surgery or last follow-up.[5]

In this chapter, we have provided a brief overview of the postoperative management of patients undergoing systemic to pulmonary artery shunt.

■ MONITORING

In the first 24–48 hours, very vigilant monitoring is mandatory because catastrophic events in the ICU occur with very little warning. The following areas need close attention:

Systemic Perfusion

- Clinical signs (capillary return, skin color, temperature of extremities)
- *Arterial pressure*: Systolic, diastolic and mean pressures
- Urine output
- Lactate levels.

Gas Exchange

- Oxygen saturation (SaO_2)
- Arterial blood gas analysis (ABG)
- End-tidal carbon dioxide ($EtCO_2$).

Shunt Patency

Murmur [sometimes best heard via the endotracheal (ET) tube]: A baseline assessment of the shunt murmur has to be made by the bedside nurse and ICU physician as soon as the infant arrives from the operating room.

HEMODYNAMIC AND INOTROPE MANAGEMENT

Choice of Inotrope and Hemoglobin Target

The goal of postoperative hemodynamic management should be to ensure shunt patency and to maintain a balance between systemic and PBF. Blood pressure is usually maintained 10–20% greater than normal to facilitate good flow through the shunt. Inotrope strategy differs among institutions and sometimes varies from patient to patient depending on the physiology. However, it is rational to use an agent or agents which will provide inotropic support with some degree of peripheral vasodilation to promote a low systemic vascular resistance. A combination of low dose epinephrine with milrinone at 0.5–0.7 µg/kg/min is a reasonable choice. As the incidence of shunt block is particularly higher in the early hours after surgery, maintenance of adequate systemic blood pressure seems intuitive. The optimum hematocrit that has to be maintained in these patients is inconclusive. It is speculated that fluid shifts and hemoconcentration might sometimes predispose to shunt occlusion. In a retrospective study of neonates undergoing systemic to pulmonary artery shunt for single ventricle palliation, early shunt occlusion within first 24 hours was significantly associated with first postoperative hematocrit. For every five additional points of hematocrit, the odds of early shunt occlusion was more than doubled.[6] A hemoglobin target of 12–13 g% seems reasonable in most patients though evidence for this is sparse.

Anticoagulation

Early postoperative phase with a fresh anastomosis, phases of low systemic pressures, pulmonary hypertension, external compression and resulting stasis, can all predispose to thrombus formation. Hence, it is rational to initiate early anticoagulation.[3] A continuous infusion of heparin is usually started in these patients soon after arrival in ICU at 10–20 unit/kg/hour to target activated partial thromboplastin time (APTT) values twice normal. Antiplatelet therapy with aspirin is initiated at a dose of 3–5 mg/kg once daily, on postoperative day 1. Heparin infusion is continued till two doses of aspirin are administered. Platelet counts have to be carefully monitored while on heparin and aspirin therapy. The protective roles of aspirin to lower shunt thrombosis and to decrease mortality in patients with systemic to pulmonary artery shunts have been previously elucidated.[7]

How to Diagnose Pulmonary Overcirculation?

The simplest bedside tool is to follow the peripheral arterial oxygen saturation (SaO_2). Typically, an SaO_2 of 75–85% represents a balanced Qp/Qs (pulmonary to systemic blood flow ratio) of 1. Oxygen saturation consistently >90% indicates increased PBF. A low diastolic blood pressure <25 mm Hg is also suggestive of a high "run off" into the pulmonary artery. Clinical signs of low cardiac output such as cool extremities, diminished pedal pulses, decreased urine output and metabolic acidosis with increased lactate in arterial blood gas should be meticulously sought for, if there is suspicion of reduced systemic blood flow. Coronary perfusion is likely to be compromised if diastolic blood pressure decreases below 20 mm Hg and sometimes manifest as ST-depression on ECG, along with rapidly developing hemodynamic instability. Patients with pulmonary atresia and intact ventricular septum with coronary sinusoids are especially vulnerable. Chest X-ray often shows congested lung fields.

This is a potentially alarming situation as this can eventually lead to a sudden cardiovascular collapse.

Management

- Reduce fraction of inspired oxygen (FiO_2) to titrate SaO_2 between 75 and 85%. In many patients, ventilation in room air is adequate.
- Ventilator settings to titrate PCO_2 to around 40–45 mm Hg
- Addition of a systemic vasodilator such as milrinone or levosimendan is reasonable for improving systemic perfusion.
- If pulmonary overcirculation is due to competing PDA flows consider surgical ligation of PDA or coil closure.
- Continue mechanical ventilation as controlled ventilation helps to regulate PBF.

How to Diagnose Decreased Pulmonary Blood Flow?

This is indicated by a peripheral arterial saturation <75%. Arterial blood gases often show a PO_2 lower than 35 mm Hg. A narrow pulse pressure is also suggestive. Reduction in PBF can be potentially due to a shunt block or high pulmonary vascular resistance (PVR) impeding PBF. Confirm shunt patency by auscultating for shunt murmur. A bedside screening echocardiogram is reasonable to demonstrate unobstructed shunt flows. If shunt is patent, low saturation may be due to pulmonary causes (atelectasis, retained secretions, etc.), increased PVR or decreased arterial oxygen content. Sometimes, there may be preferential circulation to one lung (see later).

Management of Shunt Occlusion

This is a surgical emergency, which might require emergent reintervention to establish PBF. The operating room/ICU has to prepare for emergent resternotomy. Administer

heparin bolus of 1 mg/kg and maintain continuous heparin infusion at 10–20 units/kg/h. Fluid boluses in aliquots of 5 mL/kg should be administered to improve blood pressure and facilitate forward flow through the shunt. Increasing the systemic arterial pressure through vasoconstrictors such as phenylephrine may help to maintain oxygen saturation in patients with partially occluded shunts. Choosing a higher FiO_2, and titrating the PCO_2 between 30 and 35 mm Hg might be useful to reduce PVR. Pulmonary and mechanical causes (blocked ET tube, displaced ET tube, and pneumothorax) for desaturation should be equally sought for and promptly addressed. Pulmonary toileting should be done if necessary, to remove any retained secretions.

Asymmetric Pulmonary Blood Flow

Abnormal distribution of PBF results from stenosis of one of the pulmonary artery branches. Often it is the left pulmonary artery that is stenotic. The implication of preferential flow to one lung is often not intuitive. The patients are especially vulnerable to ventilation perfusion mismatch from parenchymal lesions or airway issues involving the well-perfused lung that can result in catastrophic hypoxia. Radiologically, increased opacification of the ipsilateral lung field is suggestive of preferential increased flow to ipsilateral pulmonary artery. Asymmetric flow can be identified on echocardiogram by looking at the flows in individual pulmonary arteries.

■ VENTILATION MANAGEMENT

Ventilation Goals

The key goal of mechanical ventilation is to facilitate the balance between systemic and pulmonary blood flow. Typically, peripheral oxygen saturation between 75 and 85%

indicates a Qp/Qs of 1. A consistent increase in SaO_2 > 90% will imply pulmonary over circulation. Pulmonary hyperperfusion may be associated with signs of poor systemic perfusion including metabolic acidosis and reduced urine output. Ventilator strategies should aim to avoid factors that further decrease the PVR. This includes using lowest possible FiO_2 to target a PO_2 ranging from 40–45 mm Hg and adjusting the ventilator rate to achieve a PCO_2 45–50 mm Hg. In instances where a high PVR is suspected to be the cause of poor shunt flow, ventilator settings should be optimized to deliver higher FiO_2 to maintain PO_2 around 40–45 mm Hg and to target a PCO_2 ranging from 30 to 35 mm Hg.

Weaning and Extubation

Weaning and extubation can be considered once the patient sustains a stable hemo-dynamics. In well-balanced shunts, hemo-dynamics usually stabilize in 24–48 hours. Caution should be exercised, when spon-taneous breathing is allowed in these patients. The fall in intrathoracic pressure, change in lung volume, as well as a "washout" of carbon dioxide can facilitate increased PBF by altering PVR. Monitor for signs of low cardiac output while initiating spontaneous breathing in these patients. Most patients will benefit from a short course of noninvasive ventilation as it will help control FiO_2 and decrease work of breathing in patients with increased PBF. Extubation can sometimes be quite stormy in these patients. Hence, it is often executed in the presence of ICU physician after ensuring availability of necessary resuscitation equip-ment and drugs.

Special Nursing Considerations in Ventilated Patients

1. Endotracheal suctioning is a high-risk procedure in these infants and hence should be restricted to only when it is absolutely necessary.

2. It is reasonable to pre-oxygenate these patients with an FiO_2 10% higher than the current ventilator set FiO_2 before suctioning. Using 100% FiO_2 during Ambu ventilation can cause sudden changes in shunt flow, which can precipitate a cardiac event.

3. The presence of a physician is mandatory while performing ET suctioning especially in the first 48 hours of surgery.

4. Routine use of inline nebulizations should be avoided in the first 48 hours as the inadvertent variations in ventilator flow rates during a nebulizer flow may jeopardize the fine balance between systemic and PBF.

5. Adequate pain relief should be ensured with physician consultation before any stressful procedures such as ET suctioning, intercostal drain insertion, etc., to avoid potential triggers for increasing PVR.

◼ FLUID MANAGEMENT

Fluid management strategies should focus on maintaining adequate intravascular volume while carefully avoiding large nega-tive fluid balances in the postoperative period. The standard daily fluid prescriptions based on body surface area method will suffice for calculation of maintenance fluid requirements for shunts performed on CPB while higher maintenance rates (60–100 mL/kg/day) are allowable in patients who underwent surgery without CPB. The use of blood components in the immediate post-operative period for volume replacement is not desirable as the procoagulant effects can predispose to shunt thrombosis. Periopera-tive platelet transfusion has been previously identified as a risk factor for shunt failure related mortality.[8]

■ DIURETIC THERAPY

Diuretic therapy is typically avoided in the first 24 hours after surgery as sudden fluid shifts can lead to changes in hematocrit or blood pressure which may affect the flows through the shunt. However, a continuous infusion of furosemide may be administered cautiously in the later postoperative period in patients who have clinical evidence of fluid overload.

■ PAIN AND SEDATION MANAGEMENT

Standard pain and sedation protocol with fentanyl and/or dexmedetomidine is used. Midazolam should be used cautiously due to concerns of profound hypotension and precipitous drop in diastolic blood pressure which can be detrimental to shunt flows in the postoperative period.

■ FEEDING AND NUTRITION

It is prudent to initiate feeds cautiously in neonates with a large arterial duct pre-operatively/or in patients with signs of pulmonary over circulation postsurgery, to minimize gastrointestinal complications due to systemic hypoperfusion. Preferably trophic feeds are initiated first and cautiously escalated to goal volumes over 24–48 hours. Monitor for feed intolerance by periodic checking for abdominal distension, gastric residual volumes and vomiting. Feeds should be withheld in patients with significant systemic hypoperfusion as evidenced by metabolic acidosis or high lactate levels >4 mmol/L. It is also justifiable to withhold feeds in neonates on high doses of vasoconstricting agents (vasopressin, noradrenaline, etc.). In patients whom enteral feeds are withheld for more than 72 hours, parenteral nutrition should be considered to meet energy and protein requirements.

■ COMMON POSTOPERATIVE COMPLICATIONS

Shunt Occlusion

This is probably the most life-threatening complication in the postoperative period. The unobstructed flow through the shunt is obligatory for pulmonary circulation and survival. Shunt block is diagnosed by profound desaturation, hemodynamic instability including bradycardia, hypotension, and rapid progression to cardiac arrest. Clinical evaluation reveals loss of shunt murmur and echocardiographic evidence of poor/absent shunt flow. In a retrospective review of 207 cases undergoing modified BT shunt, in-hospital shunt occlusion occurred in 6.8% patients.[9] Pulmonary atresia/ventricular septal defect with or without major aortopulmonary collaterals and size of the pulmonary artery being shunted had a significant impact in predicting shunt occlusion. Pulmonary artery diameter <4 mm had also been implicated in previous studies to contribute to postoperative shunt failure.[10] Shunt occlusion is a surgical emergency and requires reintervention or revision of the shunt to re-establish PBF.

Low Cardiac Output

This is most often due to a compromised systemic circulation secondary to increased PBF. This is diagnosed by cool extremities, poor pedal pulses, decreased urine output, and metabolic acidosis with rising blood lactate level. Treatment is by titrating ventilator settings to decrease PBF (detailed in section *Ventilation Goals* earlier) and systemic vasodilators such as milrinone or levosimendan to improve systemic perfusion. Other cardiac cause for low cardiac output such as ventricular dysfunction or significant atrioventricular (AV) valve regurgitation should also be ruled out systematically by bedside echocardiography.

Gastrointestinal Complications

Neonates with duct dependent circulation preoperatively or those having reduced systemic blood flow secondary to an over-flowing shunt in the post-operative period are sometimes likely to develop gastro-intestinal complications such as necrotizing enterocolitis. Disruption of gut mucosal integrity can predispose to bacterial sepsis and contribute to substantial postoperative morbidity. Surgical intervention is usually not required and most patients respond to conservative management with continuous gastric aspiration, broad-spectrum antimicrobial therapy, and total parenteral nutrition. Multidisciplinary collaboration with inputs from the pediatric surgery team is valuable in the management of these critically ill patients and for planning any emergent surgical intervention if required.

■ DEINTENSIFICATION

Typically, these patients have a stormy postoperative period due to the difficulty in achieving an optimum balance between systemic and pulmonary blood flow. Usually these patients require prolonged ventilation and intensive care. Careful monitoring is required 24 hours postextubation before initiating deintensification measures. Invasive lines can be removed after inotropes are tapered off. An orally administered systemic vasodilator agent such as enalapril may be required in patients with shunt overflow, but this needs to be used with great caution in neonates who are vulnerable to renal failure. Antiplatelet therapy with aspirin should also be continued in the postoperative period. Adequate hydration should be maintained to prevent hemoconcentration and compromise of the shunt flow. While advancing feeds, meticulous attention should be focused on signs of intolerance. Diuretic dose should be carefully titrated before discharge especially in patients on enalapril due to high risk for renal dysfunction. Patients with shunt dependent PBF are vulnerable for postoperative attrition due to shunt thrombosis, shunt stenosis or pulmonary artery distortion.[11] Therefore, meticulous parent education is required before transition to the ward care and discharge. Importance of preventing inadvertent dehydration (during NPO for procedures, diarrheal diseases, excessive diuretic dosage, etc.), monitoring for feed intolerance, continuation of aspirin therapy and periodic monitoring of peripheral oxygen saturation at a local medical facility should be clearly communicated to the ward nurse and parents while planning discharge. In most situations, a reasonable balance between systemic and pulmonary circulation is achieved before discharge. Very rarely, patients may remain over-circulated with high saturations at discharge and these patients may receive once daily dose of oral furosemide for a limited period (typically 2 weeks).

■ DISCHARGE MEDICATIONS

- Aspirin at a dose of 3–5 mg/kg administered once daily. Clopidogrel is an alternative to aspirin when aspirin is not tolerated (often because of gastritis)
- *Oral iron supplements*: Maintenance dose of iron supplement is typically initiated once the infants are 2–3 months of age.

■ REFERENCES

1. Talwar S, Kumar MV, Muthukkumaran S, Airan B. Is sternotomy superior to thoracotomy for modified Blalock-Taussig shunt? Interact Cardiovasc Thorac Surg. 2014;18:371-5.
2. Dorobandu DM, Pandey R, Sharabiani MT, Mahani AS, Angelini GD, Martin RP, et al. Indications and results of a systemic to pulmonary shunts: results from a national database. Eur J Cardiothorac Surg. 2016;49:1553-63.
3. Dirks V, Pretre R, Knirsch W, Valsangiacomo Buechel ER, Seifert B, Scweiger M, et al.

Modified Blalock Taussig shunt: a not so simple palliative procedure. Eur J Cardiothorac Surg. 2013;44:1096-102.

4. Petrucci O, O'Brien SM, Jacobs ML, Jacobs JP, Manning PB, Eghtesady P. Risk factors for mortality and morbidity after the neonatal Blalock-Taussig shunt procedure. Ann Thorac Surg. 2011;92:642-52.

5. Glatz AC, Petit CJ, Goldstein BH, Kelleman MS, McCracken CE, McDonnell A, et al. Comparison between patent ductus arteriosus stent and modified Blalock-Taussig shunt as palliation for infants with ductal dependent pulmonary blood flow. Insights from the Congenital Catheterisation Research Collaborative. Circulation. 2018;137:589-601.

6. Anderson BR, Blancha VL, Duchon JM, Chai P, Kalfa D, Bacha EA, et al. The effects of post-operative haematocrit on shunt occlusion for neonates undergoing single ventricle palliation. J Thorac Cardiovasc Surg. 2017;153:947-55.

7. Li Js, Yow E, Berezny KY, Rhodes JF, Bokesch PM, Charpie JR, et al. Clinical outcomes of palliative surgery including a systemic to pulmonary artery shunt in infants with cyanotic congenital heart disease: does aspirin make a difference? Circulation. 2007;116:293-7.

8. Vitanova K, Leopold C, von Ohain JP, Wolf C, Beran E, Lange R, et al. Risk factors for failure of systemic to pulmonary artery shunts in biventricular circulation. Pediatr Cardiol. 2018;39:1323-9.

9. Guzetta NA, Foster GS, Mruthinti N, Kilgore PD, Miller BE, Kanter KR, et al. In-hospital shunt occlusion in infants undergoing a modified Blalock-Taussig shunt. Ann Thorac Surg. 2013;96:176-82.

10. Al Jubair KA, Al Fagih MR, Al Jarallah AS, Al Yousef S, Ashmeg A, Al Faraidy Y, et al. Results of 546 Blalock-Taussig shunts performed in 478 patients. Cardiol Young. 1998;8:486-90.

11. O'Connor MJ, Ravishankar C, Ballweg JA, Gillespie MJ, Gaynor JW, Tabbutt S, et al. Early systemic to pulmonary artery shunt intervention in neonates with congenital heart disease. J Thorac Cardiovasc Surg. 2011;142:106-12.

Pulmonary Artery Banding

Rakhi Balachandran

Illustration: Balaji Srimurugan
Reviewed by: R Krishna Kumar

■ INTRODUCTION

Pulmonary artery (PA) banding is a palliative procedure performed in congenital heart defects with excessive pulmonary blood flow. It is performed in situations where the primary repair is not imminently feasible or as the first stage operation in staged palliations for single ventricle with excessive pulmonary blood flow. The broad objectives of PA banding includes ameliorating symptoms of overt cardiac failure, protecting the pulmonary vascular bed from progression of hypertensive pulmonary vascular disease [e.g., single ventricle lesions with high pulmonary blood flow, children with large ventricular septal defects (VSD)/multiple VSD] and serving as a bridge to staged correction for lesions initially not amenable to two ventricle repair.[1] PA banding is also done in those infants presenting late with transposition of great arteries (TGA), to "train" the left ventricle to support the systemic circulation.[2] PA banding is now increasingly used in corrected transpositions with intact ventricular septum as a strategy to address severe regurgitation of the left atrioventricular valve (i.e., morphologically tricuspid valve). The surgical procedure involves placement of a constricting band around the proximal pulmonary artery trunk **(Fig. 1)**. The key surgical challenge is in ascertaining the correct circumference of the band. This is because, according to the Poiseuille's law, the blood flow is related to fourth power of the radius of the vessel. Therefore, a small change in diameter can have a large impact on blood flow and resistance. The appropriate circumferential length of the band is calculated based on existing formulae. According to Trusler and Mustard formula, the expected circumference of the band in inch was approximated to 20 mm +1 mm/kg of the child's body weight in single ventricle palliations and 24 mm +1 mm/kg in infants for eventual two ventricle repairs.[3] Pre-established perimeters offer only an initial starting point for surgical decision making and the final adjustment of the band is fine-tuned according to individuals' physiologic situation and hemodynamic parameters. Placement of the band should typically result in elevation of aortic systolic pressure by 10–20 mm Hg. For a patient who will eventually have a biventricular repair, PA systolic pressure should be decreased to at least 30–50% of the measured aortic systolic blood pressure. The changes in oxygen saturation after a PA band are dependent on the underlying anatomy. For multiple VSDs and normally related great arteries, saturations post band remain high. For conditions that allow some mixing such as double outlet right ventricle, oxygen saturation can drop to below 85–90% at $FiO_2 < 0.5$. For patients for eventual single

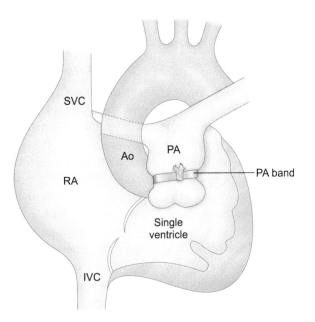

Fig. 1: First stage palliation of a univentricular heart by pulmonary artery (PA) banding. A constricting band is placed around the proximal PA trunk to reduce the pulmonary blood flow.

(IVC: inferior vena cava; RA: right atrium; SVC: superior vena cava; Ao: aorta)

ventricle palliation, the lowest possible distal main PA pressures that can be achieved with an oxygen saturation of 75–85% is desired at FiO$_2$ < 0.5. For patients with arterial transposition who require a PA band, the saturations can fall substantially and may be in the high 60s and low 70s in the early postoperative period.

It is important to distinguish between PA band for multiple VSDs from other conditions. Those with multiple VSDs maintain better saturations in general because there is little mixing of blood in the heart. The postoperative course is relatively straightforward in comparison to babies with single ventricle. The surgeons do not necessarily endeavor to reduce PA pressures to near normal levels.

Though this is seemingly a simple operation, it is often difficult to achieve an accurate constriction of the band in the operating room because of the effects of general anesthesia, controlled ventilation and open chest on the patients' cardiopulmonary physiology.[4] Most of the postoperative morbidity stems from this difficulty in establishing optimum band size for each patient given the impact of the various factors on pulmonary blood flow. Operations in the early era were associated with a mortality nearing 30%.[5] The surgical indications of PA banding has declined in established pediatric heart programs in current era because of early corrective surgery of most two ventricle lesions. With improvement in surgical expertise and careful selection of patients expected mortality in the current era is less than 5%.[6,7]

■ MONITORING

Standard hemodynamic monitoring with invasive arterial blood pressure, continuous ECG monitoring, central venous pressure (CVP) monitoring, pulse oximetry and capnography.

■ HEMODYNAMIC MANAGEMENT

Meticulous hemodynamic monitoring is very essential after PA banding because of the potential consequences related to alterations in systemic and pulmonary blood flow and changes in the loading conditions of the heart imposed by the band. Postoperative management after the banding is dictated by the degree of tightness of the band. The band produces a fixed obstruction to pulmonary blood flow. A tight band can cause acute pressure overload to the subpulmonary ventricle or to the systemic ventricle in a single ventricle physiology and may contribute to ventricular dysfunction, low systemic oxygen saturation and a low cardiac output state. A loose band on the other hand will still allow excessive pulmonary blood flow and may result in persistent heart failure and ineffective protection to the pulmonary circulation.

Clinical Recognition of Optimum Band

Ideally, an optimum band should allow a Qp/Qs (pulmonary to systemic blood flow ratio) of 1–1.5 and typically produce a peripheral oxygen saturation of 75–85% at an $FiO_2 < 0.5$ in patients with a single ventricle physiology. Adequate systemic perfusion is evident by warm extremities, good pedal pulses, and a capillary refill time of less than 2 seconds. An arterial blood gas usually demonstrates normal pH without acidosis and serum lactate levels <2 mmol/L. A long systolic murmur should be easily heard and the second heart sound should ideally have an identifiable split. Expected optimal band Doppler gradient in the postoperative period is 40–70 mm Hg. Patients with optimal band size are usually hemodynamically stable and require minimal inotropic supports. For those with multiple VSDs the adequacy of the PA band can be best assessed by the gradient across the band. A gradient of 50 mm Hg or more is desirable.

Clinical Recognition of Loose Band

A loose band is associated with increased pulmonary blood flow with a Qp/Qs >1. This is identified by an increase in peripheral oxygen saturation >90% at an $FiO_2 <0.5$ in children with single ventricle physiology. Inadequate systemic perfusion is associated with clinical signs such as cold extremities, poor pedal pulses and decreased urine output. Compromised tissue oxygen delivery results in metabolic acidosis and elevated serum lactate levels. Auscultation may reveal a relatively soft and a relatively short pulmonary outflow murmur. Ventilator strategies to increase pulmonary vascular resistance (PVR) such as decreasing inspired oxygen concentration, reducing respiratory rate to increase arterial PCO_2 levels and maintaining mild respiratory acidosis might help to control pulmonary blood flow. Afterload reducing agents such as milrinone or levosimendan may be beneficial to maximize systemic perfusion and optimize tissue oxygen delivery.

Clinical Recognition of Tight Band

A tight band may be associated with unacceptable hypoxia with saturations consistently below 75% in those with a single ventricle physiology. Significant hemodynamic instability may sometimes be seen. The acute increase in afterload may precipitate ventricular dysfunction or low cardiac output state. Sudden onset bradycardia or arrhythmias are not uncommon. Band gradient typically exceeds 60 mm Hg. Ventilator strategies should aim to decrease PVR by allowing higher inspired oxygen concentrations (>0.5), avoiding hypercarbia and permitting mild respiratory alkalosis. Inotropic support with epinephrine and milrinone is often needed. Endotracheal suctioning and tracheal extubation are important events that are likely to precipitate bradycardia and sudden cardiovascular collapse. Extreme vigil should be exerted during this procedures and emergency drugs and resuscitation equipment should be available at the bedside. Bradycardia and cardiovascular collapse from a tight band merit emergent chest opening in the intensive care unit (ICU) along with loosening of the band.

Special Challenges

PA Band in the Presence of Elevated Pulmonary Vascular Resistance

Occasionally, patients with single ventricle physiology can present late, with elevated PVR. PA band is offered only after considerable thought and discussion. These children may be quite hypoxic, despite a relatively low band gradient. They are especially prone to adverse events in the early postoperative period and often need selective pulmonary vasodilators.

PA Band in Patients with Congenital Mitral Valve Stenosis or Atresia

Here the PA band is performed together with atrial septectomy under cardiopulmonary bypass. The chronically elevated pulmonary venous pressure results in substantial elevation of PVR that often takes time to resolve. The surgeon often chooses to place a loose band initially and leave the chest open for the initial few days. The band is usually tightened to the final size at the time of chest closure. The oxygen saturations often tend to be lower than acceptable levels for the initial 48 hours.

PA Band for Training the Left Ventricle

Two situations where this operation is undertaken are in TGA with regressed left ventricle (LV) and in corrected transposition.

This is an especially challenging situation because the ventricular septum is intact. In the absence of a VSD, the untrained LV is particularly vulnerable to small changes in afterload. The band gradients are often much lower here. Treatment protocols have to be individualized to the specific situation.

■ VENTILATOR MANAGEMENT

Pulmonary artery banding, results in important alterations in the quantum of pulmonary and systemic blood flow. The adaptation to the post banding circulatory physiology may take up to 24–48 hours. Typically, most centers allow a conservative ventilator strategy using elective ventilation for 24 hours to enable adaptation to the new circulatory physiology and also to allow postoperative adjustments in the size of the band if required. The circulatory changes in the postoperative period, are due to variations in pulmonary and systemic vascular resistances or due to changes in the blood vessel diameter because of opening of folds within the vessel wall. Consequently, a band, which initially appears to be tight, might become loose in the postoperative period. Since the pulmonary vascular bed is extremely sensitive to changes in arterial PO_2 and PCO_2, the regulation of these gases plays a substantial role in adjusting pulmonary blood flow after PA banding. The ventilator management is tailored to the degree of tightness of the band **(Table 1)**.

■ FLUID MANAGEMENT

Restricted fluid strategy is preferred in view of preoperative congestive cardiac failure. Body surface area method of calculating fluid requirement is utilized for those undergoing surgery under cardiopulmonary bypass (CPB) (when combined with atrial septectomy). Volume boluses should be administered

TABLE 1: Ventilatory management (single ventricle physiology).

Type of the band	Clinical diagnosis	Management
Optimum band	Qp/Qs = 1, SaO_2 between 75 and 85%, PO_2 = 40–45 mm Hg, no acidosis, normal lactate level, band gradient = 40–70 mm Hg	• FiO_2 between 0.3 and 0.5 • RR to target PCO_2 of 35–40 mm Hg • Minimal inotropic supports • Aim to extubate within 24 hours
Loose band	Qp/Qs >1, SaO_2 >90%, PO_2 >50 mm Hg, if systemic circulation is compromised may have metabolic acidosis, lactate level >2 mmol/L, band gradient <40 mm Hg	• Decrease FiO_2 to 21% • Maintain PCO_2 at 45–50 mm Hg • Diuresis (to decrease pulmonary congestion) • Consider milrinone (to improve systemic perfusion) • Consider extubation once clinical signs improve
Tight band	Qp/Qs <1, SaO_2 < 75%, PO_2<35 mm Hg, band gradient > 60 mm Hg Lactate may be elevated if associated ventricular dysfunction	• Increase FiO_2 >0.5 • Maintain PCO_2 at 30–35 mm Hg • Mild respiratory alkalosis • Inotropes such as epinephrine and milrinone may be used if associated ventricular dysfunction • Adjustment of band size if cardiovascular instability occurs • Usually ventilated electively for 24–48 hours or until clinical stability is achieved

(Qp/Qs: pulmonary to systemic blood flow ratio; SaO_2: arterial oxygen saturation; RR: respiratory rate)

with extreme caution, as this may precipitate bradycardia and hemodynamic compromise in patients with ventricular dysfunction following the band.

PAIN AND SEDATION MANAGEMENT

Standard pain and sedation policy using fentanyl infusion and intermittent doses of midazolam is appropriate. Additional top-up doses of analgesics or sedatives are reasonable before endotracheal suctioning or painful interventions in ICU to minimize stress response and avoid sudden fluctuations in PVR.

DIURETIC THERAPY

Most patients are initiated on furosemide infusion of 1–2 mg/kg/day to promote diuresis. A negative fluid balance of 25–50 mL/kg is reasonable to minimize pulmonary congestion and to facilitate successful extubation.

FEEDING AND NUTRITION

Standard feeding protocol is followed. Patients, who require prolonged ventilation and intensive care unit stay due to suboptimal band size, require meticulous attention to calorie intake and optimal nutrition management.

COMMON POSTOPERATIVE COMPLICATIONS

Bradycardia and Sudden Cardiovascular Collapse

This is typically seen in a tight band. A tight band may acutely increase ventricular afterload and precipitate ventricular failure. Also, an acute increase in PVR especially in neonates can precipitate cardiovascular collapse following a pulmonary hypertensive crisis. Endotracheal suctioning, patient ventilator asynchrony/agitation, and pain are the usual postoperative triggers for elevated PVR.

Low Cardiac Output State

This often results from a tight band, causing ventricular dysfunction or from a loose band causing increased pulmonary blood flow with a compromised systemic perfusion. Treatment is often dictated by the cause of low cardiac output and is usually managed by ventilator maneuvers to modify pulmonary blood flow and inotrope therapy. Peritoneal dialysis should be initiated to support renal function if required.

Failed Extubation

This is commonly seen with a loose band with increased pulmonary blood flow. The potential causes include pulmonary congestion resulting from increased pulmonary blood flow, poor nutritional reserves due to pre-existing heart failure, low cardiac output state or importantly, atrioventricular (AV) valve regurgitation. Tachypnea during spontaneous breathing on weaning attempts can result in increased CO_2 washout, decreasing PVR and further increasing pulmonary blood flow. Management includes optimizing pulmonary blood flow by ventilator maneuvers to increase PVR, use of vasodilators to improve systemic perfusion, optimizing nutritional status and aggressive diuretic therapy. Increasing hematocrit to increase blood viscosity may also be beneficial in patients with admixture physiology to decrease pulmonary overcirculation. A hemoglobin level of 12–14 g/dL may be reasonable in neonates.

Late Complications

PA Band Migration

This complication can occur if the band is not anchored to adventitia of the pulmonary artery. It can lead to branch pulmonary artery distortion and may create technical problems in future surgical corrections.

Subaortic Obstruction

The ventricular hypertrophy and remodeling that follows PA banding can sometimes precipitate important subaortic obstruction in selected patients with specific anatomic substrates.[8] This subset includes patients with tricuspid atresia and transposition where the aorta arises from the right ventricle. PA band provokes ventricular hypertrophy that results in subaortic obstruction. Additionally, patients with single ventricle and a systemic (aortic) outflow dependent on a potentially restrictive bulbo-ventricular foramen are also prone to developing subaortic stenosis. Progressive subaortic obstruction can adversely affect outcomes after Fontan operation by exaggerating ventricular hypertrophy, leading to subendocardial ischemia and ventricular dysfunction.[9]

■ DEINTENSIFICATION

Postoperatively, these patients are generally ventilated for at least 24 hours to facilitate proper assessment of effective band size, gradient and hemodynamic stability. This enables hemodynamic adjustment to the altered pulmonary and systemic blood flows after banding. The child has to be observed carefully on ventilator in the spontaneous breathing mode before extubation for any evidence of hemodynamic instability, desaturation or bradycardia. Neonates and young infants may require a short period of continuous positive airway pressure (CPAP) support after extubation to decrease work of breathing and reduce ventricular afterload. Inotropes can be tapered off, if stable for 24 hours after extubation. Oral vasodilators such as enalapril may have a role in patients with increased pulmonary blood flow but they should be used carefully in neonates and young infants. The invasive lines are removed once inotropes are discontinued.

Discharge from the ICU is planned after establishing oral feeding.

DISCHARGE MEDICATIONS

Discharge medications are typically dictated by clinical condition. Diuretics need to be administered for a variable period of time. Loose bands may require extended administration of diuretics and vasodilators.

REFERENCES

1. Sharma R. Pulmonary artery banding: rationale and possible indications in the current era. Ann Pediatr Card. 2012;5:40-3.
2. Ma K, Hua Z, Yang K, Hu S, Lacour-Gayet F, Yan J, et al. Arterial switch for transposed great vessels with intact ventricular septum beyond one month of age. Ann Thorac Surg. 2014;97:189-95.
3. Trussler GA, Mustard WT. A method of banding the pulmonary artery for large isolated ventricular septal defect with and without transposition of great arteries. Ann Thorac Surg. 1972;13:351-5.
4. Valente AS, Mesquita F, Mejia JA, Maia IC, Maior MS, Branco KC, et al. Pulmonary artery banding: a simple procedure? A critical analysis at a tertiary centre. Rev Bras Cir. 2009;24:327-33.
5. Goldblatt A, Bernhard WF, Nadas AS, Gross RE. Pulmonary artery banding: indications and results in infants and children. Circulation. 1965;32:172-84.
6. Takayama H, Sekiguchi A, Chikada M, Nomo M, Ishihawa A, Takamoto S. Mortality of pulmonary artery banding in the current era: recent mortality of PA banding. Ann Thorac Surg. 2002;74:1219-24.
7. Kouchukos NT, Blackstone EH, Hanley FL, Kirklin JK. Tricuspid atresia and single ventricle physiology. In: Kirklin Barrat-Boyes Cardiac Surgery, 4th edition. Philadelphia: Elsevier Saunders; 2013. pp. 1507-74.
8. Freedom RM, Benson LN, Smallhorn JF, Williams WG, Trusler GA, Rowe RD. Subaortic stenosis, the univentricular heart, and banding of the pulmonary artery: an analysis of the courses of 43 patients with univentricular heart palliated by pulmonary artery banding. Circulation. 1986;4:758-64.
9. Freedom RM. Subaortic obstruction and the Fontan operation. Ann Thorac Surg. 1998;66:649-52.

Norwood Procedure

Aveek Jayant

Illustrations: Balaji Srimurugan

Reviewed by: R Krishna Kumar

■ INTRODUCTION

Hypoplastic left heart syndrome (HLHS) is a relatively rare cardiac anomaly and incidence rates are estimated to be only 0.016–0.036% of all live births. The importance of diagnosis, however, lies in the fact that this condition accounts for a very large proportion of cardiac deaths in the neonatal period; 23% of deaths within the first week of life and 15% of all deaths due to congenital heart disease within the first month are attributable to this condition.[1] Although most would argue that in resource rich settings the standard management of this condition would be staged palliation toward a Fontan procedure,[2] this approach should be tempered by the inevitable presence of periventricular leukomalacia at birth and the demonstrated poor quality of life when compared to children in health, or with other illnesses on follow-up.[3] Calibrated improvement in outcomes following the Norwood operation should also be measured by the fact that this surgery continues to demand and consumes a very large proportion of resources in intensive care; this operation constitutes the most common indication for post-cardiotomy extracorporeal membrane oxygenation (ECMO) use in neonates today.[4] The anatomic spectrum of this condition ranges from atresia of both aortic and mitral valves to atresia of one or the other of these valves and stenosis of the other (**Fig. 1A**). Of particular interest to those caring for these neonates is the HLHS subtype in which mitral patency accompanies aortic atresia—such neonates are at risk of developing tricuspid insufficiency (with its effects on the putative systemic right ventricle), and, understandably are at higher risk of attrition during the Norwood procedure.[1] In the current era, the Norwood operation has two distinct (yet analogous) variants which differ only in the source of pulmonary blood flow. In the classic prototype this is accomplished using a systemic–pulmonary artery shunt (**Fig. 1B**) whereas in the Sano modification this is achieved using a separate right ventricle to pulmonary artery conduit. The Sano modification was believed to achieve more stable hemodynamics, particularly in the vulnerable coronary circulation where retrograde coronary flow is demonstrable as an unavoidable correlate of the systemic-pulmonary artery shunt; this is however not without controversy and the approach to the operation seems to be institution and surgeon based.[5]

At our own institution the Norwood operation is usually accomplished at a temperature of 20–22°C with selective antegrade cerebral perfusion and the use of a weight appropriate systemic–pulmonary artery shunt.

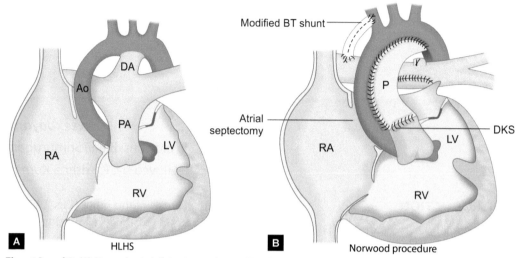

Figs. 1A and B: (A) Hypoplastic left heart syndrome (HLHS); (B) Stage I Norwood palliation for HLHS. Pulmonary blood flow is established through a modified Blalock-Taussig (BT) shunt.

[PA: pulmonary artery; RA: right atrium; RV: right ventricle; LV: left ventricle; DKS: Damus–Kaye–Stanzel anastomosis (pulmonary artery to aorta connection); P: pericardium; DA: ductus arteriosus; Ao: aorta]

MONITORING THE NEONATE AFTER NORWOOD OPERATION

Institutions performing this operation make local protocols on monitoring modalities and parameters. This is often based on availability, evidence and cost. While monitoring of invasive arterial and venous pressures, urine output, estimates of core (and sometimes peripheral) temperature and continuous electrocardiographic monitoring is probably universal and standard, other adjuncts are also sometimes used. The two particular monitors of topical interest are cerebral and flank near infrared spectroscopy (NIRS) and the continuous venous oximetry catheters that some institutions use. While our institution currently uses neither, it is exploring the option of using NIRS (single or dual site) as an option to continuously monitor oxygen delivery to the brain and the splanchnic circulation.

It is important to appreciate the principles behind using these monitors in order to understand the dynamic nature of the parallel circulation. In patients with series circulation, at constant cardiac output increased oxygen requirements (VO_2) translate to a fall in mixed venous oxygen. In the parallel circulation increased VO_2 (systemic oxygen demand) translates to a simultaneous decline in both the venous and arterial oxygen tensions (since arterial oxygen tension is intrinsically a mixture of the returned venous admixture and the pulmonary capillary blood). As such, SaO_2 (systemic arterial saturation) can therefore only be improved by increasing total cardiac output (this leads to less venous desaturation and therefore overall higher arterial oxygen tension). Most early approaches to the management of HLHS, post-Norwood procedure, have had a fixation on keeping a fixed SaO_2, typically around 80% and guessing (wrongly) that this led to a balanced Q_p/Q_s. Solving the Fick equation for SaO_2 in patients with a parallel circulation leads to the following result:

$$SaO_2 = Q_p \left(S_{pv}O_2\right) + Q_p \left(S_vO_2\right)/Q_p + Q_s$$

(where SaO_2 = systemic arterial oxygen saturation, Q_p = pulmonary blood flow, Q_s = systemic blood flow, $S_{pv}O_2$ = pulmonary venous oxygen saturation, and S_vO_2 is the mixed systemic venous oxygen saturation)

As a learning example, low systemic arterial saturations could result from a low PvO_2 because of a deliberate reduction of inspired oxygen tension *or* decreased overall Q and low SvO_2. Without a measurement of SvO_2 (or a surrogate measure such as NIRS) no treatment plan can be made. This is borne out by the early work of Twedell et al.[6] and its continuous refinement over the years.[7] While continuous oximetry catheters are available NIRS has also been used as a surrogate measure of tissue oxygen delivery and composite oxygen balance. Neither NIRS nor continuous oximetry catheters are used at our center but this protocol is in evolution.

HEMODYNAMIC MANAGEMENT AND INOTROPES

Our center typically uses small boluses of phenoxybenzamine at the initiation of cardiopulmonary bypass (doses of 0.5–1 mg/kg) leaning on the initial experience of the Wisconsin group who have foundationally changed the management of this condition in the post Norwood period.[7] Phenoxybenzamine, a nonselective α-blocker that irreversibly binds the α-adrenoceptor prevents the sudden surges in systemic vascular resistance that can occur secondary to noxious stimuli ranging from pain to endotracheal suction. Acute dramatic rises in SVR can potentially skew the Q_p/Q_s ratio toward excessive pulmonary blood flow and precipitous declines in systemic perfusion including the coronary circulation setting the stage for acute and sudden cardiovascular collapse. As such, at our center the potential for this dramatic turn of events is often negotiated by delayed sternal closure post Norwood to facilitate a need to initiate extracorporeal circulation in event of this potential crisis.

Although there is a poor evidence base to choose an inotrope over another and particularly with respect to specific disease or pathophysiology at our institution, it is usual to use titrated dose of milrinone and adrenaline to facilitate separation from cardiopulmonary bypass and for the initial postoperative period. Vasopressors are usually not initiated except when mean arterial pressures fall below 30–35 mm Hg.

FLUID MANAGEMENT

At our center fluid management is primarily dictated by the age of the neonate and whether or not the patient was born at term. It is also titrated to the daily average fluid balance as determined by weight or semi-quantitative assessment of the functional ventricle on periodic transthoracic echocardiography. Typically, the immediate postoperative period could lead to fluid prescriptions of 500 mL/m^2 with gradual titration upward to 1,000 mL/m^2 even as stabilization of hemodynamics allows early enteral nutrition and full caloric goals are sought to be obtained. Qualitative reviews[8] of the literature on this condition have suggested obtaining hemoglobin concentrations of 14–16 g/dL, and anecdotally, this approach maximizes pulmonary vascular resistance over systemic vascular resistance. However, this approach is tempered by more recent expert opinion[9] on the subject of targeting hemoglobin concentrations at no more than 10 g/dL in the presence of stable cardiovascular status. The former approach may still be considered by some in the event of runaway over circulation but the overwhelming consensus on managing the ratio of Q_p/Q_s is based on titration of inspired gas concentrations and focus on changing the total cardiac output and minimizing the SVR.[10]

Adjunct component use is virtually restricted to clinical bleeding or abnormal results on thromboelastography; use may have also been curtailed by the higher temperatures that are now maintained when using selective antegrade cerebral perfusion.

■ VENTILATORY MANAGEMENT

A short summary of the ventilatory goals post-Norwood surgery can be summarized as follows[8]:

- $PaCO_2$: 35–45 mm Hg
- PaO_2: 30–45 mm Hg
- pH: 7.35–7.40
- SaO_2: 70–85%

A cursory examination of the above prescription shows that the main aim of ventilatory management should be to prevent runaway drops in PVR that allow a skewed Q_p/Q_s ratio. This approach therefore begins with initiating ventilation with low fractional concentrations of inspired oxygen and targeting normocapnia. Adjunctive therapies (as described earlier) include carefully titrated pharmacotherapy to drop SVR to the lowest extent possible.

While emphasizing the above approach, it is also important to remember that in all patients with systemic – pulmonary arterial shunts in situ, and with particular reference to those patients with a functional single ventricle the $S_{pv}O_2$ is often overestimated. This leads to consistently underestimating the Q_p/Q_s ratio. This can be actually guessed clinically not by the SaO_2 in isolation but correlating this value to the SvO_2. The SvO_2 is often measured directly from a venous blood sample, by a continuous oximetric catheter or by a surrogate such as NIRS. This exercise should always be carried out when clinicians read a subnormal diastolic blood pressure, a wide pulse pressure as a corollary, cooling of the peripheries and oliguria. Use of advanced monitoring allows clinicians to pre-empt this downward spiral and prevent a sudden hemodynamic catastrophe in a previously normal infant. When encountering this situation, the literature advice that works consistently seems to be to add carbon dioxide to the inspired mixture as this alone improves oxygen delivery which per contra is not achieved by turning down FiO_2.[11,12] The other important therapeutic intervention is to reduce SVR maximally; in practice, when the downward spiral has already set in, using a deliberate vasodilator in the face of low coronary perfusion pressures can be tricky and counter intuitive, therefore this situation is ideally treated pre-emptively rather than post hoc.

In our unit since delayed sternal closure is the usual strategy immediate post Norwood surgery neonates can be on mechanical ventilation for several days after the procedure. Usual precautions such as standard preventive measures to prevent postextubation croup are therefore routinely employed. Even after extubation children are often receiving nasal continuous positive airway pressure (CPAP) for a further period of 24–48 hours.

■ COMMON COMPLICATIONS

The most dramatic complications after the operation result from precipitous shifts in Q_p/Q_s favoring Q_p. This could lead to a downward spiral of retrograde coronary flows away from the subendocardium, coronary ischemia and eventual cardiovascular collapse. Less extreme perturbances can lead to oliguria and splanchnic hypoperfusion (with potential for necrotizing enterocolitis). Many neonates in anticipation of a period of renal ischemia and with a view to facilitate clearance of excess body water receive peritoneal dialysis within the first few post-operative hours, usually as prophylaxis.

Although uncommon in the current era with the level of surgical skill and planning, modified BT shunts can be blocked. In our unit heparin is infused initially after control of surgical bleeding and aspirin is started latest by the second postoperative day.

Long intensive care unit stays and prolonged indwelling of central venous catheters can lead to life threatening bacterial sepsis. This is mostly gram negative and endotoxic shock can often be confounded by the presence of overcirculation leading to missed diagnoses.

On rare occasions, there is a need for rescue extracorporeal life support due to a crash in systemic hemodynamics and resultant electrical instability; or even less commonly due to a blocked BT shunt.

■ SUMMARY

The management of the Norwood operation in the postoperative phase is a continuous and exhausting challenge for pediatric cardiac intensive care.

■ REFERENCES

1. Twedell JS, Hoffman GM, Ghanayem NS, Frommelt MA, Mussatto KA, Berger S. Hypoplastic left heart syndrome. In: Allen HD, Shaddy RE, Driscoll DJ, Feltes TF (Eds). Moss and Adam's Heart Disease in Infants, Children and Adolescents, 8th edition. Philadelphia: Wolters Kluwer; 2008.
2. Wernovsky G. The paradigm shift towards surgical intervention for neonates with hypoplastic left heart syndrome Arch Pediatr Adolesc Med. 2008;162:849-53.
3. Dempster N, Cua CL, Wernovsky G, Caris E, Neely T, Allen R, et al. Children with hypoplastic left heart syndrome have lower quality of life than healthy children and children with other illnesses. Cardiol Young. 2018;28:21-6.
4. Mesher AL, McMullan DM Extracorporeal life support for the neonatal cardiac patient: outcomes and new directions. Semin Perinatol. 2014;38:97-103.
5. Ohye RG, Schranz D, D'Udekem Y. Current therapy for hypoplastic left heart syndrome and related single ventricle lesions. Circulation. 2016;134:1265-79.
6. Twedell JS, Hoffman GM, Fedderley RT, Berger S, Thomas JP, Ghanayem NS, et al. Phenoxybenzamine improves systemic oxygen delivery after the Norwood procedure. Ann Thorac Surg. 1997;67:161-8.
7. Tweddell JS, Ghanayem NS, Mussatto KA, Mitchell ME, Lemmers LJ, Musa NL, et al. Mixed venous oxygen saturation monitoring after Stage 1 palliation for hypoplastic left heart syndrome. Ann Thorac Surg. 2007;84: 1301-11.
8. Theilen U, Shekerdemian L. The intensive care of children with hypoplastic left heart syndrome. Arch Dis Child Fetal Neonatal Ed. 2005;90:F97-102.
9. Cholette JM, Willems A, Valentine SL, Bateman ST, Schwartz SM. Recommendations on RBC transfusions in infants and children with acquired and congenital heart disease from the pediatric critical care transfusion and anemia expertise initiative. Ped Crit Care Med. 2018;19:S137-48.
10. Tabbutt S, Tweddell JS, Ghanayem N. Hypoplastic left heart syndrome and other shunt dependent single ventricles. Ped Crit Care Med. 2016;17: S318-22.
11. Tabbutt S, Ramamoorthy C, Montenegro LM. Impact of inspired gas mixtures on preoperative patients with hypoplastic left heart syndrome during controlled ventilation. Circulation. 2001;104:1159-64.
12. Bradley SM, Atz AM, Simsic JM. Redefining the impact of oxygen and hyperventilation after the Norwood procedure. J Thorac Cardiovasc Surg. 2004;127:473-80.

Bidirectional Glenn Shunt

Rakhi Balachandran

Illustration: Balaji Srimurugan
Reviewed by: R Krishna Kumar

■ INTRODUCTION

Bidirectional Glenn shunt (BDGS) is a commonly performed procedure for staged palliation of patients with univentricular hearts. Patients with univentricular physiology are those in whom the cardiac anatomy is unsuitable for surgical creation of a two-ventricle circulation. Though typically, it is performed as a second stage palliation after a systemic to pulmonary artery shunt or pulmonary artery banding, in selected instances, it may be the first operation undertaken for an infant or child with single ventricle physiology. It is also used to palliate patients with difficult two-ventricle physiology until they are old enough to undergo a complex repair. Surgically, Glenn shunt involves end to side anastomosis of transected superior vena cava (SVC) to ipsilateral branch pulmonary artery **(Fig. 1)**. Blood draining from the SVC can flow into both right and left pulmonary artery and hence this is called a "bidirectional" Glenn shunt. This surgery often involves ligation of the main pulmonary artery, to abolish the antegrade pulmonary blood flow. In selected situations, some antegrade flow is deliberately left behind. This is known as a pulsatile Glenn. Additional pulmonary blood flow improves oxygen saturation, prevents formation of pulmonary arteriovenous malformations, and stimulates pulmonary artery growth.[1]

However, it may increase pulmonary artery pressures and lead to development of pleural effusions. Hemodynamic benefits of Glenn shunt include reduction of volume work of the single ventricle, a predictable Qp:Qs (pulmonary to systemic blood flow ratio) of 0.6–0.7, potential preservation of atrioventricular (AV) valve function, and long-term preservation of the myocardium by avoiding volume overload.[2] The Glenn shunt can be considered a more efficient way of improving systemic oxygen saturation when compared to the aortopulmonary shunt. This is because the Glenn shunt sends desaturated systemic venous blood from the upper half of the body directly into pulmonary circulation. This is unlike an aortopulmonary shunt (such as the Blalock–Taussig Shunt) where aortic blood (this includes the pulmonary venous return) is directed to the pulmonary circulation.

An important physiological consideration for the Glenn shunt is the fact that the pulmonary blood flow is maintained by passive forces. Therefore, the pulmonary vascular resistance (PVR) needs to be low for effective pulmonary blood flow. The neonate or young infant (<3 months) is not ideally suited to undergo the Glenn shunt because the pulmonary vascular bed is not fully developed. The number of vessels, and therefore the total cross-sectional

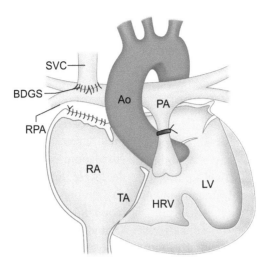

Fig. 1: Stage II palliation of single ventricle–bidirectional Glenn shunt (BDGS): Superior vena cava (SVC) is transected and anastomosed end-side to the ipsilateral, often right pulmonary artery (RPA). This is usually combined with ligation of the main pulmonary artery (PA).

(Ao: aorta; HRV: hypoplastic right ventricle; LV: left ventricle; RA: right atrium; TA: tricuspid atresia)

area of the pulmonary vascular bed of the neonate, cannot optimally support a passive pulmonary blood flow. While the ideal age at which this surgery should be performed is uncertain, younger infants undergoing Glenn tend to spend longer times in the intensive care unit (ICU). The systemic oxygen saturations in the first 48 hours are often lower with visible congestion and edema of the head. In a study comparing early (<3 months of age) and later (>3 months of age) bidirectional cavopulmonary shunts, the duration of ventilation, ICU stay and hospital stay was prolonged in the younger patient group, while the mortality, room air oxygen saturation at discharge and time to Fontan procedure remained similar between the two groups.[3] Potential causes of early morbidity in younger infants has been speculated to be poor ventilation perfusion matching, exaggerated responses of the infant lung to cardiopulmonary bypass (CPB) or elevated PVR.

MONITORING

Standard monitoring include invasive arterial blood pressure, central venous pressure (CVP) (monitored via femoral vein), continuous ECG monitoring, pulse oximetry and capnography. CVP monitored via femoral vein reflects left atrial pressure in the presence of a wide interatrial communication. Pressure monitored through a jugular venous line reflects the pulmonary artery pressure. While using femoral venous catheters for CVP monitoring or for intravenous injections, meticulous attention is required to avoid accidental introduction of air bubbles as there is a small, but important risk of paradoxical embolism and stroke in patients who have an unrestrictive interatrial communication. For the same reason, it is also prudent to avoid peripheral venous lines in the lower extremity in patients with Glenn shunts. Internal jugular vein cannulation is best avoided in patients with superior cavopulmonary anastomosis to minimize the risk of SVC thrombosis.

However if internal jugular vein is cannulated in the operating room (OR) for monitoring pulmonary artery pressures, it is removed soon after arrival in the ICU.

HEMODYNAMIC AND INOTROPE MANAGEMENT

These patients require minimal/no inotropic supports after surgery. Usually, dopamine/dobutamine at 5 µg/kg/min will suffice. In infants with important AV valve regurgitation or dysfunction of the systemic ventricle, milrinone or levosimendan may be considered. Pressure monitored through femoral venous line reflects the preload to the systemic ventricle when a liberal interatrial communication is present or when atrial septectomy is performed. The difference between the superior venacaval pressure (measured via a jugular venous catheter) and femoral venous pressure is a surrogate for the transpulmonary gradient that determines the obligatory pulmonary blood flow. A transpulmonary gradient of 5–10 mm Hg is appropriate in the postoperative period. The arterial oxygen saturation after a BDGS operation is influenced by a number of factors. It tends to be very low (70–80%) in young infants because of an immature lung vascular bed. In older infants (>6 months till about 3 years) saturations are much better, usually 85% or more. Here the high proportion of systemic venous return from the upper half of the body maintains good pulmonary blood flow. On rare occasions, where BDGS operation is performed for older children, the saturations are not very impressive (75–80%) because SVC contributes to a relatively smaller proportion of systemic venous return in older children and adults.

Postoperatively, patients should be positioned with head end of bed elevated to 30–45°. This is done to improve venous drainage from head and neck region by gravity thereby increasing SVC flows and pulmonary blood flow. Mechanical ventilation produces important hemodynamic alterations due to cardiopulmonary interactions in patients with Glenn shunts. Positive pressure ventilation increases mean airway pressure and PVR, thus decreasing forward flow in pulmonary circulation. In contrast, spontaneous breathing decreases intrathoracic pressure and mean airway pressure, and improves pulmonary blood flow. Therefore, there is a significant hemodynamic benefit to early extubation strategy in improving oxygenation after Glenn shunt.

ANTICOAGULATION

Heparin infusion at 5–20 units/kg/hour is initiated once postoperative bleeding settles as a prophylaxis against thrombosis related to the cavopulmonary anastomosis. In clinical practice, heparin infusion is often titrated to keep postoperative activated partial thromboplastin time (APTT) 1.5–2 times of the normal value. Antiplatelet therapy with aspirin is commenced on postoperative day (POD) 1 and continued at discharge.

FLUID MANAGEMENT

Standard restricted fluid strategy according to body surface area method is followed for maintenance fluids. However, maintenance of adequate intravascular volume is important as the passive pulmonary blood flow is dependent on adequate preload and a low mean airway pressure. Administration of fluid bolus is appropriate if femoral venous pressure or atrial pressure is low. If there is clinical evidence of hypovolemia or decreased oxygen saturation due to a low preload in the early postoperative period, additional fluid requirements are provided in the form of crystalloids such as ringer lactate or normal saline.

DIURETIC THERAPY

Aggressive diuretic therapy is not indicated in patients after cavopulmonary shunts. However, in patients with evidence of post-operative fluid overload or increased upper body edema and/or facial swelling, it is reasonable to start an infusion of furosemide at 1–2 mg/kg/day.

PAIN AND SEDATION MANAGEMENT

These patients benefit from early liberation from mechanical ventilation and therefore it is important to titrate analgesics and sedatives to maintain a reasonable level of consciousness. High dose of opioids can cause excessive sedation or respiratory depression that can interfere with early extubation. Therefore, agents such as dexmedetomidine along with nonsteroidal anti-inflammatory drugs (NSAIDs) are usually preferred. Regional anesthetic techniques such as caudal epidural blockade are particularly useful for adjuvant analgesia in the operating room.

VENTILATION MANAGEMENT

Early extubation in the operating room or in postoperative ICU is the common practice because of the beneficial effects of sponta-neous breathing on pulmonary blood flow. However, if the infant requires a brief period of ventilation in the postoperative period, a ventilator mode that avoids high inflation pressure and maintains good oxygenation is recommended. Modes with a decelerating flow waveform allow lower peak inspiratory pressure and facilitate homogeneous oxygena-tion than other waveforms. Therefore, pressure regulated volume control (PRVC) or pressure

controlled ventilation–volume guarantee (PCV-VG) mode where the set tidal volume is delivered at the lowest inspiratory pressure with a decelerating flow waveform is optimal during mechanical ventilation.[4] High levels of positive end-expiratory pressure (PEEP) should be avoided as it can impede forward flow of blood in the pulmonary arteries. However, a physiological level of PEEP at 3–5 cm H_2O prevents atelectasis and maintains lung volumes at functional residual capacity (FRC). Spontaneous ventilation should be encouraged at the earliest. Once the infant is breathing regularly, and hemodynamically stable, extubation is attempted after a pressure support trial.

Spontaneous breathing with negative intrathoracic pressure encourages maximum transpulmonary flow of blood. The benefits of spontaneous breathing include improved cerebral blood flow, increased pulmonary blood flow, and an increase in systemic oxygen saturation.[5] In a study of 24 patients who underwent BDGS by Huang et al. a decrease in CVP (measured from central venous cathe-ter in SVC) and increase in cerebral oxygen saturation measured by near infrared spectro-scopy (NIRS) was observed after extubation indicating the improvement in cardiac index and regional oxygen saturation with establishment of spontaneous respiration.[5] Pulmonary blood flow after BDGS is also influenced by the delicate interplay between cerebral and pulmonary vascular beds which has opposite responses to CO_2 and acid base status. Hyperventilation by lowering PCO_2, can reduce PVR and increase the cerebral vascular resistance. Bradley and colleagues showed that after BDGS, hyperventilation resulted in a significant decrease in arterial PO_2, reduction in systemic arterial oxygen saturation and reduction in transpulmonary gradient.[6] Mean cerebral blood flow velocity was reduced. They postulated that hyperventilation lowers arterial PCO_2 and increases cerebral vascular resistance. The reduction in cerebral blood flow, in turn, decreases the amount of blood returning through the SVC into the pulmonary circulation. This accounted for the reduction in systemic arterial oxygen saturation. In a study of nine infants undergoing BDGS, higher PCO_2 levels of 45 and 55 mm Hg with mild respiratory acidosis was associated with better oxygenation, Qs (cardiac output) and Qp (pulmonary blood flow) without increasing PVR.[7] Thus, a permissive hypercapnia is likely to improve the postoperative course of young infants by decreasing cerebral vascular resistance, improving cerebral blood flow, and thereby increasing the quantum of pulmonary blood flow.

COMMON POSTOPERATIVE COMPLICATIONS

Hypoxia

Patients after superior cavopulmonary anastomosis typically have a peripheral oxygen saturation between 75 and 85%. However, an oxygen saturation <75% should be evaluated for probable causes. The probable cause of post Glenn desaturation include the following:[2]

- *Pulmonary venous desaturation*: Pneumothorax, pleural effusion, pulmonary edema pneumonia, pulmonary arteriovenous malformation.
- *Systemic venous desaturation*: Anemia, high oxygen consumption states, low systemic cardiac output.
- *Decreased pulmonary blood flow*: Elevated PVR, pulmonary venous hypertension, anatomic obstruction of the Glenn pathway, increased left atrial pressure due to ventricular dysfunction or AV valve regurgitation.
- *Venovenous collaterals*: An uncommon cause of desaturation after Glenn shunt is

the development of venovenous collaterals secondary to elevated SVC pressure in early postoperative period or a previously undiagnosed left superior vena cava.

The systematic way of troubleshooting the various causes of post-Glenn hypoxia is given in **Table 1**.

Hypertension

Transient hypertension and bradycardia is a frequent postoperative finding in patients after BDGS.[2] The exact etiology is unclear. Potential causes include pain, catecholamine surge, or raised intracranial pressure due to incorporation of the Glenn circuit to cerebral venous outflow. Systemic hypertension is also likely to be a compensatory mechanism to maintain cerebral perfusion when there is an acute elevation of cerebral venous pressure after the cavopulmonary anastomosis. Additionally, acute reduction of the volume load to the single ventricle may also lead to a hypercontractile state of the myocardium contributing to hypertension. Aggressive lowering of the blood pressure is usually not warranted as it may compromise cerebral perfusion.

Sinus bradycardia is occasionally seen in the postoperative period. In a retrospective review of 60 patients with congenital heart disease undergoing BDGS, sinus bradycardia was observed in 27% patients.[8] The increased risk of sinus node dysfunction and bradycardia after Glenn have been attributed to the proximity of SVC suture lines to the sino-atrial (SA) node.

High SVC Pressures

Jugular vein catheters are generally avoided in Glenn shunts to avoid the risk of thrombosis due to residence of indwelling catheters and potential compromise of the anastomotic pathway. However, a transient

TABLE 1: Post bidirectional Glenn shunt (BDGS) desaturation checklist.

Causes of post BDGS desaturation	Investigation
1. Pulmonary venous desaturation (pleural effusion, pneumothorax, pneumonia, pulmonary edema)	Chest X-ray, screening ECHO
2. Systemic venous desaturation	
• Anemia	• Check hemoglobin
• High oxygen consumption states, e.g., sepsis	• Blood culture, CRP, blood counts
• Low cardiac output	• Serum lactate, ECHO
3. Decreased pulmonary blood flow	Cardiac catheterization, measurement of PAP, PVR, ECHO
• Increased PVR	
• AV valve regurgitation	
• Ventricular dysfunction	
• Obstruction of Glenn pathway	
4. Venovenous collateral	Bedside contrast ECHO, cardiac catheterization

(AV: atrioventricular; BDGS: bidirectional Glenn shunt; CRP: C-reactive protein; ECHO: echocardiography; PVR: pulmonary vascular resistance; PAP: pulmonary artery pressure)

neck vein pressure measurement may be obtained immediately post bypass, during intraoperative period, using needle insertion by the surgeon. This reflects the pulmonary artery pressure. An elevated jugular vein pressure recording >18 mm Hg (if available) should be considered a reflection of high SVC pressure and the probable causes should be investigated. This may be due to high PVR, anastomotic obstruction, branch pulmonary artery distortion or small sized distal pulmonary arteries. In the postoperative period, in the absence of an indwelling catheter clinical features such as facial and upper body edema is typically suggestive of high SVC pressures/SVC obstruction. Treatment should be directed at the cause. Elevated PVR may require treatment with inhaled nitric oxide or sildenafil in the postoperative period to optimize pulmonary blood flow and improve oxygen saturation.

Irritability and Altered Mentation

Following the cavopulmonary anastomosis, SVC is no longer draining to the compliant right atrium. This can potentially lead to cerebral venous congestion and raised intracranial pressure. This response is particularly exaggerated in infants with high SVC pressure and often manifests as irritability or altered mentation in the early postoperative period. This usually resolves spontaneously as the infant adapts to the circulation. Diuretic therapy with furosemide or osmotic diuretics such as mannitol may be beneficial by decreasing fluid overload states after CPB and reducing venous congestion.

Persistent Pleural Effusions and Chylothorax

Creation of a superior cavopulmonary anastomosis may result in venous congestion of the upper half of the body especially in young infants with elevated pulmonary artery pressure. This can result in increased propensity for postoperative pleural effusion and prolonged chest tube drainage.[9] Postoperative chylothorax can be a potential complication after surgery for congenital heart disease and data shows that patients with Glenn and Fontan circuits are particularly at risk.[10] Abnormal lymphatic flow from the thoracic duct toward the lung parenchyma with lymphatic perfusion of the mediastinum in patients with single ventricle physiology has been one of the proposed mechanisms.[10] Persistent pleural effusion merits detailed evaluation to rule out elevated pulmonary artery pressure, significant AV valve regurgitation or anatomical obstruction to the cavopulmonary pathway. The diagnosis and treatment of postoperative chylothorax is dealt as a separate chapter.

DEINTENSIFICATION

Inotropic supports can be tapered off shortly after extubation. Femoral venous catheter is removed as soon as inotropes are tapered off. Intercostal drains may be retained on postoperative day 1 in patients with suspicion of high SVC pressure due to concern of pleural effusion. Heparin infusion can be discontinued after initiating aspirin therapy.

DISCHARGE MEDICATIONS

- Antiplatelet therapy with aspirin
- Diuretic therapy with furosemide
- Iron prophylaxis to prevent iron deficiency anemia may be appropriate.

REFERENCES

1. Berdat PA, Belli E, Lacour-Gayet F, Planche C, Serraf A. Additional pulmonary blood flow has no adverse effect on outcome after bidirectional cavopulmonary anastomosis. Ann Thorac Surg. 2005;79:29-37.
2. Wernovsky G, Bove EL. Single ventricle lesions. In: Chang AC, Hanley FL, Wernovsky G, Wessel DL (Eds). Pediatric Cardiac Intensive Care. Philadelphia: Williams and Wilkins; 1998. pp. 271-87.
3. Petrucci O, Khoury PR, Manning PB, Eghtesady P. Outcomes of bidirectional Glenn procedure in patients less than 3 months of age. J Cardiovasc Surg. 2010;139:562-8.
4. Kocis CK, Dekeon MK, Rosen HK, Bandy KP, Croley DC, Bove EL, et al. Pressure regulated volume control vs volume controlled ventilation in infants after surgery for congenital heart disease. Pediatr Cardiol. 2001;22:233-7.
5. Huang J, Zhou Y, Zhu D. Systemic hemodynamics and regional tissue oxygen saturation after bidirectional cavopulmonary shunt: positive pressure ventilation versus spontaneous breathing. Interact Cardiovasc Thoracic Surg. 2016;23:235-9.
6. Bradley SM, Simsic JM, Mulvihill DM. Hyperventilation impairs oxygenation after bidirectional superior cavopulmonary connection. Circulation. 1998;98:1372-6.
7. Hoskote A, Li J, Hickey C, Erickson S, Van Arsdell G, Stephens D, et al. The effects of carbon dioxide on oxygenation and systemic, cerebral, and pulmonary vascular hemodynamics after the bidirectional superior cavopulmonary anastomosis. J Am Coll Cardiol. 2004;44:1501-9.
8. Reichlin A, Pretre R, Dave H, Hug MI, Gass M, Balmer C. Postoperative arrhythmia in patients with bidirectional cavopulmonary anastomosis. Eur J Cardiothorac Surg 2014;45:620-4.
9. Freedom RM, Nykanen D, Benson LN. The physiology of bidirectional cavopulmonary connection. Ann Thorac Surg. 1998;66:664-7.
10. Savla JJ, Itkin M, Rosano JW, Dori Y. Postoperative chylothorax in patients with congenital heart disease. J Am Coll Cardiol. 2017;69:2410-22.

Extracardiac Fontan Operation

Rakhi Balachandran

Illustrations: Balaji Srimurugan
Reviewed by: R Krishna Kumar

■ INTRODUCTION

A univentricular physiology exists in congenital heart defects where the anatomy is unsuitable for a biventricular repair. Fontan procedure is the final surgical palliation for congenital heart diseases (CHD) with a functionally univentricular heart. The first surgery described by Fontan and Baudet in 1971 included, a classic Glenn shunt with a valved homograft between right atrial appendage and the main pulmonary artery (PA) using right atrium as a pump to the PA.[1] The surgical technique has evolved thereafter to improve flow dynamics and to minimize complications resulting in two modifications that are currently used. These are the intracardiac lateral tunnel Fontan and the extracardiac conduit Fontan operations. The extracardiac Fontan involves directing the inferior vena caval blood flow into the pulmonary circulation by a tube graft between the inferior vena cava (IVC) and inferior surface of the right pulmonary artery (RPA) and the central PA (**Fig. 1**). A fenestration is usually created between the conduit and right atrial wall to permit decompression of the systemic venous circuit after the anastomosis. The intracardiac lateral tunnel modification uses an intracardiac baffle to direct the IVC blood into the pulmonary circulation. The final palliation thus results in a total cavopulmonary connection where both superior vena cava (SVC) and IVC blood

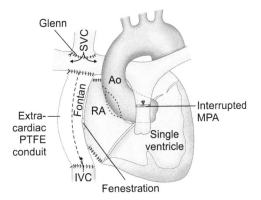

Fig. 1: Fontan procedure: The inferior vena cava (IVC) is connected to inferior aspect of right pulmonary artery by an extracardiac polytetrafluoroethylene (PTFE) conduit. A Glenn shunt performed as second stage palliation directs superior vena cava (SVC) blood into the pulmonary circulation. The final palliation thus results in both IVC and SVC blood draining into the pulmonary circulation. A fenestration is created between the conduit and right atrial wall to decompress the venous circuit.

(Ao: aorta; RA: right atrium; MPA: main pulmonary artery)

is flowing into the pulmonary circulation. The Fontan pathway exists as a single circuit with the pulmonary and systemic circulation connected in series and powered by a single ventricle. A low-pulmonary vascular resistance (PVR) and systemic venous hypertension is obligatory for driving the pulmonary blood flow (PBF). Survival to adulthood is expected in the current era with advancement of surgical techniques and modifications to prevent complications.[2] In a large single center cohort of 1,052 patients who had a modified Fontan operation 10, 20, and 30 years survival rates were 74%, 61%, and 43%, respectively.[3] Risk factors associated with reduced survival in this cohort included preoperative PA pressure >17 mm Hg, use of preoperative diuretics, asplenia, longer bypass time, absence of intra-operative sinus rhythm, elevated post bypass Fontan pressure > 20 mm Hg or operation in early era prior to 1991.[3] The management of patients with Fontan circulatory physiology comes with substantial challenges to the patient, physicians, and caretakers and it is necessary to be cognizant of various aspects of postoperative care in these unique population to facilitate optimal survival.

■ MONITORING

Standard hemodynamic monitoring with arterial blood pressure, central venous pressure (CVP), continuous ECG monitoring, pulse oximetry, and capnography is recommended. The venous pressure tracing obtained from a catheter in the femoral vein reflects the PA pressure as the IVC is now connected to the PA. A small single-lumen cannula occasionally inserted into the internal jugular vein to monitor the SVC pressure also reflects the PA pressure because of the superior cavopulmonary anastomosis. However, this catheter, if used intraoperatively, is removed soon after arrival in the ICU to prevent SVC thrombosis. The filling pressure of the functioning single ventricle can be accurately measured only by a left atrial line placed intraoperatively; however, this is not common practice in most centers.

■ HEMODYNAMIC AND INOTROPE MANAGEMENT

Circulatory Physiology after Fontan Procedure

In a patient with univentricular heart, the systemic and pulmonary venous circuits are connected in parallel resulting in volume overload to the single ventricle. Fontan operation achieves the separation of systemic circulation from the pulmonary circulation by connecting the systemic venous circuit directly to the PA. PBF and therefore cardiac output, thus becomes dependent on non-pulsatile flow of the returning systemic venous blood. In the absence of a subpulmonary pumping chamber, the driving force for PBF is the pressure gradient between the central systemic veins (i.e., CVP) and left atrial pressure (LAP) together with maintenance of a low PVR. The difference between CVP and LAP is known as the transpulmonary gradient. The systemic ventricle also acts as a suction pump during diastole adding to the forward driving force, and hence optimal ventricular diastolic function is important to maintain cardiac output in the context of a Fontan circuit.[4] The principal hemodynamic consequence of the unique circulatory physiology in the post-Fontan state includes systemic venous hypertension and chronic low cardiac output. The chronic low cardiac output despite a normal ventricular function often arises from preload deprivation of the single ventricle due to a nonpulsatile PBF in the absence of a pumping chamber, and the inability to raise the preload in response to increased metabolic demands. It also becomes intuitive, that the PVR has to remain low for the efficient functioning of the circuit. The circulatory physiology in Fontan circulation in comparison with normal biventricular circulation and single ventricle parallel circulation as illustrated by Gewillig[5] is depicted in **Figures 2A to C**.

Key Hemodynamic Goals

- *Maintain systemic venous pressure*: This is by maintenance of adequate intravascular volume. The CVP measured by the femoral venous catheter typically ranges

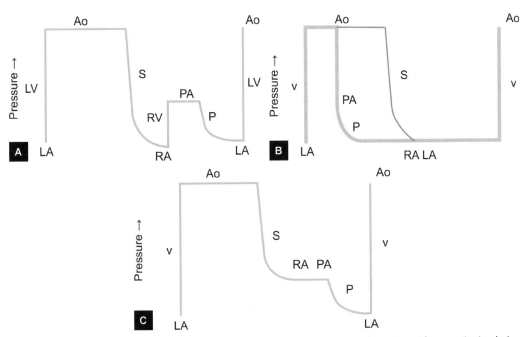

Figs. 2A to C: (A) Normal circulation. The pulmonary circulation (P) is connected in series with systemic circulation (S). The right ventricle maintains the energy to drive the pulmonary circulation against the pulmonary vascular resistance; (B) Parallel circulation in single ventricle physiology. Systemic and pulmonary circuits are connected in parallel, with volume overload of single ventricle (v). This is shown by thicker line. Admixture of systemic and pulmonary venous blood leading to arterial desaturation; (C) Fontan circulation. The systemic and pulmonary circulation is connected in series without subpulmonary pump. The volume overload to single ventricle is now less than expected for body surface area. This circulation elevates the systemic venous pressure, which can be minimized by the use of a fenestration.

(Ao: aorta; LA: left atrium; LV: left ventricle; RA: right atrium; RV: right ventricle; PA: pulmonary artery)

Source: Gewillig M. The Fontan circulation. Heart. 2005;91:839-46.[5]

from 14 to 17 mm Hg in the immediate postoperative period. Pressure gradient between the central systemic veins and the left atrium represents the transpulmonary gradient, which is the driving force for PBF (**Fig. 3**). Ideal transpulmonary gradient ranges between 5 and 10 mm Hg and can be monitored only if an indwelling LA line is available. A low femoral venous pressure, as in the case of hypovolemia, will thus decrease the transpulmonary gradient and decrease PBF. Postoperative fluid losses should be replaced to maintain adequate intravascular volume and hence the venous pressure, as guided

by hemodynamic monitoring. At our center, fresh frozen plasma or colloids like hydroxyethyl starches are used for fluid replacement if there is increased pleural drainage in the immediate post-operative phase. Transfusion of packed red cells is reasonable, if the hemoglobin concentration is less than 9 g/dL with clinical evidence of impaired tissue perfusion. It is important to recognize that most of the multisystem complications after Fontan operation are consequent to chronic systemic venous hypertension inherent to the unique circulatory physiology; and therefore, one should

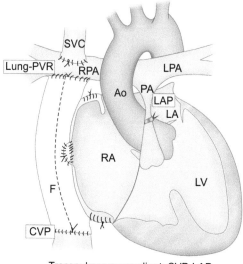

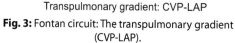

Transpulmonary gradient: CVP-LAP

Fig. 3: Fontan circuit: The transpulmonary gradient (CVP-LAP).

(CVP: central venous pressure shown by femoral vein pressure; LAP: left atrial pressure; PVR: pulmonary vascular resistance ; RPA: right pulmonary artery; LPA: left pulmonary artery; LV: left ventricle; RA: right atrium; Ao: aorta; PA: pulmonary artery; F: Fontan circuit; CVP, LAP and PVR indicate the pressure and resistances in the Fontan circuit)

endeavor to maintain cardiac output at the lowest feasible CVP.

- *Maintain a negative intrathoracic pressure*: Forward flow into the pulmonary arteries after cavopulmonary connection is encouraged by low PVR and a low mean airway pressure. Therefore, early extubation and establishment of spontaneous respiration with negative intrathoracic pressure adds to the efficiency of the Fontan circulation.
- *Preserve the function of the single ventricle*: Ventricular dysfunction can occur due to altered loading conditions of the single ventricle at various stages of palliation.[5] The reduction in preload after creation of Fontan circuit can induce remodeling and reduced compliance of the functioning

single ventricle contributing to diastolic dysfunction in the postoperative period.

- *Maintain sinus rhythm and AV synchrony*: Maintenance of sinus rhythm is necessary to maintain AV (atrioventricular) synchrony. This is important to provide the atrial kick that augments ventricular filling and maintain the preload to the lesser compliant single ventricle.
- *Minimize AV valve regurgitation (AVVR)*: AV valve regurgitation can increase LAP and decrease the transpulmonary gradient thus reducing the forward PBF. Afterload reducing agents may be beneficial if significant AV valve regurgitation coexist.
- *Minimize PVR*: A low PVR is essential for the efficiency of the circuit. An elevated PVR may exist in the postoperative period as a result of effect of cardiopulmonary bypass (CPB), presence of atelectasis or due to effects of positive pressure ventilation. A low positive end-expiratory pressure (PEEP) of 3–5 cmH$_2$O is generally well-tolerated during ventilation and helps to maintain the lungs at optimum functional residual capacity (FRC) without increasing PVR. It is reasonable to consider pulmonary vasodilators if the PA pressures remain elevated despite optimizing hemodynamic and ventilatory parameters in the postoperative period.

Inotrope Management

These patients usually do not require high dose of inotropes after separation from bypass. The most critical determinant of cardiac output in the Fontan circuit is maintenance of low PVR and adequate ventricular preload. Ventricular diastolic function and systemic vascular resistance (SVR) are not as important in comparison. While milrinone is often used to reduce SVR and in the belief that it improves diastolic function, it is important to recognize that vasodilators are not perhaps likely to help the Fontan physiology very much. The reduction in cardiac output in the post-Fontan state is primarily due to the deprived preload that leads to ventricular remodeling and reduced compliance.[5] However, milrinone may be used in combination with a low dose of epinephrine, if there is important systolic dysfunction or AV valve regurgitation. A defined perioperative management strategy incorporating peripheral vasodilators like milrinone along with anticoagulation, fluid restriction, diuretic therapy, and early extubation has been found to be beneficial in improving early outcomes after Fontan procedure.[6]

Anticoagulation

The Fontan circuit presents a substrate for increased thrombosis due to increased venous pressure, a nonpulsatile PBF, chronic low cardiac output, and use of prosthetic conduits for redirecting IVC flows. Generally, these patients are started on a heparin drip at 10–15 units/kg/hr, once the drains settle in early postoperative period. A vitamin K antagonist (Warfarin) is started on first postoperative day (POD) and titrated to target an INR 2–3. Some centers also combine aspirin for prevention of thromboembolic complications.

■ VENTILATION MANAGEMENT

The mode of ventilation has a significant impact on post-Fontan patients where the transpulmonary blood flow is obligatory and relies heavily on low PVR. A ventilator mode that avoids high inflation pressure and ensures adequate gas exchange is beneficial. Ventilation modes with a decelerating waveform offers lowest peak inspiratory pressures and ensures better oxygenation. The pressure regulated volume controlled (PRVC) mode achieves these goals as the tidal volume is guaranteed

at lowest mean airway pressure. Optimal level of PEEP (3–5 cmH$_2$O) helps to prevent atelectasis and maintain lungs at FRC without elevating PVR. Spontaneous respiration has to be encouraged at the earliest because of the obvious benefits of reduced intrathoracic pressure on the forward PBF. Hence, these patients are candidates for extubation on table or in the immediate postoperative period.[7]

Atelectasis in the postextubation phase can be detrimental as it can contribute to increased PVR, decreased PBF and eventually low cardiac output. Hence, adequate pulmonary toileting has to be ensured to prevent atelectasis by gentle chest physiotherapy and mobilization of secretions.

■ FLUID MANAGEMENT

- Standard fluid management protocol according to body surface area method is usually adopted in the postoperative period for maintenance of fluid calculation.
- As the Fontan circulation relies on venous pressure for PBF adequate intravascular volume should be maintained. Colloids or balanced electrolyte solutions may be used as replacement fluids for losses contributing to hypovolemia and low CVP in the postoperative period. Though, fresh frozen plasma (FFP) is not recommended as a volume expander, it may be used in the immediate postoperative period to correct hypovolemia with coexisting coagulopathy. Packed red cells can be administered to correct hemoglobin less than 9 g/dL in the presence of low oxygen saturation or clinical evidence of poor tissue perfusion.

■ DIURETIC THERAPY

Diuretic therapy should be cautiously used in these patients as the circulatory physiology requires maintenance of adequate preload. However, in patients who have signs of fluid overload, infusion of frusemide may be initiated at 1 mg/kg/day after an initial bolus of 0.5–1 mg/kg. Electrolyte imbalances such as hypokalemia/hypomagnesemia should be quickly identified and vigorously treated as it can trigger arrhythmias, detrimental to cardiac output in a Fontan circulation.

PAIN AND SEDATION MANAGEMENT

Standard pain and sedation protocol with fentanyl and/or dexmedetomidine is used with intermittent doses of midazolam. Nonsteroidal anti-inflammatory agents like ketorolac or paracetamol may be supplemented to facilitate pain control and ensure comfortable breathing after extubation.

FEEDING AND NUTRITION

These patients are generally kept nil per orally after surgery as they are prepared for early extubation. Nasogastric or oral feeds are initiated 4 hours after extubation, if deemed stable. In patients planned for overnight ventilation nasogastric feeds are typically started 4–6 hours after surgery and withheld thereafter in the periextubation period.

CHEST PHYSIOTHERAPY AND INCENTIVE SPIROMETRY

An often-neglected part in the postoperative care of Fontan patients is ensuring aggressive lung toileting and physiotherapy. The PBF after Fontan conversion necessitates maintenance of optimal pulmonary function, with avoidance of lung parenchymal complications such as atelectasis, consolidation, and retained secretions. This is important to maintain lungs at optimal functional residual capacity to keep PVR as low as possible. A focused respiratory care employing gentle chest physiotherapy, incentive spirometry, and clearance of secretions is important to achieve this goal. Older children can be familiarized

with breathing exercises and tools for incentive spirometry in the preoperative phase itself so as to ensure better comfort levels while using these in the postoperative period. Postoperative pain relief is important to prevent respiratory compromise and facilitate patient participation in breathing exercises. Parental presence and encouragement are important factors that ensure patient cooperation while performing respiratory care maneuvers after extubation.

COMMON POSTOPERATIVE COMPLICATIONS

Low Cardiac Output

Low cardiac output in the immediate postoperative period after Fontan is not uncommon. The Fontan physiology results in limitation of the preload reserve of the single ventricle, an elevation in systemic venous pressure, and a nonpulsatile PBF dependent on pressure gradient between central systemic veins and LA. A low cardiac output state can arise from factors affecting any component of this circuit.[8] These are discussed here:

- *Inadequate preload*: This often results from hypovolemia which can occur commonly after surgery. This is diagnosed by a low CVP and a low LAP (if available for monitoring). Treatment is by maintenance of adequate intravascular volume with colloids.

- *Elevated PVR*: A high CVP measured by femoral venous pressure reflects increased PA pressure, which can be due to an elevated PVR. This can potentially occur in post bypass state due to the effects of CPB, lung collapse, increased extravascular lung water, suboptimal ventilator settings, or anatomical concerns such as poor arborization of pulmonary vascular bed. This can impede forward flow in Fontan circuit and decrease cardiac output. The presence of a fenestration between the conduit and right atrial free wall can decompress the venous circuit and facilitate shunting into right atrium and thus maintain cardiac output in such settings, but at the cost of systemic desaturation.

- *Ventricular dysfunction*: Both systolic and diastolic dysfunction can occur in the postoperative period. Diastolic dysfunction is more common due to the altered loading conditions after the Fontan creation resulting in a relatively volume underloaded single ventricle with poor compliance. This can be suspected when there is a combination of high CVP and high LAP.
- *AV valve regurgitation*: This will result in a high CVP and a high LAP and compromise the efficiency Fontan circuit.
- *Arrhythmias*: Hemodynamically significant arrhythmias with loss of AV synchrony can impair ventricular filling and precipitate low cardiac output.
- *Anatomic obstruction in the Fontan pathway*: Any anastomotic obstruction at the level of the conduit, branch PAs, or pulmonary veins can interfere with Fontan circulation and contribute to low cardiac output state. This can present as a high CVP and low LAP.
- *Cardiac tamponade*: This can potentially occur if there is excessive bleeding after cardiac surgery.

The differential diagnosis of postoperative low cardiac output after Fontan operation is depicted in **Table 1**. The treatment is directed at the cause of low cardiac output after diagnosis.

Arrhythmias

Early and late arrhythmias can complicate postoperative period after Fontan. In a large cohort of 1,052 patients incidence of atrial

TABLE 1: Differential diagnosis of low cardiac output in Fontan circulation.

Cause of low cardiac output	CVP	LAP
Hypovolemia	Low	Low
Increased PVR	High	Low
Ventricular dysfunction	High	High
AV valve regurgitation	High	High
Fontan circuit obstruction	High	Low

(CVP: central venous pressure (typically femoral venous pressure for practical purposes); LAP: left atrial pressure; PVR: pulmonary vascular resistance; AV: atrioventricular)

arrhythmias and ventricular arrhythmias prior to hospital discharge after Fontan operation were 21% and 8%, respectively.[3] Intra-atrial re-entrant tachycardia was the most common type of supraventricular tachycardia particularly observed with early atriopulmonary connections.[9] With increasing use of extracardiac Fontan, this has become rare. Sinus node dysfunction can also occur after surgery, which merits pacemaker implantation. The extracardiac conduit modification had been introduced to reduce the arrhythmia burden compared to earlier version of Fontan circuits. The extracardiac modification avoids sinus node manipulation, does not involve extensive suture lines in the atria and avoids atrial distension. In a large meta-analysis including 3,499 patients comparing the incidence of arrhythmias between the extracardiac and intra-atrial lateral tunnel variants of the Fontan circuit, no difference was observed in the incidence of early arrhythmias or need for pacemaker therapy. However, the lateral tunnel group had a significantly higher incidence of late arrhythmias.[10] Single ventricle patients are particularly dependent on AV synchrony for the maintenance of ventricular preload and hence cardiac output. Prompt recognition and management of arrhythmias is therefore vital in the postoperative period.

TABLE 2: Causes of cyanosis after Fontan operation.

Causes of cyanosis in post Fontan physiology	Investigation
Pulmonary venous desaturation (pleural effusion, pneumothorax, pneumonia, pulmonary edema or pulmonary AV malformations in longstanding Glenn or Kawashima operation)	Chest X-ray, screening echo with contrast
Systemic venous desaturation • Anemia • High oxygen consumption states, e.g., sepsis • Low cardiac output	 • Check hemoglobin • Blood culture, CRP, blood counts • Serum lactate, echocardiography
Decreased pulmonary blood flow • Increased PVR • Atrio-ventricular valve regurgitation • Ventricular dysfunction • Obstruction of Fontan pathway	Cardiac catheterization (measurement of PAP, PVR) echocardiography
Veno-venous collaterals	Bedside contrast echo, cardiac catheterization
Too large fenestration with right to left shunt	Echocardiography
Pulmonary AV malformations	Often suspected preoperatively during the cardiac catheterization; especially common in patients with interrupted IVC after the Kawashima operation

(PVR: pulmonary vascular resistance; PAP: pulmonary artery pressure; AV: arterio-venous; CRP: C-reactive protein; IVC: inferior vena cava)

General Guidelines

- In the event of an intraoperative arrhythmia or sinus node dysfunction, placement of two atrial and two ventricular epicardial pacing wires are rational while weaning from CPB.
- Continuous ECG monitoring is recommended in pediatric cardiac intensive care unit (PCICU). It is reasonable to obtain a baseline six lead ECG upon arrival in PCICU for comparison.
- Dual chamber pacemaker with cables should be available at the bed side.
- In patients who are already being paced for complete heart block, the settings and intrinsic rhythm should be evaluated daily with documentation as and when required.
- Serum potassium, magnesium and calcium levels should be maintained within normal limits in the postoperative period.

Cyanosis

Cyanosis is an important postoperative concern after Fontan surgery. Typical oxygen saturation after a fenestrated Fontan surgery ranges from 85 to 95%. A systematic evaluation is essential to identify the cause and to institute appropriate corrective measures when hypoxia is more than anticipated.[8] The probable causes of cyanosis after Fontan operation and its troubleshooting is listed in **Table 2**.

Postoperative Effusions

Prolonged pleural drainage is a challenging problem after Fontan in some patients and can increase morbidity in the postoperative period.[11] Acute elevation of systemic venous pressure, elevated PVR, and anatomical obstruction in the Fontan pathway are potential etiological factors. In a retrospective analysis by Mascio et al., prolonged pleural effusion in Fontan patients was associated with higher preoperative mean PA pressure.[12] It is common practice to create a fenestration to decompress the systemic venous circuit to mitigate the effects of high systemic venous pressure. The beneficial effects of leaving a fenestration to decompress the venous circuit included lower mortality, significantly less pleural effusion, and shorter hospitalization among high risk patients having modified Fontan operation.[13] The decline in systemic venous pressure usually comes at the expense of some desaturation in the postoperative period.

Chylothorax

This is a potential complication after Fontan operation. The elevated systemic venous pressures after Fontan can impede thoracic duct drainage and increase lymphatic system pressures, resulting in leakage of chyle into the pleural or peritoneal cavity. In a recent review of 324 patients undergoing extracardiac fenestrated Fontan, the incidence of chylothorax was 24%.[14] Patients with chylothorax had a longer duration of chest tube requirement, longer hospital stay, and lower freedom from death and composite adverse events.[14] The diagnostic tests and management of chylothorax is dealt with in a separate chapter.

Thrombosis

Patients after Fontan surgery are vulnerable to thromboembolic complications.[2] Atrial arrhythmias, postoperative nonpulsatile blood flow to pulmonary circulation, elevated PVR are all potential risk factors for thrombosis. Pulmonary thrombi can lead to acute elevation in PVR and Fontan failure. Systemic thrombi can predispose to postoperative stroke or seizures. These patients generally receive anticoagulants after surgery. Patients are initially started on a heparin drip and later transitioned to vitamin K antagonists and/or aspirin therapy to prevent thrombotic sequelae after Fontan circulation.

Long-term Complications

Protein Losing Enteropathy

Protein losing enteropathy (PLE) is a known complication after Fontan operation. The risk for development of this complication varies depending on the study period. Some studies have reported a cumulative risk as high as 13.4% at 10 years and usually associated with poor survival.[15] The elevated systemic venous pressures in the SVC can impair thoracic duct drainage and increase lymphatic system pressures. This can result in intestinal protein loss through lymph leakage. Chronic lymphatic congestion and protein leakage will also trigger an inflammatory response. The enteric loss of proteins such as albumin, immunoglobulins, and clotting factors manifests as peripheral edema, ascites, diarrhea, malabsorption, and weight loss. This is usually diagnosed by low serum albumin and elevated fecal alpha 1 antitrypsin level. PLE is an indicator of Fontan failure and usually difficult to treat.

Plastic Bronchitis

Chronically elevated systemic venous pressures/lymphatic leakage can predispose to hypersecretion of mucus into tracheobronchial tree predisposing to formation of casts. Poor airway clearance with ciliary dysfunction is also seen in a subset of patients with heterotaxy syndrome. It is a debilitating condition often refractory to conventional treatment. Recently, identification of leakage from pulmonary lymphatic channels and selective occlusion of abnormal lymphatic channels have been reported to cause resolution of symptoms.[16] Prolonged chest tube output, postoperative chylothorax occuring after staged palliation and postoperative ascites are some of the risk factors that predict this complication.[17]

Early Fontan Failure

The creation of Fontan circuit results in systemic venous hypertension and chronic low cardiac output due to limitation of preload reserve. Careful selection of patients, better understanding of preoperative anatomy, advances in the treatment of pulmonary hypertension, superior surgical techniques and fenestration of the Fontan circuit have enabled most of the patients to adapt to the new circulatory physiology reasonably well. However, a subset of patients fails to adapt to this circulatory condition in early postoperative period. They manifest with refractory low cardiac output, persistently elevated systemic venous pressures, prolonged third space effusions and pulmonary hypertension. These patients also manifest varying degrees of end-organ dysfunction. Treatment of Fontan failure in the early postoperative period includes measures to decrease systemic venous pressure by diuretic therapy, drainage of effusions, and measures to reduce the PVR. This should be coupled with supportive therapy for end-organ dysfunction. "Take down" of Fontan circuit should be considered if conventional medical management is not successful.

■ DEINTENSIFICATION

Patients who are extubated early can be quickly weaned off inotropes and invasive lines. Intercostal drains may be retained longer in patients with high CVP to facilitate drainage of postoperative pleural effusions. Patients with high PVR may require pulmonary vasodilators and continuation of supplemental oxygen. Patient is prepared for transfer after establishing oral feeds.

■ DISCHARGE MEDICATIONS

- Furosemide is often prescribed for a variable period after discharge.
- Aldactone may be given along with Furosemide to maintain potassium levels
- Warfarin alone or in combination with Aspirin is continued at discharge.

■ REFERENCES

1. Fontan F, Baudet E. Surgical repair of tricuspid atresia. Thorax. 1971;26:240-8.
2. Clift P, Celermajer D. Managing adult Fontan patients. Where do we stand? Eur Respir Rev. 2016;25:438-50.
3. Pundi KN, Johnson JN, Dearani JA, Pundi KN, Li Z, Hinck CA, et al. 40 year follow-up after Fontan operation: longterm outcome of 1,052 patients. J Am Coll Cardiol. 2015;66: 1700-10.
4. Kheiwa A, Agarwal A, John A. Fontan circulation: contemporary review of ongoing challenges and management strategies. Cardiovasc Innovat Appl. 2018;3:107-22.
5. Gewillig M. The Fontan circulation. Heart. 2005;91:839-46.
6. Sunstrom RE, Muralidharan A, Gerrah R, Reed RD, Good MK, Armsby LR, et al. A defined management strategy improves early outcomes after the Fontan procedure: the Portland Protocol. Ann Thorac Surg. 2015;99:148-55.
7. Fiorito B, Checchia PA. A review of mechanical ventilation strategies in children following the Fontan procedure. Images Pediatr Cardiol. 2002;4:4-11.
8. Wernovsky G, Bove EL. Single ventricle lesions. In: Chang AC, Hanley FL, Wernovsky G, Wessel DL (Eds). Pediatric Cardiac Intensive Care. Pennsylvania: Williams and Wilkins; 1998. pp. 271-87.
9. Stephenson EA, Lu M, Berul CI, Etheridge SP, Idriss SF, Margossian R, et al. Arrythmias in a contemporary Fontan cohort: prevalence and clinical associations in a multicentre cross sectional study. J Am Coll Cardiol. 2010;56:890-6.
10. Li D, Fan Q, Hirata Y, Ono M, An Q. Arrythmias after Fontan operation with intra atrial lateral tunnel versus extracardiac conduit: a systematic review and meta-analysis. Pediatr Cardiol. 2017;38:873-80.

11. Mascio CE, Austin EH. Pleural effusions following the Fontan procedure. Curr Opin Pulm Med. 2010;16:362-6.

12. Mascio CE, Wayment M, Colaizy TT, Mahoney LT, Burkhart HM. The modified Fontan procedure and prolonged pleural effusions. Am Surg. 2009;75:175-7.

13. Bridges ND, Mayer JE, Lock JE, Jonas RA, Hanley FL, Keane JF, et al. Effect of baffle fenestration on outcome of modified Fontan operation. Circulation. 1992;86:1762-9.

14. Lo Rito M, O Al-Radi O, Saedi A, Kotani Y, Sivarajan BV, Russell JL, et al. Chylothorax and pleural effusion in contemporary extracrdaic fenestrated Fontan completion. J Thorac Cardiovasc Surg. 2018;155: 2069-77.

15. Feldt RH, Driscoll DJ, Offord KP, Cha RH, Perrault J, Schaff HV, et al. Protein losing enteropathy after the Fontan operation. J Thorac Cardiovasc Surg. 1996;112:672-80.

16. Itkin MG, McCormack FX, Dori Y. Diagnosis and treatment of lymphatic plastic bronchitis in adults using advanced lymphatic imaging and percutaneous embolization. Ann Am Thorac Soc. 2016;13:1689-96.

17. Schumacher KR, Singh TP, Kuebler J, Aprile K, O'Brien M, Blume ED. Risk factors and outcome of Fontan associated plastic bronchitis: a case-control study. J Am Heart Assoc. 2014;3:e000865.

Repair of Anomalous Origin of Left Coronary Artery from Pulmonary Artery

Aveek Jayant, Sreelakshmi P Leeladharan

Illustrations: Balaji Srimurugan
Reviewed by: R Krishna Kumar

■ INTRODUCTION

Anomalous origin of left coronary artery from pulmonary artery (ALCAPA) is a rare, usually isolated congenital anomaly characterized by anomalous origin of the left main coronary artery (LMCA) from the pulmonary artery (PA). Nevertheless, it is the most common serious congenital coronary anomaly.[1] If uncorrected, 90% of patients will die within a year of birth. Isolated and scattered reports of survival until into late adulthood do exist, likely on account of extensive collaterals supplying the left coronary territory. Even in such survivors attrition due to a sudden cardiac event could still supervene in a large number of patients. Contrarily, ALCAPA diagnosed in infancy and managed with coronary translocation in the current era has excellent results. Infantile circulation has little or no collateral development making the myocardium more susceptible to severe myocardial ischemia. Most patients present in early infancy with failure to thrive and overt congestive heart failure; as they transition from the neonatal circulation. This occurs typically when the pulmonary vascular resistance falls and the abnormal coronary origin leads to a left to right shunt, with the additional burden of coronary steal.

Advancements in surgical and anesthetic techniques have resulted in excellent outcomes. Direct reimplantation of the anomalous left coronary artery (LCA) into the aorta remains the choice of surgical technique and is the standard of care (Figs. 1A and B). LCA ligation is no more practiced. Other surgical options include Takeuchi repair, using the subclavian artery to lengthen the LCA, and, bypass grafting using the left internal mammary artery as a conduit. The latter options are inevitably used only when the origin of the anomalous LCA is not easily translocated. Patients usually have accompanying mitral regurgitation, which is secondary to chronic ischemia of the papillary muscles and/or left ventricular dilation. Although this is identified as a risk factor for mortality in some series, others disagree.[2] Younger age at operation (as a surrogate marker for disease severity) increases risks for a more turbulent perioperative course, but the silver lining is that ventricular function recovery is more complete the earlier the intervention is made.

■ HEMODYNAMIC MONITORING

At present our institution uses a central venous catheter, invasive arterial pressure monitoring, continuous electrocardiography and pulse oximetry. Transthoracic invasive left atrial pressure monitoring although used in some institutions as a standard of care, is only occasionally used at our institution. Periodic transthoracic echocardiograms are

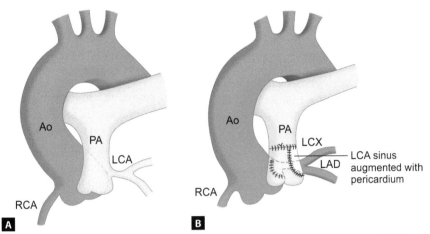

Figs. 1A and B: Anomalous origin of left coronary artery from pulmonary artery (ALCAPA). (A) Preoperative anatomy showing the origin of left main coronary artery (LCA) from the pulmonary artery (PA); (B) Anatomy after surgical repair. LCA button is translocated to aorta and the corresponding defect in PA is repaired wih pericardial patch.

(Ao: aorta; RCA: right coronary artery; LCX: left circumflex artery; LAD: left anterior descending branch)

routinely performed to assess alterations in ventricular function, degree of mitral regurgitation and volume status.

HEMODYNAMIC AND INOTROPE MANAGEMENT

Preoperative state of the patient is an important determinant of hemodynamic status of the patient. Although most infants with ALCAPA present with some severity of left ventricular dysfunction, they can have a spectrum of clinical presentation ranging from being asymptomatic to shock or cardiac arrest. Infants who are preoperatively ventilated on inotropic/mechanical circulatory support might need stiff inotropic support or extra-corporeal circulatory support (ECC) while weaning off cardiopulmonary bypass.

Phenoxybenzamine is either used before institution of cardiopulmonary bypass, or in the immediate postoperative period, to provide a milieu of very low systemic vascular resistance for the failed left ventricle. Its use is by no means universal and its opponents

cite the low ease of titration (on account of long half-life) as the principal reason for avoiding its use. The lowest tolerable limit of mean blood pressure appropriate for age is sometimes the target of drug titration. Milrinone is the typical inodilator of choice at our institution and sometimes small doses of adrenaline are used to supplement milrinone. During the period of cardiopulmonary bypass and a short period thereafter, adjunctive nitro vasodilators may also be used to aid temperature management and to achieve a target low blood pressure. Delayed sternal closure is often resorted to, as this allows for emergency institution of ECC, should there be an electrical event in postoperative intensive care. ECC[3] is a distinct part of the armamentarium for management of postoperative ALCAPA, but there is also a case made out for the management of this condition to manage the postoperative course without the use of ECC; that this emanates from a group with one of the largest experience in management of this condition should be a sign of reassurance for practitioners from low resource settings.[4]

FLUID AND BLOOD MANAGEMENT

At our center fluid management is primarily dictated by the age of the infant. It is also titrated to the daily average fluid balance as determined by weight or semiquantitative assessment of the functional ventricle on periodic transthoracic echocardiography. Typically, the immediate postoperative period could lead to daily fluid prescriptions of 500 mL/m^2 with gradual titration upwards to 1,000 mL/m^2 even as stabilization of hemodynamics allows early enteral nutrition; and full caloric goals are sought to be obtained. Qualitative reviews of the literature on this condition have suggested obtaining hemoglobin concentrations of 14–16 g/dL. However, this approach is tempered by more recent expert opinion on the subject of targeting hemoglobin concentrations at no more than 10 g/dL in the presence of stable cardiovascular status.

Adjunctive blood component use is virtually restricted to clinical bleeding or abnormal results on thromboelastography; use may have also been curtailed by the higher temperatures that are now maintained when using selective antegrade cerebral perfusion.

Furosemide infusion is started at 1–2 mg/kg/day aiming at urine output 1–2 mL/kg/hour.

Bolus doses of furosemide are avoided to prevent sudden fluid loss and hypotension.

Negative fluid balance is aimed for gradually. Adjunct peritoneal dialysis is sometimes initiated when cardiovascular status is borderline in the immediate postoperative period or prior to sternal closure.

Heparin infusion at 5–10 units/kg/hour is often initiated after ruling out bleeding from suture lines in the early postoperative period, due to concerns of LCA occlusion post repair.

However, this is purely institution based and practice variations exist across centers.

PAIN AND SEDATION MANAGEMENT

At our center, the mainstay of pain management is intravenous fentanyl as an infusion titrated to effect. Dexmedetomidine is also typically an adjunct, as lightening of sedation is planned prior to extubation. Caudal opioid doses are occasionally used (typically caudal morphine) so as to maintain a baseline analgesic state for the first 24 hours post-procedure. Nonsteroidal anti-inflammatory drugs (NSAIDs) are contraindicated in this subset and aliquots of paracetamol are often added for the initial period. Increasingly, midazolam and benzodiazepine has been used less and less.

VENTILATORY MANAGEMENT AND EXTUBATION

The patient is electively ventilated for 48 hours or more depending on clinical recovery, gradually weaned off ventilator support, and transitioned to noninvasive mode of ventilation such as nasal continuous positive airway pressure (CPAP) or high flow nasal cannula. Tidal volume of 8–10 mL/kg with positive end-expiratory pressure (PEEP) of 5 cmH$_2$O may be used, PEEP application could help prevent atelectasis and reduce pulmonary congestion. Ventilation weaning is particularly tricky as cardiopulmonary interactions (via oxygen demand supply balance, effective circulating volume and the support ventilation itself provides to an ailing ventricle) may mean a patient often successfully passes a trial of spontaneous breathing, but then is immediately borderline postextubation of the trachea. It should also be emphasized that in low resource settings, ventilation is often used as an adjunct for prolonged cardiac support, although the evidence base for this in terms of the global literature emanating from the resource rich clinical practice settings is per contra.

COMMON POSTOPERATIVE COMPLICATIONS

- Immediate complications include bleeding from suture line and poor flow in the translocated coronary artery. Adequate heparin reversal/use of antifibrinolytics may aid bleeding control. Tranexamic acid bolus dose of 10–25 mg/kg followed by infusion of 10 mg/kg/hour may be initiated
- Low cardiac output syndrome
- Prolonged mechanical ventilation
- Prolonged ICU stay
- Supravalvular pulmonary stenosis is a late complication of surgery for anomalous coronary origin.

All in all, excellent outcomes for surgery in ALCAPA can be obtained across the world even as the use of ECC as a support adjunct continues to decline in the postoperative period.[5,6]

DISCHARGE MEDICATIONS

Most patients with moderate to severe ventricular dysfunction are stabilized on a course of oral angiotensin-converting enzyme (ACE) inhibitors (enalapril) to facilitate myocardial recovery by afterload reduction after repair. Carvedilol is sometimes used in those patients with significant resting tachycardia. It might be also prudent to continue diuretic therapy with furosemide for at least 3–6 months post repair when the infant preoperatively presents with severe heart failure. Though the evidence related to the use of antiplatelet agents are sparse, our institutional practice is to initiate antiplatelet therapy with aspirin when the postoperative heparin infusion is discontinued.

REFERENCES

1. Mavroudis C, Dodge-Khatami A, Backer C, Lorber R. Coronary artery anomalies. In: Mavroudis C, Backer C, Idriss RF (Eds). Pediatric Cardiac Surgery, 4th edition. West Sussex: Wiley Blackwell; 2013.
2. Brown JW, Ruzmetov M, Parent JJ, Rodefeld MD, Turrentine MW. Does the degree of preoperative mitral regurgitation predict survival or the need for mitral valve repair or replacement in patients with anomalous origin of the left coronary artery from the pulmonary artery? J Thorac Cardiovasc Surg. 2008;136:743-8.
3. Del Nido PJ, Duncan BW, Mayer JE, Wessel DL, LaPierre RA, Jonas RA. Left ventricular assist device improves survival in children with left ventricular dysfunction after repair of anomalous origin of the left coronary artery from the pulmonary artery. Ann Thorac Surg. 1999;67:169-72.
4. Backer CL, Hillman N, Dodge-Khatami A. Anomalous origin of the left coronary artery from the pulmonary artery: successful surgical strategy without assist devices. Semin Thorac Cardiovasc Surg Pediatr Card Surg Annu. 2000;3:165-72.
5. Weigand J, Marshall CD, Bacha EA, Chen JM, Richmond ME. Repair of anomalous left coronary artery from the pulmonary artery in the modern era: preoperative predictors of immediate postoperative outcomes and long-term cardiac follow-up. Pediatr Cardiol. 2015;36(3):489-97.
6. Patra C, Singh NG, Manjunatha N, Bhatt A. The anesthetic management and physiologic implications in infants with anomalous left coronary artery arising from the pulmonary artery. J Cardiothorac Vasc Anesth. 2012;26(2):286-90.

Repair of Truncus Arteriosus

Aveek Jayant

Illustrations: Balaji Srimurugan
Reviewed by: R Krishna Kumar

■ INTRODUCTION[1-3]

Truncus arteriosus (TA) is a rare congenital heart malformation in which a single common arterial trunk (CAT) exits the heart guarded by a single common valve; this overrides the interventricular septum and supplies the coronary, pulmonary and systemic circulations **(Figs. 1 and 2)**. Although historically, the Collett Edwards, and, later the Van Praagh classification have held sway, a more functional approach is to view *truncus arteriosus or common arterial trunk* from the point of view of aortic or pulmonary dominance.[4] When there is aortic dominance the pulmonary arteries typically originate close to each other from the dorsal portion of the CAT. When there is pulmonary dominance the ductus continues as the descending thoracic aorta with consequent associated interruption of the aortic arch (IAA). This schema also allows clinical risk stratification. Most series, until recently, have demonstrated higher surgical mortality in the presence of arch interruption.[5] No scheme is complete as variants continue to be described such as sinusal origin of pulmonary arteries.[6]

Other important lesion modifiers are the location of the CAT in relation to the interventricular septum with resultant changes in location of the ventricular septal defect (VSD). The VSD can occasionally be restrictive. The status of the truncal valve in terms of leaflet numbers and dysplasia, truncal valvar stenosis or insufficiency and, finally, the pattern of pulmonary artery branching are also of considerable import. Coronary artery anomalies are not uncommon as is the presence of abnormal aortic branch arborization; all of these features are naturally of importance to the perioperative care team.

Embryologically, there is failure of spiral septation in the truncus (which causes normal division of the truncus into the aorta and proximal pulmonary arteries). Of particular interest to intensive care unit (ICU) physicians, ablation of the neural crest in chick embryos does result in TA; since the neural crest also gives rise to the pharyngeal pouches which in turn are precursors to the thymus and parathyroid glands it is no surprise that the DiGeorge (22q11.2 microdeletion) syndrome has an association with TA (and other conotruncal anomalies, as is well known). DiGeorge syndrome increases risks of airway bleeding and hyperreactivity aside from neonatal hypocalcemia, but also can be associated with varying degrees of micrognathia and a possibility of laryngeal webs. Its presence mandates the need for irradiated blood products.[1-3]

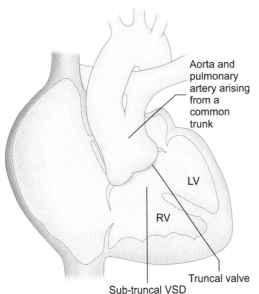

Fig. 1: Note the aorta and pulmonary artery arising from a common trunk, the truncal valve overriding the interventricular septum and the subtruncal ventricular septal defect (VSD).

(RV: right ventricle; LV: left ventricle)

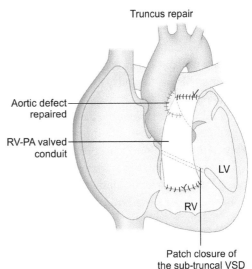

Fig. 2: Anatomy after truncus arteriosus repair: Patch closure of ventricular septal defect (VSD) and right ventricle (RV) to pulmonary artery (PA) continuity established by a conduit.

With reference to the presence of noncardiac anomalies and genetic abnormalities/syndromes children with TA often have these associated problems. In the constellation of congenital heart disease the most common lesion with noncardiac or genetic accompaniments is atrioventricular septal defect (~60%), TA has a fair share too (~40%).[7] The other major risk accruing to neonates with CAT is the risk of necrotizing enterocolitis (NEC) in the period awaiting surgical correction; TA confers an odds ratio of 2.6 (95% CI 1.9–3.5) second only to hypoplastic left heart syndrome.[8]

While this description refers only to the great arteries it is important to remember that this defect can coexist with other defects such as differences in segmentation, or defects in atrial, ventricular or atrioventricular septation.

HEMODYNAMIC MONITORING AND PATHOPHYSIOLOGIC CONSIDERATIONS

The physiology of unrepaired CAT is that of a cyanotic heart disease with pulmonary overcirculation most commonly; as such there is complete admixture with equal systemic and pulmonary saturations.

More severe cyanosis can result from the elevated pulmonary vascular resistance (PVR) in the immediate perinatal period, or from significantly and consistently elevated PVR later in life or from branch pulmonary artery (PA) stenoses. Though branch PA stenoses are rare in the Collett Edwards types 1-2, it is a frequent association in type 3 TA. As PVR declines (in the more common subtypes of CAT) over the first few postnatal days, the stage is set for gross pulmonary overcirculation with some but not marked cyanosis on presentation.

The presence of truncal valvular stenosis has been linked to sudden cardiac death. Truncal valve regurgitation tends to increase predisposition to congestive heart failure and low forward systemic cardiac output. Excessive diastolic runoff when PVR is still labile and unfixed could precipitate a state of systemic steal and coronary ischemia; it is the substrate likely for the excessive risks of NEC. Untreated CAT is a lesion that has low survival beyond the first year of life though sporadic survival into adulthood is not unknown. The occurrence of ventricular arrhythmia as a mode of sudden cardiac death has led to some focus on coronary ischemia as a precipitant: both diastolic runoff and concomitant anatomic variants are contributory.

Preoperative stabilization therefore focuses on controlling excessive fluid status, promoting urinary loss of retained fluid and, sometimes supportive ventilation with lowest tolerated fractional concentration of oxygen (FiO_2) and mild hypercapnia. Invariably, the sickest patients would be at a low threshold to temporarily withhold enteral feeding in fear of concomitant NEC. There is a case for continuously monitoring the electrocardiogram for hints of coronary ischemia secondary to steal. Although expensive, somatic and cerebral near infrared spectroscopy (NIRS) offer theoretically a method of continuously monitoring somatic oxygen delivery and guidance toward titrating therapies such as inodilators or ventilatory adjustments.

Sometimes patients have grossly elevated right ventricular afterload from anatomic stenosis or long- standing pulmonary arterial hypertension (PAH). In such patients, stabilization might involve increasing inspired oxygen and inducing alkalosis in the short term. When IAA accompanies CAT invariably there is a need for maintaining ductal patency using titrated doses of prostaglandin E1. When such patients are encountered it is possible that some centers would exclusively offer parenteral nutrition to these neonates.

At our center, most infants presenting for surgery are monitored with invasive central venous pressure and arterial pressure measurements; select cases such as those with relatively late presentation or with preoperative compromise could receive an invasive pulmonary arterial (PA) line placed transcutaneously before chest closure. Such lines are invariably retained till full stability is obtained and removal performed in the ICU with serial echocardiograms post removal to rule out bleeding or cardiac tamponade.

HEMODYNAMIC AND INOTROPE MANAGEMENT[9–13]

As delineated earlier the primary focus in most patients before surgical correction (in the operating room for surgery or in preoperative intensive care for stabilization) focuses on preventing excessive pulmonary runoff (with resultant coronary ischemia). NIRS although available is not routinely used primarily because of resource constraints; increasingly, preoperative compromise would lead us to use them in some cases. NIRS is also invariably used when Type B IAA necessitates a period of deep hypothermia with selective antegrade cerebral perfusion.

In the operating room, perilous hemodynamic conditions most importantly evidence of myocardial ischemia on ECG, could warrant emergency institution of cardiopulmonary bypass (CPB). It is also vital to pay attention to fluid status as chronic diuretic therapy, baseline elevated PVR and the increase in right ventricular afterload could actually lead to an overall decrease in cardiac output with resultant low systemic oxygen saturations. This situation would typically respond to a judicious fluid bolus and temporary measures to reduce PVR. Excessive reductions in systemic vascular resistance (SVR) too need to be avoided as the existing systemic steal could be worsened by hypotension and this in turn could exacerbate coronary ischemia. Hypotension prior to institution of CPB may necessitate treatment with epinephrine rather than a vasopressor as vasopressors could further increase systemic steal by raising SVR.

Most patients at our center would receive a balanced anesthetic which tilts toward a higher dose of opioids as CAT is not deemed eligible for early extubation at our center.

The procedure is typically performed under hypothermic CPB with some periods of low flow bypass and some form of both conventional and modified ultrafiltration. Most patients would achieve bypass separation on a combination of milrinone with epinephrine. Increasingly levosimendan use is touted as a viable alternative to milrinone use; comparative efficacy is largely unknown and therefore a matter of physician preference.

Epicardial echo would usually be performed to determine biventricular function and truncal valve function prior to bypass separation. Depending on the location of the VSD some patients might need temporary epicardial pacing, typically dual chamber synchronous pacing. The DiGeorge phenotype would invariably receive adjunct infusions of calcium. When truncal valve regurgitation is present SVR is titrated to the lowest appropriate mean arterial pressure for age.

At our center, difficult bypass separation would immediately give consideration toward keeping the chest open for delayed sternal closure once hemodynamics normalize and there is less myocardial edema with stable ventricular function. Such patients would invariably also receive a peritoneal dialysis catheter for fluid management including expedited fluid removal that would allow a shorter time to sternal closure and recovery. Although rarely used, some patients might warrant use of inhaled nitric oxide (iNO),

and, less commonly intravenous sildenafil to achieve bypass separation and hemodynamic optimization due to acute on chronic elevated PVR. Patients instituted on iNO invariably receive sildenafil to prevent rebound PAH post weaning of iNO.

Since CAT is second only to hypoplastic left heart syndrome in terms of threat to life postcardiac surgery, the usually elevated threshold in placing transthoracic invasive PA line can sometimes be lowered in these cases. This is particularly important in the sickest cases such as those involving IAA as they allow intensive care physicians to preempt sudden rises in PVR that might occur during noxious stimulation such as tracheal suction. However, at our center most children would usually be monitored with periodic transthoracic echocardiography at times of hemodynamic perturbation and placement of PA/left atrial (LA) lines is unusual, as already mentioned.

A subset of patients could develop junctional ectopic tachycardia that then jeopardizes hemodynamics. In addition to standard therapies such as cooling, rationalizing adrenergic drug therapy and overdrive pacing occasional patients do need amiodarone administered per Brisbane protocol. The use of dexmedetomidine as protective and of ivabradine as therapeutic, are utilized at our institution though it is arguable as to the robustness of currently available evidence.

■ FLUID AND BLOOD MANAGEMENT

On account of somewhat long operating times and the need for a fair degree of hypothermia most patients at our center would receive prophylactic hemostatic blood component therapy in the form of pooled platelets and cryoprecipitate. Further prescriptions such as additional doses or the use of plasma are typically decided based on point of care anticoagulation. Most patients would also receive standard but evolving doses of tranexamic acid. Given the perilous ventricular function that can often follow this surgery it is important to avoid sudden increases in cardiac preload; this is particularly important if epicardial echo or surgical communication points to a compromise in truncal valvar function and some regurgitation after repair, if necessitated by baseline valve anatomy. Once stable it is usual to pursue a net negative daily fluid balance in anticipation of either sternal closure or separation from mechanical ventilation. Fluid therapy prescriptions would therefore begin with a conservative 500 mL m^2/day eventually liberalizing as these end points are achieved based on clinical assessment and, when, necessary weight measurements.

PAIN AND SEDATION MANAGEMENT

Most patients would receive intravenous infusions of fentanyl and dexmedetomidine in our ICU. Sedations are tapered toward extubation, which currently is variable as early as the first postoperative day to sometimes up to 3–5 days after surgery. It is usual for patients to receive a bolus of fentanyl before tracheal toilet in the first few hours after surgery or depending on the behavior of pulmonary artery pressure (PAP) when available post stimulation. Although anecdotally the levels of PAH observed in a previous era are rare, the potential for paroxysmal PAH should not be ignored. Critically ill children might also occasionally receive adjunct neuromuscular blockade in the early hours after surgery primarily with a view to minimize systemic oxygen requirements.

VENTILATION AND EXTUBATION

Prior to correction as suggested above the focus is on maintaining adequate PVR so as to prevent systemic steal. Post correction the focus shifts to alleviating any reactive increases in PVR by ventilating close to functional residual capacity, in addition to producing relative hyperoxia and inducing a degree of alkalosis. Most patients will receive a period of supplemental continuous positive airway pressure (CPAP) after extubation.

COMMON POSTOPERATIVE COMPLICATIONS

- Low cardiac output after correction
- Paroxysmal pulmonary artery hypertension
- Heart block and junctional ectopic tachycardia/other tachyarrhythmias
- Truncal valvar dysfunction
- Bleeding due to long procedural times, need for hypothermia during repair
- Conduit compression during sternal closure or external chest compression such as echocardiography.

REFERENCES

1. Mavroudis C, Backer CL. Truncus arteriosus. In: Mavroudis C, Backer CL (Eds). Pediatric Heart Surgery, 4th edition. Chichester: Wiley-Blackwell; 2013. pp. 361-75.
2. Ziolkowska L, Kawalec W, Kmiec-Turska A, Walasek-Krajewska M. Chromosome 22q11.2 microdeletion in children with conotruncal heart defects: frequency, associated cardiovascular anomalies and outcome following cardiac surgery. Eur J Pediatr. 2008;167;1135-40.
3. Kyburz A, Bauersfeld U, Schinzel A, Riegel M, Hug M, Tomaske M, et al. The fate of children with microdeletion 22q11.2 syndrome and congenital heart defect: clinical course and outcome. Pediatr Cardiol. 2008;29:76-83.
4. Russell HM, Jacobs ML, Anderson RH, Mavroudis C, Spicer D, Corcrain E, et al. A simplified categorisation for common arterial trunk. J Thorac Cardiovasc Surg. 2011;141: 645-53.
5. Jacobs ML, Anderson RH. Rationalising the nomenclature of common arterial trunk. Cardiol Young. 2012;22:639-46.
6. Sharma A, Pandey NN, Kumar S. Atypical variant of truncus arteriosus: sinusal origin of pulmonary artery segment with non confluent pulmonary arteries. BMJ Case Rep. 2019;12e229547.

7. Patel A, Costello JM, Backer CL, Pasquali SK, Hill KD, Wallace AS, et al. Prevalence of noncardiac and genetic abnormalities in neonates undergoing cardiac surgery: analysis of the Society of Thoracic Surgeons Congenital Heart Surgery Database Ann Thorac Surg. 2016;102:1607-14.

8. Spinner JA, Morris SA, Nandi D, Costarino AT, Marino BS, Rossano JW, et al. Necrotising enterocolitis and associated mortality in neonates with congenital heart disease: a multi institutional study. Pediatric Crit Care Med. 2020;21:228-34.

9. Shamszad P, Moore RA, Ghanayem N, Cooper DS. Intensive care management of neonates with d-transposition of the great arteries and common arterial trunk. Cardiol Young. 2012;22:755-60.

10. Jean Martin B, Karamlou TB, Tabbutt S. Shunt lesions part II: anomalous pulmonary venous connections and truncus arteriosus. Pediatr Crit Care Med. 2016;17:S310-14.

11. Parikh S, Eisses M, Latham GJ, Joffe DC, Ross FJ. Perioperative and anaesthetic considerations in truncus arteriosus. Semin Cardiothorac Vasc Anaesth. 2018;22:285-93.

12. Chikkabyrappa S, Mahadevaiah G, Buddhe S, Alsaied T, Tretter J. Common arterial trunk: physiology, imaging and assessment. Semin Cardiothorac Vasc Anaesth. 2019;23:225-36.

13. Bibevski S, Friedland-Little J, Ohye RG, Thor T, Gaies MG. Truncus arteriosus. In: Da Cruz EM, Ivy D, Jaggers J (Eds). Pediatric and Congenital Cardiology, Cardiac Surgery and Intensive Care, 1st edition. London: Springer; 2013. pp. 1983-2001.

33

CHAPTER

Repair of Ebstein Anomaly

Aveek Jayant

Illustrations: Balaji Srimurugan
Reviewed by: R Krishna Kumar

■ INTRODUCTION[1-4]

The Ebstein malformation is the most common congenital abnormality afflicting the tricuspid valve. In essence, there is—(1) variable failure of the tricuspid valve leaflets to delaminate from the right ventricle (RV); and (2) the tricuspid valvar orifice is rotated away from the true atrioventricular junction to a region that is the junction between the right ventricular inlet and the rest of the RV **(Figs. 1 and 2)**. The anterior tricuspid leaflet (ATL) is described as sail-like with abnormal chordal attachments to the ventricular wall; the degree of ATL abnormality is likely to be more pronounced the younger the presentation. This directly causes varying degrees of tricuspid valve incompetence and "atrializes" the RV contributing to some form of chamber dysfunction. As an extension of this concept the degree of atrialization is a clear correlator to the impact of this condition and predicts clinical course beginning in utero. This is captured by the Celermajer Index[5] and is described as a ratio: **[right atrium (RA) + atrialized RV/functional RV + left atrium (LA) + left ventricle (LV)]** ; measured at end diastole. The aberrant tricuspid valve attachments can putatively obstruct RV outflow. Some form of interatrial communication is usually present; ventricular septal defects and pulmonary valvar atresia/stenosis are other associations. Up to 20% could have accessory conduction

abnormalities including some arising from compression of the normal conducting pathway. Cardiac magnetic resonance data[6,7] further clarifies that there is some form of right ventricular myopathy. At the very least, abnormal left ventricular function and depressed size are also present attributable to interventricular dependence in most cases but myopathy and non-compaction of the LV[8] has been described in a scattered fashion.

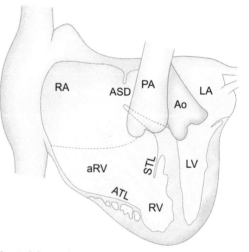

Fig. 1: Schematic representation of the tricuspid valve leaflet morphology in Ebstein malformation: Sail-like anterior tricuspid leaflet (ATL) with abnormal chordal attachment to right ventricular (RV) wall resulting in "atrialization" of right ventricle (aRV). Origin of septal tricuspid leaflet (STL) is displaced from the atrioventricular (AV) ring (dotted line). Atrial septal defect (ASD) is usually present.

(RA: right atrium; LA: left atrium; LV: left ventricle; PA: pulmonary artery; Ao: aorta)

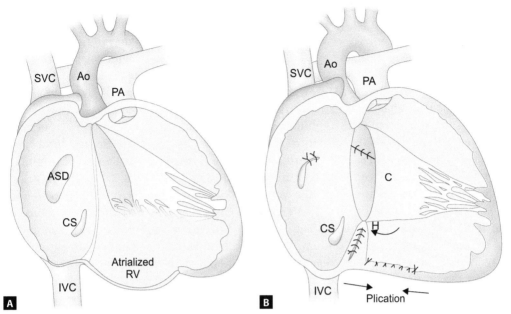

Figs. 2A and B: Diagrammatic representation of the Ebstein anomaly before (A) and after the cone repair (B).

(Ao: aorta; ASD: atrial septal defect; C refers to the newly formed "Cone" of the tricuspid valve; H: hinge point; CS: coronary sinus orifice; IVC: inferior vena cava; PA: pulmonary artery; RV: right ventricle; SVC: superior vena cava)

TABLE 1: Carpentier subtypes of the Ebstein anomaly.[33]

Type	Right ventricle	Tricuspid valve
A	Small contractile atrialized right ventricle. Adequate-size right ventricle	Moderate displacement of septal and posterior leaflets. Normal anterior leaflet
B	Large noncontractile atrialized right ventricle. Small right ventricle	Marked displacement of septal and posterior leaflets. Hypoplastic adherent septal leaflet. Normal anterior leaflet
C	Large noncontractile atrialized right ventricle. Very small right ventricle	Marked displacement of septal and posterior leaflets. Hypoplastic adherent septal and posterior leaflets. Restricted anterior leaflet motion
D	Almost completely noncontractile atrialized right ventricle (except for infundibulum)	Marked displacement of septal, posterior and anterior leaflets. Hypoplastic adherent septal and posterior leaflets. Anterior leaflet is adherent to ventricular wall

In patients admitted to the surgical pathway, the Carpentier classification of the condition and the Celermajer Index [also called the Great Ormond Street Echocardiography (GOSE) score] is useful for overall risk stratification **(Tables 1 and 2)**. A composite classification from the Mayo Clinic

TABLE 2: Great Ormond Street Echocardiography (GOSE) score.[5]

Grade I	0.5
Grade II	0.5–0.99
Grade III	1–1.49
Grade IV	>1.5

attempts to synthesize echocardiography with surgical anatomy. Fetal groups use their own scoring systems adding finer elements to in utero assessment of the fetal heart.[9]

The overall right heart dysfunction is secondary to loss of functional RV, myopathy and tricuspid regurgitation. In extreme cases, this leads to a functional form of pulmonary atresia [contributed to also by the natural pulmonary vascular resistance (PVR) at birth]. In such neonates the only source of pulmonary blood flow is the ductus arteriosus. The worst subsets also show impairment of left sided function (the reverse Bernheim effect) due to extreme interventricular septum shifts. When in addition, pulmonary regurgitation is also present there can be a circular shunt (aorta-ductus-pulmonary artery-RV-patent foramen ovale-left atrium-left ventricle-aorta). Respiratory insufficiency can also be present secondary to a grossly dilated heart (cardiothoracic ratio >80%). This reverses with surgery or as the RV decompresses gradually when PVR falls over time in the early neonatal period.

Clinical presentation occurs at all ages ranging from intrauterine death (due to hydrops fetalis) to symptoms primarily presenting well into adolescence or later in adulthood. Milder forms may remain asymptomatic altogether. Neonates can present with varying severity of illness such as clinically important cyanosis to cardiovascular collapse requiring extracorporeal support. Older children typically present with limitation of exercise capacity or sometimes with palpitations resulting from associated electrophysiologic abnormalities inherent to the Ebstein phenotype.

The initial management of the intermediate cohort (Carpentier C and D phenotypes and presenting with clinical distress) often entails oxygen and alprostadil infusions to tide over the high PVR at birth. Sicker neonates (Carpentier C and D with

GOSE scores >3) need neonatal surgical interventions. The surgical interventions are broadly either targeted at univentricular pathways or an attempt to biventricular repair: this is decided by the size of the functional RV (fRV), the substrate for tricuspid valvuloplasty and, if present, anatomic pulmonary atresia.

Univentricular pathway operations include the modified Starnes procedure[10] or, more recently, the Sano right ventricular exclusion technique.[11] The biventricular pathway, (revolutionary as it is in the pantheon of neonatal surgical interventions) was pioneered by the Knott-Craig[12] monocusp technique. Some patients though initially committed to the single ventricle pathway can go on to receive 1.5 ventricle repairs[13] or even biventricular repair. It seems reasonable to state that in the centers with the largest experience most neonates committed to surgery for Ebstein would more often than not, receive a biventricular repair. When older children are operated most would now receive the cone repair[14] or its iterations pioneered by the Mayo group.[15] Select patients are not deemed eligible for definitive surgery: in these times this is typically when they have associated severe left ventricular dysfunction. A small proportion of patients might also receive additional measures to tackle an evident electrophysiologic abnormality.

A contemporary cohort from SickKids where this diagnosis was made in utero is revealing;[9] a specially fashioned SickKids score predicted fetal outcomes better than other scores. In their cohort, subjects diagnosed perinatally and surviving to term did reach 5-year survival rates of ~80% and that therefore is the most contemporary benchmark for the worst subsets of this condition. Older children and adolescents achieve excellent functional outcomes even as the valvuloplasty techniques evolve from the original versions[16,17] with some thoughts about not always obliterating the atrialized portion of the RV as was considered gospel earlier.[18]

Most of the description that follows applies to the postoperative care of children after a cone repair of the Ebstein valve in early childhood or adolescence **(Fig. 2B)**. A small proportion of this cohort could potentially be treated with a 1.5 ventricle repair, but at the ages typically performed at our center the natural history of the condition rarely includes this subset of patients. However, surgical groups report addition of a bidirectional cavopulmonary anastomosis to the surgical plan can dramatically alter the clinical course of patients with the highest risk of right ventricular dysfunction.[19] Ebstein anomaly is a rare anomaly (<1%) and, the neonatal surgical cohort of this condition is at present rare at our center.

HEMODYNAMIC MONITORING

Since in the Ebstein anomaly the primary dysfunctional chamber is the RV, the usual monitoring consists of right sided filling pressures [central venous pressure (CVP)], invasive arterial blood pressure, temperature, continuous electrocardiography, pulse oximetry and, in very select cases tissue or brain near infrared spectroscopy (NIRS). Most patients would receive intraoperative transesophageal echocardiography always and functional transthoracic echocardiography in the postoperative period as required.

HEMODYNAMIC AND INOTROPE MANAGEMENT

The principles of management of the post repair patient are similar to other patient subsets with precarious right ventricular function. At our center most patients would receive small doses of adrenaline (0.02–0.04 μg/kg/min) and some patients with baseline impairment of RV function, additional milrinone or levosimendan adjunctively.

FLUID AND BLOOD MANAGEMENT

Fluids and/or blood is titrated to clinical end points and the CVP. However, it is moot to point out that while it has been traditionally believed that right-sided ventricular dysfunction should always be treated with liberal fluid therapy this is increasingly questioned as elevated CVP is now recognized as a key factor for acute kidney injury.[20] Most patients would leave the operating room with a fenestrated defect in the interatrial septum that would allow the right heart to decompress via this in the face of acute deterioration over baseline impairment in right ventricular function. Thus, it seems logical to administer clinically appropriate fluids depending on assessment of fluid balance, chamber function on echocardiograms and the CVP as a continuous trending parameter.

SEDATION AND PAIN MANAGEMENT

At present, most patients usually receive modest amounts of fentanyl intraoperatively and infusions of fentanyl and dexmedetomidine postoperatively. If permitted, most patients also receive central neuraxial morphine that allows lower doses of opioids to be administered perioperatively. This means that from the sedation perspective, most patients are free to be weaned from mechanical ventilation as soon as their clinical status permits.

VENTILATION AND EXTUBATION

The ventilatory management should focus on reducing PVR to allow unimpeded right ventricular forward flow. This typically entails a tidal volume just adequate to cause normocapnia, probably mild hyperoxia [given the current controversies about oxygen therapy in the intensive care unit (ICU) population[21] and cautious titration of positive end expiratory pressure. All intensivists are enjoined to remember that the relationship of PVR to lung volume is parabolic with both lung collapse and hyperinflation increasing this key parameter. It has been a dogma that all patients with a predominant right heart problem are liberated from mechanical ventilation as soon as feasible as spontaneous respiration promotes more harmonious cardiopulmonary interaction, and, by extension, interventricular dependence.[22] This said, those with the worst impairment of right ventricular function do benefit from mechanical ventilatory assistance for somewhat extended periods as this allows precarious oxygen delivery to be reallocated to critical tissue beds such as the splanchnic circulation. In such patients overzealous weaning from ventilation sets the stage for tilting a precarious oxygen delivery metric in favor of the respiratory apparatus in preference to other tissue beds. Such patients show clinical distress in the form of abnormal monitored metrics in heart rate, blood pressure and elevations in CVP and if allowed to persist, congestive hepatomegaly eventually sets in. Therefore, this situation merits:

- Less dogmatic and more individualized weaning protocols
- Assessment for resumed mechanical ventilatory support before the patient is in extremis.

COMMON POSTOPERATIVE COMPLICATIONS

In the contemporary era and particularly with reference to the predominant subset discussed here (older children with Ebstein anomaly and therefore with a survival bias that allows them to survive beyond early infancy) surgical repair outcomes are excellent. The sickest patients within this group can expect to have somewhat prolonged durations of mechanical ventilation and correspondingly longer stay in the intensive care unit. Complications therefore result, if at all from long stays in the ICU environment such as increased infectious risk, nutritional depletion, impairment of muscle tone and strength etc. A small proportion of patients can develop both tachyarrhythmias secondary to underlying substrate such as accessory tracts superimposed on the risks posed by inotrope therapy; transient or more permanent heart blocks can happen but are not common. Residual tricuspid regurgitation from suboptimal repair can happen but is rare and can be addressed with replacement although, justifiably, with intraoperative imaging full attention is given to addressing the valve in the repair pathway itself intraoperatively. For operations other than cone repair, a subset will likely receive reoperative tricuspid valvuloplasty using the cone approach.[4]

■ REFERENCES

1. Sainathan S, Silva L da F da, Silva JP da. Ebstein's anomaly: contemporary management strategies. J Thorac Dis. 2020;12(3):1161-73.
2. O'Leary P, Dearani J, Anderson RH, Spicer DE, Srivastava D. Diseases of the tricuspid valve. In: Anderson R, Kumar K, Mussato K, Redington A, Twedell JS, Tretter J, Wernovsky G (Eds). Anderson's Pediatric Cardiology, 4th edition. New York: Elsevier Inc.; 2019.
3. Ross FJ, Latham GJ, Richards M, Geiduschek J, Thompson D, Joffe D. Perioperative and anesthetic considerations in Ebstein's anomaly. Semin Cardiothorac Vasc Anesth. 2016;20(1):82-92.
4. Morray B. Preoperative physiology, imaging, and management of Ebstein's anomaly of the tricuspid valve. Semin Cardiothorac Vasc Anesth. 2016;20(1):74-81.
5. Celermajer DS, Dodd SM, Greenwald SE, Wyse RKH, Deanfield JE. Morbid anatomy in neonates with Ebstein's anomaly of the tricuspid valve: pathophysiologic and clinical implications. J Am Coll Cardiol. 1992;19(5):1049-53.

6. Liu X, Zhang Q, Yang Z, Guo Y, Shi K, Xu H, et al. Morphologic and functional abnormalities in patients with Ebstein's anomaly with cardiac magnetic resonance imaging: correlation with tricuspid regurgitation. Eur J Radiol. 2016;85(9):1601-6.

7. Ciepłucha A, Trojnarska O, Kociemba A, Łanocha M, Barczynski M, Rozmiarek S, et al. Clinical aspects of myocardial fibrosis in adults with Ebstein's anomaly. Heart Vessels. 2018;33(9):1076-85.

8. Chitturi KR, Cavazos MC, Singh R, Heredia CP, Chebrolu L. Left ventricular noncompaction with Ebstein anomaly secondary to MYH7 mutation. J Am Coll Cardiol. 2020;75(11):3078.

9. Wertaschnigg D, Manlhiot C, Jaeggi M, Seed M, Dragulescu A, Schwartz SM, et al. Contemporary outcomes and factors associated with mortality after a fetal or neonatal diagnosis of ebstein anomaly and tricuspid valve disease. Can J Cardiol. 2016;32(12):1500-6.

10. Kumar SR, Kung G, Noh N, Castillo N, Fagan B, Wells WJ, et al. Single-ventricle outcomes after neonatal palliation of severe ebstein anomaly with modified starnes procedure. Circulation. 2016;134(17):1257-64.

11. Sano S, Fujii Y, Kasahara S, Kuroko Y, Tateishi A, Yoshizumi K, et al. Repair of Ebstein's anomaly in neonates and small infants: impact of right ventricular exclusion and its indications†. Eur J Cardiothorac Surg. 2014;45(3):549-55.

12. Knott-Craig CJ, Overholt ED, Ward KE, Razook JD. Neonatal repair of Ebstein's anomaly: indications, surgical technique, and medium-term follow-up. Ann Thoracic Surg. 2000;69(5):1505-10.

13. Liu J, Qiu L, Zhu Z, Chen H, Hong H. Cone reconstruction of the tricuspid valve in Ebstein anomaly with or without one and a half ventricle repair. J Thoracic Cardiovasc Surg. 2011;141(5):1178-83.

14. da Silva JP, Baumgratz JF, da Fonseca L, Franchi SM, Lopes LM, Tavares GMP, et al. The cone reconstruction of the tricuspid valve in Ebstein's anomaly. The operation: early and midterm results. J Thorac Cardiovasc Surg. 2007;133(1):215-23.

15. Dearani JA, Bacha E, da Silva JP. Cone reconstruction of the tricuspid valve for Ebstein's anomaly: anatomic repair. Oper Tech Thorac Cardiovasc Surg. 2008;13(2):109-25.

16. Carpentier A, Chauvaud S, Macé L, Relland J, Mihaileanu S, Marino JP, et al. A new reconstructive operation for Ebstein's anomaly of the tricuspid valve. J Thorac Cardiovasc Surg. 1988;96(1):92-101.

17. Danielson GK, Fuster V. Surgical repair of Ebstein's anomaly. Ann Surg. 1982;196(4):499-504.

18. Hetzer R, Hacke P, Javier M, Miera O, Schmitt K, Weng Y, et al. The long-term impact of various techniques for tricuspid repair in Ebstein's anomaly. J Thorac Cardiovasc Surg. 2015;150(5):1212-9.

19. Chauvaud S. Bidirectional cavopulmonary shunt associated with ventriculo and valvuloplasty in Ebstein's anomaly: benefits in high risk patients. Eur J Cardiothorac Surg. 1998;13(5):514-9.

20. Chen CY, Zhou Y, Wang P, Qi EY, Gu WJ. Elevated central venous pressure is associated with increased mortality and acute kidney injury in critically ill patients: a meta-analysis. Crit Care. 2020;24(1):80.

21. Girardis M, Alhazzani W, Rasmussen BS. What's new in oxygen therapy? Intens Care Med. 2019;45(7):1009-11.

22. Bronicki RA, Penny DJ, Anas NG, Fuhrman B. Cardiopulmonary interactions. Pediatr Crit Care Med. 2016;17:S182-93.

23. Muthiah R. Ebstein anomaly—an overview. Case Rep Clin Med. 2018;7(2):90-125.

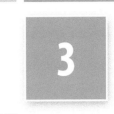

SECTION

Common Postoperative Complications

Management of Low Cardiac Output Syndrome after Pediatric Cardiac Surgery

Rakhi Balachandran, R Krishna Kumar

Reviewed by: R Krishna Kumar

■ INTRODUCTION

Maintaining adequate cardiac output (CO) and providing systemic oxygen delivery is the key component of postoperative cardiovascular support after congenital heart surgery. Precise hemodynamic tools for measuring CO and the various hemodynamic variables determining it are available in adult patients, but the assessment of CO in pediatric patients is largely by bedside clinical assessment, monitoring of atrial filling pressures, and echocardiography. Low cardiac output syndrome (LCOS), after pediatric cardiac surgery, is a pathophysiological state, which can significantly impact postoperative outcomes with increased morbidity and mortality.[1] The reported incidence of LCOS in pediatric cardiac surgery ranges from 10 to 57%.[1-3] The proposed causes of low CO state and myocardial dysfunction after cardiac surgery include inflammatory response to cardiopulmonary bypass (CPB), myocardial ischemia during cross clamping, reperfusion injury, hypothermia, suboptimal myocardial protection, and ventriculotomy during surgery.[4] In the absence of hemodynamic monitors in small children to accurately measure CO, the recognition of this clinical state is a real challenge to the pediatric intensivist and one has to heavily rely on clinical evaluation and surrogate markers for diagnosing this condition. The crux of managing LCOS in postoperative intensive care unit (ICU) is anticipatory care, early recognition of the condition, and appropriate pharmacological/critical care interventions. This chapter has attempted to provide a brief overview of the diagnosis and management of LCOS after pediatric cardiac surgery.

■ DEFINITION OF LCOS

The LCOS refers to a reduction in CO that may occur in the postoperative period after correction or palliation for congenital heart disease. Wernovsky et al. in an elegant study in postoperative arterial switch patients observed an incidence of 25% in the postoperative period with measurable drops in CO to less than $2 \ L/min/m^2$, with the nadir occurring between 9 and 12 hours following admission into the ICU.[2,5]

■ PHYSIOLOGICAL CONSIDERATIONS

What is Cardiac Output?

Cardiac output is the quantity of blood delivered to systemic circulation per unit time.

(CO = Stroke volume × Heart rate)

Cardiac output is usually indexed to body surface area (BSA) and is expressed as cardiac index (CI).

Cardiac output varies inversely with age so that CI in children at rest is 4.0–5.0 $L/min/m^2$ while for a 70-year-old adult CI is 2.5 $L/min/m^2$.[6-8]

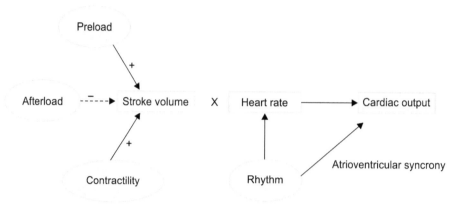

Fig. 1: Determinants of cardiac output.

What Determines Cardiac Output?

- Venous return (preload)
- Myocardial contractility
- Resistance to blood exiting the left ventricle (afterload)
- Heart rate
- Rhythm, particularly the maintenance of atrioventricular (AV) synchrony.

The determinants of CO are depicted in **Figure 1**. Besides these five important factors, there are several other determinants of adequacy of CO. They either increase the demands or underutilize the substrate for energy metabolism thus placing greater demand on the heart to pump. Alterations to any of these factors will lead to a syndrome of low CO.

WHAT ARE THE INDICATORS OF LOW CARDIAC OUTPUT SYNDROME AFTER CARDIAC SURGERY?

There are various studies, which have investigated the best predictors of mortality or morbidity in patients with LCOS. In a single center cohort of 257 patients undergoing pediatric cardiac surgery, cyanotic heart disease, longer duration of CPB, high inotropes on leaving the operating room, and increase in blood lactate were associated with major complications including LCOS

after cardiac surgery.[9] Since, vasoactive agents such as inotropes or vasodilators are routinely used for the treatment of low CO after cardiac surgery in infants, a vasoactive-inotrope score has often been tested for its ability to predict adverse outcomes including mortality. Vasoactive-inotropic score has been derived from dosages of vasoactive-inotropic drugs as described by Gaies et al.[10]

Vasoactive-inotropic score = 1 × Dopamine (μg/kg/min) + 1 × Dobutamine (μg/kg/min) + 100 × Epinephrine (μg/kg/min) + 100 × Norepinephrine (μg/kg/min) + 10 × Milrinone (μg/kg/min) + 10,000 × Vasopressin (U/kg/min).

In a single center study of 174 infants undergoing cardiac surgery high maximum vasoactive inotropic score was strongly associated with poor clinical outcomes of death, cardiac arrest, mechanical support, renal replacement therapy and neurologic injury.[10] Following are the most frequent signs that potentially aid the recognition of LCOS in the pediatric cardiac ICU.[11,12] One should also realize that most of the factors contributing to LCOS are interdependent and can be due to various reasons in a given patient.

Clinical Signs

- *Mental state*: Lethargy or excessive irritability.

- *Vital signs*: Hypo or hyperthermia, tachy or bradycardia, tachypnea, hypotension, and narrow pulse pressure.
- *Peripheral perfusion*: Cool or pale peripheries, toe temperature <30°C, prolonged capillary refill time (>3 seconds), poorly palpable pulses.
- Hepatomegaly.
- *Arterial wave form*: Blunted upstroke, narrow pulse pressure.
- *Atrial pressure and central venous pressure (CVP)*: Low in hypovolemia, high with ventricular diastolic dysfunction, decreased ventricular compliance, and cardiac tamponade.
- *Low urine output*: Less than 1.0 mL/kg/hr.

Investigations

- *Mixed venous oxygen saturation*: Mixed venous samples are typically obtained from blood drawn from pulmonary artery (PA) catheters in adult patients. However, due to the nonavailability of PA catheters suitable for use in infants and children oximetry from central venous catheters have been used as a reasonable surrogate. A mixed venous oxygen saturation >70% in two ventricle physiology and >55% in single ventricle palliations are typically suggestive of adequate CO.[13]
- Metabolic acidosis in arterial blood gas.
- Hyperkalemia.
- Elevated or increasing trends in the serum lactate (>2 mmol/L).
- Elevated blood urea and serum creatinine.

Echocardiography

- Systolic dysfunction is readily identified by poor ventricular contractility
- *Diastolic dysfunction*: This is difficult to diagnose with certainty. Systolic function is preserved, but there is evidence of elevated filling pressures and late diastolic flow reversal in systemic or pulmonary veins

- AV valve regurgitation
- *Residual lesions*: Ventricular septal defect (VSD), left ventricular (LV) outflow tract obstruction, right ventricular (RV) outflow tract obstruction, branch PA stenosis, aortopulmonary collaterals, aortic regurgitation, and pulmonary regurgitation
- Pulmonary artery hypertension (PAH)
- Pericardial effusion.

In a prospective observational study, Ulate et al. utilized a LCOS score as a clinical assessment tool to evaluate the association of low CO to clinical outcomes after congenital heart surgery.[14] The score was calculated by assigning one point each for the following parameters; tachycardia, oliguria, toe temperature < 30°C, need for volume administration > 30 mL/kg/day, decreased near infrared spectroscopy (NIRS) measurements, hyperlactatemia, and need for vasoactive agents/inotropes in excess of milrinone at 0.5 µg/kg/min. Patients with cumulative LCOS score >7 had higher morbidity, longer period of ventilation, and longer ICU as well as hospital stay. The authors concluded that higher peak and cumulative LCOS scores were independently associated with composite morbidity.[14]

WHAT ARE THE COMMON CAUSES OF LOW CARDIAC OUTPUT IN POSTOPERATIVE PATIENTS?

Again it is helpful to have a checklist to identify and treat the cause.

Preload

- Is the preload optimal for the given setting? Typically, in most situations this information is derived from the CVP recording. However, in a patient with congenital heart disease, CVP measurements have several pitfalls.
- Generally, in most patients CVP is optimized around 5–8 mm Hg. Some of the

exceptions include patients after tetralogy of Fallot (TOF) repair with significant RV hypertrophy/congenital heart disease with LV outflow tract obstructions and LV hypertrophy who require higher CVP to maintain adequate preload to the stiff noncompliant ventricles. The traditional approach included maintaining higher CVP targets of 10–14 mm Hg in patients with TOF and significant RV hypertrophy. However with the current practice of early primary repair, valve sparing techniques and better understanding of the adverse outcomes related to postoperative fluid overload, aggressive volume loading is avoided and the optimal atrial filling pressure is largely decided based on clinical indicators of adequate tissue perfusion.

- In patients with cavopulmonary connections such as Glenn or Fontan, who depend on venous pressure for maintaining pulmonary blood flow, higher CVP targets and maintenance of adequate intravascular volume is crucial. Typically, if femoral venous pressure (which reflects PA pressure) is used to guide volume management, e.g., in Fontan circulation, this is maintained between 10 and 14 mm Hg in the early postoperative period.
- Falsely higher CVP can be due to either higher positive end expiratory pressure (PEEP) or an inappropriately longer inspiratory time setting during mechanical ventilation, which is transmitted to the right atrium. An inadvertent high-ventilator setting in this circumstance can impede the venous return to the heart and contribute to decreased preload.
- It is also prudent to check for technical errors in measurement of CVP such as zeroing of transducers, checking the level of transducers, and maintaining appropriate pressure limits in the transducer flush bags.

Problems with the Pump

Myocardial Dysfunction

- As an effect of prolonged CPB
- Possible after many operations such as:
  - ALCAPA (anomalous origin of left coronary artery from PA) repair
  - Surgeries, which involve ventriculotomy
  - Arterial switch operation
- Secondary to metabolic or respiratory acidosis, which depresses the myocardial function
- PAH.

Residual/Previously Unrecognized Cardiac Lesions

- Residual/additional VSD
- Residual outflow obstructions
- AV valve regurgitation
- Aortopulmonary collaterals.

Cardiac Tamponade

This can occur in the postoperative period secondary to increased postoperative bleeding or serous/chylous pericardial effusions. Large effusions can cause decrease in CO due to cardiac tamponade.

Abnormalities of Cardiac Rhythm

Disturbance in cardiac rhythm is not uncommon in any unit caring for patients with complex congenital heart disease. Since, CO is directly proportional to heart rate, it is important to maintain a normal heart rate that is appropriate for the age. AV dyssynchrony does not result in LCOS in a normal situation. However, in certain situations where the ventricular filling pressures are elevated (e.g., TOF, LV dysfunction, single-ventricle physiology) atrial kick has significant contribution to the ventricular filling. In such circumstances, it is desirable to maintain AV synchrony. It is also possible to pace the heart in an AV sequential mode to re-establish AV synchrony. Tachyarrhythmias decrease stroke volume (due to reduced diastolic filling) and increase myocardial oxygen demand. They should be recognized and appropriately treated.

Problems with the Afterload

Afterload Mismatch

This is possible in patients after mitral valve replacement, VSD closure and patent ductus arteriosus (PDA) ligation. In patients with severe mitral regurgitation before surgery, the left ventricle pumps blood into two chambers, the systemic circulation and the low pressure left atrium. Hence, the overall after load is much less. After the surgery, the ventricle no longer pumps into the low pressure chamber. The LV now faces the relative increase (mismatch) in the afterload. Same holds true for selected patients with VSD and PDA. They can have various degrees of LV dysfunction, which recovers over time. If these patients manifest signs of low CO, they need inotropes with additional vasodilatory properties to reduce afterload till the LV function recovers.

Increased Systemic Vascular Resistance

Certain patients may have increased systemic vascular resistance (SVR). This can be recognized by cool peripheries, increased capillary refill time, and supported by increasing lactate levels in arterial blood gas. If a PA line is inserted, SVR can be calculated by thermodilution technique. These patients benefit from afterload reducing agents.

Decreased Systemic Vascular Resistance

This occurs because of vasodilatation and can lead to capillary leak. Sepsis/post-CPB vasoplegic states are the primary reasons for peripheral vasodilatation in a postoperative patient. It can be clinically recognized by warm peripheries, low CVP, increased requirement of fluids to maintain a reasonable CVP, and generalized tissue edema. These patients may benefit from a small dose of vasoconstrictor drugs to tide over the crisis.

Other Factors

Lungs

They are the organs for central gas exchange. Any parenchymal lung disease will hamper gas exchange and may result in reduced oxygen saturation. Hypoxia is a potent trigger for pulmonary vasoconstriction which in turn increases pulmonary vascular resistance and right ventricular afterload. Apart from acting as the organs for gas exchange, there exists a complex interaction between the lung mechanics and the heart. In a normally breathing person the inspiration is active and is achieved by negative intrathoracic pressure, which facilitates the right heart filling. In a patient on positive pressure ventilation the same is counterproductive and positive pressure increases the right heart filling pressures and the CVP. Positive pressure ventilation and parenchymal lung disease thus increase the RV afterload. This reduces the efficacy of RV by 20%. This is particularly true with pre-existing RV dysfunction in patients with TOF. In these situations, patients benefit from early transition to negative pressure ventilation (spontaneous breathing) as soon as the cardiac function starts recovering.

Sepsis

Sepsis and systemic inflammatory response have complex interactions with the circulatory system and affect the efficacy of circulation in many ways due the inflammatory cytokines and direct effect on peripheral vasculature.

It is important to recognize and treat sepsis in these patients as the signs of low CO and sepsis can masquerade each other.

Hyperthermia or Hypothermia

Nonshivering thermogenesis in patients with cold stress is an unrecognized factor responsible for "sudden deterioration" in many neonates in the ICU setting. Cold stress or hypothermia has varied presentation, which cannot often be differentiated with that of sepsis and LCOS in a sick neonate.

Hyperthermia due to intense peripheral vasoconstriction on the other hand is a sign of LCOS and is counterproductive by increasing the basal metabolic rate in a baby who has very minimal cardiac reserves. Utmost importance should be given to maintain normothermia. Infants should not be "cooled" or "warmed" in an ICU. They should be maintained in a thermoneutral environment.

Electrolyte, Acid Base and Glucose Disturbance

A common cause of sudden deaths and cardiac events in a postoperative ICU is electrolyte disturbance. They should be best avoided and should be looked for in an infant who is "not doing well".

It is mandatory to supplement 40–60% of the calorie requirement in any sick infant to meet the basal metabolic demands and avoid catabolism. Nutritional supplements either enteral or parenteral, need to be planned based on the individual cases. There are conflicting evidences of benefit in pediatric literature regarding tight control of blood sugars in the postoperative patients.[15-17] However, it is reasonable to avoid rapid fluctuations in the blood sugar levels.

◼ THERAPEUTIC STRATEGIES

The key to managing LCOS is anticipatory care, early recognition, and appropriate intervention. The various management strategies include pharmacological agents, mechanical ventilation, support of end-organ function, and addressing the residual defects.[4,18,19]

Pharmacological Agents

Inotropes

These are drugs, which improve myocardial contractility by modifying calcium handling and calcium-protein interactions. Commonly used inotropes include catecholamines and inodilators. Choice of inotrope is dictated by the patient's pathophysiology and the relevant hemodynamic goals.

Dopamine: This drug has action on dopaminergic receptors as well as direct action on alpha and beta-receptors. Inotropic effect is mediated by stimulation of β-1 receptors in the heart and indirectly by promoting norepinephrine release at the presynaptic terminal. Dopamine is typically used in cardiac surgical settings in dose ranges between 5 and 10 µg/kg/min.

It is a widely used catecholamine to treat systemic hypotension and low CO in neonates, infants, and children. In a study of 14 patients undergoing open heart surgery dopamine significantly increased CO and renal plasma flow.[20] The role of low dose dopamine as a renal protective agent is disputed.[21] Tachycardia occurs at high doses and can predispose to tachyarrhythmia. Alpha receptor stimulation at high doses can provoke increases in pulmonary vascular resistance in patients predisposed to pulmonary hypertension.

Epinephrine: This endogenous catecholamine acts via both α and β adrenergic receptors. Predominant effect depends on the dose given. Low doses stimulate β1 receptor and increases contractility. High doses can cause α receptor-mediated vasoconstriction. Typical dose range to achieve maximal physiological benefit is 0.01–0.05 µg/kg/min, as higher doses promote vasoconstriction mediated increase in afterload. Epinephrine is administered as a continuous intravenous infusion in critically ill children with systemic hypotension, myocardial dysfunction or low CO. It is also the first line drug in the management of cardiac arrest.

Administration at very high doses > 0.2 µg/kg/min can cause significant vasoconstriction and compromise end organ perfusion. It can cause glycogenolysis leading to hyperglycemia and hyperkalemia due to its β2 receptor-mediated effects.

Inodilators

These are pharmacological agents that combine inotropic and peripheral vasodilator properties.

Dobutamine: This is a synthetic catecholamine with predominantly β-agonist effects. Inotropic effect is mediated via the β1 receptor of the heart. β2 receptor stimulation promotes pulmonary and systemic vasodilation. Normal dose range include 1–10 µg/kg/min. Typically, a dose of 3–5 µg/kg/min is preferred in postoperative patients to facilitate myocardial contractility and to achieve additional benefit of vasodilation in increased afterload states. Doses > 5 µg/kg/min can predispose to undesirable tachyarrhythmias and hence should be restricted. A recent study comparing dobutamine and milrinone has demonstrated that both dobutamine and milrinone are safe, well-tolerated, and equally effective in preventing LCOS after pediatric cardiac surgery.[22]

Milrinone: This is a phosphodiesterase enzyme-3 (PDE 3) inhibitor, which combines gentle inotropy, peripheral, and coronary vasodilatation. It improves contractility by increasing intracellular concentration of cyclic adenosine monophosphate (cAMP). Due to long half-life its clinical effects last up to 6–24 hours after stopping infusion. Milrinone has become a popular cardiovascular drug after the PRIMACORP study, which demonstrated its efficacy in preventing LCOS after infant heart surgery.[5] The other proposed clinical benefits include pulmonary vasodilator effects and lusitropic effect facilitating ventricular relaxation. The most common clinical settings likely to benefit from milrinone therapy include patients after arterial switch operation, ALCAPA repair, and patients with significant AV valve regurgitation in postoperative period. It is administered as a bolus dose of 25–50 µg/kg initially over 1 hour followed by an infusion ranging from 0.2 to 0.75 µg/kg/min. As hypotension is often expected with the bolus dose, it is usually administered on CPB, in situations where the drug is pre-emptively started for treating post-bypass cardiac dysfunction. If started in the postoperative ICU, continuous infusion is initiated without the bolus titrated to the hemodynamic parameters. Potential adverse effects include hypotension with higher doses, thrombocytopenia, and tachyarrhythmias.

Levosimendan: Levosimendan improves myocardial performance by increasing the sensitivity of the contractile apparatus to intracellular calcium. It also opens cardiac mitochondrial ATP dependent K^+ channels linked to cardioprotective ischemic preconditioning in response to oxidative stress. It also opens the ATP sensitive K^+ channels of vascular smooth muscle producing coronary and peripheral vasodilatation.[23] It is recommended as an initial bolus of 6–12 µg/kg over 10 minutes followed by an infusion of 0.05–0.2 µg/kg/min. The infusion is continued for 24–48 hours. Persistent effect is observed after stopping the infusion due to the presence of active metabolites in the circulation. This can last as long as a week.

Vasoconstrictors

These are the drugs specifically intended for use in vasoplegic states contributing to low CO. The commonly used agents are vasopressin and norepinephrine.

Norepinephrine: This is a potent adrenergic agent that acts primarily on α receptors producing vasoconstriction. SVR is elevated and perfusion to vital organs may be impaired in high doses. Hence, its dose is titrated to achieve specific hemodynamic targets like mean arterial pressure or diastolic blood pressure. Recommended doses are in the range of 0.01–0.05 μg/kg/min.

Vasopressin: This is an endogenous hormone produced by hypothalamus. Vasopressin exerts its vasoconstrictor effects by acting on V1 receptors in peripheral vasculature to cause intense vasoconstriction. The typical dose ranges from 0.0003 to 0.002 units/kg/min. This drug has adverse effects due to the intense vasoconstriction that may compromise blood flow to vital organs in high doses leading to gut ischemia/peripheral vascular complications. Careful monitoring for signs of peripheral limb ischemia (ecchymosis, gangrene, etc.) and gut ischemia (feed intolerance, blood in stools, and paralytic ileus) is important in patients on vasopressin. It should be stopped as soon as the primary condition resolves. Additionally, vasopressin while improving the mean arterial pressure by augmenting the SVR may cause a reduction in stroke volume in patients with systolic ventricular dysfunction. Hence, its use should be restricted to specific clinical situations like catecholamine-resistant septic shock or post-CPB vasoplegic states.[24,25]

Vasodilators

These groups of drugs augment systemic oxygen delivery by improving CO in patients with low CO due to increased SVR. The agents commonly used in clinical practice include sodium nitroprusside and phenoxybenzamine. Sodium nitroprusside does not have any inotropic effects, but it dilates peripheral arterial vessels decreasing vascular resistance. It has a short half-life and is easily titratable when used as an infusion. Generally, it is used in doses of 0.5–5 μg/kg/min. Phenoxybenzamine is a nonselective alpha adrenergic receptor antagonist, which is used in single ventricle palliations like Norwood procedure for maximizing systemic blood flow.[26] This drug has a prolonged effect and might cause decrease in preload. Hence, it has to be used while being mindful of maintaining adequate intravascular volume. Typical dose ranges from 1 to 2 mg/kg/day as an intravenous infusion.

Pharmacotherapy alone may be insufficient to maintain adequate CO in the presence of severe ventricular dysfunction. In these circumstances, mechanical support of cardiac function may be required. There is limited experience with the use of intra-aortic balloon pump (IABP) in children. Additionally, arterial access and indwelling arterial catheters can be a challenge. Use of LV assist devices or extracorporeal membrane oxygenation (ECMO) can be resorted to provide successful hemodynamic support and allow recovery in selected cases. In established pediatric heart centers with an ECMO program, use of mechanical circulatory support is considered when pharmacological therapy is unable to restore adequate tissue perfusion. Complete discussion of this topic is beyond the scope of this chapter.

Other Supportive Measures in Low Cardiac Output State

Mechanical Ventilation

This predominantly supports myocardial recovery by decreasing LV afterload and decreasing work of breathing. However, cardiopulmonary interactions on RV preload and function need to be carefully considered while adjusting the ventilator settings. Ventilator settings have to be also tailored in patients with PAH to minimize increase in RV afterload, if the lungs are inflated above functional residual capacity (FRC) producing increased PVR.

Keeping the Sternum Open

This is an accepted strategy in early post-operative period with beneficial effects in neonates with myocardial edema and dysfunction. Keeping sternum open prevents myocardial compression, which occurs during closure, augments diastolic filling, and improves CO.[27,28] This also facilitates improved pulmonary function by improved thoracic cage compliance and better gas exchange.

Sedation and Paralysis

Sedation and paralysis is often beneficial in patients with low CO states to decrease stress response, improve patient ventilator synchrony during mechanical ventilation and to reduce myocardial work and oxygen consumption.

Aggressive Management of Hyperthermia

This can promote recovery of cardiac function. Keeping a lower core temperature of 35°C can reduce myocardial oxygen consumption and minimize the risk of tachyarrhythmias like junctional ectopic tachycardia, which can further compromise CO.

Supporting End Organ Function

In the event of end organ injury [renal, hepatic, central nervous system (CNS), gastrointestinal dysfunction], appropriate organ protection measures has to be instituted.

Treatment of Residual Defects

Residual lesions can sometimes complicate postoperative recovery after cardiac surgery by leading to low CO states. Some of the residual lesions that are identified in the postoperative period include VSDs, outflow tract obstructions, PA stenosis, aortopulmonary collaterals, significant AV valve regurgitation, etc. Focused echocardiography should be performed to rule out significant lesions, which might require reinterventions or pharmacological manipulations.

Besides the above strategies, post-operative complications like pulmonary artery hypertension or arrhythmias need to be addressed by specific pharmacological interventions to facilitate optimal outcomes.

■ SUMMARY

The LCOS often complicates postoperative course after congenital heart surgery. A proactive approach and anticipatory care targeted toward expected complications will be beneficial. In the absence of well-validated tools to measure CO in infants and children, clinical indicators and hemodynamic variables, remain the best diagnostic modalities. A systematic approach to identification of the cause and targeted therapy will help to optimize CO in most clinical settings. Pharmacological agents and other supportive strategies should be judiciously used for the best perioperative outcomes.

■ REFERENCES

1. Du X, Chen H, Song X, Wang S, Hao Z, Yin L, et al. Risk factors for low cardiac output syndrome in children with congenital heart disease undergoing cardiac surgery: A retrospective cohort study. BMC Pediatr. 2020;20:87.
2. Wernovsky G, Wypij D, Jonas RA, Mayer JE Jr, Hanley FL, Hickey PR, et al. Postoperative course and hemodynamic profile after the arterial switch operation in neonates and infants. A comparison of low flow cardiopulmonary bypass and circulatory arrest. Circulation. 1995;92:2226-35.
3. Robert SM, Borasino S, Dabal RJ, Cleveland DC, Hock KM, Alten JA. Postoperative hydrocortisone reduces the prevalence of low

cardiac output syndrome after neonatal cardio-pulmonary bypass. Pediatr Crit Care Med. 2015;16:629-36.

4. Wessel DL. Managing low cardiac output syndrome after congenital heart surgery. Crit Care Med. 2001;29:S220-30.

5. Hoffman TM, Wernovsky G, Atz AM, Kulik TJ, Nelson DP, Chang AC, et al. Efficacy and safety of milrinone in preventing low flow cardiopulmonary bypass and circulatory arrest. Circulation. 2003;107:996-1002.

6. Brandfonbrener M, Landowne M, Shock NW. Changes in cardiac output with age. Circulation. 1955;12:557-66.

7. Sproul A, Simpson E. Stroke volume and related hemodynamic data in normal children. Pediatrics. 1964;33:912-8.

8. Krovetz LJ, McLoughlin TG, Mitchell MB, Schebler GL. Hemodynamic findings in normal children. Pediat Res. 1967;1:122-30.

9. Murni IK, Djer MM, Yanuarso PB, Putra ST, Advani N, Rachmat J, et al. Outcome of pediatric cardiac surgery and predictors of major complications in a developing country. Ann Pediatr Card. 2019;12:38-44.

10. Gaies MG, Gurney JG, Yen AH, Napoli ML, Gajarski RJ, Ohye RG, et al. Vasoactive-inotropic score as a predictor of morbidity and mortality in infants after cardiopulmonary bypass. Pediatr Crit Care Med. 2010;11:234-8.

11. Roth SJ. Postoperative care. In: Chang AC, Hanley FL, Wernovsky G, Wessel DL (Eds). Pediatric Cardiac Intensive Care. Philadelphia: Lippincott Williams & Wilkins; 1998. pp. 151-87.

12. Heitmiller EH, Wetzel RC. Hemodynamic monitoring considerations in pediatric critical care. In: Rogers MC, Nichols DG (Eds). Textbook of Pediatric Intensive Care, 3rd edition. Baltimore: Williams & Wilkins; 1996. pp. 607-41.

13. Tweddell JS, Ghanayem NS, Mussatto KA, Mitchell ME, Lamers LJ, Musa NL, et al. Mixed venous oxygen saturation monitoring after stage one palliation for hypoplastic left heart syndrome. Ann Thorac Surg. 2007;84:1301-11.

14. Ulate K, Yanay O, Jeffries H, Baden H, Di Gennaro JL, Zimmerman J. An elevated low cardiac output syndrome score is associated with morbidity in infants after congenital heart surgery. Pediatr Crit Care Med. 2017;18:26-33.

15. Vlasselaers D, Milants I, Desmet L, Wouters PJ, Vanhorebeek I, van den Heuvel I, et al. Intensive insulin therapy for patients in pediatric intensive care: a prospective randomized controlled study. Lancet. 2009;373:547-56.

16. Agus MS, Steil GM, Wypij D, Costello JM, Laussen PC, Langer M, et al. Tight glycemic control versus standard care after pediatric cardiac surgery. N Engl J Med. 2012;367:1208-19.

17. Macrae D, Grieve R, Allen E, Sadique Z, Morris K, Pappachan J, et al. A randomized trial of hyperglycemic control in pediatric cardiac intensive care. N Engl J Med. 2014;370:107-18.

18. Shekerdemian L. Perioperative manipulation of the circulation in children with congenital heart disease. Heart. 2009;95:1286-96.

19. Chandler HK, Kirsch R. Management of low cardiac output syndrome following surgery for congenital heart disease. Curr Cardiol Rev. 2016;12:107-11.

20. Girardin E, Berner M, Rouge JC, Rivest RW, Friedli B, Paunier L. Effect of low dose dopamine on hemodynamic and renal function in children. Pediatr Res. 1989;26:200-3.

21. Schenarts PJ, Sagraves SG, Bard MR, Toschlog EA, Goettler CE, Newell MA, et al. Low dose dopamine: a physiologically based review. Curr Surg. 2006;63:219-25.

22. Brunner AC, Hug MI, Dave H, Baenziger O, Buerki C, Bettex D, et al. Prevention of low cardiac output syndrome after pediatric cardiac surgery: a double blind randomised clinical pilot study comparing dobutamine and milrinone. Pediatr Crit Care Med. 2018;19(7):619-25.

23. Choudhary M, Hote MP. Levosimendan in pediatric cardiac surgery. An evidence based review. J Pharmacol Clin Res. 2016;1:1-4.

24. Singh VK, Sharma R, Varma A. Vasopressin in the pediatric cardiac intensive care unit: myth or reality. Ann Pediatr Cardiol. 2009;2:65-73.

25. Zhongyuan L, Xu W, Juxian Y, Shoujun L, Jun Y. Vasopressin in vasodilatory shock for both left and right heart anomalous pediatric patients after cardiac surgery. Shock. 2018;50:173-7.

26. Guzetta NA. Phenoxybenzamine in the treatment of hypoplastic left heart syndrome. A core review. Anaesth Analg. 2007;105:312-5.

27. Riahi M, Tomatis LA, Schlosser RJ, Bertolozzi E, Johnston DW. Cardiac compression due to closure of the median sternotomy in open heart surgery. Chest. 1975;67:113-4.

28. Riphagen S, McDougall M, Tibby SM, Alphonso N, Anderson D, Austin C, et al. Early delayed sternal closure following pediatric cardiac surgery. Ann Thorac Surg. 2005;80:678-85.

Arrhythmias in Pediatric Cardiac Intensive Care Unit

Mani Ram Krishna

Reviewed by: R Krishna Kumar

■ INTRODUCTION

The incidence of arrhythmias in a child with congenital heart disease (CHD) is highest in the early postoperative period while they are still in the postoperative intensive care unit (ICU). It is estimated that more than 70% of infants and children who undergo cardiac surgery will experience an abnormal rhythm in the first 24 hours after surgery although benign atrial and ventricular extra-systoles constitute a majority of these episodes.[1] However, approximately 15% of these arrhythmias can be hemodynamically detrimental.[2] This is attributed to a number of factors including myocardial injury secondary to cardiopulmonary bypass (CPB), suture lines in the atrium, hypoxia, increased catecholamine levels (both intrinsic and extrinsic), electrolyte abnormalities and presence of central venous lines.[3,4] Extra-systoles are usually benign. They do not require any treatment beyond correction of any existing electrolyte abnormality. Both tachyarrhythmias and bradyarrhythmias occur in the postoperative period. The most common hemodynamically significant bradyarrhythmia is complete heart block (CHB) while the most common tachyarrhythmia is junctional ectopic tachycardia (JET). Early recognition of the arrhythmia and appropriate management helps in reducing morbidity as well as mortality. In this chapter, we discuss the common arrhythmias in the postoperative period and present the management protocol in our ICU.

■ ELECTROCARDIOGRAM

The electrocardiogram (ECG) remains the only investigation necessary to diagnose arrhythmias in the ICU. Identification of atrial (P wave) and ventricular (QRS) activities is the first step in identifying the specific rhythm abnormality. However, this can be a challenge in the immediate postoperative period because of high heart rates and prolongation in atrioventricular (AV) conduction secondary to myocardial edema or injury. Most surgeons place temporary atrial and/or ventricular pacing wires after CPB. These can be utilized to obtain an atrial electrogram (A-wire study) which conclusively identify atrial activity when there is uncertainty. When the technology is available, this can be obtained by using a separate amplifier channel which records the atrial activity on the same paper as the surface ECG. Alternatively, they can be obtained by connecting the atrial electrode to the left arm. This ensures a pure surface lead II with atrial deflections in leads I and III. In our unit, we connect the atrial electrode to the right arm ensuring a surface ECG in lead III and atrial deflections in leads I and II **(Figs. 1A and B)**. This allows us to match the ventricular deflection with the surface lead and reliably establish AV relationships.

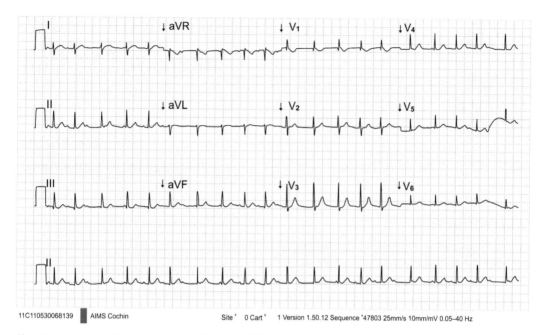

Fig. 1A: A standard 12-lead electrocardiogram (ECG) of a child who underwent cardiac surgery. There QRS complexes are irregular and there appears to be no consistent relationship between the P wave and QRS complexes. This suggests atrioventricular (AV) dissociation.

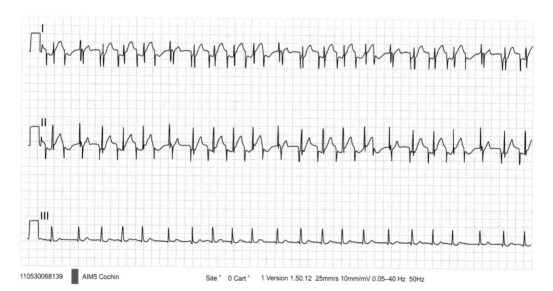

Fig. 1B: A unipolar atrial electrogram of the same patient demonstrating AV dissociation. A unipolar atrial electrogram ensures retention of a surface electrogram in one of the leads (Lead III in this case). This makes differentiation of atrial and ventricular activity easier in the other leads.

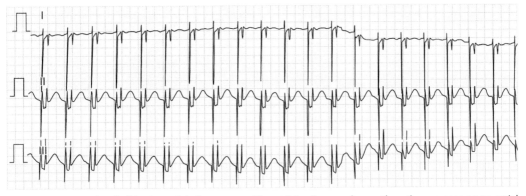

Fig. 1C: An example of a bipolar atrial electrogram. The atrial spikes are larger than they appear on an atrial electrogram. However, the absence of a surface ECG makes differentiation of atrial and ventricular activities difficult in some cases.

When two atrial pacing wires are available, both unipolar and bipolar atrial tracings can be obtained. Unipolar leads will have smaller atrial tracings but will allow simultaneous surface lead recording **(Fig. 1B)**. Bipolar leads meanwhile provide larger atrial deflections but will not permit simultaneous surface recordings, which make it difficult to establish AV relationship **(Fig. 1C)**. Atrial wires help in differentiating JET from sinus tachycardia. The atrial deflection has a consistent relationship with the QRS interval, and the R-P interval is longer than the P-R interval. In JET, there is either no consistent AV relationship (AV dissociation) or a short R-P interval.[5]

BASIC PRINCIPLES OF IDENTI-FICATION OF ARRHYTHMIA IN THE PEDIATRIC CARDIAC ICU

- A baseline 12-lead ECG should be mandatory for all children undergoing surgery with CPB. This should be performed as soon as the handover is completed, and the bedside nurse has checked on the infusions and ventilatory settings. This serves as a baseline study. Changes in the atrial axis or QRS morphology when compared to the baseline will enable accurate diagnosis of the arrhythmia.

- Whenever an arrhythmia is suspected, it is important to get an ECG. The ECG on the cardiac monitor is not standardized and errors may occur if treatment is based on the monitor **(Figs. 2A and B)**.
- All postoperative electrocardiograms should include a standard 12 lead or 6 lead as well as atrial wire recordings. This simplifies the process of interpretation.
- Whenever adenosine or any other therapy is attempted, it is important to document the response to therapy. This can provide useful diagnostic information.

BRADYARRHYTHMIA

The most common bradyarrhythmia in the postoperative period is sinus bradycardia. The causes include the use of sedation and hypothermia.[3] Sinus bradycardia is commonly noted after closure of large shunt lesions and may represent a physiological adaptation to improved systemic output. While sinus bradycardia rarely causes hemodynamic instability in older children, infants can augment their cardiac output only by a chronotropic response. Hence, when bradycardia is associated with some hemodynamic instability, temporary atrial pacing in the early postoperative period will

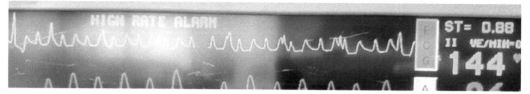

Fig. 2A: Screenshot from a cardiac monitor in a postoperative child. This was incorrectly interpreted as atrial flutter based on the tracings by a trained pediatric cardiac intensivist.

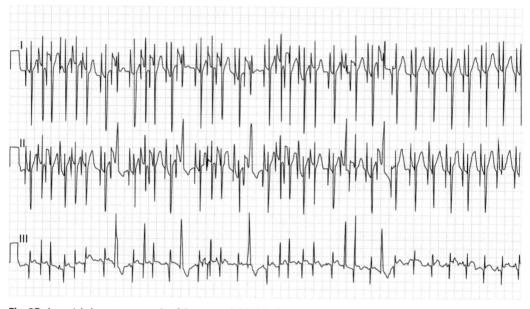

Fig. 2B: An atrial electrogram study of the same child. This demonstrates an irregular rhythm. A careful analysis of the atrial electrogram confirms premature atrial contractions (atrial ectopics) as the cause of the irregular rhythm.

aid in augmentation of cardiac output. Sinus node dysfunction occurs rarely after extensive surgery involving the atria (atrial baffling or correction of partial anomalous pulmonary venous drainage) and is managed using the same principles as CHB.

Complete Heart Block

Complete heart block as a postoperative complication has been recognized from the earliest days of congenital heart surgery.[6] The incidence of this complication has come down dramatically with improved surgical understanding of the AV nodal anatomy.

But even in contemporary surgical reviews, there remains a 1–3% risk of postoperative heart block.[7] The ECG shows evidence of AV dissociation with the atrial rate higher than the ventricular rate **(Fig. 3)**.

Complete heart block was believed to be secondary to an inflammatory reaction or surgical damage to conduction tissue in the vicinity of the AV node. It was presumed that inflammation would subside and result in recovery of conduction, while surgical damage necessitated pacemaker implantation. Recently, a genetic predisposition to CHB and a possible "two-hit" hypothesis has

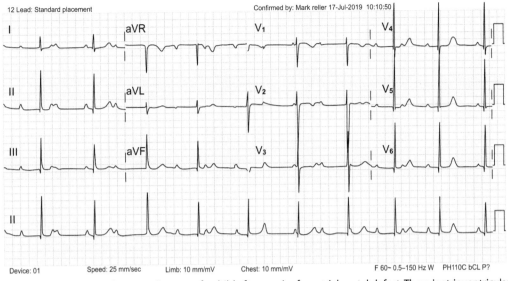

Fig. 3: A postoperative electrocardiogram of a child after repair of an atrial septal defect. There is atrioventricular dissociation with a low ventricular rate. The child developed postoperative congenital heart block.

been postulated.[8] Among 1,199 prospectively enrolled patients of a postoperative arrhythmia study, there were 56 incidences of CHB with 21 requiring pacemakers (1.7%). Certain genetic polymorphisms of the connexin-40 gene (which plays an important role in propagation of the action potential) were independently noted to confer a higher risk for development of postoperative heart block after congenital heart surgery. However, it is important to note that the study utilized a candidate gene approach and not a genome wide association approach which is considered appropriate while searching for genetic causes of a disease and the results should hence be interpreted with caution.

The perioperative risk factors for CHB include longer CPB and aortic cross-clamp times and the type of surgery [especially those involving closure of a ventricular septal defect (VSD)]. The retrospective analysis of the Pediatric Health Information System (PHIS) database which comprises 45 largest pediatric cardiac programs in the United States, identified 4,176 incidences of CHB among 101,006 surgeries with 990 permanent pacemaker (PPM) implantations (1% of all surgeries).[9] While the most common surgery requiring PPM implantation was VSD closure, the surgeries with the maximal risk of PPM implantation included the double switch operation (13.6%) and tricuspid as well as mitral valve replacements (approximately 8%). However, the PHIS was an administrative database and data recording was not adequately audited or according to stringent criteria.

A retrospective analysis was performed from the Pediatric Cardiac Critical Care Consortium (PC4) database of surgeries performed between 2014 and 2017. The PC4 database was specifically created as a quality improvement initiative. The data entry was performed by a certified data manager and rigorously audited. This hence represents the best quality of data available for a retrospective review. There were 15,901 surgeries during the study period with 422 (2.7%) instances of CHB of which 162 (1%) required a pacemaker. Among those who recovered, 50% recovered

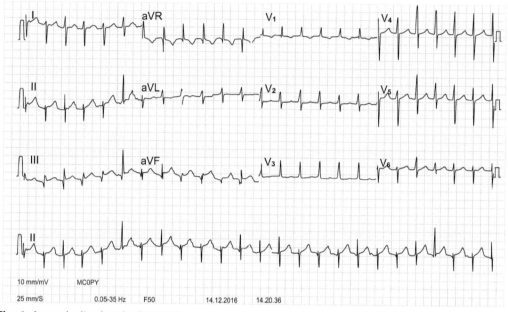

Fig. 4: A standardized 12-lead ECG of a postoperative neonate in complete heart block. There is a narrow QRS escape rhythm with a heart rate of 140 per minute suggesting an accelerated junctional rhythm. Normal atrioventricular conduction was restored by 24 hours.

by 2 days (Median recovery time – 1.9 days) and 94% by 10 days.[7] The risk factors included longer bypass time and higher surgical risk category. This is the most contemporary evidence on CHB after congenital heart surgery and suggests that the conduction recovers in two-thirds of children with postoperative CHB in approximately 10 days and the risk of PPM implementation in a contemporary cohort is 1%. The findings interestingly mirror a single center retrospective review from two decades earlier.[10]

One factor which predicts recovery of AV conduction is the presence of an accelerated junctional rhythm (AJR).[8,11] When invasive electrophysiological studies were performed on 14 children with postoperative CHB, it was recognized that 60% of those with a supra-Hisian block recovered while only 16% of those with a block at a lower level recovered.[12] A narrow complex escape rhythm at a rate higher than the normal heart rate for age (i.e., AJR) represents a supra-Hisian block (**Fig. 4**). It is speculated that the preserved automaticity of the proximal His bundle as well as its chronotropic response to the elevated catecholamines represents less severe damage to the conduction system. The presence of intermittent AV conduction in the early postoperative stage also favors recovery. In fact, the combination of intermittent AV conduction and AJR was found to have a positive predictive value of 86% for recovery in one study.[8]

Late recovery after pacemaker implantation is less common. Reports suggest that late recovery can occur in 9–30% of cases[13,14] with recovery reported as late as 20 years after surgery. However, no particular factor was shown to predict late recovery. Of greater concern, is the occurrence of late CHB after initial recovery and discharge from hospital. This could potentially result in syncope or even sudden death. When a cohort of patients operated for tetralogy of Fallot (TOF) were followed over a mean period of 28 years, transient postoperative CHB was noticed to have a strong association with sudden unexpected death.[15] When children with transient postoperative CHB were followed over a 9 year period, CHB recurred in 15% (7/44). Late recovery of CHB more than 7 days after surgery was shown to increase the risk of recurrence 13-fold.[16]

All patients with CHB should undergo synchronized AV pacing through temporary epicardial leads in the early postoperative period to ensure optimal cardiac output. There is no evidence to support anti-inflammatory therapy for postoperative CHB.[17] Recent guidelines recommend implantation of a PPM if AV block persists beyond the 7th postoperative day as a class I recommendation.[18] Current evidence suggests that it is reasonable to wait till 10 days to look for recovery. Indeed, even in the West, only two-thirds of pacemaker implantations happen by the 10th postoperative day.[7] The choice of pacemaker is usually determined by the anatomy and ventricular function. In a completely corrected heart with normal ventricular contractility, a single chamber ventricular pacemaker will be adequate to meet the cardiac output demands.[17] However, in children with functional single ventricle and in those with more than mild ventricular dysfunction, maintenance of AV synchrony and the additional filling volume provided by atrial systole becomes paramount and this subset will require dual chamber (atrial and ventricular) pacemakers.[19]

Amrita Institute of Medical Sciences (AIMS) Protocol for Management of CHB

- A baseline ECG (including atrial wire recordings) is obtained to confirm diagnosis.
- AV sequential pacing is initiated at a rate of 100–140/minute and a paced AV delay of 150 ms.

- An ECG without pacing is obtained every morning before the combined cardiac rounds to confirm the rhythm.
- Pacing is discontinued when spontaneous AV conduction returns, and the sinus rate is normal [atrial pacing (AAI) is utilized for sinus bradycardia].
- PPM implantation is recommended if there is no return of spontaneous rhythm in 7 days (with a broad complex escape rhythm or escape rate is <100/minute) or in 10 days (with a narrow complex escape rhythm and an escape rate of >100/minute).
- A dual chamber pacemaker is preferred in children undergoing staged single ventricle palliation or in the presence of severe left ventricular systolic dysfunction. In all other children, a single chamber pacemaker (VVI) is implanted.
- We do not use corticosteroids or other immunosuppressive therapy routinely for postoperative CHB.

◼ TACHYARRHYTHMIA

Sinus tachycardia is common in the postoperative ICU. It could potentially be due to a number of causes including fever, pain, low cardiac output, inotrope therapy and a systemic immune response.[3] It subsides with treatment of the underlying cause and drug therapy is seldom required. As discussed earlier, JET is the most common hemodynamically important tachyarrhythmia in the postoperative period.

Junctional Ectopic Tachycardia

The incidence of this arrhythmia in contemporary surgical series has been reported to be around 15%.[20] In the past, postoperative JET was thought to be due to injury or edema in the region of the AV node. However, it is now thought that JET is a result of ischemia-reperfusion injury of the conduction tissue which is exacerbated by inotrope use.[20,21] Alterations in action potential timings have been demonstrated in the AV node in response to ischemia-reperfusion on cellular lines tested in the laboratory. JET has been shown to occur even during surgeries not involving VSD closure[20] and a greater troponin levels have been reported in children with postoperative JET suggesting a role for ischemia.[22] Although a self-limiting arrhythmia, JET can result in significant hemodynamic instability. JET is defined as a narrow complex tachycardia with a heart rate greater than 170/minute and either AV dissociation **(Fig. 5A)** or 1:1 ventriculo-atrial (V-A) conduction **(Fig. 5B)**. The differentiation from sinus tachycardia may be difficult at high heart rates as the P wave may not be readily seen. The use of atrial wire ECG helps in the recognition of atrial activity and confirmation of the diagnosis. JET is an automatic tachycardia arising from the bundle of His. Animal studies have documented an important role for the funny current channels (involved in sinus node depolarization) in the genesis of junctional tachycardia.[23] The increased heart rate and resultant decreased diastolic filling in addition to the loss of AV synchrony results in hemodynamic instability.

A number of pre and perioperative factors have been reported to increase the risk of postoperative JET.[2,20,22] Younger age, long CPB time, repair of conotruncal defects and increased inotrope use in the immediate postoperative period have been associated with an increased incidence of JET. Among the individual drugs, dopamine and milrinone have the highest association with postoperative JET. Milrinone which is commonly used for prevention of a low cardiac output state has been shown to be associated with a 3-fold risk for tachyarrhythmias.[24] The phosphodiesterase inhibitory action of milrinone results in increased intracellular calcium and this is believed to increase the risk of tachyarrhythmias. A possible genetic predisposition to JET has also been proposed with a particular polymorphism in the angiotensin-converting enzyme (ACE) implicated. Indeed, some studies have shown

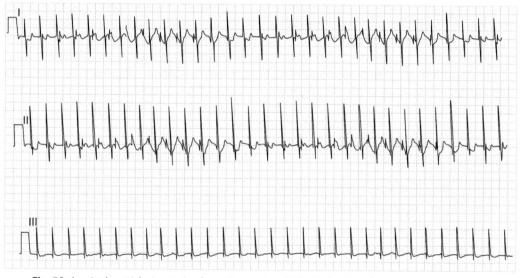

Fig. 5A: A unipolar atrial wire study of a postoperative child with junctional ectopic tachycardia with atrioventricular dissociation.

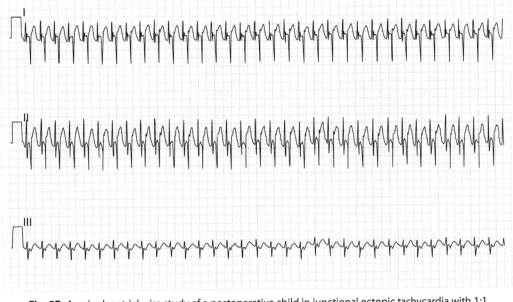

Fig. 5B: A unipolar atrial wire study of a postoperative child in junctional ectopic tachycardia with 1:1 ventriculoatrial conduction.

a protective effect of postoperative ACE inhibitor use against tachyarrhythmias, but this warrants further study.

A number of perioperative factors have been shown to reduce the incidence of JET. Addition of magnesium to the CPB circuit has been shown to reduce the incidence of JET in one study.[25] The effect was shown to be dose-dependent and was not related to preoperative hypomagnesemia. However, this effect was not shown by other investigators. Dexmedetomidine is a centrally acting sedative which is being used more commonly. It has been shown to have vagal stimulatory and sympatholytic activity through its action on central imidazoline and alpha-2 receptors, respectively. The use of dexmedetomidine in the early postoperative period has been shown to reduce the incidence of JET.[26]

The conventional treatment of JET includes cooling, correction of electrolyte abnormalities, moderation of inotrope therapy and pain relief.[21] These serve to reduce the adrenergic stimulus to the heart and help control the arrhythmia. Despite early initiation of therapy, nonpharmacological management is successful in only a minority of patients.[27] The most widely used drug in the postoperative period is amiodarone. The approach reported by Haas et al. with repeated boluses to achieve a response followed by an infusion to maintain rate or rhythm control (popularly dubbed as the Brisbane protocol) is widely used.[28] The protocol is described in **Flowchart 1**. The major concern with amiodarone use in the postoperative patient is its propensity to cause hypotension. With our recent understanding of the molecular origin of JET, ivabradine a selective inhibitor of the funny channels has emerged as a possible candidate drug in JET. We have used ivabradine for postoperative JET in a small number of patients with reasonable success.[29] Ivabradine is hemodynamically neutral and has been shown to be safe. However, it is available only as an oral preparation and this

Flowchart. 1: The protocol for use of amiodarone in postoperative junctional ectopic tachycardia.

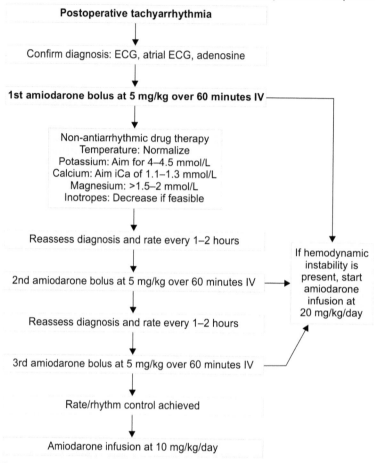

Source: Adapted from Haas NA, Plumpton K, Justo R, Jalali H, Pohlner P. Postoperative junctional ectopic tachycardia (JET). Z Kardiol. 2004;93(5):371-80.[28]

might limit its utility in a subset of patient who are not fed orally and those with poor enteric absorption. Despite early initiation of treatment, a small number of patients do not respond to nonpharmacological therapy or antiarrhythmic therapy. Initiation of extracorporeal support has been shown to be lifesaving in this subset of patients.[30]

The AIMS Protocol for Treatment of JET

- The diagnosis is confirmed by obtaining a standard ECG and atrial wire recordings.

- Blood samples are sent for blood gas analysis as well as serum electrolyte levels (potassium, calcium and magnesium).
- Nonpharmacological therapy is initiated including cooling to 35°C (if feasible and appropriate) and correction of electrolyte abnormalities.
- Attempts are made to rationalize inotrope therapy. In particular, adrenaline and dopamine are tapered to the lowest possible dose and consideration is given toward switching milrinone to levosimendan.

- If the rhythm continues to be JET, pharmacological therapy is instituted. Our preferred drug was amiodarone. However, recently ivabradine has emerged as the first-line pharmacological agent unless contraindications exist.
- When the ventricular rate falls below 140/minute, overdrive atrial pacing (AAI) at a rate of 140/minute is started to provide AV synchrony.

Ivabradine Dosage in Postoperative JET

The dose range of ivabradine is 0.05–0.15 mg/kg twice daily. Our protocol for ivabradine use in postoperative JET has been as follows:

- A first dose of ivabradine at 0.05 mg/kg is administered through the nasogastric tube.
- If there is no response at the end of 2 hours, an additional dose of ivabradine at 0.05 mg/kg is administered through the nasogastric tube.
- If there is response to therapy, then ivabradine is continued at a dose of 0.05 mg/kg twice daily for 2 days (4 doses).

Other Tachyarrhythmias

Other supraventricular tachyarrhythmias to occur in the postoperative period include paroxysmal supraventricular tachycardia (SVT), atrial flutter and atrial fibrillation. When the diagnosis is unclear, atrial electrograms can be obtained or adenosine administered to understand the mechanism of tachyarrhythmia better. Most SVT in the pediatric cardiac surgical ICU have an underlying accessory pathway. In particular, children with Ebstein anomaly and congenitally corrected transposition of great arteries have underlying accessory pathways and are at a higher risk for SVT and adenosine can be used therapeutically to terminate the arrhythmia. Atrial flutter and fibrillation can be converted to sinus rhythm by direct current (DC) cardioversion. Atrial fibrillation, especially in adults with CHD, who have large, scarred atria has a high recurrence rate and frequently requires antiarrhythmic therapy to maintain sinus rhythm. The risk of atrial fibrillation is maximum in older patients and those with pulmonary hypertension.[31] Amiodarone is the most frequently used antiarrhythmic agent.

Ventricular tachycardia (VT) is a rare arrhythmia in the postoperative period. Its incidence is believed to be less than 5%[2] although transient ventricular arrhythmias not requiring treatment may be more common.[32] The risk factors include longer CPB time and more complex cardiac surgeries. VT requiring treatment has been shown to be associated with an increased risk of in-hospital mortality.[32] They frequently cause hemodynamic instability and will need to be addressed rapidly. Regular broad complex tachyarrhythmias with hemodynamic instability are best treated by synchronized cardioversion with 0.5–1 Joule per kg. Amiodarone is a reasonable pharmacological alternative. Polymorphic ventricular tachycardia and Torsades de pointes (TdP) can occur in the early postoperative period due to a combination of electrolyte abnormalities and drugs resulting in QTc prolongation. This can be treated with intravenous magnesium at a dose of 25 mg/kg as an infusion over 10 minutes. Children who develop VT in the postoperative period may be at an increased risk for recurrence and should be subjected to a detailed evaluation before discharge from hospital.

■ REFERENCES

1. Grosse-Wortmann L, Kreitz S, Grabitz RG, Vazquez-Jimenez JF, Messmer BJ, von Bernuth G, et al. Prevalence of and risk factors for perioperative arrhythmias in neonates and children after

cardiopulmonary bypass: continuous holter monitoring before and for three days after surgery. J Cardiothorac Surg. 2010;5:85.

2. Delaney JW, Moltedo JM, Dziura JD, Kopf GS, Snyder CS. Early postoperative arrhythmias after pediatric cardiac surgery. J Thorac Cardiovasc Surg. 2006;131(6):1296-300.

3. Kabbani MS, Al Taweel H, Kabbani N, Al Ghamdi S. Critical arrhythmia in post-operative cardiac children: recognition and management. Avicenna J Med. 2017;7(3):88-95.

4. Valsangiacomo E, Schmid ER, Schupbach RW, Schmidlin D, Molinari L, Waldvogel K, et al. Early postoperative arrhythmias after cardiac operation in children. Ann Thorac Surg. 2002;74(3):792-6.

5. Batra AS, Balaji S. Post operative temporary epicardial pacing: when, how and why? Ann Pediatr Cardiol. 2008;1(2):120-5.

6. Lillehei CW, Sellers RD, Bonnabeau RC, Eliot RS. Chronic postsurgical complete heart block. With particular reference to prognosis, management, and a new P-wave pacemaker. J Thorac Cardiovasc Surg. 1963;46:436-56.

7. Romer AJ, Tabbutt S, Etheridge SP, Fischbach P, Ghanayem NS, Reddy VM, et al. Atrioventricular block after congenital heart surgery: analysis from the Pediatric Cardiac Critical Care Consortium. J Thorac Cardiovasc Surg. 2019;157(3):1168-77 e2.

8. Murray LE, Smith AH, Flack EC, Crum K, Owen J, Kannankeril PJ. Genotypic and phenotypic predictors of complete heart block and recovery of conduction after surgical repair of congenital heart disease. Heart Rhythm. 2017;14(3):402-9.

9. Liberman L, Silver ES, Chai PJ, Anderson BR. Incidence and characteristics of heart block after heart surgery in pediatric patients: a multicenter study. J Thorac Cardiovasc Surg. 2016;152(1):197-202.

10. Weindling SN, Saul JP, Gamble WJ, Mayer JE, Wessel D, Walsh EP. Duration of complete atrioventricular block after congenital heart disease surgery. Am J Cardiol. 1998;82(4):525-7.

11. Paech C, Dahnert I, Kostelka M, Mende M, Gebauer R. Association of temporary complete AV block and junctional ectopic tachycardia after surgery for congenital heart disease. Ann Pediatr Cardiol. 2015;8(1):14-9.

12. Driscoll DJ, Gillette PC, Hallman GL, Cooley DA, McNamara DG. Management of surgical complete atrioventricular block in children. Am J Cardiol. 1979;43(6):1175-80.

13. Batra AS, Wells WJ, Hinoki KW, Stanton RA, Silka MJ. Late recovery of atrioventricular conduction after pacemaker implantation for complete heart block associated with surgery for congenital heart disease. J Thorac Cardiovasc Surg. 2003;125(6):1291-3.

14. Bruckheimer E, Berul CI, Kopf GS, Hill SL, Warner KA, Kleinman CS, et al. Late recovery of surgically-induced atrioventricular block in patients with congenital heart disease. J Interv Card Electrophysiol. 2002;6(2):191-5.

15. Hokanson JS, Moller JH. Significance of early transient complete heart block as a predictor of sudden death late after operative correction of tetralogy of Fallot. Am J Cardiol. 2001;87(11):1271-7.

16. Aziz PF, Serwer GA, Bradley DJ, LaPage MJ, Hirsch JC, Bove EL, et al. Pattern of recovery for transient complete heart block after open heart surgery for congenital heart disease: duration alone predicts risk of late complete heart block. Pediatr Cardiol. 2013;34(4):999-1005.

17. Garcia RU, Safa R, Karpawich PP. Postoperative complete heart block among congenital heart disease patients: contributing risk factors, therapies and long-term sequelae in the current era. Prog Pediatr Cardiol. 2018;49:66-70.

18. Epstein AE, DiMarco JP, Ellenbogen KA, Estes NA, 3rd, Freedman RA, Gettes LS, et al. 2012 ACCF/AHA/HRS focused update incorporated into the ACCF/AHA/HRS 2008 guidelines for device-based therapy of cardiac rhythm abnormalities: a report of the American College of Cardiology Foundation/American Heart Association Task Force on Practice Guidelines and the Heart Rhythm Society. J Am Coll Cardiol. 2013;61(3):e6-75.

19. Bulic A, Zimmerman FJ, Ceresnak SR, Shetty I, Motonaga KS, Freter A, et al. Ventricular pacing in single ventricles–a bad combination. Heart Rhythm. 2017;14(6):853-7.

20. Moak JP, Arias P, Kaltman JR, Cheng Y, McCarter R, Hanumanthaiah S, et al. Post-operative junctional ectopic tachycardia: risk factors for occurrence in the modern surgical era. Pacing Clin Electrophysiol. 2013;36(9):1156-68.

21. Tharakan JA, Sukulal K. Postcardiac surgery junctional ectopic tachycardia: a 'Hit and Run' tachyarrhythmia as yet unchecked. Ann Pediatr Cardiol. 2014;7(1):25-8.

22. Mildh L, Hiippala A, Rautiainen P, Pettila V, Sairanen H, Happonen JM. Junctional ectopic tachycardia after surgery for congenital heart

disease: incidence, risk factors and outcome. Eur J Cardiothorac Surg. 2011;39(1):75-80.

23. Dobrzynski H, Nikolski VP, Sambelashvili AT, Greener ID, Yamamoto M, Boyett MR, et al. Site of origin and molecular substrate of atrioventricular junctional rhythm in the rabbit heart. Circ Res. 2003;93(11):1102-10.

24. Smith AH, Owen J, Borgman KY, Fish FA, Kannankeril PJ. Relation of milrinone after surgery for congenital heart disease to significant postoperative tachyarrhythmias. Am J Cardiol. 2011;108(11):1620-4.

25. Manrique AM, Arroyo M, Lin Y, El Khoudary SR, Colvin E, Lichtenstein S, et al. Magnesium supplementation during cardiopulmonary bypass to prevent junctional ectopic tachycardia after pediatric cardiac surgery: a randomized controlled study. J Thorac Cardiovasc Surg. 2010;139(1):162-9 e2.

26. Chrysostomou C, Sanchez-de-Toledo J, Wearden P, Jooste EH, Lichtenstein SE, Callahan PM, et al. Perioperative use of dexmedetomidine is associated with decreased incidence of ventricular and supraventricular tachyarrhythmias after congenital cardiac operations. Ann Thorac Surg. 2011;92(3):964-72.

27. Walsh EP, Saul JP, Sholler GF, Triedman JK, Jonas RA, Mayer JE, et al. Evaluation of a staged treatment protocol for rapid automatic junctional tachycardia after operation for congenital heart disease. J Am Coll Cardiol. 1997;29(5):1046-53.

28. Haas NA, Plumpton K, Justo R, Jalali H, Pohlner P. Postoperative junctional ectopic tachycardia (JET). Z Kardiol. 2004;93(5):371-80.

29. Krishna MR, Kunde MF, Kumar RK, Balaji S. Ivabradine in post-operative junctional ectopic tachycardia (JET): breaking new ground. Pediatr Cardiol. 2019;40(6):1284-88.

30. Cools E, Missant C. Junctional ectopic tachycardia after congenital heart surgery. Acta Anaesthesiol Belg. 2014;65(1):1-8.

31. Brock MA, Coppola JA, Reid J, Moguillansky D. Atrial fibrillation in adults with congenital heart disease following cardiac surgery in a single center: analysis of incidence and risk factors. Congenit Heart Dis. 2019;14(6):924-30.

32. Fuchs SR, Smith AH, Van Driest SL, Crum KF, Edwards TL, Kannankeril PJ. Incidence and effect of early postoperative ventricular arrhythmias after congenital heart surgery. Heart Rhythm. 2019;16(5):710-6.

Pulmonary Hypertension in the Postoperative Period

R Krishna Kumar

■ BACKGROUND

Pulmonary hypertension is a feared complication of surgery for certain forms of congenital heart disease (CHD). In the early postoperative period, this complication may become sufficiently severe to be labeled as a crisis that has the potential of becoming life-threatening.[1] This brief chapter will discuss the definitions, predispositions, pathophysiology, and diagnosis of pulmonary hypertension and pulmonary hypertensive (PH) crisis in the postoperative period after congenital heart surgery.

■ DEFINITIONS

Pulmonary hypertension: The most consistently accepted definition of pulmonary hypertension in the intensive care unit (ICU) setting is mean pulmonary artery (PA) pressure greater than 25 mm Hg. However, the mean PA pressure is only obtained by a monitoring line or catheter placed in the PA. In situations where only, echocardiographic estimation of PA pressure is feasible, pulmonary hypertension may be defined as estimated PA systolic pressure of more than ½ systemic systolic pressure.[1] In the postoperative period, PA pressures should always be viewed in the context of systemic arterial pressures. Mild pulmonary hypertension (PA mean < 30 mm Hg or ≤½ systemic mean pressures) is commonly encountered in the postoperative period after CHD surgery and does not require specific treatment. Higher PA pressures merit concern

and PA pressures >¾ systemic often require prompt treatment.

Pulmonary hypertensive crisis: The definition of PH crisis has been somewhat arbitrary. Episodes where pulmonary/systemic artery pressure ratio rises to more than 0.75 are labeled as PH crisis.[2,3] Episodes are classified as major PH crisis if there is an associated fall in the systemic artery pressure of at least 20% or a fall in transcutaneous oxygen saturation to <90% or both. Episodes are labeled as minor if the systemic artery pressure and oxygen saturation remain stable.

■ POPULATION AT RISK

The occurrence of PH crisis in the postoperative period can often be anticipated if one is aware of the population at risk. If PH crisis is anticipated before the operation it is valuable to place an indwelling PA line at the time of operation. The following situations predispose to the development of PH crisis in children after congenital heart surgery and are described here.

Conditions

Left to right shunts: If heart surgery is undertaken when early pulmonary vascular obstructive disease has set in PH crisis can be expected. It is often possible to suspect occurrence of early pulmonary vascular disease. The clues to the development of early pulmonary vascular disease in children with large left to right shunts include:

- Absence of obvious clinical or noninvasive evidence of a large left to right shunt
- If a cardiac catheterization is undertaken and pulmonary vascular resistance index (PVRI) measures more than 3.5 wood units.m^2.

The common left to right shunts where PH crisis can occur include: large or unrestrictive ventricular septal defects (VSD) with some elevation in PVRI. Aortopulmonary windows and origin of one PA from the aorta are also associated with some elevation in PVRI and consequently PH crisis can be expected after surgery. Secundum atrial septal defects (ASD) do not usually have elevation in pulmonary vascular resistance (PVR) early in life. However, PH crisis is known to occur after surgery for certain forms of primum ASD especially if associated with a relatively small left ventricle (LV) size (the unbalanced form of primum ASD) or if associated with Down syndrome.

Common atrioventricular (AV) septal defects have a rapid progression of pulmonary vascular changes, particularly if associated with Down syndrome and PH crisis is not uncommon if operation is performed after the age of 6 months.

Admixture lesions with increased pulmonary blood flow: Here the pulmonary vascular disease occurs much earlier than in left to right shunts because these conditions have considerable pulmonary blood flows. The most rapid progression to pulmonary vascular obstructive disease occurs in transposition with VSD or a large patent ductus and persistent truncus arteriosus. Rapid progression can also be expected in patients with total anomalous pulmonary venous connection (TAPVC) even if the venous return is unobstructed and, lesions with single ventricle physiology and unprotected pulmonary blood flow. In these conditions PH crisis can be expected in the postoperative period particularly if beyond the first 3 or 4 months of life.

Pulmonary venous obstruction: Obstruction to pulmonary venous return results in a markedly increased PVR. The pulmonary arteries of these patients are extremely reactive because of marked arteriolar smooth muscle hypertrophy and hyperplasia. These patients are particularly prone to PH crisis and PA lines should be considered at the time of surgical repair. Examples of conditions associated with pulmonary venous obstruction include: obstructed TAPVC, VSD with congenital mitral stenosis, cor triatriatum and, pulmonary vein stenosis.

Newborns: Newborns have a greater tendency for development of PH crisis after surgery because pulmonary arterioles accompanying the terminal bronchiole have a relatively higher smooth muscle content in their vessel wall. This normally regresses over the next few months.

Associated pulmonary disease: Associated congenital lung conditions such as lung hypoplasia can markedly reduce the number of small peripheral pulmonary arteries. This makes them prone to pulmonary hypertension. Parenchymal lung disease increases the propensity toward PH crisis through a variety of mechanisms that include impaired gas exchange.

Associated conditions and upper airway obstruction: Down syndrome appears to increase the rate of progression of pulmonary vascular disease. This is, in part, related to upper airway obstruction and hypoventilation with hypoxia and hypercarbia. Other conditions known to be associated with upper airway obstruction include laryngotracheomalacia, subglottic stenosis secondary to congenital causes or trauma during endotracheal intubation, Pierre-Robin syndrome and, post cleft palate repair.

■ PATHOPHYSIOLOGY

The occurrence of pulmonary hypertension in the postoperative period is as a result of combination of the following three fundamental changes:

1. *A substrate for intense pulmonary vasoconstriction*: This includes vessel wall changes in the pulmonary arterioles in high flow lesions. There is increase in the smooth muscle content and wall thickness of the pulmonary arterioles as well as an abnormal extension of muscle into the arterioles accompanying the distal respiratory bronchi and alveoli. There is also a relative paucity of the number of small vessels in the lung parenchyma. This is measurable as a reduction in alveolar to arterial ratio. At an ultrastructural level there is increase in the permeability of the endothelial cell with excessive proliferation of the extracellular matrix.

2. *Changes in the vascular endothelium after exposure to cardiopulmonary bypass (CPB)*: The endothelium is injured by exposure to CPB. The synthesis of endogenous nitric oxide (NO) is markedly diminished. The injured endothelium attracts platelets and this releases a variety of vasoconstrictors. As a result, the arteriole has a strong tendency to constrict. The progressive reduction in bypass duration and cross clamp time in recent years has possibly contributed to the reduced incidence of PH crisis after infant and newborn heart surgery.

3. *Postoperative triggers*: Common postoperative triggers for pulmonary vasoconstriction include sudden changes in airway pressures, airway stimulation from vigorous suctioning, lung parenchymal lesions and, excessive sympathetic drive. There are neuroendocrine bodies located in the smaller airways that release vasoconstrictors in response to stimulation.

■ MEASUREMENT OF PA PRESSURE IN ICU[3,4]

Indwelling pulmonary arterial lines: Most modern centers now place PA lines whenever there is an anticipated possibility of PH crisis developing in the postoperative period. Systolic, diastolic, and mean pressures are continuously displayed. Sources of error in recording include partial occlusion from clots or kinks in the line, distal placement in the PA wedge position, air-locks in the system and, errors in zeroing. Simultaneous systemic pressure should always be available. The PA pressure trends serve as useful indicators of progress after congenital heart surgery. PH crisis is typically anticipated to occur as the child awakens from the effects of anesthesia and paralysis, during suctioning of airways, during periods of rapid swings in airway pressure and, following withdrawal from NO. However, many episodes of PH crisis occur without warning in absence of any of the known precipitants. Apart from monitoring the PA pressures the PA line can be used for vasodilator infusion. Phenoxybenzamine can be administered directly via the PA line.

In recent times, the incidence of PH crisis has declined considerably even for patients with substrates for vasoconstriction, such as obstructed TAPVC in the newborn. As a result, many ICUs seldom use PA lines.

Echocardiography: In the event that PA pressure is not available (malfunction of the PA line or when PA lines have not been placed), indirect echocardiographic estimation of PA pressure is the best alternative. Doppler estimation of velocity of the tricuspid regurgitation (TR) jet is considered the most reliable of all the noninvasive estimates of PA pressure. The Doppler velocity of the TR

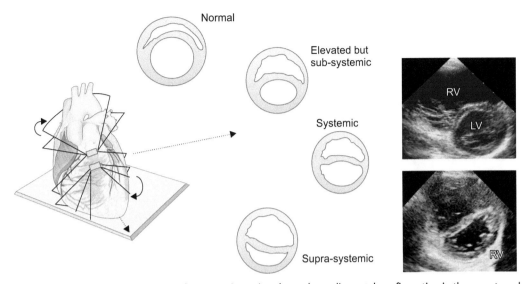

Fig. 1: Echo assessment of pulmonary hypertension using the end systolic septal configuration in the parasternal short axis views. Various septal configurations along with two representative echo images are shown here.

(LV: left ventricle; RV: right ventricle)

essentially measures the instantaneous peak systolic pressure difference between right ventricle (RV) and right atrium (RA). In the absence of a pressure gradient between RV and PA, the PA systolic pressure is assumed to be equal to the RV systolic pressure.

Unfortunately, TR may be absent altogether or not sufficient to generate a good quality signal. In such situations, the end systolic configuration of interventricular septum can help indirectly determine the RV systolic pressure in relation to the systemic pressure **(Fig. 1)**.

■ DIAGNOSIS OF PH CRISIS

As indicated under "definition" the term "PH crisis" is a somewhat arbitrary one and there are differences in thresholds for diagnosis. Whenever PH crisis is anticipated, close observation of the PA pressure trend is often mandated in the postoperative period. Progressive increases in PA pressures over a few hours should be viewed with seriousness. Treatment measures need to be instituted if PA pressures reach 75% of systemic pressures.

Once systemic pressures start to decline, it should be considered as an emergency and aggressive measures should be instituted to reduce PA pressures. Patients with intracardiac communications such as a patent foramen ovale or a fenestration of the VSD patch are likely to have a drop in the monitored oxygen saturation without a significant fall in systemic arterial pressures. Suspecting PH crisis when PA pressures are not monitored is difficult. However, episodes of hypotension and/or desaturation should be viewed with seriousness especially if the patients are potential candidates for episodes of PH crisis. Often an emergency echocardiogram performed during these episodes will reveal a high TR velocity or a septal configuration suggestive of elevated RV systolic pressures.

■ MANAGEMENT OF PULMONARY HYPERTENSION AND HYPERTENSIVE CRISIS

Measures to prevent episodes of PH crisis should be incorporated into routine postoperative care if there is a substrate for PH crisis. In addition, the likelihood of PH crisis can be anticipated if high PA pressures are recorded as the patient comes off CPB after complete correction of the heart defect.

Following operation for conditions such as obstructed TAPVC, PH crisis is almost inevitable if specific measures are not instituted. Measures to prevent PH crisis include the following:

- *Minimizing the influence of common triggers*: Use of deep sedation, analgesia and muscle relaxation
- Hyperventilation to induce mild respiratory alkalosis (PCO_2 <35 mm Hg, pH: 7.4–7.5, PaO_2 100–150 mm Hg)
- Cautious tracheal suction after preoxygenation, premedication with sedation or analgesic
- *Pulmonary vasodilators*: Phenoxybenzamine, inhaled NO and sildenafil as appropriate
- Delayed sternal closure in selected cases; typically these are very sick neonates, often a few hours old, with obstructed total anomalous pulmonary venous return
- Avoiding extubation for at least 6–12 hours after the last crisis.

In spite of all preventive measures, some children develop a crisis. Treatment measures should be rapidly instituted if a rapidly rising trend in PA pressures is observed, preferably well before the systemic pressures start to decline. Hand ventilation with hyperventilation to a $PaCO_2$ of 30–35 mm Hg should be initiated. Nebulized salbutamol in older infants may help. Deeper levels of sedation or anesthesia together with muscle relaxation should be instituted when appropriate. Inhaled NO and phenoxybenzamine should be administered if these initial measures are ineffective. Occurrence of a crisis merits an even sharper vigil to prevent further episodes. Careful and

slow weaning from the ventilator should be planned once the episodes are controlled and the PA pressures return to normal.

Selective Pulmonary Vasodilators

Inhaled Nitric Oxide

Nitric oxide is a potent endogenous, endothelium derived vasodilator that directly relaxes vascular smooth muscle through stimulation of soluble guanylate cyclase and increased production of intracellular cyclic guanosine monophosphate (cGMP). Since pulmonary arterial hypertension is associated with a defect in the production of NO and, by inference, with decreased nitric oxide-induced vasodilatation, NO has been proposed as a potential therapy. Short-term inhalation of NO has substantial pulmonary specific vasodilator effects in humans. Long-term inhaled NO therapy, while showing a benefit in small series and case reports, is very cumbersome to use, so it is unlikely to be given to a large number of patients. In addition, an interruption in its administration can cause hemodynamic deterioration. Anecdotal reports suggest that treatment with L-arginine, the substrate of NO synthase, reduces PA pressure and increases exercise tolerance in patients with pulmonary arterial hypertension. Inhaled NO is perhaps a useful adjunct to critical care settings where pulmonary hypertension occurs frequently. Examples of such settings include tertiary level neonatal ICUs and centers with a large pediatric cardiac surgical volume. Following pediatric cardiac surgery, inhaled NO is often initiated in the operation room and patients are typically transferred to the ICU on it. It is prudent to use the lowest possible dose of inhaled NO. High doses (>40 ppm) are associated with methemoglobinemia. The need for inhaled NO has declined in most units in recent times with improvements in case selection, surgical support times, perfusion strategies, and with the availability of less expensive selective pulmonary vasodilators. Additionally, there is no demonstrable improvement in outcomes with inhaled NO.[5]

Sildenafil

Another strategy for increasing the activity of endogenous NO in pulmonary arterial hypertension is to enhance nitric oxide dependent, cGMP-mediated pulmonary vasodilatation through inhibition of the breakdown of cGMP by phosphodiesterase type 5. Phosphodiesterase type 5 inhibitors, such as sildenafil, have an acute pulmonary vasodilator effect. In a study involving patients with pulmonary arterial hypertension, short-term intravenous administration of sildenafil during right heart catheterization reduced PVR in a dose-dependent manner. Sildenafil is commonly administered in the ICU in patients who are candidates for PH crisis or persistent pulmonary artery hypertension (PAH).[6] Sildenafil is typically administered in doses ranging from 0.2 to 0.5 mg/kg/dose orally via the nasogastric tube. Intravenous sildenafil is also available and can be used in situations when nasogastric feeding is completely withheld. The loading dose is 0.1 mg/kg as a bolus followed by 0.03 mg/kg/hour.[7]

Bosentan

Bosentan is traditionally used for chronic situations such as in idiopathic PAH and Eisenmenger syndrome. Its use in acute care settings, such as for postoperative PAH is largely reserved for refractory situations when sildenafil alone is not effective. Bosentan can only be administered orally. The usual starting dose is 2 mg/kg/dose every 12 hours, often in combination with sildenafil. Liver function tests must be obtained after a week of therapy and enzyme elevations (>2 times basal levels) warrant discontinuation.

Nonselective Vasodilators

With the advent of specific pulmonary vasodilators, the role of nonselective vasodilators such as phenoxybenzamine and milrinone has declined. Indeed, in patients with PH crisis, systemic vasodilators may cause the blood pressure to fall critically in those with a fixed low cardiac output state as a result of elevated PVR.

■ REFERENCES

1. Shah S, Szmuszkovicz JR. Pediatric perioperative pulmonary arterial hypertension: a case-based primer. Children (Basel). 2017;4(10):92.
2. Del Pizzo J, Hanna B. Emergency management of pediatric pulmonary hypertension. Pediatr Emerg Care. 2016;32(1):49-55.
3. Brunner N, de Jesus Perez VA, Richter A, Haddad F, Denault A, Rojas V, et al. Perioperative pharmacological management of pulmonary hypertensive crisis during congenital heart surgery. Pulm Circ. 2014;4(1):10-24.
4. Gorenflo M, Gu H, Xu Z. Perioperative pulmonary hypertension in paediatric patients: current strategies in children with congenital heart disease. Cardiology. 2010;116(1):10-7.
5. Wong J, Loomba RS, Evey L, Bronicki RA, Flores S. Postoperative inhaled nitric oxide does not decrease length of stay in pediatric cardiac surgery admissions. Pediatr Cardiol. 2019c;40(8): 1559-68.
6. El Midany AA, Mostafa EA, Azab S, Hassan GA. Perioperative sildenafil therapy for pulmonary hypertension in infants undergoing congenital cardiac defect closure. Interact Cardiovasc Thorac Surg. 2013;17(6):963-8.
7. Fraisse A, Butrous G, Taylor MB, Oakes M, Dilleen M, Wessel DL. Intravenous sildenafil for postoperative pulmonary hypertension in children with congenital heart disease. Intensive Care Med. 2011;37(3):502-9.

Postoperative Chylothorax in Patients with Congenital Heart Disease

Balaganesh Karmegaraj, Balaji Srimurugan

Illustrations: Balaji Srimurugan
Reviewed by: R Krishna Kumar

■ INTRODUCTION

The lymphatic system has three cardinal functions that include maintenance of interstitial fluid balance, immune surveillance and absorption of fat. The retention of plasma in the interstitial space is a "safety valve" to the circulation defending the failing heart from volume load.[1] If the lymphatic pressure increases, the safety function is activated and the system responds by increasing the amount of lymph contained within and transported by the system. The system functions as a reservoir, "protecting the failing heart" from volume overload (the Starling resistor effect).

The incidence of postoperative chylothorax in patients with congenital heart disease (CHD) is between 0.85 and 6.6%.[2] It is commonly seen in cavopulmonary anastomoses (Glenn and Fontan surgeries) where there is a sudden increase in the central venous pressure. Additionally, it is also seen in a variety of other cardiac operations where there is a possibility of direct injury to the large lymphatic channels inside the thoracic cavity. Postoperative chylothorax is associated with longer length of hospital stay, increased risk of in-hospital mortality and higher cost of hospitalization. Multiple diagnostic algorithms for chylothorax have been developed and theories have been proposed to suggest the etiologies of traumatic and nontraumatic chylothorax.

■ CAUSES

The cause of traumatic chylothorax is direct injury or surgical laceration of the central thoracic duct (TD) or one of its lymphatic tributaries. The causes of non-traumatic chylothorax have been reported in congenital genetic syndromes (e.g., Down, Noonan, or Turner syndromes) and postcongenital cardiac surgery patients with high central venous pressure. This is most common after cavopulmonary anastomoses. However, a rise in central venous pressure may also happen with other operations such as after repair of tetralogy of Fallot, stage I Norwood and situations where there is right ventricular dysfunction or tricuspid valve regurgitation resulting in high right atrial pressure.

■ MECHANISM OF CHYLOTHORAX

In the normal lung, both the pulmonary arteriolar pressure and pulmonary capillary wedge pressures are higher than the central venous pressure, resulting in normal reabsorption of fluid **(Figs. 1 and 2)**.

In Glenn and Fontan circulations, the lung is exposed to a paradox in which lymph from the lung is required to drain at a higher pressure than it is created. After the superior cavopulmonary anastomosis, the lung interstitium is subjected to a normal hydrostatic pressure, because more than 80% of the total lung arterial flow returns to

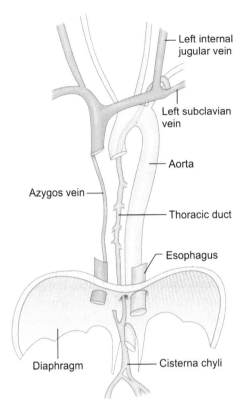

Fig. 1: Anatomy of the thoracic lymphatic circulation. Thoracic duct originates in the cisterna chyli and ascends anterior to the vertebrae and it ends by opening into the angle of junction of the left subclavian vein with the left internal jugular vein.

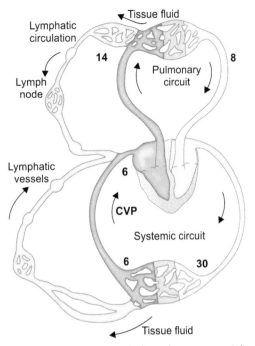

Fig. 2: In normal lung, both the pulmonary arteriolar and capillary wedge pressures are higher than the central venous pressure (CVP), resulting in normal reabsorption of fluid. The numerical values denote pressure in mm Hg.

the heart via pulmonary veins. However, there is a constant propensity toward fluid accumulation in the lung, because the lymphatic circulation drains to a higher pressure compared with normal. The increase in resistance to lymphatic drainage results in lymphatic endothelial cells adherence and lymph cannot be effectively removed from the interstitium. In contrast with pulmonary edema resulting from increased pulmonary capillary wedge pressure as a result of left heart pump failure or left-sided obstruction, the congested lung commonly seen in the early Glenn/Fontan patient is often related to lymph formation and accumulation, with

pleural effusions as a manifestation of this imbalance **(Fig. 3)**.[3,4]

■ MODES OF LYMPHATIC FAILURE

Lymphatic imaging and selective catheterization as reported by Dori et al. now allow understanding lymphodynamics and identification of three modes of lymphatic failure:[3]

1. *Traumatic leak*
2. *Pulmonary lymphatic perfusion syndrome* (when retrograde flow occurs from the thoracic duct to the lung or mediastinum)
3. *Central lymphatic flow disorder*: It is characterized by abnormally low or absent central lymphatic flow, effusions in more than 1 compartment, and dermal backflow through abdominal lymphatic collaterals.

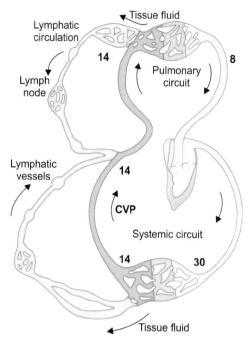

Fig. 3: After superior cavopulmonary anastomosis, the lymphatic circulation drains to a higher pressure compared with normal. The numerical values denote pressure in mm Hg.

(CVP: central venous pressure)

[Seen in syndromic children with CHD (Noonan, Down, Turners), hypoplastic left heart syndrome with intact atrial septum and rarely with transposition of great arteries and complete atrioventricular septal defects.][3]

MEDICAL MANAGEMENT OF CHYLOTHORAX[5]

Management of chylothorax includes conservative, interventional or surgical treatments **(Flowchart 1)**.

Confirmation of Diagnosis

The initial step requires confirmation of chylothorax—pleural fluid triglyceride level >110 mg/dL, pleural fluid cholesterol/serum cholesterol ratio <1.0 and, presence of chylomicrons.

Goals of Management

1. Relief of respiratory symptoms by removal of the pleural fluid by intercostal drainage
2. Prevention of recurrence by treatment of the underlying cause
3. Prevention/treatment of coexisting malnutrition and immunodeficiency.

Strategies to Reduce the Flow of Chyle through the Thoracic Duct

Typically, this is managed in three stages depending on quantity of drainage. When chylous accumulation is copious, for the first 2–5 days, nothing is administered orally and all nutrition is administered parenterally. This often dramatically reduces the quantity of drainage. Once fluid accumulation stops altogether, a fat-free diet is initiated first for a variable period of time. Again, the duration is dictated by the quantity of chyle that accumulates and by the nutritional status of the child as well as the feasibility of supplementation with parenteral nutrition. At some point, typically after about 4–5 days, medium chain triglyceride (MCT) may be added to the diet.

While it is true that MCTs are absorbed directly into the portal venous system, bypassing lymphatic drainage, we have often seen that early initiation of MCT often results in reaccumulation of chyle. MCT formulas lack essential fatty acids (EFA), so adjunctive EFA supplements are beneficial if these formulas are used for > 3 weeks.

Somatostatin/Octreotide cause a reduction in intestinal blood flow by vasoconstriction of the splanchnic circulation, with reduction of lymphatic fluid production. In comparison with somatostatin, octreotide has a longer half-life, greater potency, and the option of subcutaneous administration. The starting dose of somatostatin is 3.5 µg/kg/hour, which can be increased to 10 µg/kg/hour. The dose

Flowchart 1: Approach to chylothorax.

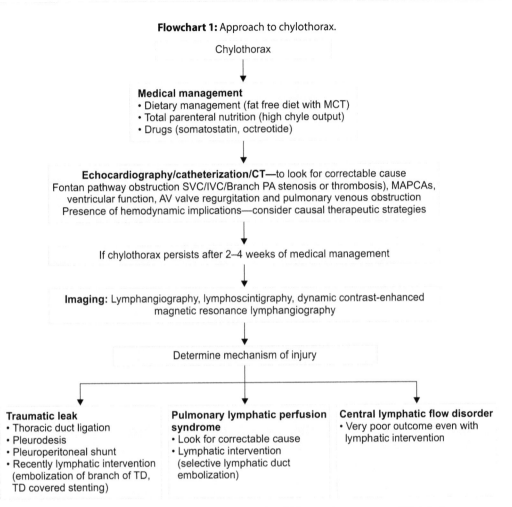

(MCT: medium chain triglyceride; CT: computed tomography; SVC: superior vena cava; IVC: inferior vena cava; PA: pulmonary artery; MAPCA: major aortopulmonary collateral; AV: atrioventricular; TD: thoracic duct)

for octreotide in children has ranged from 0.3 to 1.0 µg/kg/hour. The most common therapeutic scheme used in the available literature is intravenous infusion at a starting dose of 1 µg/kg/h, gradually increasing to 10 µg/kg/h according to the therapeutic response.[7] It is generally believed that somatostatin or octreotide need to be initiated early and are not very effective once chylous drainage is established for a few days.

Till date there are no randomized controlled trials on efficacy of octreotide in children with chylothorax. Nineteen isolated case reports of neonates with chylothorax in whom octreotide was used either subcutaneously or intravenously were available. Fourteen case reports described successful use (resolution of chylothorax), four reported failure (no resolution) and one reported equivocal results following use of octreotide. The timing of initiation, dose, duration and frequency of doses varied markedly. Gastrointestinal intolerance and clinical presentations suggestive of necrotizing enterocolitis and transient hypothyroidism were reported as side effects.[8] In a retrospective study, where somatostatin was used predominantly (11/14 cases) as treatment, this modality reduced the pleural drainage and need for respiratory support without significant side effects.[9] Another 12-year single-center retrospective cohort study assessed the safety and efficacy of octreotide as a therapeutic option in clinical setting. It showed that management of post-cardiac surgery induced chylothorax with octreotide shows promising benefits with an acceptable safety profile.[10]

▍ DEFINITION OF CLINICAL IMPROVEMENT OR FAILURE

Improvement is generally defined as a daily drainage <10 mL/kg/day, while daily drainage >10 mL/kg/day after 4 weeks of conservative management is classified as failure. Generally, a 2–4-week trial of nonsurgical therapy is reasonable before surgery is considered.[6]

Conservative management of chylothorax in children is successful in >80% of cases. The likelihood of failure is high in children who have syndromes that are associated with poor lymphatic system function (e.g., Noonan's syndrome), copious drainage and persistent elevation of central venous pressure. If conservative management fails, then surgical procedures such as thoracic duct ligation, pleurodesis, and pleuroperitoneal shunts may be considered. More recently, percutaneous embolization of the thoracic duct has emerged as a minimally invasive alternative for the treatment of chylothorax.[4] Dynamic contrast enhanced magnetic resonance lymphangiography[4] is a new imaging technique that uses an intranodal injection of gadolinium-based contrast agents to visualize the anatomy and flow characteristics of the central lymphatic system.

▍ COMPLICATIONS OF CHYLOTHORAX

- Malnutrition, hyponatremia, loss of selenium, fluid imbalance, respiratory distress, increased risk of thrombosis as a result of loss of nutrients
- Because of this secondary immunodeficiency, children with chylothorax are at risk for development of infections.

▍ REFERENCES

1. Foldi M, Papp N. The role of lymph circulation in congestive heart failure. Jap Circ J. 1961;25:703.
2. Shuyan C, Wendy L, Wilfred HS, Lik-cheung C, Adolphus KT, Yiu-fai C. Chylothorax in children after congenital heart surgery. Ann Thorac Surg. 2006;82(5):1650-6.
3. Savla JJ, Itkin M, Rossano JW, Dori Y. Post-operative chylothorax in patients with congenital heart disease. J Am Coll Cardiol. 2017;69(19):2410-22.
4. Kreutzer J, Kreutzer C. Lymphodynamics in congenital heart disease: the forgotten circulation. J Am Coll Cardiol. 2017;69(19):2423-7.
5. Tutor JD. Chylothorax in infants and children. Pediatrics. 2014;133(4):722-33.
6. Soto-Martinez M, Massie J. Chylothorax: diagnosis and management in children. Paediatr Respir Rev. 2009;10(4):199-207.
7. Bellini C, Cabano R, De Angelis LC, Bellini T, Calevo MG, Gandullia P, et al. Octreotide for congenital and acquired chylothorax in newborns: a systematic review. J Paediatr Child Health. 2018;54(8):840-7.
8. Das A, Shah PS. Octreotide for the treatment of chylothorax in neonates. Cochrane Database Syst Rev. 2010;9:CD006388.
9. Yin R, Zhang R, Wang J, Yuan L, Hu L, Jiang S, et al. Effects of somatostatin/octreotide treatment in neonates with congenital chylothorax. Medicine (Baltimore). 2017;96(29):e7594.
10. Aljazairi AS, Bhuiyan TA, Alwadai AH, Almehizia RA. Octreotide use in post-cardiac surgery chylothorax: a 12-year perspective. Asian Cardiovasc Thorac Ann. 2017;25(1):6-12.

Neurological Complications after Pediatric Cardiac Surgery

Sudheer Babu Vanga

Reviewed by: Aveek Jayant

■ INTRODUCTION

The mortality associated with the surgical repair of congenital heart defects has improved considerably in the last two decades and is now less than 10% in most major units.[1] Subsequently quality of life has become a point of focus as a significant proportion of neonates (25–90%) could have impairments in the neurodevelopmental domain. While many factors may not be modifiable such as existing abnormalities at birth, genetic factors and so on, there is naturally effort to control modifiable factors to the extent possible.

■ MECHANISM OF INTRAOPERATIVE CEREBRAL INJURY

The etiology of brain damage is multifactorial and preoperative abnormalities (hyper/hypotonia, difficulty in feeding, choreoathetosis, spasticity, macro/microcephaly) are identified in 50% of neonates with congenital heart disease (CHD). These are in themselves predictive for neurodevelopmental disability after heart surgery. Intraoperative hypoxia/ischemia or the reperfusion that follows is probably the principal mechanism responsible for neurological injury. However, the risk of intraoperative hypoxic-ischemic/reperfusion injury extends into the postoperative period when cardiorespiratory instability, together with cerebral autoregulatory dysfunction, predisposes to further cerebral hypoxic-ischemic injury.[1]

■ PREDICTORS OF CEREBRAL INJURY

- Prematurity
- Lower brain maturity scores
- Perinatal hypoxia
- Cyanotic heart lesions
- Preoperative hemodynamic instability and mechanical ventilation
- Complex open heart procedures, particularly those performed under deep hypothermic circulatory arrest (DHCA)
- Postoperative low cardiac output syndrome (LCOS).

■ FACTORS RESPONSIBLE FOR CEREBRAL INJURY DURING CARDIAC SURGERY

- Hypoxic-ischemic insult
- *Embolism*: Gaseous or particulate
- Hyperthermia
- Systemic inflammatory response
- Hypo/hyperglycemia
- Low hematocrit
- Biventricular dysfunction
- Intracranial hemorrhage.

Based on the circulatory arrest studies published from Children's Hospital, Boston on DHCA versus low flow bypass for arterial switch operations, the following intraoperative strategies can be done during cardiopulmonary bypass (CPB) to prevent brain injury after neonatal congenital heart surgery.[2]

- Maintain hematocrit >24%
- Avoid/limit DHCA to < 40 minutes

- Use some form of cerebral perfusion with neuromonitoring instead of DHCA; this typically takes the form of selective antegrade cerebral perfusion
- Maintain mean arterial pressure (MAP) of 40–45 mm Hg on CPB
- Limit volatile anesthetic exposure
- Maintain serum glucose levels between 100 and 200 mg/dL
- Avoid hypoglycemia (blood glucose <50 mg%).

MANIFESTATIONS OF POSTOPERATIVE NEUROLOGICAL DYSFUNCTION

- Delayed recovery of consciousness
- Postoperative seizures
- Periventricular white matter injury.
- Stroke
- Movement disorders
- Spinal cord injury
- Brachial plexus and peripheral nerve injury
- Critical illness myopathy.

Delayed Recovery of Consciousness

Delayed recovery of consciousness in the pediatric postcardiac surgical unit would normally call for the following steps:
- Follow the standard approach for assessing impaired consciousness in any patient.
- Exclude hepatic or renal impairment which can cause impaired metabolism and excretion of sedative drugs resulting in altered mental state.
- Prolonged usage of neuromuscular blocking agents—delays recovery of motor function and mimics as impaired consciousness. It can be confirmed with peripheral nerve stimulator and nerve conduction studies.
- Postoperative seizures manifests as prolonged postictal state.

Electroencephalogram (EEG) may be helpful to exclude this condition.
- Perioperative stroke can cause delayed awakening.
- An exact cause of an impaired postoperative mental status is not established quickly in most cases and many of these children ultimately demonstrate features suggestive of hypoxic-ischemic/reperfusion injury.
- Consider imaging as soon as feasible when recovery is unusually delayed; in most units this takes the form of head computed tomograms in the early postoperative period and magnetic resonance imaging (MRI) scans of the brain as soon as feasible.

Postoperative Seizures

- Most common neurological injury after cardiac surgery with an incidence of 19%.[3]
- As per experience from Boston Circulatory Arrest Study, incidence of EEG-only and electroclinical seizures were 20% and 6%, respectively.[4]
- Risk factors for seizures are increased duration of DHCA, the presence of a ventricular septal defect, and older age at the time of surgery.
- Avoidance of DHCA does not prevent seizures.
- Most seizures occurred 13–36 hours after surgery and are associated with worse neuropsychological outcomes.
- Bedside clinical assessment for seizures is unreliable and EEG monitoring is warranted.
- The only risk factors for electrographic seizures were delayed sternal closure and longer DHCA duration, neonates who subsequently required extracorporeal membrane oxygenation (ECMO) or those who have experienced cardiac arrest.[4]

- Since seizures are associated with worse neurological outcome, postoperative continuous EEG is mandatory especially in high risk patients and almost always when there are extreme events such as cardiac arrest.

Etiology of postoperative seizures are:

- Idiopathic
- Cerebral dysgenesis
- Metabolic factors such as hypoglycemia, hypocalcemia, hypomagnesemia
- Postoperative stroke
- Hypoxic-ischemic/reperfusion injury due to diffuse cerebral hypoperfusion or focal vaso-occlusive insult
- Cryptogenic seizures
- Long-term outcome depends on etiology
- Infants with seizures due to postoperative stroke are at 20–30% risk of developing subsequent epilepsy[5].

Cryptogenic seizures:

- Also called postpump seizures
- This occur due to hypoxic-ischemic/reperfusion injury[6]
- Risk factors were younger age at presentation, the use and duration of DHCA and the type of heart defect in addition to genetic vulnerability[7]
- Differs from perinatal seizures by delayed onset and favorable outcome
- Clinical course is typical with onset typically 24–48 hours after surgery
- It can be focal or multifocal and often evolves to status epilepticus and then rapidly wanes off
- Sometimes only confined to paroxysmal autonomic changes
- Responds to lorazepam, phenobarbital or phenytoin
- Short course of postpump seizures allows for early withdrawal of anticonvulsants
- West syndrome (infantile spasms, mental retardation, and epilepsy) has been described following a course of intractable postpump seizures[8].

Periventricular White Matter Injury (Periventricular Leukomalacia)

- White matter injury (WMI) is the most common type of brain injury in newborn infants undergoing surgery for CHD.
- Prematurity further enhances the risk of periventricular leukomalacia (PVL).[9]
- Its incidence is 20% before surgery and is associated with brain immaturity, and 42% after cardiac surgery.
- The target for diffuse WMI in PVL is immature oligodendrocytes which are highly susceptible to the preoperative ischemic insult as well as reduced white matter blood supply even after reperfusion compared to other brain regions in the perioperative period. Not only cytotoxic, even the maturation of oligodendrocytes is affected.
- It occurs at similar rates after non-bypass and bypass surgery.[9]
- Prolonged exposure to CPB (with or without DHCA) is a risk factor for PVL, possibly secondary to the systemic inflammatory response to CPB.
- The strongest associated clinical factor is diagnostic group, occurring at higher rates in infants having either single ventricle or arch surgery.
- Hypotension and hypoxemia in the early postoperative period, especially diastolic hypotension, significantly increase the risk of PVL, possibly secondary to cerebral ischemia.[9]
- The new onset of WMI was associated with the duration of CPB, postoperative lactate level, brain maturity, and WMI before surgery.
- As PVL damages white matter tracts that are deeper/more medial in location that

control the lower extremity, it presents as spastic diplegia (most common sign).[10]

- Initially, infants may have generalized low muscle tone with hypertonia in the neck extensors, apnea, bradycardia, irritability, and pseudobulbar palsy with poor feeding.
- Later as characteristic features of spastic diplegia evolve – all the stigmata of upper motor neuron involvement such as hypertonia, brisk deep tendon reflexes, scissoring of lower extremities, contractures and abnormal gross and fine motor coordination appear.
- Upper extremity function can also be impaired.
- Extensive white matter involvement may result in quadriplegia.
- Cerebral visual impairment is an important sequel of PVL.
- It is important for prognostication to subject patients to MRI scans; these scans have a prognostic value not only for neurodevelopmental outcome, but also for epilepsy.[10]
- A comparison between the preoperative and follow-up MRI images in children with CHD reveals recovery, if any and potential for later diffuse cerebral atrophy.
- No specific treatment exists for PVL.
- WMI is associated with increased mortality after discharge from intensive care but was not associated with neuro-development at 2 years of age. Brain immaturity on MRI was associated with adverse neurodevelopmental outcomes in all domains.
- Infants with PVL require close neuro-developmental follow-up at high-risk clinics that particularly include reha-bilitation physicians and specialists, in addition to core clinical staff.

Stroke

- Incidence of stroke in CHD is 25–30%.[11]
- Stroke associated with heart disease may be related to a number of mechanisms including: (1) embolic occlusion of some or the other branches of the arterial tree, (2) paradoxical (i.e., a cardiac anatomy that permits an embolus of systemic venous origin access to the cerebral circulation) and (3) venous occlusion.
- Focal arterial occlusive and watershed infarcts are the most common patterns of stroke seen, suggesting thromboembolism and hypoperfusion as the mechanisms of injury.
- Two types of arterial ischemic stroke (AIS) exist based on the timing of occurrence—periprocedural and spontaneous.[11]
  - *Periprocedural AIS*: This typically occurs during or within 72 hours of the target procedure such as surgery, catheterization, or extracorporeal support.
  - *Spontaneous AIS*: This occurs more than 72 hours after procedure. Periprocedural AIS is more common than spontaneous AIS.
- Strokes which occur during or imme-diately following cardiac surgery are under recognized due to the effects of postoperative sedative and paralyzing agents.
- Risk factors for stroke include lower birth weight, preoperative mechanical ventilation, lower hematocrit during CPB, and high blood pressure at the time of ICU admission.[12] Importantly, other operative variables, such as duration of CPB and the use of DHCA, were not shown to be associated with an increased risk of stroke. Neither did postoperative hypoxemia and hypotension increase the risk of stroke

suggesting that PVL and stroke were caused by different pathways.[12]

Stroke could therefore result from air embolism due to accidental injection of air into invasive lines. Thrombus can occur from stasis or paradoxical venous embolism in case of ventricular assist devices, or ECMO Alternatively, intracardiac stasis resulting from localized areas of low flow or global ventricular dysfunction could predispose to local thrombosis. Prosthetic material in areas of disturbed flow also increases the chance of thrombus formation. Elevated right atrial pressure transmitted to the cerebral venous circulation can predispose to central venous thrombosis. In those with a Fontan circulation systemic venous hypertension could trigger a procoagulant pathway.[13] It is uncertain as to what is the exact role of a patent foramen ovale (PFO) or arrhythmias.

Diagnostic challenges of stroke in children:
- Stroke is mostly under-recognized and leads to marked delays in diagnosis. Presentation is highly dependent on the age of the child and may not be specific.[14]
- Toddlers and infants present with nonspecific symptoms such as irritability, somnolence, lethargy, feeding difficulty, apneic spells and hypotonia or sometimes with focal seizures. Older children may present with more specific complaints such as a speech defect, localized weakness, visual disturbances and so on. Functionally, the aim of clinical and imaging triage is to differentiate ischemic, hemorrhagic and nonvascular etiologies, triggering different management cascades.[11]
- *Management of stroke in pediatric patients*: Ischemic stroke is managed with long-term anticoagulation provided in the form of antiplatelet agents such as aspirin, clopidogrel or anticoagulants such as low molecular weight heparin (LMWH), and

warfarin. The role of thrombolytic therapy is not defined as hemorrhagic complications are not uncommon.
- *Stroke prophylaxis*: Universally accepted guidelines for both primary and secondary stroke prophylaxis in children are lacking as the guidelines seem to be extensions of adult experience. Primary stroke prophylaxis might include prosthetic heart valves, dilated cardiomyopathy, or intracardiac thrombus.

Neurologic manifestations of infective endocarditis:
- *Clinical manifestations are*: Meningitis, brain abscess, seizures, septic embolism and hemorrhage.
- One-third of the children with infective endocarditis develop neurological complications even with appropriate antibiotics.
- Causes highest mortality, 80–90% primarily due to intracranial hemorrhage.
- In cases of cardiogenic stroke, the possibility of septic embolism should be considered prior to initiating anticoagulant therapy.

Movement Disorders

- Choreoathetosis is the most common movement disorder after pediatric cardiac surgery
- It has an incidence of around 20%
- Other rarer postoperative movement disorders include oculogyric crises and parkinsonism.

Risk Factors[15]

- Cyanotic CHD, particularly with systemic-to-pulmonary collaterals from the head and neck
- Age at surgery older than 9 months
- Excessively short cooling periods prior to attenuation of intraoperative blood flow
- Deep hypothermic circulatory arrest
- Alpha-stat pH management strategy

- Pre-existing developmental delay
- Prolonged use of fentanyl and midazolam (mild and transient).

Typical Course

- Some patients have subacute delirium. Involuntary movements start on day 2–7 in the distal extremities and orofacial muscles, progressing proximally to involve the girdle muscles and trunk; these could then intensify and be present all through the period children are awake. Oculomotor and oromotor apraxia, gaze abnormalities, feeding problems, language deficits may be present.

Diagnosis

- Neuroimaging studies are nonspecific, seldom focal, and most commonly consist of diffuse cerebral atrophy
- Helpful in excluding other disorders
- EEG is usually normal or diffusely slow with no ictal changes.

Management

- Refractory to treatment
- Successful movement control is achieved only at the expense of excessive sedation
- Judicious use of sedation should aim to restore a fragmented sleep-wakefulness cycle which contributes to delirium
- Focus on the severe agitation and insomnia that accompanies them
- Decreasing the level of external (e.g., noise, light) and internal (e.g., pain) stimuli is useful in limiting the intensity of the involuntary movements.

Antidyskinetic medication such as:
- Dopamine receptor blockers (e.g., phenothiazines, butyrophenones)
- Dopamine-depleting agents (e.g., reserpine, tetrabenazine)
- Dopamine agonists (e.g., levodopa, pramipexole)

- GABAergic agents (benzodiazepines, barbiturates, baclofen)
- Valproate, carbamazepine, phenytoin, diphenhydramine, and chloral hydrate
- Oromotor dyskinesia is often severe enough to impair feeding and predispose to aspiration
- Nasogastric or even gastrostomy tube feedings may be necessary to meet the high caloric demands of the constant involuntary movements.

Recovery

- Recovery is highly variable in duration and may be determined by severity of presentation with severe cases having a high incidence of persistent dyskinesia. When severe there are global neurodevelopmental deficits.

Spinal Cord Injury

- Rare complication following pediatric cardiac surgery
- Usually occurs after aortic coarctation repair (0.4–1.5%)[16]
- Due to hypoxic-ischemic/reperfusion injury to watershed territories
- Most commonly in the lower thoracic cord, where transverse infarction results in postoperative paraplegia
- Ischemia between the territories of the anterior and posterior spinal circulations; results in predominant anterior spinal cord involvement.

Brachial Plexus and Peripheral Nerve Injury

- Pressure and traction injury occurs following prolonged immobility following surgery
- Pressure palsies mostly involves the fibular (peroneal) and ulnar nerves.

Brachial plexus injury:

- Prolonged traction during the extreme and sustained arm abduction during cardiac catheterization – injures lower brachial plexus
- Internal jugular vein catheterization may injure upper brachial plexus by direct physical trauma or extravasation of blood into the plexus
- Symptoms usually resolve gradually and completely.

Critical Illness Myopathy

- Occurs due to prolonged use of nondepolarizing neuromuscular blocking drugs
- Prolonged usage leads to a condition ranging from necrotizing myopathy to an axonal motor neuropathy with variable sensory involvement
- Occurs most commonly with the steroidal muscle relaxants such as vecuronium and pancuronium
- Concomitant use of corticosteroids may increase the risk.

▌SUMMARY OF MAJOR RECOMMENDATIONS

Prenatal period:

- Achieve accurate prenatal cardiac diagnosis
- Avoid premature delivery (deliver in or near tertiary cardiac center).

Presurgical period:

- Limit the time presurgery to 3–4 days if possible in cyanotic patients
- Consider MRI to assess baseline brain injury status.

Intraoperative period:

- Maintain hematocrit on bypass 25% or greater
- Do not practice tight glucose control
- Avoid or limit DHCA to 30 minutes

- Use near infrared spectroscopy (NIRS) monitoring and treat low regional oxygen saturation (rSO_2) less than 50%
- Maintain MAP on CPB at 40–45 mm Hg.

Postoperative period:

- Monitor EEG in high-risk patients and treat seizures
- Limit ICU stay with early extubation and discharge protocols
- Obtain postoperative MRI
- Ensure longer term follow-up.

▌REFERENCES

1. Brossard-Racine M, duPlessis AJ, Vezina G, Robertson R, Bulas D, Evangelou IE et al. Prevalence and spectrum of in utero structural brain abnormalities in fetuses with complex congenital heart disease. AJNR Am J Neuroradiol 2014; 35:1593-9.
2. Andropoulos DB, Easley RB, Gottlieb EA, Brady K. Neurologic injury in neonates undergoing cardiac surgery. Clin Perinatol. 2019; 46(4):657-71.
3. Clancy RR, McGaurn SA, Wernovsky G, Gaynor JW, Spray TL, Norwood WI, et al. Risk of seizures in survivors of newborn heart surgery using deep hypothermic circulatory arrest. Pediatrics. 2003;111(3):592-601.
4. Naim MY, Gaynor JW, Chen J, Nicolson SC, Fuller S, Spray TL, et al. Subclinical seizures identified by postoperative electroencephalographic monitoring are common after neonatal cardiac surgery. J Thorac Cardiovasc Surg. 2015;150(1):169-80.
5. Chadehumbe MA, Khatri P, Khoury JC, Alwell K, Szaflarski JP, Broderick JP, et al. Seizures are common in the acute setting of childhood stroke: a population-based study. J Child Neurol. 2009;24(1):9-12.
6. Kinney HC, Panigrahy A, Newburger JW, Jonas RA, Sleeper LA. Hypoxic-ischemic brain injury in infants with congenital heart disease dying after cardiac surgery. Acta Neuropathol. 2005;110(6):563-78.
7. Clancy RR, Sharif U, Ichord R, Spray TL, Nicolson S, Tabbutt S, et al. Electrographic neonatal seizures after infant heart surgery. Epilepsia. 2005;46(1):84-90.
8. du Plessis AJ, Kramer U, Jonas RA, Wessel DL, Riviello JJ. Case report West syndrome following

deep hypothermic infant cardiac surgery. Pediatr Neurol. 1994;11(3):246-51.

9. Beca J, Gunn JK, Coleman L, Hope A, Reed PW, Hunt RW, et al. New white matter brain injury after infant heart surgery is associated with diagnostic group and the use of circulatory arrest. Circulation. 2013;127(9): 971-9.

10. Ahya K, Suryawanshi P. Neonatal periventricular leukomalacia: current perspectives. Res Reports Neonatol. 2018;8:1-8.

11. Nowak-Göttl U, Günther G, Kurnik K, Sträter R, Kirkham F. Arterial ischemic stroke in neonates, infants, and children: an overview of underlying conditions, imaging methods, and treatment modalities. Semin Thromb Hemost. 2003;29(4):405-14.

12. Chen J, Zimmerman RA, Jarvik GP, Nord AS, Clancy RR, Wernovsky G, et al. Perioperative stroke in infants undergoing open heart operations for congenital heart disease. Ann Thorac Surg. 2009;88(3):823-9.

13. Barker PC, Nowak C, King K, Mosca RS, Bove EL, Goldberg CS. Risk factors for cerebrovascular events following fontan palliation in patients with a functional single ventricle. Am J Cardiol. 2005;96(4):587-91.

14. Jordan LC, Hillis AE. Challenges in the diagnosis and treatment of pediatric stroke. Nat Rev Neurol. 2011;7(4):199-208.

15. Levin DA, Seay AR, Fullerton DA, Simoes EA, Sondheimer HM. Profound hypothermia with alpha-stat pH management during open-heart surgery is associated with choreoathetosis. Pediatr Cardiol. 2005;26(1):34-8.

16. Christenson JT, Sierra J, Didier D, Beghetti M, Kalangos A. Repair of aortic coarctation using temporary ascending to descending aortic bypass in children with poor collateral circulation. Cardiol Young. 2004;14(1):39-45.

Acute Kidney Injury after Pediatric Cardiac Surgery

Aveek Jayant

Reviewed by: R Krishna Kumar

■ BACKGROUND

Acute kidney injury (AKI) is not uncommon in children postcardiac surgery. The incidence can be as high as 40–60% in certain high risk patients who undergo surgical correction of congenital heart disease (CHD). Yet others show that the risk of AKI decreases with older children and are highest in the neonatal cohort undergoing cardiac surgery.[1] AKI mirrored by even small and subclinical rises in serum creatinine is associated with longer durations of mechanical ventilation, inotrope use and stay in the intensive care unit (ICU) besides aggravating mortality risk.[2,3] There is also some evidence akin to adults, that AKI confers long-term risks for chronic kidney impairment and its consequences such as development of systemic hypertension.[4,5]

In view of the intense focus on kidney as a key target organ, for global clinical outcome, a mix of new and old risk factors continue to emerge. It has been shown recently that preoperative caloric status and inability to achieve full caloric feeds before surgery is an independent risk factor of AKI after cardiac surgery in neonates.[6] Other well-known risk factors include but not limited to are, younger age, higher complexity of cardiac surgery, concomitant long cardiopulmonary bypass (CPB) duration, and preoperative renal impairment/need for renal replacement.[7-9] Composite risk scores are developed to predict AKI postcardiac surgery.[10] While

inotrope scores (as surrogate for degree of postoperative cardiac functional impairment) are logically risks for AKI, the role of albumin and avoidance of milrinone are not as clearly understandable.[9,11] Finally, a clear paradigm has emerged in fluid management, that fluid overload (FO) is clearly both causative and contributory to the development of AKI after heart surgery.[12] Fluids, therefore, are equally important therapeutic targets and should be treated as drugs with a potential for harm.

■ DIAGNOSIS

The three diagnostic models of AKI in the pediatric population are Pediatric Risk Injury Failure Loss End-Stage (P-RIFLE), Acute Kidney Injury Network (AKIN) and Kidney Diseases Improving Global Outcomes (KDIGO). These scoring systems are detailed in the **Table 1**.

As such AKIN and KDIGO show closer agreement to each other than to P-RIFLE.

Accordingly, calibration of the incidence and risk models differ, based on which of these diagnostic criteria are being applied. Many pediatric intensive care units seem to have a bias toward using P-RIFLE, as it is probably more sensitive in picking up stage 1 events.

Calculation of Estimated GFR

As a practical tool, it is important for clinicians to know in some detail how to calculate the

TABLE 1: Diagnostic criteria for acute kidney injury.

P-RIFLE	Criteria—serum creatinine	Criteria—urine output
Stage 1 (Risk)	eGFR decreased by 25%	<0.5 mL/kg/h for 8 hours
Stage 2 (Injury)	eGFR decreased by 50%	<0.5 mL/kg/h for 16 hours
Stage 3 (Failure)	eGFR decreased by 75%	<0.3 mL/kg/h for 24 hours or anuria >12 hours
Stage 4 (Loss)	Persistent failure >4 weeks	
Stage 5 (End Stage)	ESRD persistent failure >3 months	
AKIN	**Criteria—serum creatinine**	**Criteria—urine output**
Stage 1	Increase SCr >50% or >0.3 mg/dL	<0.5 ml/kg/h for 6 hours
Stage 2	Increase SCr >100%	<0.5 mL/kg/h for 12 hours
Stage 3	Increase SCr >200%	<0.3 mL/kg/h for 24 hours or anuria >12 hours
KDIGO	**Criteria—serum creatinine**	**Criteria—urine output**
Stage 1	Increase SCr >50–99% or >0.3 mg/dL	<0.5 mL/kg/h for 6–12 hours
Stage 2	Increase SCr >100–199%	<0.5 mL/kg/h for more than 12 hours
Stage 3	Increase SCr >200% or eGFR <35 mL/min/1.73 m² (Age <18 years)	<0.3 mL/kg/h for at least 24 hours or anuria >24 hours

(AKIN: acute kidney injury network; eGFR: estimated glomerular filtration rate; ESRD: end stage renal disease; KDIGO: kidney disease—improving global outcomes; P-RIFLE: pediatric version of risk, injury, failure, loss, and end-stage; SCr: serum creatinine)

estimated glomerular filtration rate (eGFR). The Schwartz formula is traditionally used, to calculate eGFR in children but is based on the serum creatinine (SCr) by the Jaffe method:

GFR (mL/min/1.73 m²) = K × (height)/(SCr in mg/dL)

K=muscle factor; in preterm infants up to 1 year of age 0.33; term infants up to 1 year of age 0.45; child or adolescent girl 0.55; adolescent boy 0.7.

With the gradual migration to measure creatinine using the enzymatic method: The Chronic Kidney Disease in Children (CKiD) formula is used:

GFR (mL/min/1.73 m²) = 0.431 (height/SCr)

The reference values are:

>2 years: 110–120 mL/min/1.73 m²
Preterm infants: <10 mL/min/1.73 m²
Term infants: 10–40 mL/min/1.73m²

Of topical relevance to the pediatric cardiac intensive care units (PCICU), some groups correct for fluid balance[13,14] where the adjusted Serum creatinine = measured SCr [1 + cumulative net fluid balance (L)]/ total body water (kg), where total body water = 0.6 × body weight in kg. As an extension, progressive positive fluid balance has been shown to correlate to AKI after cardiac surgery and has also been a key element of the concept of renal angina[15] (with incremental risk of FO in relation to overall risk; thus tolerance of relative amounts of overload is closely linked to the baseline risk with even 5% FO increasing risk in the high risk cohorts) and has specifically been validated in the PCICU population.[12]

There has also been enormous interest in migrating diagnosis of AKI, particularly preclinical AKI, on the basis of biomarkers—typically these markers either are signatures of tubular injury, inflammatory markers or those that denote cell cycle arrest—cystatin C and neutrophil gelatinase associated lipocalin. Use of these markers in the immediate post bypass period, significantly

TABLE 2: Investigations for acute kidney injury (AKI).

Urine	General analysis, sodium, creatinine
Blood	Urea, creatinine, blood urea nitrogen (BUN), electrolytes, phosphorous, albumin
Renal ultrasound	Post renal causes of AKI

enhances the diagnosis of AKI. Based on this, some studies initiate fenoldopam which has been shown to confer some protection on AKI progression when used pre-emptively.[8] Once a definitive diagnosis of AKI is made, the investigations, which are given in **Table 2** need to be considered.

Differentiating Prerenal or Intrinsic AKI

For postoperative cardiac critical care, the main point of discrimination is often between prerenal and intrinsic AKI. The absence of proteinuria or hematuria, a high specific gravity and urine osmolality >500 mOsm/kg in addition to urine Na < 10 mEq/L (20–30 meq/L in neonates) suggest a strong prerenal component.

A very high BUN/creatinine ratio (>20) should suggest a prerenal etiology. It is reasonable to calculate the fractional excretion of sodium (FENa):

$$FENa = \frac{Urine\ Na \times (SCr)}{Urine\ Cr \times (Serum\ Na)} \times (100)$$

The FENa is <1% in prerenal AKI and >2% in intrinsic and postrenal AKI. The ratio is somewhat higher in neonates. It is not routinely used in our unit as measurement is confounded by diuretic use (which is routine in our practice).

■ MANAGEMENT

When clinical suspicion and laboratory features suggest pre-renal AKI, the primary goals are to eradicate predisposing factors such as depleted circulating volume, poor

chamber function, nephrotoxic medications, and sepsis. Although some units do advocate Fenoldopam use, it is not available in our practice.

Diuretic use has reached some form of equipoise and when there is established AKI, it is reasonable to withhold diuretics. Diuretics do not contribute to renal recovery and could potentially cause ototoxicity. The only putative advantage of using diuretics in AKI is in volume management but it is important to emphasize that they neither prevent nor treat AKI.

Fluids

Following a diagnosis of AKI, it is important to use volume status, although the best method and their controversies elude easy solution. In our unit this is based on composite assessment of fluid balance, ventricular volumes on echocardiography, complemented by assessments of invasive filling pressure at their extreme ends. Invasive filling pressure alone should be deemphasized in the overall assessment of fluid status. Volume resuscitation is usually accomplished using isotonic crystalloids, and colloids including albumin are generally avoided. When intrinsic renal AKI is established, fluids are restricted as they contribute to AKI and fluids are titrated to insensible water losses, typically one-third Holliday Segar levels given as D5W or D10W.

Hyperkalemia Management

Standard therapies are instituted for hyperkalemia when present.

Nutrition

Patient energy requirements are calculated as age appropriate and usual amounts of protein are added with a provision for supplementing protein in patients on renal replacement therapy (RRT). Enteral nutrition that is low on potassium and phosphate and tailored by the clinical dietitian is usual.

Renal Replacement Therapy

At our unit, hyperkalemia and anuria >2 hours is generally taken to trigger renal replacement therapies. However others strongly suggest (based on the RENAL study) that RRT should be considered when fluid overload is >15% of body weight. Other common indications for initiating RRT are enumerated in **Box 1**.

There are three major modalities for providing RRT in children[16] **(Table 3)**.

Although in principle, extracorporeal therapies such as intermittent hemodialysis and continuous renal replacement therapy (CRRT) are theoretically possible in the smallest of patients including neonates, other considerations such as need for complex vascular access, hemodynamic instability and anticoagulation, significantly limit their use in the immediate postoperative period.

Peritoneal dialysis (PD) is the mainstay of RRT in our unit. In PD, the peritoneal membrane and its large surface serve as the membrane separating blood from the dialysate. However, the abdomen, as a body cavity, is rich in lymphatics and, as a result a large proportion (estimated 50%) can be reabsorbed via the lymphatics limiting the efficacy of solute and fluid removal. PD is performed by running a prescribed dialysis solution into the abdominal cavity (via a surgically placed catheter), allowing it to "dwell" for a certain period of time and then cause it to "drain". As general rules, ultrafiltration and solute clearance is dependent on the volume and osmolality of dialysate fluid, the dwell time and permeability of the peritoneal membrane to a particular substance. Fluid is removed due to an osmotic gradient which diminishes over the dwell cycle, therefore for fluid removal the primary determinants are a high osmotic

---

BOX 1: Renal indications for renal replacement therapy.

- Oliguria or anuria
- Metabolic acidosis
- Hyperkalemia
- Fluid overload
- Azotemia
- Uremic symptoms such as bleeding or encephalopathy

TABLE 3: Comparison of various modes of renal replacement therapy.

Method specificities	PD	IHD	CRRT
Vascular access	No	Yes	Yes
Complexity	No	High	Moderate
Systemic or regional anticoagulation	No	Yes	Yes
Dialysis dose			
Solute removal	Moderate	High	High
Fluid removal	Moderate	Moderate	High
Clinical situation			
Hemodynamic instability	Yes	No	Yes
Respiratory failure	+/−	Yes	Yes
Abdominal sepsis/surgery	No	Yes	Yes

(CRRT: continuous renal replacement therapy; IHD: intermittent hemodialysis; PD: peritoneal dialysis)

Source: Adapted from Roger's Textbook of Pediatric Intensive Care.[16]

gradient (typically achieved by increasing the concentration of glucose in the dialysate) and a short dwell cycle. Solute clearance, on the other hand is predominantly decided by the volume of dialysate (as it recruits a larger surface for exchange) as also longer dwell times. Among the many mechanical complications that can occur with catheters placed into hollow cavities, of topical importance to cardiac surgical patients is the presence of a potential thoracoabdominal communication (typical when catheters are placed during chest closure via the diaphragm)—this allows PD fluid to leak out of chest tubes and disallowing adequate exchange times and should be avoided.

Numerous PD fluid prescriptions are available and could be tailored to the individual needs of patients. As such, lactate containing PD solutions are preferably avoided in children with profound metabolic acidosis. The typical volume instilled is 10–20 mL/kg although in our unit the usual cycles would employ the lower range of volumes due to the potential for cardiopulmonary interactions. Dwell times can range from 30 to 240 minutes though during initiation, dwell times are usually deliberately short as primacy is given to ultrafiltration. In case of doubt as to the hemodynamic effects of PD in postoperative patients via cardiopulmonary interaction and the potential for intra-abdominal hypertension the usual strategy is to use smaller volumes of dialysate; abdominal pressure can also be measured using a bladder catheter with the balloon filled with a volume of 1 mL/kg. Technical details of PD kinetics can be found in this technical review.[14] PD is terminated and catheter removed when clearance goals are met and there is resumption of native renal function. PD however is contraindicated, if there are defects in the diaphragm or abdominal wall, abdominal sepsis, suspected necrotizing enterocolitis and pre-existing intra-abdominal hypertension.

In sum, despite PD being a suboptimal modality for RRT it remains the most feasible and technically simple modality of use in postoperative pediatric cardiac surgical intensive care.

FUTURE DIRECTIONS

There seems to be path breaking evidence from adult cardiac surgery that pre-emptive diagnosis using a basket of biomarkers and a focused bundle thereafter can reduce the frequency and severity of AKI.[17] At the same time device applications focused on the pediatric population to deliver CRRT and other blood based RRT are gaining traction: at least one, CARPE DIEM™ is a machine that can deliver CRRT to neonates.[18] There is also some push to monitor renal oxygen status using near infrared spectroscopy (NIRS) in the most vulnerable neonates.[19] While practitioners doubtless need to be aware of these developments they cannot be unaware of practice variation between centers in the low- and middle-income countries (LMIC) to those in high resource settings and adapt the emerging literature to their practice patterns and resources.

REFERENCES

1. Kaddourah A, Basu RK, Bagshaw SM, Goldstein SL. Epidemiology of acute kidney injury in critically ill children and young adults. N Engl J Med. 2017;376:11-20.
2. Morgan CJ, Zappitelli M, Robertson CM, Alton GY, Sauve RS, Joffe AR, et al. Risk factors for and outcomes of acute kidney injury in neonates undergoing complex cardiac surgery. J Pediatr. 2013;162:120-7.
3. Blinder JJ, Goldstein SL, Lee VV, Baycroft A, Fraser CD, Nelson D, et al. Congenital heart surgery in infants: effects of acute kidney injury on outcomes. J Thor Cardiovasc Surg. 2012;143:368-74.

4. Askenazi DJ, Ambalavanan N, Goldstein SL. Acute kidney injury in critically ill newborns: what do we know? What do we need to learn? Pediatr Nephrol. 2009;24:265-74.

5. Shaw NJ, Brocklebank JT, Dickinson DF, Wilson N, Walker DR. Long-term outcome for children with acute renal failure following cardiac surgery. Int J Cardiol. 1991;31:161-5.

6. Piggott KD, Liu A, Monczka J, Fakioglu H, Narasimhulu SS, Pourmoghadam K, et al. Inadequate preoperative nutrition might be associated with acute kidney injury and greater illness severity postoperatively. J Thorac Cardiovasc Surg. 2018;155:2104-9.

7. Webb TN, Goldstein SL. Congenital heart surgery and acute kidney injury. Curr Opin Anesthesiol. 2017; 30:105-12.

8. Gist KM, Kwiatkowski DM, Cooper DS. Acute kidney injury in congenital heart disease. Curr Opin Cardiol. 2017;32:101-7.

9. Yuan SM. Acute kidney injury after pediatric cardiac surgery. Pediatrics Neonatol. 2019; 60:3-11.

10. Cardoso B, Laranjo S, Gomes I, Freitas I, Trigo C, Fragata I, et al. Acute kidney injury after pediatric cardiac surgery: risk factors and outcomes proposal for a predictive model. Rev Port Cardiol. 2016;35:99-104.

11. Esch JJ, Salvin JM, Thiagarajan RR, DelNido PJ, Rajagopal SK. Acute kidney injury after Fontan completion: risk factors and outcomes. J Thorac Cardiovasc Surg. 2015;150(1):190-7.

12. Hassinger AB, Wald EL, Goodman DM. Early postoperative fluid overload precedes acute kidney injury and is associated with higher morbidity in pediatric cardiac surgery patients. Pediatr Crit Care Med. 2014;15:131-8.

13. DeSena HC, Nelson DP, Cooper DS. Cardiac intensive care for the neonate and child after cardiac surgery. Curr Opin Cardiol. 2015;30: 81-8.

14. Fischbach M, Warady BA. Peritoneal dialysis prescription in children: bedside principles for optimal practice. Pediatr Nephrol. 2009;24:1633-42.

15. Basu R, Chawla LS, Wheeler DS, Goldstein SL. Renal angina: an emerging paradigm to identify children at risk of renal injury. Pediatr Nephrol. 2012;27:1067-78.

16. Extracoporeal organ support therapy. In: Nichols DG, Shaffner DH (Eds). Roger's Textbook of Pediatric Intensive Care, 5th edition. Philadelphia: Wolters Kluwer; 2016.

17. Meersch M, Schmidt C, Hoffmeier A, Von Aken H, Wempe C, Gerss J, et al. Prevention of cardiac surgery associated AKI by implementing the KDIGO guidelines in high risk patients identified by biomarkers: the PrevAKI randomized controlled trial. Intensive Care Med. 2017;43:1551-61.

18. Goldstein SL. Pediatric acute kidney injury: the time for nihilism is over. Front Pediatr. 2020; 8:16.

19. Harer MW, Chock VY. Renal tissue oxygenation monitoring – an opportunity to improve kidney outcomes in the vulnerable neonatal population. Front Pediatr. 2020;8:241.

Management of Cardiac Arrest in Pediatric Cardiac Intensive Care Unit

Sreelakshmi P Leeladharan
Reviewed by: Aveek Jayant

■ INTRODUCTION

Cardiac arrest (CA) is a rare event in general pediatric population as compared to adults. Among CA in pediatric population, children with underlying heart disease have higher incidence of CA.[1] Managing CAs in pediatric cardiac intensive care unit (PCICU) poses different challenges owing to the diversity of anatomy and physiology among various cardiac lesions both congenital and acquired, as also the age of patients varying from infants to young adults. Pediatric basic life support (BLS) and pediatric advanced life support (PALS) focuses on cardiopulmonary resuscitation (CPR) of children with normal hearts, and substantial knowledge gaps exist when applied to children with structural cardiac abnormalities. Incidence of CA in PCICU is 3–6%,[1-3] which is almost 10 times more than in children with normal hearts.[4] Survival to hospital discharge ranges from 32 to 50%. Children with univentricular physiology have higher rates of attrition, while children postcardiac surgery had better survival rates after CA than those with medical cardiac conditions.[2] Timely identification of signs of deterioration and pre-emptive management to avert a CA are crucial in this setting.

■ MANAGEMENT OF CARDIAC ARREST

Cardiac arrest management can be divided into three phases: (1) pre-arrest, (2) arrest, and (3) post-arrest phase.

Pre-arrest Phase

Prevention of CA is the mainstay of treatment in PCICU. Various tools can be of use for this.

Pediatric Early Warning Score (PEWS) incorporates a set of early warning signs that help to identify worsening clinical and hemodynamic trends so that CA can be aborted when incipient. The Children's Hospital, Boston has modified PEWS to formulate the Cardiac-Children's Hospital Early Warning Score (C-CHEWS).[5] C-CHEWS is primarily applicable to the inpatient wards but the overall abbreviated assessment could be useful in the PCICU for patients after liberation from mechanical ventilation in high-dependency areas where nurses can alert physicians of an impending crisis (**Table 1**). The sequential approach to the management of clinical deterioration identified by C-CHEWS assessment is depicted in **Figure 1**. In the intensive care environment clinical signs are complemented by additional monitoring

TABLE 1: Cardiac-Children's Hospital Early Warning Score.[5]

	0	1	2	3	Score
Behavior/Neuro	• Playing/ sleeping appropriately • Alert, at patient's baseline	Sleepy, somnolent when not disturbed	• Irritable, difficult to console • Increase in patient's baseline seizure activity	• Lethargic, confused, floppy • Reduced response to pain • Prolonged or frequent seizures • Pupils asymmetric or sluggish	
Cardiovascular	• Skin tone appropriate for patient • Capillary refill ≤2 seconds	• Pale • Capillary refill 3–4 seconds • Mild* tachycardia • Intermittent ectopy or irregular HR (not new)	• Gray • Capillary refill 4–5 seconds • Moderate* tachycardia	• Gray and mottled • Capillary refill >5 seconds • Severe* tachycardia • New onset bradycardia • New onset/ increase in ectopy, irregular HR or heart block	
Respiratory	• Within normal parameters • No retractions	• Mild* tachypnea/ increased WOB (flaring, retracting) • Up to 40% supplemental oxygen • Up to 1 L NC > patient's baseline need • Mild desaturations < patient's baseline • Intermittent apnea self-resolving	• Moderate* tachypnea/ increased WOB (flaring, retracting, grunting, use of accessory muscles) • 40–60% oxygen via mask • 1–2 L NC > patient's baseline need • Nebs q 1–2 hours • Moderate desaturations < patient's baseline • Apnea requiring repositioning or stimulation	• Severe* tachypnea • RR < normal for age • Severe increased WOB (i.e., head bobbing, paradoxical breathing) • >60% oxygen via mask • >2 L NC > patient's baseline need • Nebs q 30 minutes—1 hour • Severe desaturations < patient's baseline • Apnea requiring interventions other than repositioning or stimulation	
Staff concern		Concerned			
Family concern		Concerned or absent			
					Total

	Mild*	Moderate*	Severe*
Infant	≥10% ↑ for age	≥15% ↑ for age	≥25% ↑ for age
Toddler and older	≥10% ↑ for age	≥25% ↑ for age	≥50% ↑ for age

(HR : heart rate; RR: respiratory rate; WOB: work of breathing; NC: nasal cannula)

Approach to the deteriorating patient on cardiac inpatient units:
Escalation of care: Cardiac -Children's Hospital Early Warning Score
(C-CHEWS) assessment algorithm

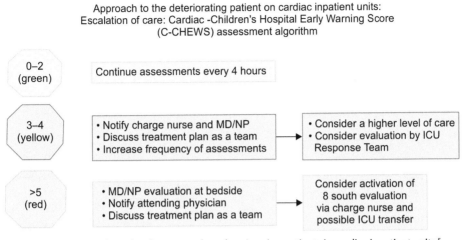

Fig. 1: C-CHEWS algorithm for approach to deteriorating patients in cardiac inpatient units.[5]
(ICU: intensive care unit; MD: doctor of medicine; NP: nurse practitioner)

such as filling pressures, invasive blood pressures, arterial blood gases, when applicable, and almost always screening transthoracic echocardiography to evaluate chamber function and filling status. PEWS has not been accorded a high-priority status in both the 2015 and 2019 Pediatric Advanced Life Support guidance.

Pediatric Advanced Life Support[6,7]

Conventional CPR is inherently inefficient with compressions providing only ≈10–30% of normal blood flow to the heart and 30–40% of normal blood flow to the brain;[8] the anatomic and physiological substrates of congenital heart defects (CHD) can further limit the effectiveness of conventional CPR finally limiting effective pulmonary blood flow (PBF), systemic blood flow (SBF), and cerebral perfusion. Hence, survival after CA can be low (41%) in infants and children with cardiac disease. Emphasis on prearrest phase to prevent CA and on arrest phase to provide high-quality CPR is important to improve resuscitation outcomes. Cardiac Advanced Life Support (CALS) modifies conventional

PALS pathways toward the postoperative cardiac period: Primarily, applied to adults, the principles of early defibrillation, first-line usage of epicardial pacing wires, which are available and emphasis on resternotomy are applicable to the PCICU setting. The treatment algorithms for pediatric CA and CA after cardiac surgery are depicted in **Flowchart 1** and **Figure 2**, respectively. Extracorporeal cardiopulmonary resuscitation (ECPR) can be used in case of failed conventional CPR in specialized environments if the underlying cause for arrest is a reversible one or as bridge to other therapy such as transplant.[9,10] The availability of expertise and equipment enables ECPR to be more readily applied to the PCICU.

The cardiac advanced life support protocol could be used in PCICU for immediate or early postoperative patients. Since, most postcardiac surgery patients have pacing wires; in case of a bradycardia the patient can be paced. In case of an arrest, if patient is already paced then the pacing should be switched off to rule out ventricular fibrillation (VF). Early postoperative period also gives the advantage

Flowchart 1: Pediatric cardiac arrest algorithm 2020.[7]

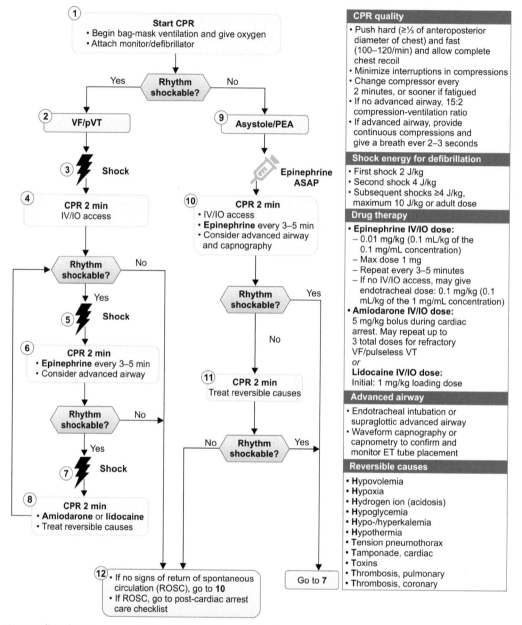

(CPR: cardiopulmonary resuscitation; PEA: pulseless electrical activity; VT: ventricular tachycardia; ASAP: as soon as possible; ET: endotracheal)

of option for resternotomy. In PCICU in case of a CA, the surgical and perfusion teams are alerted immediately to prepare for an emergent resternotomy and/or ECPR.

Special Considerations of Congenital Heart Disease in PCICU Arrest

The American Heart Association (AHA) released a scientific statement on CPR in

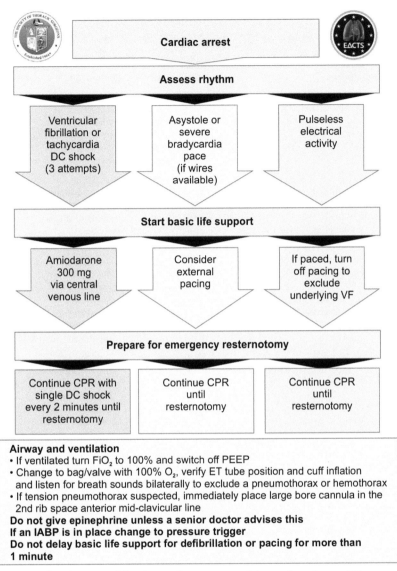

Fig. 2: Management of cardiac arrest following cardiac surgery and the cardiac advanced life support protocol.[11]
(*Drug doses not normalized to the PCICU*).

(PEEP: positive end-expiratory pressure; PCICU: pediatric cardiac intensive care unit; IABP: intra-aortic balloon pump; CPR: cardiopulmonary resuscitation; ET: endotracheal; DC: direct current; VF: ventricular fibrillation)

Infants and Children With Cardiac Disease in 2018, which discusses in detail specifics of resuscitation in various cardiac lesions.[12]

The resuscitation profiles for patients with structurally normal heart and those who have undergone single ventricle palliation are elaborated in **Table 2**. The unique challenges with respect to the type of CHD and special considerations while resuscitating these patients in PCICU are depicted in **Table 3**. The recommened energy dose for defibrillation and cardioversion is provided in **Table 4**.

TABLE 2: Resuscitation profiles for structurally normal heart and those that have undergone single ventricle palliation.[12]

Physiology	Circulation description	Circulation of blood	Chest compressions	Chest recoil	Positive-pressure ventilation
Structurally normal heart	Two-ventricle series circulation without heart disease	Systemic veins—lungs—pulmonary veins—body	• RV compression results in PBF • LV compression results in SBF	Increases the transthoracic gradient from the systemic veins to the RA, increasing RV filling	Decreases the transthoracic gradient from the systemic veins to the RA, decreasing RV filling
Stage 1 Norwood or shunted physiology	Single-ventricle parallel circulation with shunt-dependent PBF	Systemic veins—single ventricle—lungs (via shunt) or body	Single-ventricle compression results in PBF (shunt ± PVR) and SBF (SVR)	Increases filling to the preload-dependent single ventricle	Decreases filling to the preload-dependent single ventricle
Bidirectional Glenn and hemi-Fontan	Single-ventricle parallel circulation with PBF dependent on multiple arteriolar vascular beds	IVC—single ventricle—body/brain—SVC—lungs—pulmonary veins—body	Single-ventricle compression results in SBF	• Predominantly fills the RA from the IVC • SVC flow dependent on cerebral vascular resistance and PVR	Decreases filling to the single ventricle by impeding SVC flow and IVC filling
Fontan	Single-ventricle series circulation	Systemic veins—lungs—pulmonary veins—body	Single-ventricle compression results in SBF	• Predominantly fills the PAs with IVC blood flow (PVR) • SVC flow dependent on cerebral vascular resistance and PVR	Decreases filling to the single ventricle by impeding both SVC and IVC flow

(IVC: inferior vena cava; LV: left ventricle; PA: pulmonary artery; PBF: pulmonary blood flow; PVR: pulmonary vascular resistance; RA: right atrium; RV: right ventricle; SBF: systemic blood flow; SVC: superior vena cava; SVR: systemic vascular resistance).

TABLE 3: Physiology, unique challenges and recommended action for specific cardiac lesions.

Physiology	Unique challenges	Data	Recommended action[12]
Stage 1 Norwood or shunted physiology	Difficult to obtain effective PBF because: • Shunt dependent • PVR vs. SVR/DBP	62.3% of patients who developed postoperative cardiac arrest after stage 1 Norwood palliation died compared with a mortality rate of 12.5% among those patients who did not develop postoperative cardiac arrest.[13] (STS-CHSD registry data)	Conventional high-quality CPR, consider additional management within minutes of the resuscitation: • Resternotomy (immediate/early postoperative period) • Treatment of arrhythmias or use of external pacing, if indicated • Treatment of possible shunt thrombosis, and • Early activation of the ECLS team

Contd...

Contd...

Physiology	Unique challenges	Data	Recommended action[12]

Superior cavopulmonary anastomosis and Fontan	• Chest compressions create SBF but minimal PBF. Reduced PBF causes:
	  – Reduced oxygenation
	  – Reduced preload to systemic ventricle causing low cardiac output
	• Low cardiac output can worsen, if there is hemodynamically significant AVVR[14]
	• Increased risk of neurological injury due to increased SVC pressure, limiting cerebral blood flow[14]
		• Poor survival if develops cardiac arrest, increased risk of end organ injury[13]
		• 0.9% of patients (17 of 1,923) undergoing a Fontan correction developed postoperative cardiac arrest, and 41.2% of these patients died[13]
		• (STS-CHSD registry data)
			• Ventilatory strategies such as spontaneous or negative-pressure ventilation can be useful to increase cardiac output *(Class IIa; Level of Evidence C)*
			• In conditions causing hypoxemia, ventilatory strategies that target a mild respiratory acidosis and a minimum mean airway pressure without atelectasis can be useful to increase cerebral and systemic arterial oxygenation *(Class IIa; Level of Evidence B)*
			• Intervention when prearrest low cardiac output is recognized and impaired DO_2 develop. *(Class IIa; Level of Evidence C)*

Right-sided heart disease (RVOT reconstruction: TOF, double-outlet RV TOF type, truncus arteriosus)	At risk for both systolic and diastolic RV dysfunction. The risk is determined by: • Age of the patient • Degree of volume or pressure overload imposed on the RV • Duration the RV has been exposed to abnormal loading conditions • Residual or additional postoperative lesions Physiological and anatomic factors associated with an increased risk of postoperative RV systolic or diastolic dysfunction: • Preoperative RV hypertrophy with an RV that functions at systemic (or suprasystemic) pressures and decompresses through a ventricular septal defect (VSD) • An operative procedure that includes VSD closure and RV outflow tract reconstruction • Postoperative pulmonary valve insufficiency with acute RV volume loading (particularly if the RV is hypertrophied) RV dysfunction from resection of muscular obstruction (especially if the moderator band is damaged or excised) or ventriculotomy with or without insertion of an RV-to-pulmonary artery conduit	Hospital survival was 95.0% for the tetralogy of Fallot group and 90.7% for the truncus arteriosus group[15]	• Recommendations for high-quality CPR should be followed • Limited filling of the RV during chest recoil if the RV has restrictive physiology with diastolic dysfunction • Additional fluid should be administered to augment intravascular volume • Decreased PBF due to worsening pulmonary regurgitation during chest compression, LV preload and cardiac output • Minimize the time to repeat administration of epinephrine as coronary perfusion and blood flow to a hypertrophied RV can be limited during chest compressions • Hemodynamically significant supraventricular arrhythmia [i.e., supraventricular tachycardia (SVT) or JET] should be viewed as prearrest states and must be identified and treated promptly • Chest compressions can compress and obstruct the reconstructed RV outflow tract • Thus, if CPR is needed in the immediate postoperative period, opening chest to enable open-chest cardiac massage might be necessary

Contd...

Contd…

Physiology	Unique challenges	Data	Recommended action[12]

Pulmonary arterial hypertension (PAH)	• Children with PAH can develop sudden cardiac arrest[16-20]
	• Arrhythmia, pulmonary hemorrhage, left main coronary compression by the pulmonary artery, pulmonary artery dissection or embolus, spontaneous PAH crisis, or dose reduction or withdrawal of a pulmonary artery vasodilator can trigger cardiac arrest.
	• Acute RV decompensation in a patient with little reserve is usually the ultimate cause of the cardiac arrest
		Conventional resuscitation with CPR and medications is rarely effective with a 6% reported survival rate in adults with PAH developing cardiac arrest[17]	• Treat possible reversible causes of increased PVR:
			  – Inadvertent interruption in targeted pulmonary hypertension drugs
			  – Hypercarbia
			  – Hypoxia
			  – Arrhythmia
			  – Cardiac tamponade, or
			  – Drug toxicity
			• Alkali administration does not improve outcome, excessive ventilation during resuscitation is harmful[18]
			• Positive-pressure ventilation will decrease systemic venous return, RV filling, and cardiac output generated during chest compressions
			• Rapid consideration of ECLS provides best survival chance, if high-quality CPR and pulmonary hypertension specific therapy fails[19-21]

• Left-sided heart disease • Severe mitral valve stenosis and mitral regurgitation	• Elevated LA pressure and PVR limit effective PBF and ultimately the systemic cardiac output generated by chest compressions • In severe mitral stenosis, cardiac output generated by chest compressions is further limited by restriction of flow of pulmonary venous return across the mitral valve and decreased filling of the LV • In severe mitral regurgitation, cardiac output generated by chest compressions is further limited by the regurgitant blood flow from the LV across the mitral valve	In a study of >100 children undergoing mitral valve repair or replacement predominantly for mitral regurgitation, the mortality rate was nearly 10%, and 10% required mechanical circulatory support in the immediate postoperative period[21]	If high-quality CPR remains ineffective, early consideration of ECLS might offer the best chance of survival
Critical aortic valve stenosis and severe aortic valve regurgitation	• In aortic stenosis flow across the aortic valve is obstructed so the stroke volume and cardiac output generated during chest compressions are reduced • Hypertrophied LV is poorly compliant limiting LV filling further compromising stroke volume and cardiac output	Newborns with critical aortic stenosis, percutaneous aortic balloon valvuloplasty is associated with low mortality and is the preferred approach in most centers[21]	Chest compressions must generate sufficient aortic root pressure to support adequate coronary perfusion to the hypertrophied myocardium

Contd…

Contd...

Physiology	Unique challenges	Data	Recommended action[12]
	In aortic regurgitation, the regurgitant flow across the aortic valve back into the LV in aortic regurgitation, limits the stroke volume and cardiac output generated during chest compressions, compromising both cardiac output and coronary perfusion	In presence of pre-existing LV dysfunction both percutaneous and surgical interventions are associated with higher mortality[21,22]	
Total anomalous pulmonary venous connection (TAPVC)	• Neonates with obstructed TAPVC can present in a critical state immediately after birth with a combination of respiratory failure, pulmonary hypertension, and circulatory collapse; preoperative ECLS is occasionally indicated to support DO_2[23] • Poor LV diastolic function and pulmonary hypertension is common after correction of TAPVC. High-quality CPR and resuscitation drugs may be ineffective in generating PBF, LV filling, and cardiac output		• Treat possible reversible causes of increased PVR, including inadvertent interruption in targeted pulmonary hypertension drugs, hypercarbia, hypoxia, acidosis, arrhythmia, or cardiac tamponade • Provision of pulmonary hypertension–specific therapy including iNO, 100% oxygen, and establishment of adequate ventilation • ECLS can be beneficial if the above fails

(AVVR: atrioventricular valve regurgitation; DBP: diastolic blood pressure; ECLS: extracorporeal life support; iNO: inhaled nitric oxide; JET: junctional ectopic tachycardia; LV: left ventricle; LA: left atrium; PBF: pulmonary blood flow; PVR: pulmonary vascular resistance; RV: right ventricle; RVOT: right ventricular outflow tract; SVR: systemic vascular resistance; STS-CHSD: Society of thoracic surgeons-congenital heart surgery database; SBF: systemic blood flow; SVC: superior vena cava; TOF: tetralogy of Fallot; VSD: ventricular septal defect)

TABLE 4: Energy doses for cardioversion and defibrillation.[12]

Rhythm	Energy
SVT or VT/wide-complex tachycardia with a pulse	• An initial energy dose of 0.5–1 J/kg synchronized to avoid precipitating VF • Subsequent dose is increased to 2 J/kg, if initial low dose does not work; again synchronized mode
VF/pulseless VT	• Initial dose of 2–4 J/kg • Subsequent doses use 4 J/kg, and higher doses can be considered, although the dose should not exceed 10 J/kg[6] • Open sternum and internal paddles, the adult dose for defibrillation is 10–20 J, and 0.6–0.7 J/kg in children

(SVT: supraventricular tachycardia; VT: ventricular tachycardia; VF: ventricular fibrillation)

Site for Chest Compression in Single Ventricle

The AHA recommends that compressions be performed on the sternum just below the intermammary line in infants and on the lower half of the sternum in children.[24] However, there is limited data on whether there is a need to modify this position in infants and children with single ventricle (or any CHD). A recent Korean single center case series of 185 patients (median age 0.5–12.5 years) with single ventricle [73 before creation of the superior cavopulmonary anastomosis (CPA), 61 after superior CPA, and 51 after Fontan procedure)] found that in all patients, the largest cross-sectional area of the systemic ventricle [assessed by computed tomography (CT) scan] was under the lower quarter (i.e., bottom 25%) of the sternum.[25]

Mechanical Support

ECLS and ECPR

Extracorporeal life support (ECLS) also known as extracorporeal membrane oxygenation (ECMO) is used in hospitals for the treatment of CA in adults and children refractory to initial high quality CPR.[26] When ECLS is deployed during resuscitation of CA, it is referred to as ECPR. The cannulation strategy employed for ECPR is summarized in **Table 5**.

The mechanical circulatory support algorithm is depicted in **Flowchart 2**.[27]

Post-arrest Phase

The post-arrest phase is characterized into immediate, early, intermediate, and recovery stages according to the American Heart Association guidelines (**Fig. 3**). The crux of post-arrest management is to limit ongoing injury, provision of organ support and rehabilitation.

◼ MONITORING

General monitoring includes standard ICU care such as continuous electrocardiography, pulse oximetry, blood pressure measurement (typically invasive estimates in the PCICU), temperature, and urine output. Specific monitoring might be extended to end-tidal carbon dioxide, measure of core temperature, electroencephalography to (rule out seizures and for prognostication), periodic assessment of arterial blood gases

TABLE 5: Cannulation strategy for ECPR.[12]					
	Peripheral cannulation		**Central cannulation**		
Physiology	**Venous**	**Arterial**	**Venous**	**Arterial**	**Comments**
Biventricular circulation	Internal jugular or femoral	Common carotid or femoral	Systemic venous atrium	Aorta	Left atrial decompression may be required
Single ventricle or shunted physiology	Internal jugular	Common carotid	Systemic venous or common atrium	Aorta	Shunt restriction may be required; for carotid cannulation with an MBTS, cannula position can result in shunt overcirculation or occlusion
Superior cavopulmonary anastomosis	Internal jugular and/or femoral	Common carotid	SVC and/or systemic venous or common atrium	Aorta	Additional venous cannula may be required
Fontan	Internal jugular and/or femoral	Common carotid or femoral	Fontan baffle	Aorta	Additional venous cannula may be required; pulmonary venous atrial drainage may be required

(MBTS: modified Blalock-Taussig shunt; SVC: superior vena cava; ECPR: extracorporeal cardiopulmonary resuscitation

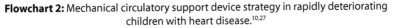

Flowchart 2: Mechanical circulatory support device strategy in rapidly deteriorating children with heart disease.[10,27]

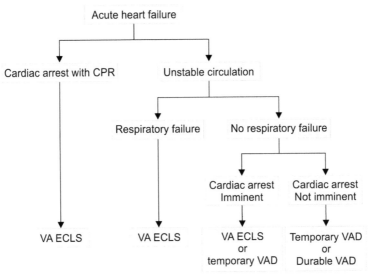

(VA ECLS: venoarterial extracorporeal life support; VAD: ventricular assist device; CPR: cardiopulmonary resuscitation)

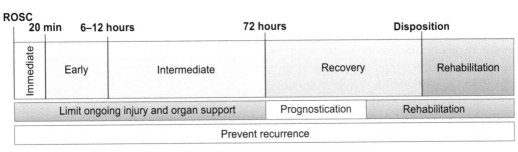

Fig. 3: Post-arrest management.
(ROSC: return of spontaneous circulation)

for ventilatory status, blood sugar and electrolytes, and some form of brain imaging typically later in the phase of postarrest for prognostication, if warranted.

Neurological Monitoring

Major goals of post–CA care are mitigating the extension of the primary ischemic brain injury and prevention of secondary brain injury. Therefore, it is important to ensure appropriate neurological monitoring in the post-arrest phase to facilitate optimal recovery. The following action items should be given careful consideration while monitoring a post-CA patient.

Electroencephalography: Electroencephalography (EEG) is important to identify and treat seizures that may not be clinically apparent. Seizures can increase cerebral metabolic demand and cause secondary injury. However, seizures can be a symptom (as opposed to the cause) of the degree of injury that is already present.[28,29] It is recommended to initiate EEG monitoring as soon as feasible, and continue monitoring for 24–48 hours (or for 24 hours after return to normothermia) whenever possible.

Hyperoxia and hypercapnea: After ROSC target PaO_2 and $PaCO_2$ value appropriate to the specific patient condition.[27] It is now typical to recommend the lowest fraction of oxygen needed for a target oxygenation of 94–99% on pulse oximetry. In patients with univentricular physiology, accepting an oxygen saturation appropriate to the cardiac physiology is reasonable. Further, ventilation should be titrated to normocapnia recognizing the harms of extreme variation in carbon dioxide levels on potentiating brain injury.

Fever > 38°C on first day of resuscitation, is a common consequence of the post-resuscitation syndrome and is considered detrimental to outcomes.[30,31] The PALS 2015 guideline recommends either 5 days of continuous normothermia or 2 days of deliberate hypothermia (32–34°C) followed by normothermia (36.5–37.5°C) for the next 3 days.[24] The potential risks of hypothermia in children with CHD, particularly, its effects on hemodynamics and on drug metabolism should be kept in mind.[32]

There is insufficient evidence to suggest a particular glucose target post ROSC. Neither is there proof of benefit from use of corticosteroids.

Finally, for those children who recover from cardiac arrest, a multidisciplinary evaluation with formulation of a comprehensive care plan (that takes into account the acute after-effects such as respiratory, nutritional, and neuromuscular insufficiency from the long stay) and a medium term plan for those who have neurologic sequeleae from the event, are important considerations to facilitate good outcomes.

■ SUMMARY

Cardiac arrest in PCICU is almost always preventable and therefore available tools for recognizing pre-arrest situations should be efficiently utilized to escalate care as appropriate. The existing knowledge gaps in cardiac arrest management should be addressed to provide high quality CPR suited to the specific circulatory physiology in children with CHD. Comprehensive post-arrest management is important to limit end-organ injury and facilitate good outcomes.

■ REFERENCES

1. Parra DA, Totapally BR, Zahn E, Jacobs J, Aldousany A, Burke RP, et al. Outcome of cardiopulmonary resuscitation in a pediatric cardiac intensive care unit. Crit Care Med. 2000;28(9):3296-300.
2. Tabbutt S, Marino BS. Cardiopulmonary resuscitation in congenital and acquired heart disease. Pediatr Crit Care Med. 2016;17: S194-200.
3. Peddy SB, Fran Hazinski M, Laussen PC, Thiagarajan RR, Hoffman GM, Nadkarni V, et al. Cardiopulmonary resuscitation: special considerations for infants and children with cardiac disease. Cardiol Young. 2007; 17(S4):116-26.
4. Lowry AW, Knudson JD, Cabrera AG, Graves DE, Morales DLS, Rossano JW. Cardiopulmonary resuscitation in hospitalized children with cardiovascular disease: estimated prevalence and outcomes from the Kids' inpatient database. Pediatr Crit Care Med. 2013;14(3):248-55.
5. McLellan MC, Connor JA. The cardiac children's hospital early warning score (C-CHEWS). J Pediatr Nurs. 2013;28(2):171-8.
6. De Caen AR, Berg MD, Chameides L, Gooden CK, Hickey RW, Scott HF, et al. Part 12: Pediatric advanced life support: 2015 American Heart Association guidelines update for cardiopulmonary resuscitation and emergency cardiovascular care. Circulation. 2015;132(18):S526-42.
7. Maconochie IK, Aickin R, Hazinski MF, Atkins DL, Bingham R, Couto TB, et al. Pediatric life support: 2020 International consensus

on cardiopulmonary resuscitation and emergency cardiovascular care science with treatment recommendations. Circulation. 2020;142:140-84.

8. Meaney PA, Bobrow BJ, Mancini ME, Christenson J, de Caen AR, Bhanji F, et al. Cardiopulmonary resuscitation quality: improving cardiac resuscitation outcomes both inside and outside the hospital. Circulation. 2013;128(4):417-35.

9. Joffe AR, Lequier L, Robertson CM. Pediatric outcomes after extracorporeal membrane oxygenation for cardiac disease and for cardiac arrest: a review. ASAIO J. 2012;58(4):297-310.

10. Kane DA, Thiagarajan RR, Wypij D, Scheurer MA, Fynn-Thompson F, Emani S, et al. Rapid-response extracorporeal membrane oxygenation to support cardiopulmonary resuscitation in children with cardiac disease. Circulation. 2010;122(11 Suppl):S241-8.

11. Brand J, McDonald A, Dunning J. Management of cardiac arrest following cardiac surgery. BJA Educ. 2018;18(1):16-22.

12. Marino BS, Tabbutt S, MacLaren G, Hazinski MF, Adatia I, Atkins DL, et al. Cardiopulmonary resuscitation in infants and children with cardiac disease: a scientific statement from the American Heart Association. Circulation. 2018;137:691-782.

13. Gupta P, Jacobs JP, Pasquali SK, Hill KD, Gaynor JW, O'Brien SM, et al. Epidemiology and outcomes after in-hospital cardiac arrest after pediatric cardiac surgery. Ann Thorac Surg. 2014;98(6):2138-43.

14. Jolley M, Thiagarajan RR, Barrett CS, Salvin JW, Cooper DS, Rycus PT, et al. Extracorporeal membrane oxygenation in patients undergoing superior cavopulmonary anastomosis. J Thorac Cardiovasc Surg. 2014;148(4):1512-8.

15. Kaza AK, Lim HG, Dibardino DJ, Bautista-Hernandez V, Robinson J, Allan C, et al. Long-term results of right ventricular outflow tract reconstruction in neonatal cardiac surgery: options and outcomes. J Thorac Cardiovasc Surg. 2009;138(4):911-6.

16. Sanatani S, Wilson G, Smith CR, Hamilton RM, Williams WG, Adatia I. Sudden unexpected death in children with heart disease. Congenit Heart Dis. 2006;1(3):89-97.

17. Hoeper MM, Galiè N, Murali S, Olschewski H, Rubenfire M, Robbins IM, et al. Outcome after cardiopulmonary resuscitation in patients with pulmonary arterial hypertension. Am J Respir Crit Care Med. 2002;165(3):341-4.

18. Aufderheide TP, Lurie KG. Death by hyperventilation: a common and life-threatening problem during cardiopulmonary resuscitation. Crit Care Med. 2004;32(9 Suppl):S345-51.

19. King R, Esmail M, Mahon S, Dingley J, Dwyer S. Use of nitric oxide for decompensated right ventricular failure and circulatory shock after cardiac arrest. Br J Anaesth. 2000;85(4):628-31.

20. Rubin LJ. Primary pulmonary hypertension. N Engl J Med. 1997;336(2):111-7.

21. Myles PS, Hall JL, Berry CB, Esmore DS. Primary pulmonary hypertension: prolonged cardiac arrest and successful resuscitation following induction of anesthesia for heart-lung transplantation. J Cardiothorac Vasc Anesth. 1994;8(6):678-81.

22. Agnoletti G, Raisky O, Boudjemline Y, Ou P, Bonnet D, Sidi D, et al. Neonatal surgical aortic commissurotomy: predictors of outcome and long-term results. Ann Thorac Surg. 2006;82(5):1585-92.

23. Ishino K, Alexi-Meskishvili V, Hetzer R. Preoperative extracorporeal membrane oxygenation in newborns with total anomalous pulmonary venous connection. Cardiovasc Surg. 1999;7(4):473-5.

24. Atkins DL, Berger S, Duff JP, Gonzales JC, Hunt EA, Joyner BL, et al. Part 11: Pediatric Basic Life Support and Cardiopulmonary Resuscitation Quality: 2015 American Heart Association Guidelines Update for Cardiopulmonary Resuscitation and Emergency Cardiovascular Care. Circulation. 2015;132(18 Suppl 2):S519-25.

25. Park JB, Song IK, Lee JH, Kim EH, Kim HS, Kim JT. Optimal chest compression position for patients with a single ventricle during cardiopulmonary resuscitation. Pediatr Crit Care Med. 2016;17(4):303-6.

26. Raymond TT, Cunnyngham CB, Thompson MT, Thomas JA, Dalton HJ, Nadkarni VM. Outcomes among neonates, infants, and children after extracorporeal cardiopulmonary resuscitation for refractory inhospital pediatric cardiac arrest: a report from the National Registry of Cardiopulmonary Resuscitation. Pediatr Crit Care Med. 2010;11(3):362-71.

27. Kleinman ME, Chameides L, Schexnayder SM, Samson RA, Hazinski MF, Atkins DL, et al. Part 14: Pediatric advanced life support:

2010 American Heart Association Guidelines for Cardiopulmonary Resuscitation and Emergency Cardiovascular Care. Circulation. 2010;122(18 Suppl 3):S876-908.

28. DeLorenzo RJ, Waterhouse EJ, Towne AR, Boggs JG, Ko D, DeLorenzo GA, et al. Persistent nonconvulsive status epilepticus after the control of convulsive status epilepticus. Epilepsia. 1998;39(8):833-40.

29. Jaitly R, Sgro JA, Towne AR, Ko D, DeLorenzo RJ. Prognostic value of EEG monitoring after status epilepticus: a prospective adult study. J Clin Neurophysiol. 1997;14(4):326-34.

30. Nolan JP, Neumar RW, Adrie C, Aibiki M, Berg RA, Böttiger BW, et al. Post-cardiac arrest syndrome: epidemiology, pathophysiology, treatment, and prognostication. A Scientific Statement from the International Liaison Committee on Resuscitation; the American Heart Association Emergency Cardiovascular Care Committee; the Council on Cardiovascular Surgery and Anesthesia; the Council on Cardiopulmonary, Perioperative, and Critical Care; the Council on Clinical Cardiology; the Council on Stroke. Resuscitation. 2008;79(3):350-79.

31. Jaskiewicz JA, McCarthy CA, Richardson AC, White KC, Fisher DJ, Dagan R, et al. Febrile infants at low risk for serious bacterial infection—an appraisal of the Rochester criteria and implications for management. Febrile Infant Collaborative Study Group. Pediatrics. 1994;94(3):390-6.

32. Polderman KH. Application of therapeutic hypo-thermia in the intensive care unit. Opportunities and pitfalls of a promising treatment modality–Part 2: Practical aspects and side effects. Intens Care Med. 2004;30(5):757-69.

41

CHAPTER

Infections after Pediatric Cardiac Surgery: A Primer for Clinicians in Low Resource Settings

Aveek Jayant

Reviewed by: R Krishna Kumar

▪ INTRODUCTION

Congenital heart disease (CHD) is the most common birth defect.[1] Access to adequate surgical expertise remains a key focus.[2] Even as efforts to improve this facet of caring for children with CHD gain momentum it is important to recognize that substantial improvements have been made in individual centers.[3] It is also vital to recognize that infectious risks pose disproportionate hazards to undoing the substantial quality improvements that have been made over the previous few years.[4] This risk applies to care processes in existence and those in evolution. While, undoubtedly, the maximum focus in relation to pediatric cardiac care should be on preventing these infections in the first place, the galloping increases in antimicrobial resistance[5-7] will do well to reinforce the tremendous urgency of the steps needed in redesigning care overall. As lower resource settings gain momentum in providing for these children they will likely shift progressively to operating on smaller children, particularly, neonates. A shift in primacy is evident in the recent guidelines from India.[8] This population faces unprecedented risks from hospital acquired infections, in general, and gram negative bacterial and fungal sepsis, in particular.[9,10] Viewed from another perspective there is an imperative need to ration and rationalize antibiotic prescriptions in the pediatric cardiac intensive care unit; the net practice toward this goal constitutes antimicrobial stewardship (AMS).[11,12] AMS coupled with rigorous infection control are the key pragmatic steps to halt the devastation wrought by hospital acquired sepsis. Yet, AMS cannot easily be sustained in a program that has poor infection control, overall. The combination of surgical stress and cardiopulmonary bypass make the clinical and preliminary laboratory diagnosis of hospital acquired infections difficult in the setting of pediatric cardiac surgery as the pan-inflammatory state owing to both share many features in common.[13] Thus, all in all, we make a case for practical and continuous infection control and antimicrobial stewardship as the key elements of the delivery of pediatric cardiac care. In this chapter, we primarily discuss infection control while the general guidelines on perioperative antibiotic use are covered in the chapter on antibiotic policy (Chapter 15).

▪ PREVENTING INFECTIONS

1. Handwashing
2. Bloodstream infections (BSI)

3. Infectious ventilator associated complications (IVAC)
4. Urinary tract infections
5. Sternal wound infections.

Handwashing

Handwashing is the cornerstone of infection control in hospitals. It was first proposed by the Hungarian physician Ignaz Semmelweis (1818–65) who is now regarded as the Father of Infection Control (although his efforts to pioneer this during his lifetime did not see the light of day).[14] While universally accepted as the key to infection control, it is still plagued by extremely patchy implementation.[15] The World Health Organization (WHO) has championed handwashing at the center of its campaign for patient safety ever since 2009.[16] The WHO has suggested this key maneuver to include 6 steps and guidance to perform each of these steps at 5 well defined time points in clinical practice.[17] From the universal experience of infection control experts this simple paradigm needs constant reinforcement and has, even till date, not achieved the uniform adherence that is expected across and within hospitals. Direct observation as a key to improving handwashing practice has been the gold standard but is confounded by the Hawthorne effect.[18] Finer analysis of the steps of handwashing practice reveals it to involve some complexity in terms of the psychomotor and cognitive skills. This results in some steps being more difficult to replicate than the others.[19] As a corollary, numerous methods have been attempted including curtailing steps[20] and using gaming based technology to improve performance.[21,22] Evidence also suggests that shortening the prescribed duration to about half in experienced nurses is as efficacious as the prescribed 30 seconds.[23] These innovations are important as diligent studies have shown that one of the crucial impediments to effective handwashing is time: in busy surgical intensive care units (ICU) as the number of opportunities increase, so does the amount of time required to be set aside for handwashing alone.[24] In surgical ICUs, conscientious handwashing could take up to an hour a shift and this crucial time element could be a failure in overall poor compliance.[24] Finally, there is the element of feedback. Observation by infection control nurses has been considered the gold standard of handwashing compliance.[25] Electronic monitoring, although probably not standardized as yet, might modify the process of feedback. Low resource settings should also consider modeling compliance based on additional methods such as handrub utilization.[26] In sum, we suggest scrupulous handwashing is still not an established practice in most hospital settings. Continuous effort is required to implement this strategy using a mix of literature proven and unit specific strategies.

Bloodstream Infections

Bloodstream infections (BSI) have a devastating impact on patients, in general, and in vulnerable patients such as neonates, in particular. In the Delhi Neonatal Infection Study (DeNIS), about 25% of the deaths in neonatal intensive care were attributable to sepsis with culture positive sepsis causing mortality rates between 12 and 15%.[9] Data from our center and other centers in low resource settings has shown that infections could increase mortality rates three fold in postoperative pediatric cardiac critical care besides lengthening duration of ventilation and length of stay in ICU.[4] Infections could derail outcomes in low risk surgical groups as well.[4] At the same time, multidrug resistance in hospital and other settings continues to increase in hospital and in the larger environment around us.[6,7] This makes preventing infections a high priority. Preventing infections has centered on key steps in preoperative, intraprocedural, and postprocedural care. This has been formulated as a bundle and the bundle approach continues to receive extended validation.[27,28] Insertion focuses on handwashing (scrubbing at our unit), full barrier precautions, chlorhexidine preparation of skin (although it is uncertain whether this should be universally implemented in children below 2 months of age[29]) and, using the least number of lumens as feasible. Site specific guidance is exceptionable for pediatric and neonatal central venous catheter (CVC) insertion unlike adults where subclavian site is chosen over others;[30] this is, above all, related to the practical difficulties in securing access in the smallest children. It is recommended to use nonsuture based methods for securing catheters;[31] however, it is uncertain how many postoperative units follow this guidance. For patients younger than 18 years there are no recommendations as to dressing methods but current Center for Disease Control and Prevention (CDC) recommendations suggest use of chlorhexidine impregnated dressings for all adults.[31] Likewise it is not routine currently to use antibiotic impregnated catheters in children presenting for cardiac surgery although there is guidance from the CDC to consider their use should the anticipated duration of catheter days exceed 5 days at the time of insertion. For arterial catheter insertions at central sites precautions similar to CVC insertion are recommended whereas for peripheral arterial lines handwashing alone might suffice. There are no recommendations as to how frequently an arterial line should be changed but CVC should have the shortest residence time in situ and consideration

to relocating the CVC to a different site might be considered on an individualized basis beyond 7 days of insertion in our unit. This is a unit specific policy given that routine replacement of CVC so as to prevent infection is not a recommended practice. For peripheral catheters a time period of 72–96 hours is typically suggested for adults, but in children catheters need only be replaced on an "as needed" basis. Guidewire exchanges in groups such as neonates have tentative approval[31] (given the overall difficulty in securing these lines) but our unit prefers to site these catheters at a different location whenever feasible. High primacy is given to removing a CVC as early as feasible: this is backed by high quality evidence and a strong recommendation from different guidelines.[29,31] For umbilical vascular access, it is generally suggested removal as soon as feasible, typically before 5 days of insertion though in exceptional circumstances these catheters may be maintained for up to 15 days.[29]

Maintenance bundles are probably more important than insertion bundles given that their efficacy is a time dependent domain and involves more than one operation. It is therefore the use of the CVC in intensive care that probably poses the highest infectious risk. Current recommendations suggest that handwashing and sterile gloves are used before accessing the device. In addition, when injection ports are accessed they should be duly disinfected with 70% alcohol that is allowed to dry before injection. Administration sets, hubs, three way stopcocks are ideally replaced every 72 hours. Daily chlorhexidine baths are also encouraged and there is fairly consistent evidence that this dents the incidence of bacteremia/Central Line Associated Bloodstream Infection (CLABSI).[32,33] Finally, in units not able to stem the CLABSI rate at acceptable levels, it is possible to consider chlorhexidine impregnated dressings (in children > 3 months) or antibiotic locks.[29]

In addition to operational efficiency in following bundle-based care, it is also important to put in place a surveillance mechanism for all infections in the ICU including BSIs. Surveillance outlines the deficits in bundle implementation and is the first step toward redirecting infection control approaches to a higher level of stringency. Bloodstream infections are commonly divided into two distinct categories: Primary and secondary, the latter due to blood seeding of infection at another body site. Focus of this section is on preventing primary BSI. BSI, in the presence of a CVC have two different surveillance definitions[34]: Central Line Related Bloodstream Infections (CRBSI) and Central Line Associated Bloodstream Infections (CLABSI). CRBSI pins down the diagnosis to the CVC as the incriminating factor and relies on an earlier time to positivity or a higher colony count in paired cultures from the CVC and another site. CRBSI operational surveillance is not implemented in many centers as paired samples are not always feasible in children and this definition does entail higher costs. CLABSI, on the other hand can only circumstantially link the CVC to the BSI by insisting on a gap of at least two calendar days from insertion/access to first diagnosis. However when using CLABSI based surveillance, reported rates are usually underestimated.[35]

Special considerations apply to the neonatal population. Preterm infants (increasingly served as health systems improve and surgical units take on this challenge) are prone to infection and have both short- and long-term consequences such as death and neurodevelopmental disability respectively.[36] Neonates operated early on in life are not immune from acquired infections from the birth passage such as group B Streptococcus. Once admitted to units caring for critical CHD, a different risk exposure begins right from insertion of peripheral venous access to discharge from a surgical critical care unit, in our unit, this occasionally does takes the form of multidrug resistant gram negative sepsis, given their preponderance in the hospital ecology[10] and in the larger community.[37] Both of the common biomarkers (C-reactive protein and procalcitonin) used to adjudicate infections are not useful early in postnatal life; in addition, of course, they are not useful immediately proximate to cardiac surgery.[13] Given that there is a significant burden of culture negative sepsis, it is important for units to make a protocol adapted from several of the guidelines[38-40] in the literature to arbitrate the need for antibiotics balancing stewardship to individual clinical risk in a systematic manner.

Infectious Ventilator Associated Complications

Prior to 2013, the diagnosis of ventilator associated pneumonia (VAP) was primarily radiologic and this was recognized as inadequate for surveillance purposes. Adult definitions were revised and defined as infectious ventilator associated complications since then. Pediatric and neonatal definitions however lagged and, to date, continue to be in some flux. While there appears to be data to suggest that developing a ventilator associated event (VAE) does alter clinical course, it is still problematic to sort patients into the three boxes that are suggested: ventilator associated complications, infectious ventilator associated complications and VAP.[41] Our unit experience is that currently applied definitions may inadequately capture these complications. Further, the developers stress that this is a surveillance

TABLE 1: Definitions of ventilator associated events (VAE).

VAE category	Requirements and criteria
A. Ventilator associated condition (VAC)	• Definitions are applied to patients on mechanical ventilation for at least 4 days • Patients are required to be stable on ventilator for ≥ 2 calendar days preceding event or showing daily decline in minimum mean airway pressure (MAP) or FiO_2 values (defined by lowest value of FiO_2 or PEEP (positive end expiratory pressure) during a calendar day that is maintained for at least 1 hour • VAC criteria – Increase $FiO_2 \geq 0.25$ or MAP > 4 cmH_2O sustained for 2 days (for definition purposes MAP 0–8 cmH_2O = 8 cmH_2O)
B. Infection related ventilator associated complications (IVAC)	• VAC criteria + Temperatures <36°C or>38°C or abnormal white blood cell (WBC) count <4,000 or >12,000 cells/mm³ AND • A new antimicrobial agent is started and continued for > 4 days within 2 days of the increase in PEEP or FiO_2
C. Possible ventilator associated pneumonia (PVAP)	Meets criteria in IVAC in B above and additionally • Positive culture from respiratory secretions [endotracheal aspirate, bronchoalveolar lavage (BAL), lung tissue or protected specimen brush] >10⁵ colony forming units (CFU)/mL • Purulent respiratory secretions (>25 polymorphonuclear cells and <10 squamous epithelial cells per low power field) and positive culture as above but not meeting the quantitative threshold OR • A positive test from pleural fluid or lung histopathology or diagnosis positive for Legionella/a respiratory virus within 2 days of meeting the IVAC criteria

TABLE 2: Clinical pulmonary infection score (for ventilated children).

Variables	Score		
	0	1	2
Temperature	36.5–38.4°C	38.5–39°C	<36° or >39°C
WBC (10⁹ L⁻¹)	4–11	<4 or >11 and absence of band forms or >11–17 with no differentiation	>11 with band forms or > 17 with no differentiation
Pulmonary secretions	Absent	Present but not purulent	Present and purulent
Chest X-ray	No infiltrate	Diffuse or patchy infiltrate	Localized infiltrate
Oxygenation (PaO_2/FiO_2)	> 240 and no ARDS		< 240 and ARDS
Microbiology	Negative		Positive

(WBC: white blood cell; ARDS: acute respiratory distress syndrome)

definition, and clinical workflow and diagnoses are not adequately defined by the current nomenclature. An overview of these definitions is provided in **Table 1** but these definitions are in evolution and often institution specific.[41,42] Although the latest National Health Systems Network (NHSN) uses mean airway pressure (MAP), other authors have used positive end expiratory pressure (PEEP) in place of MAP.[34]

Table 2 and Box 1 show other representative scoring systems.[41] However, no score is perfect and the cornerstones of diagnosis: temperature instability or chest radiological change are confounded by a range of age dependent or environment

Radiologic criteria

- New or progressive pulmonary infiltrates
- Pneumatoceles
- Consolidation or cavitation if < 1 year old. On 2 serial chest X-rays

Clinical criteria (at least 3 clinical or laboratory criteria)

- New or worsening purulent bronchial secretions
- Core temperature > 38.5°C or < 36°C
- White blood cell (WBC) counts
  - 0–1 week > 34×10^9 L^{-1}
  - 1 week to 1 month > 19.5 or < 5×10^9 L^{-1}
  - 1 month–1 year >17.5 or <5×10^9 L^{-1}
  - 2–5 years > 15.5 or <6×10^9 L^{-1}
  - 6–12 years >13.5 or < 4.5×10^9 L^{-1}
  - 13–18 years > 11 or < 4×10^9 L^{-1}
- Significant (+) culture from respiratory specimen *OR*
- Significant culture from alternate site

dependent conditions.[43] The CDC criteria stand out for their lack of including chest radiology in the diagnostic paradigm and the reasons are well known.[44]

Among pediatric patients, VAP is most common in the age group of 2–12 months and then again in children beyond 10 years of age.[45] In India, VAP rates can be as high as 38%[46] in the general pediatric intensive care units (PICU) with gram negative organisms majorly implicated; evolving epidemiology suggests *Acinetobacter* spp. *and Pseudomonas* spp predominate,[46] whereas in other practice settings *Staphylococcus, Haemophilus* and other common respiratory pathogens in the community are reported.[47] Given the epidemiology in low resource settings, chances of drug resistant Enterobacteriaceae and other multidrug resistant gram negative bugs being recovered as the causative organisms is likely common. Expectedly, VAP and other healthcare associated infections (HAIs) increase patient cost besides greatly lengthening stay in intensive care by close to a week

or more.[48] Therefore, it is only logical that high priority be accorded to VAP prevention.

The VAP prevention has many similar principles to preventing HAI in general: as in prevention of BSI handwashing by healthcare workers who provide respiratory care to children is the most primary intervention. It has been proven that this omnibus generic approach based on handwashing simultaneously decreases all categories of HAI.[45] The other key elements of VAP[49] prevention in children are: (1) Age appropriate oral care; (2) Head of bed elevation; (3) Application of aspiration precautions; (4) Proper airway suction techniques; and, (5) Maintenance of safe endotracheal cuff pressures. Other routine measures include suction only as needed and without instillation of saline whenever feasible, and avoidance of condensation of water in breathing circuits or their periodic drainage.[41] However, as with other PICU literature a lot of this evidence is extrapolated from adults and some of it, is of uncertain value when applied to the PICU. While there are structured guidelines for oral care in children[50] use of chlorhexidine in oral care for intubated children is inconsistently effective.[51] Likewise, while adults are often ventilated in semirecumbent positions to prevent gravitational aspiration of gastric contents and thus VAP, there are pediatric studies which show the lateral position to be better.[52] It is, in fact, recommended that infants are nursed supine and flat by the American Academy of Pediatrics.[53] Observational data do not support duration of enteral nutrition (EN) or use of prepyloric tubes to increase VAP rates; but they do show increased rates of VAP when universal antacid therapy is recommended.[54] Topically, a multicentric study of the use of stress ulcer prophylactic medications in children after congenital heart surgery is underway.[55] What should worry all practitioners from

BOX 2: INICC VAP prevention in PICU recommendations.

- Surveillance for VAP
- Hand hygiene
- Nursing in semirecumbent position
- Daily assessment of readiness to wean and use weaning protocols
- Regular oral care with an antiseptic solution
- Use of noninvasive ventilation whenever possible
- Preference of orotracheal over nasotracheal intubation
- Maintenance of endotracheal cuff pressures of 20 cmH$_2$O pressure
- Removal of condensate from ventilator tubings keeping the circuit closed during such removal
- Change of circuit only when circuit is visibly soiled
- Avoidance of gastric distention
- Avoidance of antacid therapies
- Use of sterile water to reuse reusable respiratory equipment

(INICC: International Nosocomial Infection Control Consortium; VAP: ventilator associated pneumonia; PICU: pediatric intensive care unit)

BOX 3: Preventing catheter associated urinary tract infections (CAUTI)—key elements.[61]

- Full barrier precautions and sterile preparation at insertion
- Avoid kinks and obstruction to allow free drainage
- Empty bag regularly
- Avoid disconnections
- Keep bag below bladder to prevent backflow
- Secure catheter to leg to avoid traction

low-middle income countries (LMIC) is the high rate of VAP reported in our practice[46] compared to the global benchmark rates for this complication, even in studies that are across countries and, therefore, more representative of the diversity of PICU settings (38% vs. 5% respectively).[56] VAP has been shown to increase the duration of ICU stay by >11 days and increase mortality risks by 3-fold.[56] The only representative evidence for VAP prophylaxis from a range of LMIC practice settings is from the International Nosocomial Infection Control Consortium (INICC);[57] this data includes data generated at the authors' hospital and is summarized in **Box 2**.

A range of the INICC recommendations however is in conflict with those of other PICUs; it is important to emphasize however one universal precept in prevention of VAP, viz. an attempt to minimize the at-risk period[56,57] by daily attempts to wean. More often than not, outside of the native cardiac condition and the attendant effects of surgery,

due attention is required for a sedoanalgesia protocol that factors this,[58] in addition, to structured assessment and protocolization.[59]

Catheter Associated Urinary Tract Infections

Catheter associated urinary tract infections (CAUTI) are less of a problem in the PICU/ pediatric cardiac intensive care unit (PCICU) setting as compared to adult intensive care.[60] Common with all the other preventable HAI the key prevention measures are, of course, avoidance of insertion and limiting the duration of use to the shortest possible time.[61] The other key elements of the bundle are summarized in **Box 3** and have high quality evidence backing them.

Sternal Wound Infections

Sternal wound infections after pediatric cardiac surgery are quoted to have an incidence ranging from 0.5 to 8%.[62-64] Traditional risk factors have been considered to be age <1 year, durations of cardiopulmonary bypass >105 minutes and exposure to multiple red cell transfusions;[65] a newly described risk factor has been preoperative length of stay in hospital preceding surgery.[64] A snapshot of the mined literature suggests there is virtually no uniformity with regard to the nature, doses and durations of surgical site infection prophylaxis in children undergoing cardiac surgery.[66,67] Interestingly, when single agent protocols using a first generation

BOX 4: Recommended actions for prevention of surgical site infections after pediatric cardiac surgery.[65,67]

Preoperative

- Screening and decontamination of the nares for MRSA, if local prevalence is high
- Chlorhexidine baths unless age and sensitivity are contraindications on the previous night and morning of surgery. Care for small children including precautions for thermal neutrality

Intraoperative

- Ensure a 2nd generation cephalosporin is administered within 60 minutes prior to skin incision; ensure repeat dosing 4 hourly and, if local protocols allow supplemental dosing into the pump prime
- Chlorhexidine skin preparation or povidone iodine skin preparation
- Minimize operating room flux

Postoperative

- Ensure barrier precautions before dressing change
- Use sterile precautions while performing echocardiograms 0–5 days after surgery
- Use an occlusive dressing for 48 hours
- Remove epicardial pacing wires as soon as feasible

(MRSA: methicillin-resistant *Staphylococcus aureus*)

cephalosporin was used there was a shift toward gram negative organisms from some reports and the overall incidence of gram negative organisms as the incriminating bacteria was around 20%. Thus, while it seems reasonable to focus on using anti-staphylococcal measures from the point of view of stewardship other measures such as diligent skin scrubs to remove such organisms from the surface also has renewed importance. In regions with high prevalence of Methicillin Resistant *Staphylococcus aureus* (MRSA) certain units routinely suggest decontamination of the nares with mupirocin ointment preoperatively. Chlorhexidine for skin preparation in all children >1,500 g is also advised.

An assortment of measures obtained from different sources is summarized in **Box 4**. A prickly issue is the use of antibiotics

as prophylaxis when the chest is not closed immediately after surgery (for surgical reasons related to cardiac function, myocardial edema, anticipated need for extracorporeal support, etc.). Here again, while the rates of usage or recommended prophylaxis is virtually non-existent in some settings[66] it could be universal in others.[68] The latter approach could be based on the high prevalence of infections in such patients in some reports (as high as 50%).[69] However, indiscriminate use of antibiotics or universal use of antibiotics should probably be considered not standard of care in the face of complete lack of evidence supporting this practice. Once deep sternal infections have set in, it is usual to prescribe antibiotics based on the culture and antibiotic sensitivity of isolates obtained from pus or tissue. It is however a point of debate as to how they are best managed: by early primary closure[62] or conservative management using vacuum assisted drainage.[63] The latter practice is slowly gaining traction[70] and, is near universally used in units such as ours.

■ SUMMARY

As can be seen from this overview of infection control and follow-up for infections after pediatric cardiac surgery, the only universal fact seems to be about enormous practice variations. It is also known that primary prevention is the way to go given that antibiotic stewardship is the only way to ration and make antibiotics available for the few children who would desperately need it when infections strike in this precarious pathway. This chapter is less about the methods (which we assume will be decided by a combination of local needs and practice and the established methods of controlling infections widely described in the literature) but more about reinforcing this imperative: of stringent infection control being a choiceless need in this surgical pathway.

■ REFERENCES

1. van der Linde D, Konings EE, Slager MA, Witsenburg M, Helbing WA, Takkenberg JJM, et al. Birth prevalence of congenital heart disease worldwide. J Am Coll Cardiol. 2011;58(21):2241-7.
2. Vervoort D, Zheleva B, Jenkins KJ, Dearani JA. Children at the heart of global cardiac surgery: an advocacy stakeholder analysis. World J Pediatr Congenit Heart Surg. 2021;12(1): 48-54.
3. Kumar R. Congenital heart disease profile: four perspectives. Ann Pediatr Cardiol. 2016; 9(3):203.
4. Sen AC, Morrow DF, Balachandran R, Du X, Gauvreau K, Jagannath BR, et al. Postoperative infection in developing world congenital heart surgery programs: data from the International Quality Improvement Collaborative. Circ Cardiovasc Qual Outcomes. 2017;10(4):2-9.
5. CDDEP. Scoping Report on Antimicrobial Resistance in India. [online] Available from: https:// cddep.org/wp-content/uploads/2017/11/scoping-report-on-antimicrobial-resistance-in-india.pdf. [Last Accessed April, 2021].
6. Taneja N, Sharma M. Antimicrobial resistance in the environment: the Indian scenario. Indian J Med Res. 2019;149(2):119.
7. Walia K, Ohri V, Madhumathi J, Ramasubramanian V. Policy document on antimicrobial stewardship practices in India. Indian J Med Res. 2019;149(2):180.
8. Saxena A, Relan J, Agarwal R, Awasthy N, Azad S, Chakrabarty M, et al. Indian guidelines for indications and timing of intervention for common congenital heart diseases: revised and updated consensus statement of the Working group on management of congenital heart diseases. Ann Pediatr Cardiol. 2019; 12(3):254.
9. Characterisation and antimicrobial resistance of sepsis pathogens in neonates born in tertiary care centres in Delhi, India: a cohort study. Lancet Glob Health. 2016;4(10):e752-60.
10. Jajoo M, Manchanda V, Chaurasia S, Sankar MJ, Gautam H, Agarwal R, et al. Alarming rates of antimicrobial resistance and fungal sepsis in outborn neonates in North India. PLOS One. 2018;13(6):e0180705.
11. Barlam TF, Cosgrove SE, Abbo LM, MacDougall C, Schuetz AN, Septimus EJ, et al. Implementing an antibiotic stewardship program: guidelines by the Infectious Diseases Society of America and the Society for Healthcare Epidemiology of America. Clin Infect Dis. 2016;62(10): e51-77.
12. CDC. Core Elements of Hospital Antibiotic Stewardship Programs 2019. [online] Available from: https://www.cdc.gov/antibiotic-use/healthcare/pdfs/hospital-core-elements-H.pdf. [Last Accessed April, 2021].
13. Zant R, Stocker C, Schlapbach LJ, Mayfield S, Karl T, Schibler A. Procalcitonin in the early course post pediatric cardiac surgery. Pediatr Crit Care Med. 2016;17(7):624-9.
14. Best M. Ignaz Semmelweis and the birth of infection control. Qual Saf Health Care. 2004;13(3):233-4.
15. The Joint Commission On Infection Prevention & Control: Experiences, case studies and news about infection prevention and control. [online] Available from: https://www.jointcommission.org/resources/news-and-multimedia/blogs/on-infection-prevention-control/2019/09/focus-on-improving-hand-hygiene-compliance-to-protect-patients-and-health-care-workers/. [Last Accessed April, 2021].
16. World Health Organization. WHO Guidelines on Hand Hygiene in Health Care: a Summary. [online] Available from: https://www.who.int/gpsc/5may/tools/who_guidelines-hand-hygiene_summary.pdf. [Last Accessed April, 2021].
17. World Health Organization. World Hand Hygiene Day. [online] Available from: https://www.who.int/campaigns/save-lives-clean-your-hands. [Last Accessed April, 2021].
18. Srigley JA, Furness CD, Baker GR, Gardam M. Quantification of the Hawthorne effect in hand hygiene compliance monitoring using an electronic monitoring system: a retrospective cohort study. BMJ Qual Saf. 2014;23(12): 974-80.
19. Widmer A. Andreas F Widmer for the Basel infection control team. BMC Proc. 2011; 5(S6):P123, 1753-6561-5-S6-P123.
20. Tschudin-Sutter S, Rotter ML, Frei R, Nogarth D, Häusermann P, Stranden A, et al. Simplifying the WHO 'how to hand rub' technique: three steps are as effective as six—results from an experimental randomized crossover trial. Clin Microbiol Infect. 2017;23(6):409.e1-409.e4.

21. Ghosh A, Ameling S, Zhou J, Lacey G, Creamer E, Dolan A, et al. Pilot evaluation of a ward-based automated hand hygiene training system. Am J Infect Control. 2013;41(4):368-70.

22. Lacey G, Zhou J, Li X, Craven C, Gush C. The impact of automatic video auditing with real-time feedback on the quality and quantity of handwash events in a hospital setting. Am J Infect Control. 2020;48(2):162-6.

23. Pires D, Soule H, Bellissimo-Rodrigues F, Gayet-Ageron A, Pittet D. Hand hygiene with alcohol-based hand rub: how long is long enough? Infect Control Hosp Epidemiol. 2017;38(5): 547-52.

24. Stahmeyer JT, Lutze B, von Lengerke T, Chaberny IF, Krauth C. Hand hygiene in intensive care units: a matter of time? J Hosp Infect. 2017;95(4):338-43.

25. World Health Organization. Guide to Implementation. [online] Available from: https://apps. who.int/iris/bitstream/handle/10665/70030/WHO_IER_PSP_2009.02_eng.pdf. [Last Accessed April, 2021].

26. Haubitz S, Atkinson A, Kaspar T, Nydegger D, Eichenberger A, Sommerstein R, et al. Handrub consumption mirrors hand hygiene compliance. Infect Control Hosp Epidemiol. 2016;37(6):707-10.

27. Tang HJ, Lin HL, Lin YH, Leung PO, Chuang YC, Lai CC. The impact of central line insertion bundle on central line-associated bloodstream infection. BMC Infect Dis. 2014;14(1):356.

28. Sun Y, Bao Z, Guo Y, Yuan X. Positive effect of care bundles on patients with central venous catheter insertions at a tertiary hospital in Beijing, China. J Int Med Res. 2020;48(7): 030006052094211.

29. Ling ML, Apisarnthanarak A, Jaggi N, Harrington G, Morikane K, Thu LT, et al. APSIC guide for prevention of Central Line Associated Bloodstream Infections (CLABSI). Antimicrob Resist Infect Control. 2016;5(1):16.

30. The Joint Commission. CVC Insertion Bundles. [online] Available from: https://www.jointcommission.org/-/media/tjc/documents/resources/clabsi/clabsi_toolkit_tool_3-18_cvc_insertion_bundles.pdf?db=web&hash=0EF50D5D763A3694D28938B3B5DED960. [Last Accessed April, 2021].

31. CDC. Guidelines for the Prevention of Intravascular Catheter-Related Infections, 2011. [online] Available from: https://www.cdc.gov/infectioncontrol/pdf/guidelines/bsi-guidelines-H.pdf. [Last Accessed April, 2021].

32. Pallotto C, Fiorio M, De Angelis V, Ripoli A, Franciosini E, Quondam Girolamo L, et al. Daily bathing with 4% chlorhexidine gluconate in intensive care settings: a randomized controlled trial. Clin Microbiol Infect. 2019;25(6): 705-10.

33. Milstone AM, Elward A, Song X, Zerr DM, Orscheln R, Speck K, et al. Daily chlorhexidine bathing to reduce bacteraemia in critically ill children: a multicentre, cluster-randomised, crossover trial. Lancet. 2013;381 (9872):1099-106.

34. CDC. National Healthcare Safety Network (NHSN): Patient Safety Component Manual. chttps://www.cdc.gov/nhsn/pdfs/pscmanual/pcsmanual_current.pdf. [Last Accessed April, 2021].

35. Larsen EN, Gavin N, Marsh N, Rickard CM, Runnegar N, Webster J. A systematic review of central-line–associated bloodstream infection (CLABSI) diagnostic reliability and error. Infect Control Hosp Epidemiol. 2019;40(10) 1100-6.

36. Stoll BJ. Neurodevelopmental and growth impairment among extremely low-birth-weight infants with neonatal infection. JAMA. 2004;292(19):2357.

37. Thacker N, Pereira N, Banavali S, Narula G, Vora T, Chinnaswamy G, et al. Alarming prevalence of community-acquired multidrug-resistant organisms colonization in children with cancer and implications for therapy: a prospective study. Indian J Cancer. 2014; 51(4):442.

38. NEO-KISS. Nosocomial infection surveillance for preterm infants with birthweight <1500g. [online] Available from: https://www.nrz-hygiene.de/fileadmin/nrz/module/neo/NEO-KISSProtocol_english_240210.pdf. [Last Accessed April, 2021].

39. The Working Group on Neonatal Infectious Diseases of the Section of Neonatology of the Dutch Paediatric Society, Heijting IE, Antonius TA, Tostmann A, de Boode WP, Hogeveen M, et al. Sustainable neonatal CLABSI surveillance: consensus towards new criteria in the Netherlands. Antimicrob Resist Infect Control. 2021;10(1):31.

40. Seale AC, Obiero CW, Berkley JA. Rational development of guidelines for management of neonatal sepsis in developing countries. Curr Opin Infect Dis. 2015;28(3):225-30.

41. Iosifidis E, Pitsava G, Roilides E. Ventilator-associated pneumonia in neonates and

children: a systematic analysis of diagnostic methods and prevention. Future Microbiol. 2018;13(12):1431-46.

42. Iosifidis E, Coffin S. Ventilator-associated events in children: controversies and research needs. Pediatr Infect Dis J. 2020;39(4):e37-9.

43. Williams L. Ventilator-associated pneumonia precautions for children: what is the evidence? AACN Adv Crit Care. 2019;30(1):68-71.

44. Willson DF. Outcomes and risk factors in pediatric ventilator-associated pneumonia: guilt by association. Pediatr Crit Care Med. 2015;16(3):299-301.

45. Haut C. Preventing pediatric ventilator-associated pneumonia. Nurs Crit Care. 2015;10(6):42-7.

46. Vijay G, Mandal A, Sankar J, Kapil A, Lodha R, Kabra SK. Ventilator associated pneumonia in pediatric intensive care unit: incidence, risk factors and etiological agents. Indian J Pediatr. 2018;85(10):861-6.

47. Roeleveld PP, Guijt D, Kuijper EJ, Hazekamp MG, de Wilde RBP, de Jonge E. Ventilator-associated pneumonia in children after cardiac surgery in The Netherlands. Intensive Care Med. 2011;37(10):1656-63.

48. Sodhi J, Satpathy S, Sharma D, Lodha R, Kapil A, Wadhwa N, et al. Healthcare associated infections in paediatric intensive care unit of a tertiary care hospital in India: hospital stay and extra costs. Indian J Med Res. 2016;143 (4):502.

49. Natale JE, McBeth C, Powne A, Montes R, Butler E, Amezquita A. Implementation of Five-element, Interprofessional Ventilator-associated Pneumonia Prevention Bundle in the Pediatric Intensive Care Unit. In: Council on Quality Improvement and Patient Safety Program [Internet]. Itasca, Illinois: American Academy of Pediatrics; 2018. pp. 118.

50. Johnstone L, Spence D, Koziol-McClain J. Oral hygiene care in the pediatric intensive care unit: practice recommendations. Pediatr Nurs. 2010;36(2):85-7.

51. Jácomo AD, Carmona F, Matsuno AK, Manso PH, Carlotti AP. Effect of oral hygiene with 0.12% Chlorhexidine gluconate on the incidence of nosocomial pneumonia in children undergoing cardiac surgery. Infect Control Hosp Epidemiol. 2011;32(6):591-6.

52. Aly H, Badawy M, El-Kholy A, Nabil R, Mohamed A. Randomized, controlled trial on tracheal colonization of ventilated infants:

53. Task Force On Sudden Infant Death Syndrome. SIDS and Other Sleep-Related Infant Deaths: Updated 2016 Recommendations for a Safe Infant Sleeping Environment. Pediatrics. 2016;138(5):e20162938.

54. Albert BD, Zurakowski D, Bechard LJ, Priebe GP, Duggan CP, Heyland DK, et al. Enteral nutrition and acid-suppressive therapy in the picu: impact on the risk of ventilator-associated pneumonia. Pediatr Crit Care Med. 2016;17(10):924-9.

55. Mills KI, Albert BD, Bechard LJ, Duggan CP, Kaza A, Rakoff-Nahoum S, et al. Stress ulcer prophylaxis versus placebo—a blinded randomized control trial to evaluate the safety of two strategies in critically ill infants with congenital heart disease (SUPPRESS-CHD). Trials. 2020;21(1):590.

56. Gupta S, Boville BM, Blanton R, Lukasiewicz G, Wincek J, Bai C, et al. A multicentered prospective analysis of diagnosis, risk factors, and outcomes associated with pediatric ventilator-associated pneumonia: Pediatr Crit Care Med. 2015;16(3):e65-73.

57. Rosenthal VD, Álvarez-Moreno C, Villamil-Gómez W, Singh S, Ramachandran B, Navoa-Ng JA, et al. Effectiveness of a multidimensional approach to reduce ventilator-associated pneumonia in pediatric intensive care units of 5 developing countries: International Nosocomial Infection Control Consortium findings. Am J Infect Control. 2012;40(6):497-501.

58. Walz A, Canter MO, Betters K. The ICU liberation bundle and strategies for implementation in pediatrics. Curr Pediatr Rep. 2020;8(3): 69-78.

59. Harris J, Ramelet AS, van Dijk M, Pokorna P, Wielenga J, Tume L, et al. Clinical recommendations for pain, sedation, withdrawal and delirium assessment in critically ill infants and children: an ESPNIC position statement for healthcare professionals. Intensive Care Med. 2016;42(6):972-86.

60. CDC. Current HAI Progress Report. [online] Available from: https://www.cdc.gov/hai/data/portal/progress-report.html. [Last Accessed April, 2021].

61. Grant M, Hardin-Reynolds T. Preventable Health Care–Associated Infections in Pediatric Critical Care. J Pediatr Intensive Care. 2015;04(02):79-86.

62. Tsuji S, Ikai A, Oyama K, Kin H, Koizumi J. Outcomes of primary sternal closure for

postoperative mediastinitis in children. Eur J Cardiothorac Surg. 2021;477.

63. Wu Y, Wang J, Dai J, Wang G, Li H, Li Y, et al. Is vacuum-assisted closure therapy feasible for children with deep sternal wound infection after cardiac surgery? The pooling results from current literature. Artif Organs. 2021;13936.

64. Storey A, MacDonald B, Rahman MA. The association between preoperative length of hospital stay and deep sternal wound infection: a scoping review. Aust Crit Care. 2021;S1036731420303702.

65. Costello JM, Graham DA, Morrow DF, Morrow J, Potter-Bynoe G, Sandora TJ, et al. Risk Factors for surgical site infection after cardiac surgery in children. Ann Thorac Surg. 2010;89(6):1833-42.

66. Kennedy JT, DiLeonardo O, Hurtado CG, Nelson JS. A systematic review of antibiotic prophylaxis for delayed sternal closure in children. World J Pediatr Congenit Heart Surg. 2021;12(1):93-102.

67. Woodward C, Taylor R, Son M, Taeed R, Husain SA. Efforts to reduce infections in delayed sternal closure patients: a survey of pediatric practice. World J Pediatr Congenit Heart Surg. 2020;11(3):310-5.

68. Hatachi T, Sofue T, Ito Y, Inata Y, Shimizu Y, Hasegawa M, et al. Antibiotic prophylaxis for open chest management after pediatric cardiac surgery. Pediatr Crit Care Med. 2019;20(9):801-8.

69. Elassal AA, Eldib OS, Dohain AM, Abdelmohsen GA, Abdalla AH, Al-Radi OO. Delayed sternal closure in congenital heart surgery: a risk-benefit analysis. Heart Surg Forum. 2019;22(5):E325-30.

70. Sherman G, Shulman-Manor O, Dagan O, Livni G, Scheuerman O, Amir G, et al. Vacuum-assisted closure for the treatment of deep sternal wound infection after pediatric cardiac surgery. Pediatr Crit Care Med. 2020;21(2):150-5.

SECTION

4

Special Considerations and Procedures

Peritoneal Dialysis in Pediatric Cardiac Intensive Care Unit

Balaji Srimurugan

Illustrations: Balaji Srimurugan

Reviewed by: Brijesh P Kottayil

■ INTRODUCTION

Peritoneal dialysis (PD) is a well-recognized mode of renal replacement therapy in pediatric cardiac surgical patients. This technique employs the basic principle of diffusion across a semipermeable membrane (i.e., peritoneum) from solution to solution, of varying osmotic gradients.[1-3] Improvement in surgical techniques with reduced cardiopulmonary bypass (CPB) duration, and improved perfusion strategies, have limited the use of postoperative peritoneal dialysis in the current era to specific circumstances. Broadly, its indications in the postcardiac surgery scenario are two-fold.

1. To facilitate solute clearance in patients with postoperative acute kidney injury. Typically acute kidney injury after cardiac surgery occurs as sequelae of postoperative low cardiac output state or due to an underlying primary renal pathology.
2. To facilitate fluid removal by ultrafiltration, in patients with fluid overload and capillary leak syndrome after CPB. Fluid overload occurs frequently after congenital heart surgery and has been linked to adverse postoperative outcomes.

■ PROCEDURE FOR PERITONEAL DIALYSIS CATHETER INSERTION

Though PD catheter insertion can be done as a blind procedure, our institutional policy is to place the PD catheter intraperitoneally by surgical dissection in the operating room (OR) or in the postoperative intensive care unit (ICU). The procedure is performed under sedation and/or paralysis after ensuring adequate analgesia. It is prudent to take special precautions to avoid iatrogenic bleeding or bowel injury, particularly in the vulnerable period after CPB where a coexisting coagulopathy or low cardiac output state can increase the morbidity related to trauma. It is worthwhile to seek assistance of the OR team with nursing expertise while performing PD insertion in the ICU.

Articles to be Kept Ready

1. Sterile gown pack with a fenestrated sterile drape (Hole towel)
2. Sterile gloves
3. Chlorhexidine gluconate with alcohol solution (Tincture)
4. No. 15 surgical blade
5. Electrocautery
6. Sterile gauze pieces: 2 × 2
7. 3 way with stop cock × 2
8. Suture material: 6-0 prolene × 1, 4-0 silk ×1
9. Iodine impregnated transparent dressing (Ioban™, 3M™, USA)
10. Peritoneal Dialysis solution
11. Measured volume burette set
12. Pediatric PD catheter [At our center a perforated wound closure suction catheter (RomoVac set®, Romsons) cut to the required length or a modified 10 Fr infant

feeding tube with additional holes is used as an alternative to conventional PD catheter].

Preinsertion

- Explain the procedure to the patient and family as appropriate
- Ensure that coagulopathies are corrected before the procedure
- Assemble all the essential equipment by the bedside before commencement of the procedure
- Ensure that appropriate monitors are in place—ECG, pulse oximetry, arterial blood pressure, temperature monitoring
- Appropriate sedation, analgesia and/or paralysis has to be ensured.

Site of Insertion

The site of choice for the insertion of the catheter is 0.5–1 cm above the level of the umbilicus.[2] The presence of both the anterior and posterior rectus sheath in this area offers good support to the PD catheter, in addition to ensuring safety at the time of insertion. It is wise to stay partly to one side of the midline, as there is increased likelihood of encountering engorged blood vessels in the midline, particularly in neonatal population.

Surgical Steps

- Skin preparation and draping of the anticipated site of insertion keeping the umbilicus and 2 cm above it exposed.
- Make a transverse incision not more than 1.5 cm, just above the umbilicus.
- Place two skin stay sutures that keep the skin retracted as one works his way through the layers of the anterior abdominal wall (each step under vision).
- The subcutaneous tissue is divided with electrocautery to expose the anterior rectus sheath.
- A linear slit is made on the anterior rectus sheath, to suit the size of the catheter.

A purse string suture using 6-0 prolene is taken around this slit on the anterior rectus sheath.

- Using a fine mosquito forceps, the rectus muscle underneath the sheath is lateralized in order to expose the posterior rectus sheath.
- Two mosquito forceps are used to pick up the posterior sheath ensuring that the held part is completely clear of bowel loops.
- Using a Pott's scissors, the held portion between the two mosquito forceps is incised to enter the peritoneal cavity (most often the peritoneum is adhered to the posterior rectus sheath). In the presence of preperitoneal fat, this step has to be done independently for the posterior rectus sheath and the peritoneum.
- The PD catheter/suction drain catheter of appropriate size is inserted through the opening made in the peritoneum directing it downward into one of the iliac fossa.
- The purse string on the anterior rectus sheath is fastened to secure the tube in place.
- The skin is closed with a horizontal mattress suture securing the catheter with it.

TECHNIQUE OF PERITONEAL DIALYSIS

Peritoneal Dialysis Fluid Prescription

This should be tailored to the patients' clinical status and the need for fluid and solute removal. Dextrose concentration contributes to the osmolality of the PD fluid. This is commercially available in concentrations of 1.5%, 2.5% and 4.5% dextrose containing formulation. The higher the dextrose concentration, the greater the osmolality.[4–6]

A typical PD prescription should indicate the following:

- *Concentration of the PD fluid*: Specify whether isotonic/hypertonic cycles

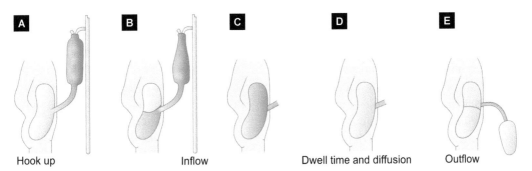

Figs. 1A to E: Schematic representation of peritoneal dialysis cycle depicting the inflow, dwell time and drain (outflow) time.

depending on need for fluid and solute removal.

- *Exchange volume*: Typically, volumes of 10 mL/kg are sufficient for fluid and solute removal in neonates and infants. However, this may be increased to 15 mL/kg for better solute removal if required.

- *Fill (inflow), dwell and drain (outflow) times*: *Fill time* is the time required for inflow of PD fluid; *dwell time* is the duration for which the fluid is allowed to remain in peritoneal cavity; *drain time* is the time allowed for drainage of the fluid out of the peritoneal cavity. Typically, an inflow time of 10 minutes, dwell time of 30 minutes and drain time of 20 minutes is allowed. This may be individualized, depending on the need for ultrafiltration or solute removal. Longer dwell time may be required for effective solute removal.

- *Frequency and duration of PD*: Typically, hourly PD cycles are prescribed, but can be tailored to the individual situation and requirement. The components of a PD cycle are depicted in **Figures 1A to E.**

NURSING CONSIDERATIONS TO ENSURE PATENCY AND OPTIMAL FUNCTIONING OF THE PERITONEAL DIALYSIS CATHETER

Maintaining patency of the catheter and ensuring optimal utility of the peritoneal drainage system is a challenging task for the bedside nurse. An hour to hour attention to the management of the dialysis catheter is therefore essential to achieve the desired targets. The bedside nurse must check the following aspects during maintenance of a PD catheter.

- At all times, ensure that the PD circuit is devoid of air bubbles, starting from the fluid reservoir to the site of entry of the catheter. Air bubbles when moved along the circuit tend to exert a negative pressure which can suck in omentum from the peritoneal cavity.

- At no point of time should a suction be exerted in a PD circuit in an attempt to relieve obstruction. A gentle flush can solve the issue whereas a suction can only make it worse. Neonates in particular have a loose omentum, which tends to get sucked into the PD catheter even with minimal suction pressures.[4]

- Maintain an upward arch of the catheter at its exit from the abdominal wall. This ensures that the tip of the catheter remains at the most dependent portion of the peritoneal cavity.

- The surgical team has to be notified if the PD catheter is blocked or the drainage is suboptimal.

- In addition to this, it is also important to observe the effect of PD on cardiovascular and respiratory system. In patients with poor lung compliance and significant ventricular dysfunction, the increase in intra-abdominal pressure and major fluid shifts associated with PD, can profoundly affect cardiopulmonary interactions. These effects have to be meticulously sought for and corrective measures should be instituted.

- *Infection control*: Meticulous aseptic precautions are to be ensured during insertion, maintenance and removal of PD catheter.

CATHETER REMOVAL

Catheter removal is done when PD is no longer required for postoperative care. Generally, in the postoperative ICU, the catheter is removed just prior to the extubation of the patient, as subtle changes in the intra-abdominal pressure can alter the respiratory mechanics in an extubated patient. If the catheter is still retained after the extubation, it is reasonable to leave it for drainage. Patient agitation has to be prevented while removing the catheter in an extubated patient by appropriate analgesia/sedation to prevent inadvertent omental prolapse.

COMPLICATIONS

- Bleeding during insertion.
- *Catheter leak*: PD catheter leak at the site of insertion most often implies that there is a block in the intraperitoneal component of the catheter.
- Hemorrhagic PD exudate results from local trauma, blood vessel injury, and coexisting uncorrected coagulopathies.

- While dissecting through the abdominal wall, care should be taken to avoid bowel injury at each step of dissection. Underlying sepsis or necrotizing enterocolitis can also increase the likelihood of bowel injury and it is prudent to avoid PD under these circumstances.[7]
- *Herniation of omentum from the insertion site*: This typically occurs if the incision in the rectus sheath is too wide, and manifests most commonly during the time of removal of the PD catheter.

REFERENCES

1. Ronco C, Crepaldi C, Cruz DN. Peritoneal Dialysis: From Basic Concepts to Clinical Excellence. Basel: Karger Medical and Scientific Publishers; 2009. pp. 244.
2. Wood M. Nephrology: Nursing Standards and Practice Recommendations. Kingston: Canadian Association of Nephrology Nurses and Technologists; 2008.
3. Daugirdas, JT, Blake PG, Ing TS. Physiology of peritoneal dialysis. In: Handbook of Dialysis. Philadelphia: Lippincott Williams & Wilkins; 2006. pp. 323.
4. Pina JS, Moghadam S, Cushner HM, Beilman GJ, McAlister VC. In-theater peritoneal dialysis for combat-related renal failure. J Trauma. 2010;68(5):1253-6.
5. Schmitt CP, Zaloszyc A, Schaefer B, Fischbach M. Peritoneal dialysis tailored to pediatric needs. Int J Nephrol. 2011;2011:940267.
6. Chan K, Patrick IP, Chiu CSW, Cheung Y. Peritoneal dialysis for congenital heart disease in infants and young children. Ann Thorac Surg. 2003;76:1443-9.
7. Kawanishi H, Moriishi M. Encapsulating peritoneal sclerosis: prevention and treatment. Perit Dial Int. 2007;27(Suppl 2):S289-92.

Cardiac Catheterization in the Postoperative Period

R Krishna Kumar

■ INTRODUCTION

The decision to catheterize a patient soon after surgery for congenital heart disease (CHD) has to be carefully undertaken. With substantial improvements in the quality of imaging, the indications for cardiac catheterization are largely limited to catheter interventions. With improving quality of congenital heart surgery, the need for catheter interventions is likely to decline. However, they cannot be avoided altogether given the enormous variety of congenital heart defects and the trend toward addressing the more complex conditions surgically. The indications for catheter interventions vary from center to center depending on the institutional profile of operations for CHD.

A number of theoretical considerations exist. There is always a concern of performing procedures at surgical sites with fresh suture lines.[1,2] Several logistic concerns exist as well. They include, transport to and from the catheterization laboratory, access, monitoring and care during the procedures. Obtaining access is sometimes challenging in these patients because of previously placed invasive lines. There are safety concerns that relate to the relatively limited hemodynamic reserves of the postoperative child with residual issues. The amount of contrast medium that can be used in these patients is limited as well. Specific improvisations are needed in situations where resources are limited.[3] This review will discuss the earlier mentioned issues, that relate to performing catheter interventions in the early postoperative period.

■ DEFINITION

For the purpose of catheter interventions the "early" postoperative period can be defined as within 6 weeks after surgery. Conventionally this is considered as the required time period for optimal tissue healing.

■ INDICATIONS

Some of the possible indications for catheter interventions in the early postoperative period are listed in the **Table 1**. This is by no means comprehensive as numerous possibilities exist, given the large variety of congenital heart lesions and operations that are performed for them.

Defects Deliberately Left behind by Surgeons

Fenestrations in the ventricular septal defect (VSD) or atrial septal defect (ASD) patch and Fontan baffle are sometimes deliberately left behind by the surgeons because the early postoperative hemodynamic concerns may not allow complete closure of these defects. These concerns include pulmonary artery pressures, size of the branch pulmonary arteries and incomplete arborization. These fenestrations

TABLE 1: Catheter interventions in the postoperative period.

Broad category	Specific defect	Catheter intervention
Residual defects deliberately left behind by the surgeon	Fenestrations in ASD and VSD patch	Closure with occlusive devices (atrial septal occluder, ventricular septal occluder or duct occluder for VSD)
	Antegrade flow in after Glenn shunts	Closure with occlusive device (Ventricular septal or duct occluder)
	Vertical vein after repair of total veins	Closure with occlusive device or vascular plug
Defects accidentally left behind by surgeons	Residual obstructive lesions in branch pulmonary arteries, outflow tracts and baffle	Balloon angioplasty or stent deployment
	Residual defects at patch margins, intramural VSD, forward flow after Fontan, pseudoaneurysms	Closure with occlusive devices
Previously unrecognized defects	Aortopulmonary and venous collaterals	Coil occlusion, occlusion with the vascular plug
	Left superior vena cava	Occlusion with coil, vascular plug or occlusive device
	Additional VSD	Closure with a ventricular septal occluder or duct occluder
	Branch PA stenosis, coarctation	Balloon angioplasty/stent placement
Indications dictated by changed physiology	Enlargement of atrial communication or Fontan fenestration	Balloon dilation
Iatrogenic problems	Vascular occlusion (SVC occlusion from neck lines)	Balloon dilation/stent placement
	Complete heart block	Pacemaker insertion
Failed surgical procedure	Blocked aortopulmonary shunts	Balloon angioplasty/stent placement, stenting the patent arterial duct

(ASD: atrial septal defect; PA: pulmonary artery; SVC: superior vena cava; VSD: ventricular septal defect)

may start shunting inappropriately in the early postoperative period.[4] Similarly the vertical vein that is sometimes deliberately left behind after repair of total anomalous pulmonary venous return (TAPVR) to allow decompression in the event of pulmonary hypertensive crisis, may start to shunt from left atrium to right atrium as the pulmonary artery pressures decline. Forward flow across the pulmonary valve after a "pulsatile" bidirectional Glenn shunt may result in adverse hemodynamics in the early postoperative period in the occasional patient.[5]

Defects Accidentally Left behind by Surgeons

With continuing refinements of surgical techniques, residual defects are increasingly uncommon. The frequent use of intra-operative transesophageal echocardiogram has contributed immensely to reducing the incidence of residual defects. However, occasionally residual VSDs at patch margins do get left behind. Following repair of double outlet right ventricle "intramural" defects are well-described and can be difficult to avoid altogether. Residual obstructive lesions can occasionally be seen after branch pulmonary artery reconstructions and in either outflow tracts. Pseudoaneurysms of the aorta or the pulmonary artery stump can potentially be closed with occlusive devices.[6] Rarely it may be difficult for the surgeon to ligate or divide the pulmonary artery in order to eliminate forward flow. This can happen if there are adhesions in the region of the main pulmonary artery. An occlusive device can be put across the pulmonary valve to interrupt flows.

Previously Unrecognized Defects

This is one of the most common indications for catheterization in the early postoperative period. With the increasing use of echocardiography for comprehensive preoperative evaluation, there are occasional patients who have unrecognized defects that are detected in the early postoperative period. The most common such defects are additional muscular VSDs, aortopulmonary collaterals, branch pulmonary artery stenosis and coarctation.

Indications Dictated by the Altered Postoperative Physiology

Examples in this category include the need to enlarge or create atrial septal opening following operations such as correction of tetralogy of Fallot and enlargement of the fenestration following the Fontan operation.

Iatrogenic Problems

With long stays in intensive care units (ICUs) and having indwelling central lines in place, occlusion of vessels are not uncommon. Occlusion of the superior vena cava has major adverse consequences. Balloon dilation or stenting may be required to relieve venous occlusion. In older patients with complete heart block after congenital heart surgery, permanent pacemaker placement may be accomplished transvenously in the cardiac catheterization laboratory.

Failed Surgery

Acute occluded aortopulmonary shunts may be relieved in the catheterization laboratory either through balloon dilation with or without stent placement[7] in the catheterization

laboratory or stenting of the patent arterial duct if feasible.[8]

■ SPECIAL CONSIDERATIONS

Catheter Manipulations

Catheter manipulations should be gentle. Glidewires® (Terumo) with soft and curved tips should be used first to negotiate regions with fresh suture lines. The catheters should be used over these wires. Balloon tipped catheters can also be used.

Ability of Sutures to Withstand Balloon Expansion

A variety of freshly sutured regions can potentially undergo angioplasty and stent implantation without resultant vascular disruption. Vascular suture lines are commonly constructed from polypropylene monofilament (Prolene). Prolene can elongate as much as 34% before the breaking. It is important to determine from the surgeons as to what was used for the suture lines. It is also important to recognize that sutures from different manufacturers may have different thresholds for disruption after balloon expansion. One of the reasons why it may be feasible to perform balloon dilation in fresh suture lines could also relate to an enlargement of the circumference of the suture line (increased distance between parallel throws) in response to balloon inflation, which prevents suture breakage within the limits of the angioplasties performed. Notwithstanding these considerations it is perhaps important to always use a pressure gauge to determine the pressure used for the balloon dilation and not exceed 3–4 atmospheres. Prolene suture lines can be safely and effectively expanded with angioplasty using balloon/stenosis ratios of approximately 2.5/1.0. Because effective angioplasty often requires higher balloon/stenosis ratios, in many instances, stent placement is preferable to angioplasty in the early postoperative period. Additionally, by limiting recoil, stents ensure a more predictable and durable result.

Hemodynamic Instability Resulting from Specific Procedures

Some interventions are associated with frequent occurrence of hemodynamic instability that is often poorly tolerated. Catheter closure of VSD in infants and small children is a good example. This is perhaps because a wire-loop in the ventricle can mechanically interfere with effective ventricular contractions. The postoperative patient may be particularly vulnerable. For the same reason balloon dilation and stent placements in branch pulmonary artery and outflow tract can be challenging. It may be necessary to leave wire loops in the right ventricle to allow stability of the balloon-stent-wire assembly. This is sometimes at the cost of patient stability. The likelihood of instability can be substantial in the very young with small ventricular cavity size.

Transport to and from the Cardiac Catheterization Laboratory

The catheterization laboratory and postoperative ICUs are often at different locations. Safe transport to and from catheterization laboratory has to be a carefully coordinated team effort often led by the anesthesiologist-interventionist. A number of small details require attention. They include airway, lines and supports, temperature maintenance, hemodynamic and rhythm monitoring.

Access

Access for cardiac catheterization can be especially challenging in the early postoperative period. Existing central venous lines may be required to keep important inotrope infusions. Arterial lines may be required

for continuous hemodynamic monitoring. Alternative access sites may not be readily available. For this reasons unconventional access sites need to be explored. These include: transhepatic and subclavian for venous access and the axillary artery for access to the left heart. In very small infants with open sternum, sheaths can be placed surgically into the main pulmonary artery or homograft directly to allow passage of the balloon stent assembly. After the procedures, it is usually necessary to leave behind reliable access (central venous and arterial) especially if the previous sites have been used for the procedure.

Altered Physiologic State and Limited Reserves

The typical patient requiring intervention after cardiac surgery has residual lesions that limit hemodynamic and respiratory reserves. The physiological state may also be altered by most palliative operations. These are important considerations. Contrast usage may be influenced by renal function which can be deranged in these circumstances. For these reasons, maximum diagnostic information should be sought through noninvasive means. Unnecessary angiograms should be avoided.

Interpreting Hemodynamic Data

The unique features in the postoperative state include positive pressure ventilation, use of high fraction of inhaled oxygen, use of inotrope and vasodilators, substantially altered physiology (especially after aorto-pulmonary shunts and single ventricle palliations). These issues should be considered while hemodynamic data is interpreted. For example: a 2 mm Hg gradient in the proximal pulmonary artery branches could be quite important after a Glenn shunt and a 20 mm Hg gradient may be acceptable after placement of a right ventricle to pulmonary artery conduit.

Challenges in the Limited Resource Environment

Many newly established centers in emerging economies and the developing countries work under substantial resource constraints. The cost of interventions can add substantially to the costs of surgery and intensive care. Innovations and improvisations are therefore required to keep costs affordable.

Extracorporeal or Cardiopulmonary Support

In institutions with resources, for patients at exceptionally high risk, a cardiopulmonary support (CPS) unit can be made available in the catheterization laboratory to allow for rapid initiation of cardiopulmonary bypass should it become necessary. Catheter-interventions have been performed under extracorporeal membrane oxygenation (ECMO) support.[9,10]

▌ PREREQUISITES FOR PERFORMING CATHETER INTERVENTIONS IN THE EARLY POSTOPERATIVE PERIOD

- Thorough noninvasive assessment of the precise anatomic and physiologic derangement: Often all this requires is a thorough transthoracic echocardiography. Occasional patients require transesophageal echo or rarely computed tomography (CT) or magnetic resonance imaging (MRI) to precisely define the problem.
- Consensus among all caregivers on the need for intervention.
- Careful planning and a clear roadmap for the procedure, including all small details.
- A detailed informed consent from the family after explanation of the risks and benefits of the procedure.

▌ OUTCOMES

While there are a few studies that have systematically discussed results after catheter interventions in consecutive patients, a substantial publication bias is likely. A number of isolated cases in many centers may not have reported their results.

Zahn et al. reported the largest series of interventions in the early postoperative period in 62 patients with a median age of 4 months (2 days to 11 years), weight 4.7 kg (2.3–45 kg), who underwent 66 catheterizations on median postoperative day 9 (0–42 days). Thirty-five cases involved 50 interventional procedures. Nine patients required extracorporeal CPS. Success rates were 100% for angioplasty and vascular occlusion and 87% for stent implantation. Complications included stent migration (one patient), cerebral vascular injury (one patient), and left pulmonary artery stenosis (one patient). Thirty procedures involved angioplasty or stent implantation, including 26 involving a recently created suture line. Suture disruption or transmural vascular tears were not observed. There was no procedural mortality. Thirty-day survival for patients undergoing intervention was 83%. Other studies have not reported such excellent results.[2]

Rosales et al. reviewed the clinical course of patients undergoing interventional catheterization for peripheral pulmonary stenosis at a surgical site <7 weeks after surgery. Successful dilation (SD) was defined as >50% increase in predilation diameter. From 1984 to 2000, 17 patients had 19 proximal pulmonary arteries dilated 1 to 46 (median 8) days postoperatively. Median age and weight were 3.1 year and 12.7 kg. Three arteries were initially occluded. Seventeen arteries had initial balloon dilation with postintervention imaging available in 15; 8 arteries had stent dilation. The arterial diameter increased from 3.9 ± 2.6 to 5.5 ± 2.8 mm (p < 0.001). Nine of these arteries had stents placed with diameter increasing to 8.7 ± 3.7 mm (p <0.001 compared with post-balloon dilation diameter).

Stents increased the diameter in all arteries and made four of four failed balloon dilation successful. In the two most recent procedures, stents were placed without prior balloon dilation with diameter increasing from 1.3 to 9 mm and 8.2 to 14 mm. A stent was placed in 1 of 7 arteries prior to 1993 and in 10 of 12 arteries thereafter (p < 0.004). Three patients prior to 1995 had catheterization-related deaths secondary to vessel rupture after balloon dilation. They concluded that stent placement increases vessel diameter substantially more than balloon dilation alone. Stents reduce the acute complication rate and avoid early reoperation in this patient group.[1]

CONCLUSION AND RECOMMENDATIONS

Catheter interventions may be required in a variety of situations in the early postoperative period. This group of patients as a whole is challenging because they are sicker with limited reserves. There are important logistic and safety issues and close attention to a number of details is necessary. In spite of concerns of performing procedures at sites with fresh suture lines, there are reports of successful balloon dilation and stent placements. There is a need for a carefully coordinated team approach for these procedures.

REFERENCES

1. Rosales AM, Lock JE, Perry SB, Geggel RL. Interventional catheterization management of perioperative peripheral pulmonary stenosis: balloon angioplasty or endovascular stenting. Cathet Cardiovasc Interv. 2002;56:272-7.
2. Zahn EM, Dobrolet NC, Nykanen DG, Ojito J, Hannan RL, Burke RP. Interventional catheterization performed in the early postoperative period after congenital heart surgery in children. J Am Coll Cardiol. 2004;43;1264-9.
3. Kumar RK, Tynan M. Catheter Interventions for congenital heart disease in the third world. Pediatr Cardiol. 2005;26:1-9.
4. Vaidyanathan B, Kannan BR, Kumar RK. Device closure of residual ventricular septal defect after repair of tetralogy of fallot using the amplatzer duct occluder. Ind Heart J. 2005;57:64-6.
5. Anil SR, Kannan BR, Kumar RK. Transcatheter closure of native pulmonary artery for elimination of accessory pulmonary blood flow after bidirectional Glenn shunt. Ind Heart J. 2003;55:373-5.
6. Vaidyanathan B, Kannan BR, Kumar RK. Catheter closure of pseudo-aneurysm of main pulmonary. Circulation. 2004;110:1709.
7. Siva Kumar K, Anil SR, Ravi Chandra M, Natarajan KU, Kamath P, Kumar RK. Emergency Transcatheter recanalization of acutely thrombosed Blalock-Taussig shunts. Ind Heart J. 2001;53:743-8.
8. Mahesh K, Kannan BR, Anil SR, Kamath P, Kumar RK. Stenting of the patent arterial duct to improve pulmonary blood flow. Ind Heart J. 2005;57:704-8.
9. desJardins SE, Crowley DC, Beekman RH, Lloyd TR. Utility of cardiac catheterization in pediatric cardiac patients on ECMO. Cathet Cardiovasc Interv. 1999;46:62-7.
10. Booth KL, Roth SJ, Perry SB, del Nido PJ, Wessel DL, Laussen PC. Cardiac catheterization of patients supported by extracorporeal membrane oxygenation. J Am Coll Cardiol. 2002;40:1681-6.

Management of Intercostal Drains in the Pediatric Cardiac Intensive Care Unit

Praveen Reddy Bayya

Illustration: Praveen Reddy Bayya

Reviewed by: Brijesh P Kottayil

◼ INTRODUCTION

Intercostal drains (ICD) are routinely placed in the operating room in most patients after pediatric cardiac surgery to facilitate the drainage of blood, fluid or air. The usual drainage tubes in a postoperative patient include pleural, mediastinal and pericardial drains. Occasionally an ICD may need to be inserted in the intensive care unit (ICU) for the treatment of pneumothorax or drainage of pleural effusion. Appropriate management of ICD is important to ensure optimal functioning of the drainage system and to avoid complications. It is essential for the caregivers in ICU to understand the common indications of ICD insertion and the management of ICD in a postoperative patient.

◼ INDICATIONS FOR POSTOPERATIVE ICD INSERTION

Pleural Effusion

Pleural effusions in the postoperative period may be serous, chylous or hemorrhagic. Their etiology can be categorized as follows:

Hemorrhagic effusions:
- An inadvertant communication between the pleura and pericardium that was not recognized during surgery can sometimes lead to postoperative blood accumulation in the pleural cavity.
- Injury to the ipsilateral internal mammary artery either during sternal closure or by

the sharp tip of a pacing wire can rarely lead to gradual bleeding into an otherwise unbreached pleural cavity.

Chylothorax:
- *Lymphatic injury during surgery*: More common in Blalock–Taussig shunt, patent ductus arteriosus ligation and coarctation repair via thoracotomy[1]
- Right ventricular (RV) failure or high right atrial pressures
- Superior vena cava (SVC) obstruction
- High SVC pressure after a Glenn anastomosis or after a Fontan operation.

Serous effusions[1]:
- RV failure or increased hydrostatic pressure
- Post Glenn or Fontan surgeries
- Fluid overload and third spacing due to an inflammatory response (increased capillary permeability)
- Hypoalbuminemia resulting in decreased oncotic pressure.

Diagnosis of a Pleural Effusion

Effusions are usually detected incidentally in the ICU on chest X-rays (CXR). Symptoms associated with larger effusions include shortness of breath, fever, chest pain, tachypnea and rarely cardiac decompensation.[1] Routine physical examination reveals decreased air entry especially in the posterior and basal lung fields with a dull percussion note. In massive effusions, mediastinal shift and therefore, a tracheal shift will occur to the opposite side. A CXR should be taken, preferably in a slight head up position to diagnose and quantify the effusion. CXR in lateral decubitus position aids in diagnosis of small pleural effusions.[1] Echocardiography can reveal even small fluid accumulations, but quantification is difficult and the decision to insert an ICD often needs a CXR too. Ultrasound evaluation of the chest is a good diagnostic tool. The gold standard for diagnosis is a computed tomography (CT) scan, but this is an expensive test associated with radiation exposure and is usually not necessary.[1]

CXR features of a pleural effusion:

- *Erect posteroanterior (PA) film*: This shows a uniform opacity, filling the costophrenic angles, obscuring the diaphragmatic shadow and extending up the chest wall with a concave upper edge. It is higher laterally than medially.
- *Supine film*: The effusion may appear as an apical cap or a generalized diffuse increase in opacification of the ipsilateral lung. A massive effusion leads to mediastinal shift.

Pneumothorax

A spontaneously occurring pneumothorax needs a high degree of suspicion and alertness to be diagnosed on time. Identification and management of pneumothorax merits critical importance, as it can be life threatening in a neonate or infant. This can occur due to an unnoticed breach in the pleura, which will manifest as a pneumothorax in the postoperative CXR. Such pneumothoraces are nonexpanding and usually small, but may need an ICD. A pneumothorax can also occur in any patient on positive pressure ventilation. Another common cause of postoperative pneumothorax is entrainment of air into the pleural cavity following the removal of an ICD.

A sudden decrease in oxygen saturation, unexplained increase in airway pressures in mechanically ventilated patients, or sudden bradycardia and hypotension are typical presenting features. Further signs to be elicited are:

1. Tracheal shift to the opposite side
2. Increased transillumination on the suspected side in neonates
3. Decreased or absent chest expansion and/or air entry
4. Resonant percussion note.

In case of a hemodynamic compromise, it is essential to drain the pneumothorax immediately, even if it means not waiting for a CXR confirmation. A 16 Fr arterial cannula (or larger in bigger kids) should be inserted into the second intercostal space just above the upper border of the third rib in the midclavicular line. The stylet is then taken out and a three-way is connected. The three-way is opened to the atmosphere to let out air and is closed once clinical improvement occurs. An intravenous tubing set may be connected to one limb of the three-way and placed in a bottle of water to confirm escape of air and achieve a water seal.

■ INTERCOSTAL DRAIN INSERTION[2-4]

Articles to be Kept Ready

- Sterile gown pack
- Linen Pack
- Sterile gloves
- Chlorhexidine tincture
- Gauze packets
- Local anesthetic: Lignocaine 1%
- 5 cc syringe
- ICD tray
- No. 11 surgical blade
- ICD underwater sealed drain system (UWSD) with bottle **(Fig. 1)**
- Irrigation fluid
- Suture material: 3-0 silk
- Suction tubings
- 18 G needle
- Appropriate size drainage tube/intercostal catheter as described later

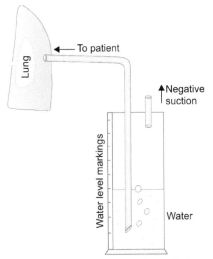

Fig. 1: Diagrammatic representation of intercostal drain (ICD) system in postoperative cardiac surgical patient.

- Adhesive tape/elastic adhesive bandage (Dynaplast)
- Crash cart/emergency intubation equipment should be readily accessible at the bedside.

Size of ICD catheter: Sizes from 8 FG upward are available in multiples of 4. Size selected depends on the weight of the patient and also the indication. Usually a smaller size is selected for pneumothorax, while larger sizes are needed for draining fluid.

Patient Position

Child is propped up to 45 degrees if conscious and off ventilator support. If on ventilator and hemodynamically stable, a slight head up and lateral rotation to bring the ipsilateral side up, would suffice. The hand on the side of procedure is raised and kept above the head.

Sedation and Analgesia

Appropriate sedation and analgesia should be given by the ICU attending physician. Nil per oral (NPO) hours should be confirmed before procedural sedation, if insertion is planned as an elective procedure.

Insertion Procedure

The preferred site is in the 4th or 5th intercostal space slightly anterior to the anterior axillary line. An appropriately sized horizontal skin incision is placed after local preparation and local anesthesia. The incision site should ensure the creation of a subcutaneous tunnel for the ICD before it enters the intercostal space. The tube is directed posteriorly for draining fluids.

After Care

The ICD is secured in place with a silk stitch and also anchored to the patient's side with plaster. The ICD in connected to an UWSD and proper swing should be ensured. Negative suction is connected. Adequate analgesia is continued post procedure.

▌ CARE OF THE INTERCOSTAL DRAIN[5,6]

The ICD site should be inspected during every ICU shift change. The key points to be noted are as follows:

Is There any Discharge from the ICD Site?

- Seropurulent discharge from the ICD suggests infection and often requires culture and sensitivity testing along with prompt removal of the drain/ICD site change.
- Fresh bleeding from the skin edge may necessitate a pressure dressing or additional suture application
- Blood/serous discharge indicates blockage of ICD lumen resulting in peritubal seepage of pleural collection. A CXR will confirm intrapleural collections. If applying a negative suction (see later) fails to drain the fluid, the ICD may have to be changed. It is prudent to avoid a pressure dressing when there is peritubal seepage

of fluid. Instead the fluid should be allowed to drain out and a loose gauze dressing applied around the drain site to soak it in.

What is the Position of the ICD Tube?

The mark on the ICD tube at the skin level should be noted. A mark of ≤ 2 cm at skin level could mean that the ICD has been displaced from the intrathoracic cavity, and one or more holes of the ICD tube are potentially lying in the subcutaneous plane. This has to be confirmed on CXR.

When one or more holes of the ICD tube lie in the subcutaneous plane, it can lead to the following problems:

- Subcutaneous emphysema in case of ongoing air leak from the lung
- Risk of pneumothorax if the tube slips out any further
- Increased risk of pneumothorax during ICD removal by an unsuspecting staff.

Hence, such ICDs should be promptly removed or replaced.

Is There a Column Swing?

A mediastinal drain has large swing of the fluid column in the tube with each breath. However, a similar swing in a pleural drain of > 2 cm is a contraindication for ICD removal. A large column swing indicates a failure of the lung to fully expand and indirectly points to the presence of an air leak from the lung, which if large enough, can be demonstrated by bubbles appearing in the underwater seal on coughing or deep inspiration.

Is There an Air Leak?

Presence of air bubbles emanating from the underwater seal suggests one of the following possibilities:

- *Damage in the tubings*: Any breach in the tubings can cause air leak and also allow air to be sucked into the chest. Therefore

any likely damage to the ICD tubing should be promptly identified and sealed.

- *Loose connectors* can cause air leak and have similar consequences necessitating prompt identification and corrective action.
- *Lung injury*: Examine the CXR to ensure lung is fully expanded. If air pockets remain despite negative suction on the ICD it suggests loculated pneumothorax or amount of air leak more than the air being drained by the ICD. Both these conditions necessitate placement of an additional ICD. Occasionally air leak from the lung may cease if the negative suction on the ICD is removed, and this may be attempted in situations of persistent air leak.

Suction Pressure and Suction Tubing

The negative suction of about 5 KPa (about 30 mm Hg) is usually applied in a pediatric patient. Occasionally, the suction tubing is connected to the water-seal bottle but suction pressure is erroneously kept at zero. This can lead to build up of positive pressure in the ICD system and accumulation of air or fluid in the chest. Alternately the suction pressure may be set correctly, but the tubing may have been disconnected from the ICD bottle, leading to pleural collections. Hence proper connection of the tubing to the ICD bottle and proper adjustment of suction pressure should be ensured at least once in 4–6 hours.

NURSING RESPONSIBILITIES IN THE IMMEDIATE POSTOPERATIVE PERIOD

- Note the number and site of drains
- Mark the operating room level of blood/fluid in the ICD bottle
- Ensure application of adequate suction as described earlier
- Do not apply negative suction in an open sternum patient

- Monitor the amount of blood loss from the intercostal drains per hour. Varying criteria have been used to define significant blood loss in the postoperative period. However, a drainage more than 10 mL/kg/hour at any point of time, can be life threatening and should be immediately informed to the surgical team
- Ensure that the tubes are kept patent by milking the tube in the early postoperative period as there is risk of clotting and obstruction to drainage from the tube. This can lead to pericardial collection and cardiac tamponade
- Sudden decline in the amount of drainage should raise the suspicion of a tube block. This can lead to cardiac tamponade and hence should be brought to the attention of the surgical team
- Observe the nature of drainage from the tube, i.e., sanguineous/serosanguineous/serous/chylous drainage
- Ensure strict aseptic precautions while handling the intercostal drainage system
- Monitor for any kinks/twisting/disconnections of the ICD tubes
- The bottles have to be emptied promptly if likely to exceed capacity
- Monitor for air leaks/breaches in the drainage system
- A semi-Fowler's position has to be ensured to facilitate optimal drainage from the tube.

TRANSPORTING PATIENT FROM ONE LOCATION TO ANOTHER

The UWSD should always be maintained upright and below the level of the patient's chest. With these precautions the patient can walk about or be transported. However, if these conditions cannot be ensured during transport then the tubing is clamped with a soft clamp for the duration of transport to prevent air from entering the chest.

INTERCOSTAL DRAIN REMOVAL

The skin wound of the ICD insertion site should be sealed immediately upon ICD removal. To do this, a preplaced silk "U-stitch" may be used. Alternatively, the ICD site is covered with a piece of gauze and sealed with transparent film dressing or elastic adhesive bandage for a period of 5–7 days.

During removal certain precautions are essential:

1. The patient has to hold the breath in end inspiration. If this is not possible due to young age, inability to follow instructions or patient being on ventilator, every attempt should be made to remove the ICD during expiration to prevent the sucking-in of air during ICD removal.
2. The tube should be removed in a single brisk attempt under the cover of a gauze and the skin incision site sealed as described earlier.
3. Physical examination and confirmation of bilateral equal air entry is important after ICD removal.
4. A chest X-ray should be obtained after removal of a pleural drain to rule out any complications (pneumothorax/lung collapse).

REFERENCES

1. Talwar T, Agarwala S, Mittal CM, Choudhary SK, Airan B. Pleural effusions in children undergoing cardiac surgery. Ann Pediatr Cardiol. 2010;3(1):58-64.
2. Kumar A, Dutta R, Jindal T, Biswas B, Dewan RK. Safe insertion of a chest tube. National Med J India. 2009;22(4):192-8.
3. Senanayake EL, Smith GD, Rooney SJ, Graham TR, Greaves I. Chest drains: an overview. Trauma. 2017;19(2): 86-93.
4. Laws D, Neville E, Duffy J. BTS guidelines for the insertion of a chest drain. Thorax. 2003;58(Suppl. 2):ii53-ii59.
5. Allibone L. Nursing management of chest drains. Nurs Standard. 2003;17(22):45-54.
6. Charnock Y, Evans D. Nursing management of chest drains: a systematic review. Aust Crit Care. 2001;14(4):156-60.

Pacing in the Pediatric Cardiac Intensive Care Unit

Mani Ram Krishna

Reviewed by: R Krishna Kumar

■ INTRODUCTION

Temporary cardiac pacing is an integral part of management of a postoperative child. Surgeons place temporary pacing wires after most surgeries involving cardiopulmonary bypass. This acts as a critical diagnostic and therapeutic tool to manage a range of arrhythmias and hemodynamic instabilities. In this chapter, we will endeavor to familiarize the readers with insertion and maintenance of temporary pacing wires, basic definitions involved in cardiac pacing, the indications, setting and troubleshooting during cardiac pacing.

■ TEMPORARY PACING WIRES

Unipolar and Bipolar Pacing Wires

The pacing wires have a small needle at the epicardial end and a longer needle which is brought out through the skin **(Fig. 1)**. There are variants available which can be clipped or screwed into the myocardium. Both unipolar and bipolar variants of the temporary epicardial wires are available and widely used. In the unipolar variant, the negative electrode (anode) is placed on the myocardium while a separate positive electrode (cathode) is sutured to the skin. In bipolar electrodes, the anode and cathode are within the same pacing wire 8 mm apart with the anode located at the distal end which is attached to the myocardium and the cathode in a more proximal position. The bipolar electrodes require a smaller current for

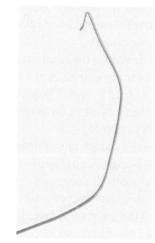

Fig. 1: The Centenial™ cFEP 13 unipolar temporary pacing wire has a simple needle design at the electrode end.

myocardial activation because of the smaller distance between the positive and negative electrodes. This, hence, results in lesser current drain compared to the unipolar electrodes. The unipolar electrodes in contrast are less expensive and hence more commonly used in resource limited settings. It is important to place a colored tag on the anode to enable differentiation between the two electrodes. The commonly available single chamber and dual chamber temporary pulse generators are shown in **Figures 2A to D**.

Inflammatory Response

Whenever the myocardium is activated by the pacing system, there is inflammation

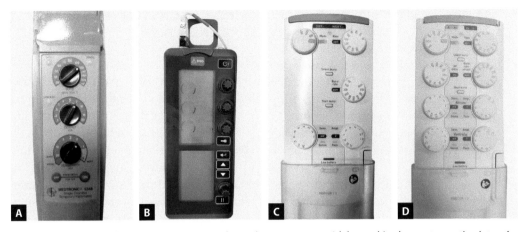

Figs. 2A to D: Some of the temporary pacemaker pulse generators widely used in the postoperative intensive care unit—(A) The Medtronic 5348 single chamber pacemaker; (B) The Medtronic 5392 dual chamber pacemaker; (C) The Biotronik Reocor S single chamber pacemaker; (D) The Biotronik Reocor D dual chamber pacemaker.

at the interface between the myocardium and the pacing wire. The inflammation is directly proportional to the amount of current and hence the quantum of inflammation is much higher in unipolar pacing systems.[1] Chronic inflammation results in the formation of a fibrous capsule around the pacing lead and an increase in pacing thresholds. Permanent pacing systems overcome this problem by steroid elution where a slow release of fluorinated corticosteroid (typically dexamethasone) limits the inflammatory response and ensures lower pacing threshold. However, steroid eluting temporary pacing wires are not available. A significant increase in pacing and sensing thresholds is noted approximately 4 days after placement in temporary pacing wires.[2] Most temporary pacing systems fail by the 7th to 10th postoperative day as a result of the inflammatory response although in exceptional circumstances, they have been used for a period of 3 months.[3]

Care of Temporary Pacing Wires

Temporary pacing wires are typically placed in the right atrium and ventricle after completion of cardiac surgery just before chest closure. By convention (albeit informal), the atrial pacing wires are brought out to the right of the sternum and the ventricular wires to the left. Negative electrodes are also identified by placing a colored tag. As the pacing wires provide a direct low resistance access to the heart, they carry a very high risk of inducing malignant ventricular arrhythmias including ventricular fibrillation.[4] It is hence important to prevent static electric forces. Nurses who handle pacing wires should always wear gloves and should touch metallic surfaces around the cot to discharge any static electric potential prior to handling the pacing wire.[4] The external end of the wires should be protected in a plastic casing at all times. In our unit, we utilize the plastic cover of sterile needles to encase temporary wires. The barrel of syringes has also been utilized in other units for this purpose.

In addition to general care, the nurse handling the baby should also carry out daily checks to ensure proper functioning of the pacing wires. In most units, this is performed by the day shift nurse soon after nursing handover is completed. The daily checks should include the following:

- The nurse should ensure that the pacemaker mode, rate, sensitivity, and output match the orders charted by the intensivist.
- The nurse should check adequacy of the pacemaker battery and ensure that additional new batteries are readily available. This is of vital importance in pacemaker dependent patients in whom a period of cessation of pacing may prove catastrophic.
- In postoperative patients who are pacemaker dependent, the underlying rhythm should be checked once a day by reducing the pacemaker rate to a very low value. It is the custom in our unit to obtain an electrocardiogram (ECG) in all pacemaker dependent patients before the morning cardiac rounds.
- The sensing and pacing thresholds should be checked once every day. In patients with no underlying rhythm however, checking pacing thresholds can occasionally result in inability to regain capture despite increasing the output.

Removal of the Temporary Pacing Wires

The temporary pacing wires can usually be dislodged from the myocardium by applying gentle traction. The movement of the heart aids dislodgement. It is important to avoid excessive force which can result in myocardial injury and pericardial effusion. In some instances, it becomes impossible to remove the wire by applying reasonable force. In such cases, an acceptable alternative is to cut the wire as close to the skin as possible. The wire then recoils into the chest cavity. Such retained metallic bits are harmless and have been shown to be safe in the long term. It is safe to perform magnetic resonance imaging in children with retained temporary pacing wires since they have no antenna to concentrate the magnetic energy from the scanner.[5]

INDICATIONS FOR TEMPORARY PACING WIRES

Diagnostic

Temporary epicardial pacing wires have both diagnostic and therapeutic utility in the pediatric postoperative intensive care unit (ICU). Their diagnostic utility stems from the ability to obtain atrial electrograms (AEG) using the atrial wires. Such electrograms are popularly referred to as "A-wire" studies and are obtained by connecting the atrial temporary pacing wire to the right arm channel of the ECG machine while obtaining a standard 6 lead ECG. This serves to augment the P wave when it is difficult to discern in a surface ECG.[6] This can help in differentiating junctional ectopic tachycardia (JET) from sinus tachycardia and other reentrant supraventricular tachycardias (SVT) when the P wave may not be clearly visible at very high fast rates. A detailed description of the atrial electrogram is provided in the chapter on postoperative arrhythmias.

Therapeutic

The main purpose of inserting temporary pacing wires after congenital heart surgery is to enable pacing of the atria and/or ventricles to manage dysrhythmias in the postoperative period. The various indications for pacing in the postoperative period may be categorized into:

Bradyarrhythmias:
- Sinus node dysfunction
- Sinus bradycardia
- Atrioventricular (AV) conduction disturbances–high degree AV block.

Tachyarrhythmias:
- Junctional ectopic tachycardia—overdrive atrial pacing is utilized to further suppress the junctional tachycardia after rate control is obtained using antiarrhythmic medications

- Re-entrant atrial tachyarrhythmias including atrial flutter and SVT—burst atrial pacing at very high heart rates can terminate the arrhythmia.

Atrial or sequential AV pacing is frequently utilized in infants with sinus bradycardia or AV dissociation with a good ventricular rate. Infants, in particular, are dependent on heart rate to augment cardiac output and atrial pacing is a superior alternative to pharmacological augmentation of heart rate in the immediate postoperative period. Restoration of AV synchrony in infants and children with AV block has also been shown to improve hemodynamics in the early postoperative period.[7]

ALTERNATIVES TO TEMPORARY CARDIAC PACING

Despite their established diagnostic and therapeutic utilities, it has been argued that temporary pacing wires need not be inserted universally after congenital heart disease surgery.[8] Temporary pacing can be reliably obtained using current generation transcutaneous pacing systems. However transcutaneous pacing can only be provided in an asynchronous mode and is uncomfortable to the patient often requiring sedation.[4] Transvenous pacing through a temporary pacing wire placed under fluoroscopic or ultrasound guidance offers more reliable capture than transcutaneous pacing but carries a higher risk of infections and lead dislodgement. The atria can be stimulated by transesophageal pacing and this modality could be utilized for atrial—only pacing as well as for burst pacing of the atria to terminate re-entrant tachyarrhythmias. However, it is not possible to pace the ventricle by transesophageal pacing wires.[6] None of these alternative modalities can replicate the diagnostic utility of temporary epicardial pacing wires in obtaining AEG. Thus, despite the availability of alternative modalities, temporary pacing wires remain the cheapest and most effective pacing modality in the postoperative patient.

■ DEFINITIONS IN PACING

Dual-chamber pacemaker: A pacemaker connected to both the atria and the ventricle. This enables sensing as well as pacing of both the chambers and helps maintain AV synchrony. This is important to optimize cardiac output in the postoperative patient.

Amplitude: This is the measurement of the output provided by the pacemaker. This is typically expressed as current (milliamperes) in temporary pacemakers and voltage (millivolts) in permanent pacemakers.

Capture: Capture is the depolarization of the cardiac chamber as a result of the electrical impulse provided by the pacemaker. During ventricular pacing, it is seen as a spike followed by a QRS complex. Loss of capture is seen as a spike which is not followed by a QRS complex **(Figs. 3A and B)**.

Intrinsic rate: This is the patient's own atrial or ventricular rate originating from the heart itself.

Intrinsic rhythm: This is the rhythm of the patient's conduction system. This can be normal (sinus rhythm) or abnormal (e.g., sinus bradycardia, complete heart block or junctional tachycardia).

Sensitivity: It is the pacemaker's ability to sense the intrinsic rhythm. The sensitivity number is the smallest electrical signal that can be detected by the pacemaker. The smaller the sensitivity number, the more sensitive the pacemaker is.

Threshold: This is the minimum electrical signal which can elicit a depolarization

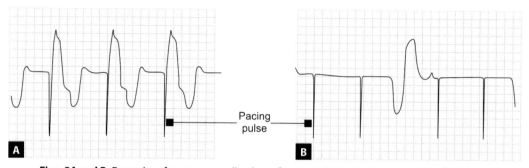

Figs. 3A and B: Examples of capture as well as loss of capture during temporary ventricular pacing.

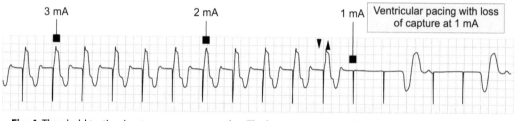

Fig. 4: Threshold testing in a temporary pacemaker. The lowest output at which there is consistent capture is 2 mA, which represents the ventricular pacing threshold.

consistently. Typically, the output of a temporary pacemaker is programmed to 2–3 times the threshold **(Fig. 4)**.

Overdrive pacing: When a postoperative patient is in an abnormal rhythm, pacing can be provided at a rate slightly higher than the patient's heart rate in order to suppress the abnormal rhythm and maintain AV synchrony. This is most frequently employed in postoperative JET when the junctional rate is less than 140/minute.

Postventricular atrial refractory period (PVARP): This is a function reserved for dual chamber pacemakers. This is the time period after ventricular depolarization when the atrial sensing is stopped temporarily. This prevents the atrial lead from inappropriately sensing ventricular activity as atrial.

■ PACEMAKER PROGRAMMING

The pacemaker settings are described utilizing the generic code devised jointly by the Heart Rhythm Society and the British Society of Pacing and Electrophysiology which was last revised in 2002.[9] The code (referred to as NBG code) consists of 5 positions. However, only the first 3 positions are relevant in temporary epicardial pacing and this is provided in **Table 1**. The commonly used pacing modes in the postoperative period and their indications have previously been described in detail[10] and are summarized in **Table 2**.

The basic steps to initiate cardiac pacing in the postoperative ICU are summarized and discussed here.

TABLE 1: Description of the first 3 positions of the Heart Rhythm Society and British Pacing and Electrophysiology Group genetic code (NBG code) for pacemaker programming.

I: Chamber paced	II: Chamber sensed	III: Response to sensing
O: None	O: None	O: None
A: Atrium	A: Atrium	T: Triggered
V: Ventricle	V: Ventricle	I: Inhibited
D: Dual	D: Dual	D: Dual

TABLE 2: Common temporary pacing modes used in the pediatric cardiac postoperative intensive care unit, their indications, and limitation.

Pacing mode	Indications	Limitation
AAI	• Sinus bradycardia • Sinus node dysfunction with preserved atrioventricular (AV) conduction • Atrial overdrive pacing in junctional ectopic tachycardia (after rate control is achieved to below 140 beats per minute)	This mode cannot be used when AV conduction abnormalities are suspected
VVI	• Sinus bradycardia (when atrial pacing wires are not available/cannot be used) • Complete Heart Block (however, DDD will remain the preferred mode)	This modality leads to loss of AV synchrony and could potentially result in hemodynamic instability in the postoperative patient with poor hemodynamic reserve
DDD	• All symptomatic bradyarrhythmia • Overdrive pacing for both supraventricular and ventricular tachyarrhythmias after adequate rate control	There is a small risk of "tracking" atrial arrhythmias resulting in very high ventricular rates. This can be prevented by setting an upper tracking rate if such a facility is available in the temporary pacemaker

Steps to Initiate Single Chamber Pacing

1. Identify the atrial and ventricular pacing wires. Typically, the atrial wires come out of the right side of the patient's chest and the ventricular wire on the left side.
2. Connect the pacing leads to the patient cable and ensure that it is locked tightly.
3. Screw the patient cable into the pacing box and ensure that you hear a click.
4. Switch the pacemaker on by pressing the ON/OFF button and holding it for 2 seconds.
5. Most single chamber pacemakers will allow you to set the pacing rate, threshold, and sensitivity.
6. First set the desired pacing rate.
7. Set the output at the maximum possible value (typically 10 mA in most temporary pacemakers) and look for capture **(Figs. 3A and B)**.
8. Slowly reduce the output of the pacemaker by 1 mA till there is loss of capture. The threshold will be the lowest output at which there is consistent capture **(Fig. 4)**.
9. Set the pacemaker output to 2–3 times the threshold.

10. If the patient is in sinus rhythm, check the intrinsic rate. Then keep the pacemaker rate at 10 bpm and check if the intrinsic rhythm is sensed accurately. If it is not sensed, reduce the sensitivity value till the intrinsic rhythm is correctly sensed.
11. Lock the pacemaker settings to ensure the settings are not changed accidentally. This provides an additional degree of safety especially when a patient is moved.

Steps to Initiate Dual Chamber Pacing

1. Identify the atrial and ventricular pacing wires
2. Connect the wires to the appropriate patient cables and the cables to the appropriate slots in the pacemaker
3. Switch the pacemaker on
4. Select the pacing mode (typically DDD)
5. Set a lower rate
6. Set an AV interval (typically this is between 150 and 200 ms)
7. Set an upper pacing rate
8. Calculate thresholds separately for the atrium and ventricle as described earlier. Next set the output for 2–3 times the threshold

9. Determine sensitivity thresholds as described earlier for atria and ventricles
10. Set PVARP
11. Lock the pacemaker.

BASIC PACEMAKER TROUBLESHOOTING

- *Failure to pace (No output)*
  No pacing spikes are discernible on the monitor and there are no paced beats. The etiology includes:
  - Battery depletion
  - Faulty cable connection/dislodgement
  - Lead displacement or fracture
  - Oversensing

  This can also be due to oversensing. If the sensitivity is kept at a very low level, the pacemaker may inappropriately sense far field potentials.

- *Loss of capture (Figs. 5A and B)*
  The electrical stimulus is delivered (as evidenced by a pacing spike on the monitor)

but does not result in atrial or ventricular depolarization. This could be due to:
  - Lead dislodgement/fracture
  - Low output setting
  - Increased resistance to conduction resulting in an increased threshold (this happens frequently in temporary pacing leads after 7–10 days)
  - Electrolyte imbalances including hyperkalemia and acidosis

- *Undersensing (Fig. 6)*
  The pacemaker fails to correctly detect intrinsic atrial or ventricular activity and inappropriately delivers an output after an intrinsic beat. The most common cause is inappropriate pacemaker programming in an asynchronous pacing mode (AOO, VOO or DOO). If this is ruled out other causes would include:
  - Low battery reserve
  - Low voltage complexes

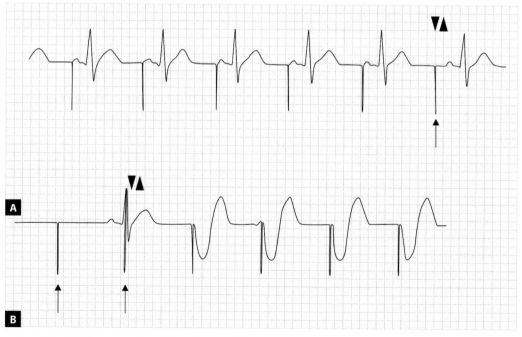

Figs. 5A and B: Two examples of loss of capture. The pacing spike indicates output from the pacemaker but there is no atrial or ventricular depolarization following the pacing spike.

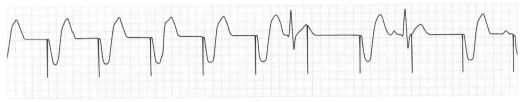

Fig. 6: ECG of a paced postoperative patient. Undersensing resulted in inappropriate pacing despite the presence of intrinsic QRS.

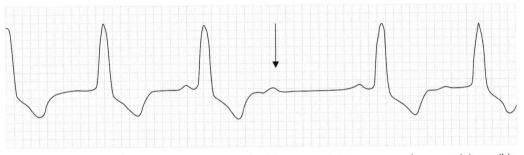

Fig. 7: Monitor tracing of a patient on temporary pacing. The arrow points to a nonpaced segment. It is possible that the P wave was inappropriately sensed as ventricular activity and pacing was inhibited.

- Low sensitivity
- Lead dislodgement or fracture
- *Oversensing* **(Fig. 7)**
  The pacemaker is inappropriately inhibited even though there is no intrinsic depolarization. The etiology would include:
  - High sensitivity
  - Low PVARP (if atrial lead is oversensing) resulting in inappropriate sensing of ventricular depolarization: This could be corrected by increasing the PVARP
- Electromechanical interference from surrounding monitors
- T wave sensing.

ECG strips for practice to understand the concepts are provided in the Quiz section with **Figures 8 and 9**.

QUIZ

Q.1A. What is happening in **Figure 8?**

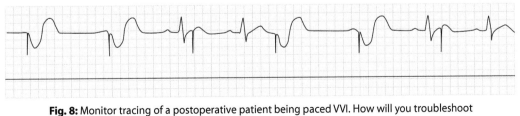

Fig. 8: Monitor tracing of a postoperative patient being paced VVI. How will you troubleshoot this pacing problem?

Q.1B. What are the next steps you should do to correct the problem?

Q.2A. What is happening in **Figure 9?**

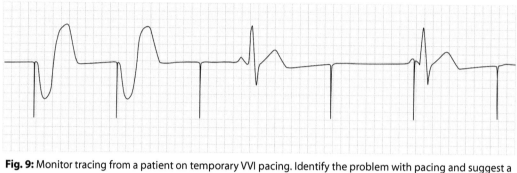

Fig. 9: Monitor tracing from a patient on temporary VVI pacing. Identify the problem with pacing and suggest a solution for the same.

Q.2B. What is the next step in management?

■ REFERENCES

1. Wirtz S, Schulte HD, Winter J, Godehardt E, Kunert J. Reliability of different temporary myocardial pacing leads. Thorac Cardiovasc Surg. 1989;37(3):163-8.
2. Elmi F, Tullo NG, Khalighi K. Natural history and predictors of temporary epicardial pacemaker wire function in patients after open heart surgery. Cardiology. 2002;98(4):175-80.
3. Filippi L, Vangi V, Murzi B, Moschetti R, Colella A. Temporary epicardial pacing in an extremely low-birth-weight infant with congenital atrioventricular block. Congenit Heart Dis. 2007;2(3):199-202.
4. Reade MC. Temporary epicardial pacing after cardiac surgery: a practical review: part 1: general considerations in the management of epicardial pacing. Anaesthesia. 2007;62(3):264-71.
5. Hartnell GG, Spence L, Hughes LA, Cohen MC, Saouaf R, Buff B. Safety of MR imaging in patients who have retained metallic materials after cardiac surgery. AJR Am J Roentgenol. 1997;168(5):1157-9.
6. Batra AS, Balaji S. Postoperative temporary epicardial pacing: when, how and why? Ann Pediatr Cardiol. 2008;1(2):120-5.
7. Janousek J, Vojtovic P, Chaloupecky V, Hucin B, Tlaskal T, Kostelka M, et al. Hemodynamically optimized temporary cardiac pacing after surgery for congenital heart defects. Pacing Clin Electrophysiol. 2000;23(8):1250-9.
8. Fishberger SB, Rossi AF, Bolivar JM, Lopez L, Hannan RL, Burke RP. Congenital cardiac surgery without routine placement of wires for temporary pacing. Cardiol Young. 2008;18(1):96-9.
9. Bernstein AD, Daubert JC, Fletcher RD, Hayes DL, Luderitz B, Reynolds DW, et al. The revised NASPE/BPEG generic code for antibradycardia, adaptive-rate, and multisite pacing. North American Society of Pacing and Electrophysiology/British Pacing and Electrophysiology Group. Pacing Clin Electrophysiol. 2002;25(2):260-4.
10. Reade MC. Temporary epicardial pacing after cardiac surgery: a practical review. Part 2: Selection of epicardial pacing modes and troubleshooting. Anaesthesia. 2007;62(4):364-73.

Inhaled Nitric Oxide: A Concise Review of its Use in the Pediatric Cardiac Intensive Care Unit

Sudheer Babu Vanga, Thushara Madathil, Aveek Jayant

Reviewed by: Aveek Jayant

■ INTRODUCTION

In 1980, Furchgott and Zawadski discovered that endothelium released a mediator that caused smooth muscle relaxation, and, by extension, vasodilation.[1] This was later identified as nitric oxide (NO)[2] and the work led to the award of a Nobel prize in medicine.[3] Nitric oxide when administered exogenously or when produced in vivo activates a cellular cascade that ultimately leads to smooth muscle relaxation and, therefore, vasodilation **(Fig. 1)**. Since then, NO has been recognized to have roles that go well beyond just vasodilation to inflammation; as a cytotoxic and cytostatic agent; its larger than life role in regulating vascular health; and its potential for adverse effects when administered or when produced in excess within the body.[4,5] Its biologic chemistry as the smallest

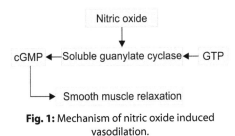

Fig. 1: Mechanism of nitric oxide induced vasodilation.

(cGMP: cyclic guanosine monophosphate; GTP: guanosine triphosphate)

Source: Edwards AD. The pharmacology of inhaled nitric oxide. Arch Dis Child Fetal Neonatal Ed. 1995;72(2): F127-30.

signaling molecule within the body has been elucidated in great detail uncovering the distinct isoforms of the enzyme nitric oxide synthase (and their roles in synthesis of NO from L-arginine and oxygen using a host of cofactors).[6] Unregulated NO systems are incriminated in the runaway vasodilation in sepsis and some of its coincident myocardial dysfunction.[7] NO is also unstable in air and undergoes spontaneous oxidation to NO_2 which is universally toxic to the respiratory tract,[8,9] and, is a key target for action in atmospheric pollution. NO also reacts with the superoxide ion to form peroxynitrate which is cytotoxic. In aqueous solution, NO degrades to nitrite and dinitrogen trioxide (NO_2^- and N_2O_3). The latter can form downstream compounds such as nitrosothiols which, by protein nitrosylation, have several cascading pluripotent effects.[8] Yet, as one of the star molecules that shows the tight connection between basic science research and clinical therapies, NO is rapidly degraded by hemoglobin (Hb)[10] to result in methemoglobin (or with deoxyHb to form iron nitrosyl Hb) making it a highly selective pulmonary vasodilator.[11] This alone probably accounts for our inability to substitute its life saving therapeutic roles across disease spectra or age groups ranging from persistent pulmonary hypertension of the newborn,[12] the prevention and treatment of other causes of respiratory distress in the neonatal period,[13] its gold standard roles in vasodilator testing across age groups,[14,15] and, as a rescue agent in pulmonary hypertension triggered right ventricular failure after congenital heart defect repair[16-19] or in the setting of heart,[20] lung[21] transplantation or ventricular assist device placement.[22] Yet, this description will be incomplete if we do not advert to the (anecdotal) drastic reduction in its historical use from units such as ours and the systematic description of such efforts to reduce its use elsewhere.[23,24] This is largely cost driven, but even otherwise, the use of an expensive therapy with a background of adverse effects does call for stringency based on evidence.

NITRIC OXIDE ADMINISTRATION

Ideally, inhaled nitric oxide (iNO) should be administered using a special purpose system that delivers nitric oxide calibrated to the flow of other respiratory gases and also continuously senses and measures the accuracy of delivery and level of nitrogen dioxide. This typically is done by one of the special purpose devices for this purpose (NOxBOX$_1$®, INOMAX® are examples). However, iNO may also be delivered directly from prefilled cylinders into the ventilator circuit using the equation given here.[25,26] Typically, the cylinders used have a concentration of 800 parts per million (ppm) with nitrogen as the diluent.[26]

Dose = (NO gas mixture cylinder concentration) (NO flow rate)/(Ventilator flow + NO flow)

Inhaled nitric oxide delivery is not as simple as it seems. The actual concentrations of iNO a patient receives is dependent on mode of ventilation, delivery point in the circuit, bias ventilatory flow, whether or not iNO is being delivered continuously or phased with inspiration, and cylinder volume status. Further, iNO has an impact on concentration

of oxygen[26] and tidal ventilation to small patients.[27] Consequently, it is important for practitioners to seek guidance from the iNO delivery system manufacturers about the extent of validation each system has undergone with respect to the patient ventilator in use, and what requirements there might be, when transitioned to spontaneous breathing, noninvasive support or high frequency ventilation. Strict adherence is required to the vendor specific instructions to ensure consistent delivery and avoid side effects from hazards such as NO_2.

It is mandatory to use an in-line monitor that continuously assesses the accuracy of iNO delivery and also measures the concentration of NO_2. Typically, doses used are in the range of 5–20 ppm, though use in the higher ranges of delivery systems (up to 80 ppm and higher with special purpose delivery systems) is also described.[28] Anecdotally, the use of iNO in doses higher than 20 ppm is usually not recommended on account of risks of methemoglobinemia; however this has also been recently questioned.[28] It would, however, be safe to obtain periodic assessment of methemoglobin, particularly if high doses are being used in a sustained fashion. The general principle remains that iNO should be used in compelling circumstances, at the lowest effective dose, and for the shortest time feasible.[23] Clinical practice guidelines[29] recommend adjunctive use of sildenafil in the pediatric cardiac intensive care unit (PCICU) to prevent rebound pulmonary hypertension based on evidence.[30] Most patients sick enough to require iNO are weaned off gradually as an effort to prevent rebound as well.

USES OF INHALED NITRIC OXIDE

- *Persistent pulmonary hypertension of the newborn*: In this setting, iNO has been suggested based on several trials[31,32] proving efficacy. Cumulative evidence extends its use to hypoxic respiratory failure in term or late preterm infants without congenital diaphragmatic hernia.[13]

- In the determination of operability (acute vasoreactivity testing) in late presenting left to right shunts and associated pulmonary arterial hypertension (APAH).[33-35]

- *In treating pulmonary hypertensive crisis in the PCICU*: It is suggested that the rationale for its use in this setting arises from the endothelial dysfunction that follows various stresses surrounding surgery. This wide-ranging decline in endothelial integrity causes a relative paucity of endogenous NO, triggering "reactive pulmonary artery hypertension". In patients at risk this is often countered using inodilator medications such as milrinone,[36] and, more recently, levosimendan.[37] Although this is often the "go to" modality in refractory pulmonary hypertension after cardiac surgery, there is uncertainty as to what is the exact nature or size of clinical benefit.[38,39] It is, however, clear that the therapy does significantly reduce mean pulmonary artery pressures (mPAP) with attendant benefits on gas exchange and may decrease duration of mechanical ventilation.[40] There is also anecdotal evidence of its utility in extreme situations such as cardiac arrest with underlying pulmonary artery hypertension (PAH).[41] It is typical to use sildenafil as an adjunct, given the compelling trial evidence,[30] to prevent NO rebound which usually occurs as iNO is weaned to low levels below 5 ppm; this seems to be the expert consensus.[34,35,42] It is also possible that practitioners might consider replacing this role of iNO with an inhaled prostacyclin[43] in locations where it is available. It may be more cost-effective than iNO;[43] however this benefit may not be sustained in the current era where iNO therapy is sought to be revolutionized using a novel technology.[44]

- *In the setting of pediatric heart transplantation with elevated pulmonary artery pressure*: Here iNO has been shown to reduce the incidence of right ventricular failure in the implanted organ.[45,46] However, use is not uniform[47] and prolonged use has been linked to worse outcome; although it could well be debated that extended use has resulted from residual severity of illness. iNO has also been used to assist the right ventricle in the setting of left ventricular assist device implantation.[48,49]

- As a rescue strategy in patients with decreased pulmonary blood flow after a bidirectional Glenn shunt/Fontan operation.[50,51] However, this is not a substitute for diligent assessment of suitability for such procedures based on hemodynamic data derived from cardiac catheterization. This role is likely a short-term measure in the face of reversible factors such as enhanced pulmonary vascular reactivity proximate to surgery or increased mPAP from reversible lung injury.

■ CONTRAINDICATIONS

Inhaled nitric oxide is contraindicated in any patient whose systemic perfusion is dependent on extrapulmonary right to left shunting such as duct dependent systemic circulation. It is also relatively contraindicated in Type II PAH until the underlying cause is treated or addressed or there has been a studied rationale to its use in this setting.[52] iNO should not be used in patients with congenital deficiency of enzymes that prevent handling of methemoglobin such as cytochrome b5 reductase deficiency or when there is baseline methemoglobinemia due to some acquired cause. In the latter case, introduction of iNO can confound the diagnosis of the originally elevated levels of methemoglobin. Methemoglobin levels of >4% should trigger suspicion of either iNO overdose or the need to anticipate discontinuation and substitution to other inhaled or parenteral therapies. Persistent methemoglobinemia even after discontinuation of iNO can be treated with either vitamin C or methylene blue.[53]

ADVERSE EFFECTS

These are some of the side effects of iNO therapy:

- Dizziness
- Dyspnea
- Headache
- Hematuria
- Hyperbilirubinemia
- Hyperglycemia
- Hypokalemia
- Hypotension
- Infection
- Methemoglobinemia
- Prolonged bleeding time
- Pulmonary edema
- Thrombocytopenia
- Withdrawal.

The most dangerous of these adverse effects is rebound PAH that tends to occur when iNO doses are reduced below 5 ppm. Sildenafil therapy has been found to decrease this outcome (as earlier).

SUMMARY

Inhaled nitric oxide remains the mainstay of life-threatening PAH in the acute setting. However, use and duration of use are steadily decreasing in real world practice due to enhanced efforts at stewardship, curtailing use to situations entailing hemodynamic compromise and the availability of other therapies such as inhaled prostanoids.

REFERENCES

1. Furchgott RF, Zawadzki JV. The obligatory role of endothelial cells in the relaxation of arterial smooth muscle by acetylcholine. Nature. 1980;288(5789):373-6.
2. Palmer RMJ, Ferrige AG, Moncada S. Nitric oxide release accounts for the biological activity of endothelium-derived relaxing factor. Nature. 1987;327(6122):524-6.
3. The Nobel Prize. (2018). Furchgott Lecture. [online] Available from: https://www.nobelprize.org/uploads/2018/06/furchgott-lecture.pdf. [Last Accessed May, 2021].
4. Epstein FH, Moncada S, Higgs A. The L-arginine-nitric oxide pathway. N Engl J Med. 1993;329(27):2002-12.
5. Moncada S, Higgs EA. The discovery of nitric oxide and its role in vascular biology: the discovery of nitric oxide and its role in vascular biology. Br J Pharmacol. 2006;147(S1):S193-201.
6. Forstermann U, Sessa WC. Nitric oxide synthases: regulation and function. Eur Heart J. 2012;33(7):829-37.
7. Vincent JL, Zhang H, Szabo C, Preiser JC. Effects of nitric oxide in septic shock. Am J Respir Crit Care Med. 2000;161(6):1781-5.
8. Weinberger B. The toxicology of inhaled nitric oxide. Toxicol Sci. 2001;59(1):5-16.
9. Petit PC, Fine DH, Vásquez GB, Gamero L, Slaughter MS, Dasse KA. The pathophysiology of nitrogen dioxide during inhaled nitric oxide therapy. ASAIO J. 2017;63(1):7-13.
10. Schechter AN, Gladwin MT. Hemoglobin and the paracrine and endocrine functions of nitric oxide. N Engl J Med. 2003;348(15):1483-5.
11. Ichinose F, Roberts JD, Zapol WM. Inhaled nitric oxide—a selective pulmonary vasodilator: current uses and therapeutic potential. Circulation. 2004;109(25):3106-11.
12. Inhaled nitric oxide in full-term and nearly full-term infants with hypoxic respiratory failure. N Engl J Med. 1997;336(9):597-604.
13. Barrington KJ, Finer N, Pennaforte T, Altit G. Nitric oxide for respiratory failure in infants born at or near term. Cochrane Database Syst Rev. 2017: CD000399.
14. Atz AM, Adatia I, Lock JE, Wessel DL. Combined effects of nitric oxide and oxygen during acute pulmonary vasodilator testing. J Am Coll Cardiol. 1999;33(3):813-9.
15. Krasuski RA, Warner JJ, Wang A, Harrison JK, Tapson VF, Bashore TM. Inhaled nitric oxide selectively dilates pulmonary vasculature in

adult patients with pulmonary hypertension, irrespective of etiology. J Am Coll Cardiol. 2000;36(7):2204-11.

16. Roberts JD, Lang P, Bigatello LM, Vlahakes GJ, Zapol WM. Inhaled nitric oxide in congenital heart disease. Circulation. 1993;87(2):447-53.

17. Hopkins R, Bull C, Haworth S, Deleval M, Stark J. Pulmonary hypertensive crises following surgery for congenital heart defects in young children. Eur J Cardiothorac Surg. 1991;5(12):628-34.

18. Miller OI, Tang SF, Keech A, Pigott NB, Beller E, Celermajer DS. Inhaled nitric oxide and prevention of pulmonary hypertension after congenital heart surgery: a randomised double-blind study. Lancet. 2000;356(9240):1464-9.

19. Russell IAM, Zwass MS, Fineman JR, Balea M, Rouine-Rapp K, Brook M, et al. The effects of inhaled nitric oxide on postoperative pulmonary hypertension in infants and children undergoing surgical repair of congenital heart disease. Anesth Analg. 1998;87(1):46-51.

20. Ardehali A, Hughes K, Sadeghi A, Esmailian F, Marelli D, Moriguchi J, et al. Inhaled nitric oxide for pulmonary hypertension after heart transplantation: Transplantation. 2001;72(4): 638-41.

21. Kao CC, Parulekar AD. Postoperative management of lung transplant recipients. J Thorac Dis. 2019;11(S14):S1782-8.

22. Antoniou T, Prokakis C, Athanasopoulos G, Thanopoulos A, Rellia P, Zarkalis D, et al. Inhaled nitric oxide plus iloprost in the setting of post-left assist device right heart dysfunction. Ann Thorac Surg. 2012;94(3):792-8.

23. Di Genova T, Sperling C, Gionfriddo A, Da Silva Z, Davidson L, Macartney J, et al. A stewardship program to optimize the use of inhaled nitric oxide in pediatric critical care. Qual Manag Health Care. 2018;27(2):74-80.

24. Rogerson CM, Tori AJ, Hole AJ, Summitt E, Allen JD, Abu-Sultaneh S, et al. Reducing unnecessary nitric oxide use: a hospital-wide, respiratory therapist-driven quality improvement project. Respir Care. 2021;66(1):18-24.

25. Edwards AD. The pharmacology of inhaled nitric oxide. Arch Dis Child Fetal Neonatal Ed. 1995;72(2):F127-30.

26. Francoe M, Troncy E, Blaise G. Inhaled nitric oxide: technical aspects of administration and monitoring. Crit Care Med. 1998;26(4):782-96.

27. Ranallo CD, Thurman TL, Holt SJ, Frank-Pearce SG, Anderson MP, Heulitt MJ. Effect of nitric oxide delivery device on tidal volume accuracy during mechanical ventilation at small tidal volumes. Respir Care. 2020; 65(11):1641-7.

28. Goldbart A, Golan-Tripto I, Pillar G, Livnat-Levanon G, Efrati O, Spiegel R, et al. Inhaled nitric oxide therapy in acute bronchiolitis: a multicenter randomized clinical trial. Sci Rep. 2020;10(1):9605.

29. Lopes AA, Barst RJ, Haworth SG, Rabinovitch M, Dabbagh MA, Cerro MJ del, et al. Repair of congenital heart disease with associated pulmonary hypertension in children: what are the minimal investigative procedures? Consensus Statement from the Congenital Heart Disease and Pediatric Task Forces, Pulmonary Vascular Research Institute (PVRI). Pulm Circ. 2014;4(2):330-41.

30. Namachivayam P, Theilen U, Butt WW, Cooper SM, Penny DJ, Shekerdemian LS. Sildenafil prevents rebound pulmonary hypertension after withdrawal of nitric oxide in children. Am J Respir Crit Care Med. 2006;174(9):1042-7.

31. Davidson D, Barefield ES, Kattwinkel J, Dudell G, Damask M, Straube R, et al. Inhaled nitric oxide for the early treatment of persistent pulmonary hypertension of the term newborn: a randomized, double-masked, placebo-controlled, dose-response, multicenter study. Pediatrics. 1998;101(3):325-34.

32. Clark RH, Kueser TJ, Walker MW, Southgate WM, Huckaby JL, Perez JA, et al. Low-dose nitric oxide therapy for persistent pulmonary hypertension of the newborn. N Engl J Med. 2000;342(7):469-74.

33. Apitz C, Hansmann G, Schranz D. Hemodynamic assessment and acute pulmonary vasoreactivity testing in the evaluation of children with pulmonary vascular disease. Expert consensus statement on the diagnosis and treatment of paediatric pulmonary hypertension. The European Paediatric Pulmonary Vascular Disease Network, endorsed by ISHLT and DGPK. Heart. 2016;102(Suppl 2):ii23-9.

34. Abman SH, Hansmann G, Archer SL, Ivy DD, Adatia I, Chung WK, et al. Pediatric pulmonary hypertension: guidelines from the American Heart Association and American Thoracic Society. Circulation. 2015;132(21):2037-99.

35. Hansmann G, Koestenberger M, Alastalo T-P, Apitz C, Austin ED, Bonnet D, et al. 2019 updated consensus statement on the diagnosis and treatment of pediatric pulmonary hypertension: The European Pediatric Pulmonary Vascular Disease Network (EPPVDN), endorsed by

AEPC, ESPR and ISHLT. J Heart Lung Transplant. 2019;38(9):879-901.

36. Burkhardt BE, Rücker G, Stiller B. Prophylactic milrinone for the prevention of low cardiac output syndrome and mortality in children undergoing surgery for congenital heart disease. Cochrane Heart Group, editor. Cochrane Database Syst Rev. 2015: CD009515.

37. Thorlacius EM, Wåhlander H, Ojala T, Ylänen K, Keski-Nisula J, Synnergren M, et al. Levosimendan versus milrinone for inotropic support in pediatric cardiac surgery: results from a randomized trial. J Cardiothorac Vasc Anesth. 2020;34(8):2072-80.

38. Bizzarro M, Gross I, Barbosa FT. Inhaled nitric oxide for the postoperative management of pulmonary hypertension in infants and children with congenital heart disease. Cochrane Anaesthesia Group, editor. Cochrane Database Syst Rev. 2014:CD005055.

39. Wong J, Loomba RS, Evey L, Bronicki RA, Flores S. Postoperative inhaled nitric oxide does not decrease length of stay in pediatric cardiac surgery admissions. Pediatr Cardiol. 2019;40(8):1559-68.

40. Villarreal EG, Aiello S, Evey LW, Flores S, Loomba RS. Effects of inhaled nitric oxide on haemodynamics and gas exchange in children after having undergone cardiac surgery utilising cardiopulmonary bypass. Cardiol Young. 2020;30(8):1151-6.

41. Bredmose PP, Buskop C, Lømo AB. Inhaled nitric oxide might be a contributing tool for successful resuscitation of cardiac arrest related to pulmonary hypertension. Scand J Trauma Resusc Emerg Med. 2019;27(1):22.

42. Molloy S, McVea S, Thompson A, Bourke T. In the child with pulmonary hypertension, does treatment with enteral sildenafil compared with a slow wean from nitric oxide alone prevent rebound pulmonary hypertension and allow for discontinuation of nitric oxide? Arch Dis Child. 2020;105(4):410-2.

43. Chen SH, Chen LK, Teng TH, Chou WH. Comparison of inhaled nitric oxide with aerosolized prostacyclin or analogues for the postoperative management of pulmonary hypertension: a systematic review and meta-analysis. Ann Med. 2020;52(3-4):120-30.

44. Medgadget. (2015). Novel Portable Nitric Oxide Generator Pulmonary Hypertension Therapy. [online] Available from: https://www.medgadget.com/2015/07/novel-portable-nitric-oxide-generator-pulmonary-hypertension-therapy.html. [Last Accessed May, 2021].

45. Ofori-Amanfo G, Hsu D, Lamour JM, Mital S, O'Byrne ML, Smerling AJ, et al. Heart transplantation in children with markedly elevated pulmonary vascular resistance: impact of right ventricular failure on outcome. J Heart Lung Transplant. 2011;30(6):659-66.

46. Daftari B, Alejos JC, Perens G. Initial experience with sildenafil, bosentan, and nitric oxide for pediatric cardiomyopathy patients with elevated pulmonary vascular resistance before and after orthotopic heart transplantation. J Transplant. 2010;2010:1-6.

47. Bearl DW, Dodd DA, Thurm C, Hall M, Soslow JH, Feingold B, et al. Practice variation, costs and outcomes associated with the use of inhaled nitric oxide in pediatric heart transplant recipients. Pediatr Cardiol. 2019;40(3):650-7.

48. Yahagi N, Kumon K, Nakatani T, Matsui J, Sasako Y, Isobe F, et al. Inhaled nitric oxide for the management of acute right ventricular failure in patients with a left ventricular assist system. Artif Organs. 1995;19(6):557-8.

49. Argenziano M, Choudhri AF, Moazami N, Rose EA, Smith CR, Levin HR, et al. Randomized, double-blind trial of inhaled nitric oxide in LVAD recipients with pulmonary hypertension. Ann Thorac Surg. 1998;65(2):340-5.

50. Gamillscheg A, Zobel G, Urlesberger B, Berger J, Dacar D, Stein JI, et al. Inhaled nitric oxide in patients with critical pulmonary perfusion after Fontan-type procedures and bidirectional glenn anastomosis. J Thorac Cardiovasc Surg. 1997;113(3):435-42.

51. Latus H, Gerstner B, Kerst G, Moysich A, Gummel K, Apitz C, et al. Effect of inhaled nitric oxide on blood flow dynamics in patients after the Fontan procedure using cardiovascular magnetic resonance flow measurements. Pediatr Cardiol. 2016;37(3):504-11.

52. Gerges C, Gerges M, Fesler P, Pistritto AM, Konowitz NP, Jakowitsch J, et al. In-depth haemodynamic phenotyping of pulmonary hypertension due to left heart disease. Eur Respir J. 2018;51(5):1800067.

53. UpToDate. (2021). Methemoglobinemia. [online] Available from: https://www.uptodate.com/contents/ methemoglobinemia?search=methemoglobinemia&source=search_result&selectedTitle=1~150&usage_type=default&display _rank=1#H2423216097. [Last Accessed May, 2021].

Praveen Reddy Bayya
Illustration: Praveen Reddy Bayya
Reviewed by: Aveek Jayant

◼ DEFINITION

Extracorporeal membrane oxygenation (ECMO) is a form of extracorporeal life support where an external circuit carries the patient's venous blood to an oxygenator for gas exchange and returns it to the patient circulation, thus augmenting or completely replacing the patient's heart and/or lung function.

The ECMO is commonly of venovenous (VV) or venoarterial (VA) modes, for respiratory and circulatory failure respectively. Congenital heart disease (CHD) (commonly for postoperative support after corrective or palliative cardiac surgery), cardiogenic shock and cardiomyopathy are the most frequent diagnoses in neonatal and pediatric ECMO and VA mode is the most common, accounting for 97%.[1] Mechanical circulatory support is an important tool in the postcardiotomy management of children as surgeons attempt to stretch the boundaries of operability of CHD. Survival to discharge from hospital is still around 50% or less according to data from the registry of the Extracorporeal Life Support Organization (ELSO). The substantial costs, equipment and expertise involved, limit the wider application of this technology. By default, ECMO is often initiated when conventional therapies fail or when cardiac arrest is imminent; this approach further limits the outcomes of this therapy. Since ECMO is often initiated in crash situations,

or rarer, in the operating room immediate to surgery, cannulation is often inevitably central. Finally, the low penetration and use overall, precludes centers from establishing and practicing care pathways including establishing ECMO as a form of extracorporeal cardiopulmonary resuscitation (ECPR). It is unknown what impact all of these factors have on outcomes, when compared to the overall registry data from ELSO. Compared to current ELSO data it also seems unlikely that centers such as ours will institute ECMO to support the univentricular heart except in rare situations (e.g., the go to modality in certain cases such as support after a bidirectional Glenn shunt where conventional CPR is futile). In contrast, ECMO use in the setting of univentricular hearts, and the Norwood operation, in particular, contributes the largest share to global use of postcardiotomy ECMO. In the absence of a broader framework that incorporates assist devices and a countrywide transplantation program, ECMO in our setting is a niche therapy for some children, who have assured surgical quality to tide over a temporary crisis in the immediate postcardiotomy period.

◼ CIRCUIT OVERVIEW

Cannulation:[2] "Central ECMO", referring to open chest ECMO with cannulation of aorta

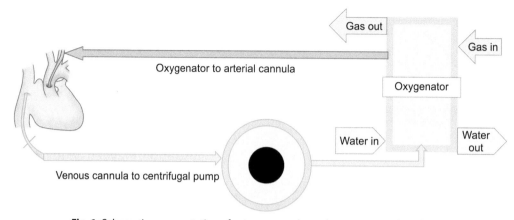

Fig. 1: Schematic representation of extracorporeal membrane oxygenation circuit.

and right atrium/vena cava, is the most common form of ECMO instituted in the cardiac intensive care unit (ICU). Alternatively ECMO can be instituted via peripheral cannulation, the sites being carotid vessels in infants and younger children (<15 kg), or femoral vessels in older children (>15 kg).[3]

The circuit used consists of a centrifugal pump and an integrated oxygenator/heat exchanger. Hemofilters are added when needed. A schematic representation of the ECMO circuit is provided in **Figure 1**.

■ ECMO RELATED CLINICAL DUTIES

ECMO Specific Routine Nursing Care

- *"Start of shift" nursing checklist*: Cannula position and position maintenance, cleanliness of cannula and line sites, peripheral pulse marked with indelible ink, protection of pressure points.
- *Monitoring and documentation*:
  - *Rhythm and heart rate*: Sinus rhythm/atrioventricular synchrony promote ventricular recovery.
  - *Vitals*: Hourly mean arterial pressure (MAP), central venous pressure (CVP), temperature, blood flow, urine output, fluid balance, pupils, warmth and color of peripheries, capillary filling and peripheral pulse when recordable.

In case of peripheral ECMO via femoral cannulae, the peripheral limb circulation should be assessed hourly with Doppler, and limb girth at calf and mid-thigh measured hourly for ensuring adequacy of venous return.

While optimal MAP has not been defined in postcardiac arrest patients, higher MAP benefits cerebral perfusion; and maintenance of low systemic vascular resistance (SVR) is critical for myocardial dysfunction.[4] Monitoring SvO_2 and lactate trends early on are important indicators of response to therapy and can identify persistent low cardiac output (inadequate ECMO flows).[4]

- Sampling
- Routine sampling:
  - 4- or 6-hourly arterial blood gases (ABGs)
  - Activated clotting time (ACT) 1–2 hourly or as needed[5]
  - Daily blood investigations
  - Activated partial thromboplastin time (APTT) 6-hourly (less accurate in neonates and children)
- Dressing and line position monitoring

- *Training*: Structured team training, of doctors as well as nurses has been found to increase the probability of post-cardiotomy ECMO weaning and survival.[6]

ECMO Specific Routine Medical Care

- *Cardiac considerations*:[3]
  - The acute loss of preload and sudden increase in afterload on ECMO initiation causes worsening of cardiac function and recovery takes 3–7 days. Hence, afterload reduction is important.
  - When left ventricular function is inadequate, the ensuing ventricular distension leads to pulmonary edema and subendocardial ischemia, onset of which is in 4–8 hours in most cases. Hence, venting the left heart is critical in these patients and the requirement for this should be assessed after ECMO initiation. Since ECMO initiation is often via central cannulation in open chest conditions, surgical options to vent the left heart are readily available and are typically applied soon after initiating ECMO based on an assumption that this is the key to facilitating early recovery.
  - *Inotrope requirements and choice*:
    - Severe cardiac dysfunction—adrenaline, dobutamine (to prevent blood stasis in ventricle and aortic root)
    - Vasodilatory shock—norepinephrine, vasopressin (for peripheral vasoconstriction)
    - Poor systemic perfusion/ventricular dysfunction-phentolamine, nitroprusside (for peripheral vasodilatation and afterload reduction)
    - Considering that the ECMO circulation is both preload and afterload dependent, maintaining adequate preload and reducing excessive afterload is obviously crucial to achieving pump output.

- *Fluid management*: While the limitations of CVP as a correlate of volume status have to be kept in mind, in combination with circuit characteristics such as low flow and circuit chatter it assists in guiding fluid management. Diagnostic value of CVP in a patient on ECMO is given in **Table 1**. Troubleshooting guide for commonly encountered scenarios in a patient on ECMO is depicted in **Table 2**.

- *Routine investigations*: Daily chest X-rays should be taken when feasible. Position of endotracheal tube, nasogastric tube, invasive lines and cannulae are to be noted. Evidence of pleural collection and pneumothorax to be looked for.

Daily blood investigations:
  - Complete blood count is done daily.
  - It is recommended practice to measure platelet counts daily and transfuse platelets to maintain levels of 80,000/mm^3.
  - Fibrinogen levels should be checked daily and fresh frozen plasma (FFP) or fibrinogen transfused to maintain levels in the normal range (250–300 mg/dL).[3]
  - Renal and hepatic functions are assessed on the first day after initiation of ECMO and thereafter, when needed.
  - In case of bleeding, prothrombin time (PT)/international normalized ratio (INR), APTT, platelet count, fibrinogen

TABLE 1: Diagnostic role of central venous pressure (CVP) in a patient on extracorporeal membrane oxygenation.

CVP	Circuit flows	Probable diagnosis
Low	Low	Hypovolemia
High	Low	Cardiac tamponade
High	High	Hypervolemia

TABLE 2: Troubleshooting guide for commonly encountered monitoring issues.

Issue	Potential corrective actions

Low flow	• Inadequate preload:
	  – Administer volume or transfuse
	  – Assess for bleeding
	  – Assess for inlet cannula kinking
	• Increased afterload:
	  – Assess for kinking of outflow cannula
	  – Assess pump for thrombus
	  – Decrease MAP with antihypertensives
	• Increase RPM

Low MAP	• Assess for bleeding, systemic infection • Administer volume or transfuse • Start vasopressor • Increase ECMO flow
Low PaO$_2$	• Increase circuit FiO$_2$ • Increase circuit flow • Assess oxygenator function • Increase ventilator support
Increased PCO$_2$	• Increase sweep gas flow • Increase ventilator support
Low SvO$_2$	• Increase ECMO flow • Ensure adequate PaO$_2$ • Transfuse blood

Increased lactate level	• Assess for local ischemia (gut, limb)
	• Increase systemic O$_2$ delivery
	  – Increase ECMO flow
	  – Transfuse
	  – Increase PaO$_2$ if low

(ECMO: extracorporeal membrane oxygenation; MAP: mean arterial pressure; RPM: rotations per minute)

levels and thromboelastography (TEG) are indicated.

- Blood culture is sent in the presence of fever or clinical evidence of infection.
- When hemolysis is suspected, plasma hemoglobin levels are measured. Normal levels are below 10 mg/dL and a raise should prompt a search for the source of hemolysis.
- *Assessing adequacy of ECMO support*[3]: Venous saturations of 70-80% are to be maintained. Peripheral tissue perfusion is assessed by monitoring peripheral temperature, color of peripheries, capillary filling, urine output, lactate levels on ABG and MAP. It is useful to periodically assess for recovery of ventricular function; patients who do not obtain this state in 48-72 hours of initiation have poor prognosis and each institution should formulate a guideline that allows withdrawal of support after a predetermined period that matches the global literature on this important milestone.

- *Anticoagulation*: The ECMO circuit is procoagulant and inadequate anticoagulation leads to circuit clots, accelerated platelet deposition and systemic fibrinolysis.[3] After initiation of ECMO, once APTT drops to twice the normal or ACT drops to 300 S, heparin infusion is started.[7] Meanwhile ACT is checked every 15-30 minutes. Heparin is started at 5-10 units/kg/hour and can be increased up to 20, titrating infusion rate to maintain an ACT of 180-220 S (180-200 in coated circuits, 200-220 in non-coated circuits).[5,6] Heparin infusion in neonates usually starts at higher rates, and increased up to 30 units/kg/hour due to their low plasma concentration of ATIII. Heparin induced thrombocytopenia is extremely rare in neonates.[5] Bolus heparin at 10-20 units/kg is administered if ACT drops to below 160 S.

Platelets are maintained at >50,000/mm³ and >80,000/mm³ in nonbleeding and bleeding patients, respectively. APTT is maintained at 50-70 S.[8] It is important to remember that APTT poorly correlates with antifactor Xa and heparin levels in neonatal and pediatric patients due to developmental differences in coagulation and the effect of acute phase reactants in critical illness, and hence does not perform reliably.[3]

- *Ventilator management*[3]: Ventilation strategies are different for VV and VA ECMO. For VA ECMO the aim of ventilation is to prevent atelectasis and maintain normal functional residual capacity (FRC) by maintaining adequate positive end expiratory pressure (PEEP). Overventilation should be avoided in a patient on full VA ECMO flows, since the pulmonary blood flow is minimal. A suggested ventilatory strategy is depicted below.
  - Pressure limited ventilation
  - Elevated PEEP (10 cmH$_2$O)
  - Tidal volume 6–8 mL/kg
  - Peak inspiratory pressures (PIP) no higher than 18–20 cmH$_2$O
  - Low respiratory rate (10/min)
  - Meticulous pulmonary hygiene.
    In neonates current ELSO guidelines recommend:[5]
  - PIP no higher than 15–22 cmH$_2$O
  - PEEP of 5–8 cmH$_2$O
  - Rate of 12–20/mm
  - Inspiratory time of 0.5 seconds
  - FiO$_2$ of 0.21–0.3.
- *Blood product transfusion*: Hemoglobin should be kept above 8–9 g/dL to optimize oxygen delivery.[9] A restrictive transfusion strategy is shown not to be harmful and packed red blood cells (PRBC) transfusion should be restricted to hematocrit <25%, the presence of bleeding or signs of inadequate oxygen delivery.[10]
  Platelets are transfused to maintain levels described earlier.
  Cryoprecipitate transfusion is reserved for patients with bleeding to maintain fibrinogen >150 mg/dL.
  Fresh frozen plasma is transfused in the presence of clinical bleeding titrated to point of care monitoring of coagulation.

- *Antibiotics*: At the time of initiation of ECMO, prophylactic antibiotics are given as per institutional policies. No routine antibiotics are required for patients on ECMO.
- *Temperature management*: The heat exchanger in the ECMO circuit is used to maintain required temperature. Normothermia is usually maintained. Cooling is needed for neuroprotection, to decrease patient metabolic demands, and for treatment of fever. If there is a concern for hypoxic ischemic brain injury, mild hypothermia (32–34°C) for the first 24–72 hours may be maintained.[5]
- *Analgesia and sedation*: Sedation should be minimized if cannulation is peripheral, in order to facilitate spontaneous movement and ventilation. In chest open patients, our unit prefers infusion of short acting muscle relaxants and fentanyl at 2 µg/kg/hour. Due to circuit adsorption and hemofiltration dosing requirements may be elevated.
- *Stress ulcer prophylaxis*: Proton pump inhibitors are recommended for all patients on ECMO at our center.
- *Hemofiltration*: This is initiated if there is progressive interstitial edema, insufficient response to pharmacological diuresis and in renal failure. It is usual to initiate some form of ultrafiltration in the early and late stages of the ECMO run: initially to correct the excessive fluid therapy that might accompany a cardiopulmonary arrest and subsequent resuscitation and later to facilitate smoother return to physiological function of lungs and other organs.
- *Nutrition*: Feeding is initiated once lactate levels normalize. Routine feeding protocols are followed. Early initiation of nutrition is recommended.[3] Total parenteral nutrition with fluid restriction

and a calorie target of 80 kcal/kg/day is preferred to enteral nutrition in neonates on ECMO.[5] Lipids are administered through a peripheral line to avoid circuit thrombosis due to lipid precipitation.[5]

ECMO COMPLICATIONS: PREVENTION AND MANAGEMENT

The most common complications are as follows (% incidence in brackets):

- Mechanical pump malfunction (1.5–1.8%)
- Mechanical oxygenator failure (6.1–7.2%)
- Cannula site hemorrhage (10.7–15.6%)
- Surgical site hemorrhage (29%)
- Pulmonary hemorrhage (5.2%)
- Central nervous system (CNS) hemorrhage (5.3–11.3%)
- CNS infarction (3.4–5%)
- Renal failure (7.2–12.3%)
- Hyperbilirubinemia (4.9–7.2%) and infection (7–11%).

The prevention and treatment of these complications are discussed here in detail.[1]

Bleeding

Bleeding can be postprocedural or spontaneous. Hypothermia and acidosis are corrected. Heparin is withheld in consultation with the surgeon and all deficiencies in clotting elements corrected. Tranexamic acid loading dose (100 mg/kg) is given and maintenance infusion at 10 mg/kg/hour is initiated for 6 hours. Infusion rate has to be reduced in renal and hepatic dysfunction. Protamine and factor VIIa are not routinely used and should be used with caution and in consultation with the surgeon. Occasionally surgical exploration may be needed; persisting bleeding of >2 mL/kg/hour for more than 4 hours or >10 mL/kg of bleeding in 1 hour should be brought to the attention of surgical team.

Intracranial Hemorrhage

Bleeding into the head or brain parenchyma is a serious ECMO complication, especially in neonates. Head ultrasound (HUS) should be performed every 24 hours for at least the first 3–5 days in stable neonates on ECMO, beyond which period they are not cost-effective.[11] If hemodynamic or coagulation instability is present in neonates on ECMO, daily HUS should be performed. Small bleeds necessitate only optimization of coagulation status and twice daily HUS. Moderate or large bleeds warrant weaning from ECMO.[5]

Cannula Dislodgement and Site Contamination

These are dangerous complications and need to be prevented.

- *Securing the cannulae*: All cannulae must be secured at least at two points, and this should be checked during every nursing shift change.
- *Cannula position*: This should be checked daily in the chest X-rays and change in position should be addressed immediately.
- *Cannula dressing*: Insertion sites must be kept unsoiled and dressings changed as and when needed, by the nursing staff.
- *Patient movement*: Moving the patient for chest X-rays, back care and position change should be done in the presence of the intensivist and perfusionist. Meticulous attention should be paid to prevent cannula dislodgement or kinking, during patient movement for these procedures.

REFERENCES

1. Thiagarajan RR, Barbara RP, Rycus PT, McMullan DM, Conrad SA, Fortenberry JD, et al. Extracorporeal Life Support Organization Registry International Report 2016. ASAIO J. 2017;63:60-7.

2. Harvey C. Cannulation for neonatal and pediatric extracoporeal membrane oxygenation for cardiac support. Front Pediatr. 2018;6:17.

3. Brown G, Deatrick KB. Paediatric Cardiac Failure. In: ECLS Guidelines 2018. Michigan: Extracorporeal Life Support Organization; 2018.

4. Marino BS, Tabbutt S, MacLaren G, Hazinski MF, Adatia I, Atkins DL, et al. Cardiopulmonary resuscitation in infants and children with cardiac disease: a scientific statement from the American Heart Association. Circulation. 2018;137:e691-e782.

5. Gray B, Rantoul N. Extracorporeal Life Support Organization Guidelines for Neonatal Respiratory Failure, version 1.4. Michigan: Extracorporeal Life Support Organization; 2017.

6. Miana LA, Caneo LF, Tanamati C, Penha JG, Guimaraes VA, Miura N, et al. Post-cardiotomy ECMO in pediatric and congenital heart surgery: impact of team training and equipment in the results. Braz J Cardiovasc Surg. 2015;30(4):409-16.

7. Lequier L, Annich G, Al-Ibrahim G, Bembea M, Brodie D. ELSO Anticoagulation guideline 2014. Michigan: Extracorporeal Life Support Organization; 2014.

8. ELSO Guidelines for Cardiopulmonary Extracorporeal Life Support Extracorporeal Life Support Organization, Version 1.3. Michigan: Extracorporeal Life Support Organization; 2013.

9. Hirose H, Pitcher HT, Baram M, Cavarocchi NC. Issues in the intensive care unit for patients with extracorporeal membrane oxygenation. Crit Care Clin. 2017;33:855-62.

10. King CS, Roy A, Ryan L, Singh R. Cardiac support. Emphasis on venoarterial ECMO. Crit Care Clin. 2017;33:777-94.

11. Allen KY, Allan CK, Su L, McBride ME. Extracorporeal membrane oxygenation in congenital heart disease. Semin Perinat. 2018;42:104-10.

48

CHAPTER

Myocardial Protection in Pediatric Cardiac Surgery

Suresh G Nair

Reviewed by: Rakhi Balachandran

■ INTRODUCTION

The objective of every cardiac surgery must be a technically perfect anatomic correction while avoiding any myocardial damage in pursuit of this goal. Despite advances in surgical and anesthetic techniques, pediatric myocardial protection remains relatively unchanged. Perioperative myocardial damage and low output syndrome remains the most common cause of morbidity and mortality following technically successful cardiac repair. Cardiac damage from inadequate myocardial protection causes low output syndrome, which prolongs hospital stay and may also result in delayed myocardial fibrosis, leading to cardiac dysfunction months to years later. Cardio-protective strategies have evolved to limit intraoperative damage during a complicated procedure. *Surgeons and anesthesiologists must refrain from using "simplistic cardioplegic solutions" for the very reason that simplicity and safety are not synonymous.* Optimal myocardial protection requires integration of various techniques to achieve the best results.

■ PREOPERATIVE CONSIDERATIONS

Pediatric hearts are more subjected to physiologic stress (pressure/volume overload and hypoxia) that is quite different from those seen in adults. It has been shown that the immature myocardium has greater tolerance to ischemia when compared with mature myocardium. There are a number of peculiarities associated with the neonatal and infant heart that needs to be understood.

- *Substrate metabolism*: In adults, up to 90% of the energy requirements are derived from the metabolism of fatty acids. In contrast, the main substrate for the neonatal heart is glucose. The transition from glucose to fatty acids as the main source of energy takes place in the first few weeks of life. The ability of the neonatal heart to utilize glucose is related to the reduced expression of the insulin sensitive glucose transporter (GLUT4) and the enhanced expression of noninsulin sensitive glucose transporter (GLUT1) at the cellular level of neonates.[1]

- *Glucose uptake and enhanced recovery*: A positive correlation has been demonstrated between enhanced glucose uptake and return of myocardial contractile function. Since, the neonatal myocardium primarily utilizes glucose as the substrate, it is conceivable that the neonatal myocardium should tolerate and recover from ischemia better.

- *Calcium overload*: The activity of the sarcoplasmic reticulum in neonate is lower than in the adult heart. Therefore, the ability to release calcium upon stimulation and its reuptake into the sarcoplasmic reticulum is also diminished. In pediatric hearts, the calcium required for contractile function is mainly supplied by influx from the extracellular space. Postischemic calcium overload may be caused by providing a perfusion medium with normal or high calcium during surgery.

- *Enzyme activities*: The antioxidant defense system in the body includes superoxide dismutase, glutathione reductase and catalase. Glutathione reductase is markedly reduced in children with tetralogy of Fallot.[2] Strategies to reduce generation of free radicals during the reperfusion period may be particularly useful in these children.

- *Enzyme activity*: 5' nucleotidase is an enzyme bound to plasma membrane and catalyzes the conversion of adenosine monophosphate to adenosine. Whereas, adenosine monophosphate cannot pass the plasma membrane, adenosine gets easily lost to the extracellular space. Loss of adenosine from the intracellular pool results in slower regeneration of ATP after establishment of reperfusion. Whereas, the ATP content of the heart is not a predictor of postischemic recovery, the size of the adenine nucleotide pool is important. If this pool is depleted significantly, immediate recovery of contractile function is impossible. The inhibition of 5' nucleotidase or lack of its activity as in the new-born has been shown to improve ischemic tolerance.[3]

In summary, the preference of immature myocardium for glucose, the abundant stores of glycogen, and the low activity of 5'nucleotidase contribute to the extensive ischemia tolerance of the pediatric heart. In contrast, the reduced enzyme activity of the free-radical scavenging system and the increased calcium sensitivity may decrease myocardial ischemia tolerance and make the heart more prone to damage during reperfusion. Although, the immature myocardium may show a certain degree of tolerance to ischemia, if the same myocardium is stressed, it shows a similar tolerance to ischemia as the adult heart.

Volume overloading of the pediatric heart occurs in many situations. The ability of the immature myocardium to compensate for this is limited, because these hearts function at high diastolic volume and therefore have limited diastolic reserve. Similarly, congenital lesions that lead to ventricular outflow obstruction or result in increased arterial resistance lead to ventricular hypertrophy. Hypertrophy also causes regional disturbances in myocardial blood flow and subendocardial ischemia.

■ CARDIOPLEGIA

Neonatal myocardial protection remains suboptimal resulting in an increased operative mortality as compared to older children and adults. Extrapolating adult cardio-protective strategies to the neonatal heart can be potentially harmful. Cardioplegic solutions may vary but the principles that underlie the composition of all solutions include:

- The ability to produce immediate arrest
- Hypothermia
- Substrate enrichment
- Appropriate pH
- High osmolarity to prevent myocardial edema
- Membrane stabilization.

We will now review some of these key features of cardioplegia.

Types of Cardioplegia

In general, cardioplegia can be divided into two types: (1) *blood cardioplegia and*

(2) *crystalloid cardioplegia. Blood cardioplegia* is probably the most popular cardioplegia used across the world. In general, autologous blood from the cardiopulmonary bypass circuit is mixed with crystalloid cardioplegia solution (commercial or prepared locally) and delivered to the patient at a low temperature with or without the use of a cardioplegia delivery system. High potassium content is generally used for immediate cardiac arrest. A number of additives including citrate-phosphate-dextrose, magnesium, lidocaine, bicarbonate, or mannitol are added to protect and prevent ischemia and reperfusion injury.

Crystalloid cardioplegia is characterized by high potassium content (10–40 mmol/L) and also have a high buffering capacity. The major advantage of crystalloid cardioplegia is that it is cheap, easy to use, and some of them can be used as a single dose for the entire duration of aortic cross clamp. Crystalloid cardioplegia is generally available as *intracellular type and extracellular* type.

- *Intracellular type crystalloid cardioplegia* is characterized by a low sodium and calcium content. The classical example of intracellular type of cardioplegia is *del Nido* cardioplegia
- *Extracellular cardioplegia* is characterized by a high sodium, magnesium and calcium content. *St Thomas cardioplegia* is an example of extracellular type cardioplegia.

Cardioplegia can also be classified based on the *type of arrest* it induces. Most cardioplegic agents induce cardiac arrest by depolarizing the myocardial membrane resulting in diastolic arrest. This includes St Thomas solution, customized cardioplegia and del Nido solutions. On the other hand, low sodium containing cardioplegic agents produce hyperpolarization of the myocardial membrane and induce cardiac arrest.

Custodial cardioplegia is the classic example of this type of cardiac arrest.

Blood Cardioplegia

Blood cardioplegia predominates in pediatric cardiac surgery. Both blood and crystalloid (St Thomas) cardioplegia provide excellent myocardial protection in the unstressed neonatal heart. However, in a hypoxic stressed heart the situation is different. Blood cardioplegic solutions not only protect the heart from further damage but also facilitate recovery from the injury caused by hypoxia and reoxygenation resulting in better preservation of myocardial and vascular function. Blood cardioplegia has several advantages over crystalloid cardioplegia:

- With blood cardioplegia, the heart is arrested in an oxygenated environment, so no loss of high-energy phosphate occurs during the short period of electro-mechanical activity between aortic cross camp and cardioplegic arrest. A significant decrease of high-energy phosphates may occur before arrest with crystalloid cardioplegia.
- Blood cardioplegia is more physiological, has high oxygen reserve due to the hemoglobin content and has physiological buffering capacity. In addition, blood cardioplegia has physiological oncotic pressure, is rich in free-radical scavenging, contains metabolic substrates and also results in less systemic hemodilution.
- Blood cardioplegia provides nutrients and oxygen during multidose infusions to enhance cellular metabolism and replenish depleted stores.
- *"Warm cardioplegic induction"* is a part of blood cardioplegic technique where a sick heart is arrested in an environment where the heart is allowed to metabolically resuscitate before cardiac arrest

is induced. The metabolic revival helps the sick myocardium to go through the subsequent period of ischemia in a better fashion.

- The hypoxic heart may be susceptible to reperfusion injury after a period of ischemia. Some centers use terminal *"hot shot"* to minimize the myocardial damage sustained during the period of ischemia. Here, before removal of cross clamp, the heart is perfused with high potassium containing warm blood. During the period of "hot shot", the ischemic myocardium recovers its metabolic activity before removal of the clamp.

- "Microplegia" is a form of blood cardioplegia that is used based on its potential advantages of reduced systemic hemodilution, reduced myocardial edema, better preservation of high-energy substrates, and better oxygen delivery. Microplegia is delivered as warm or cold blood mixed with the cardioplegia (60:1, blood:crystalloid ratio) with high (100 mmol/L) or low (40 mmol/L) dose of potassium.

It is important to understand the role of each constituent of cardioplegia in myocardial protection.

Potassium: High potassium is generally used for induction of immediate cardiac arrest. For blood cardioplegia, the potassium concentration in the induction dose is between 20 and 30 mmol/L and this reduces to 10–20 mmol/L in the maintenance dose. Very high concentrations of potassium in the cardioplegia (>40 mmol/L) can be harmful and damaging to the myocardium.

Buffering agents: Sodium bicarbonate or tris-hydroxymethyl aminomethane (THAM) is used in most cardioplegic solutions as buffering agent to counteract acidosis that occurs during the period of ischemia. THAM has an advantage, in the sense that it corrects

intracellular acidosis whereas bicarbonate corrects only extracellular acidosis.

Mannitol: Mannitol is another common constituent of cardioplegic solutions. Mannitol prevents myocardial edema by virtue of its high oncotic pressure and also exhibits antioxidant properties.

Calcium and magnesium: An important consideration regarding myocardial protection is the concentration of calcium in the cardioplegic solution. For reasons mentioned earlier, the neonatal heart is particularly sensitive to ischemia reperfusion injury when normocalcemic cardioplegia is used. Hypocalcemic cardioplegic solutions allowed repair of the injury caused by hypoxia and reoxygenation, resulting in complete preservation of myocardial and vascular endothelial cell function.[4] Transient fluxes in cardioplegic ionized calcium levels can occur because of variability in pH, hemodilution, temperature, potassium, and perhaps most importantly systemic calcium levels in the bypass circuit. The immature myocardium is particularly sensitive to this fluctuation in calcium levels as they are unable to handle a sudden increase in calcium load.

During ischemia, magnesium is lost from the intracellular space. This is associated with increased incidence of postoperative arrhythmias and loss of magnesium-mediated cellular functions. Addition of magnesium to the cardioplegic solution has been associated with reduced incidence of postoperative arrhythmias and improved myocardial function. The improved myocardial performance is primarily related to the ability of magnesium to prevent the entry of calcium into the cell during the reperfusion period as well as displace calcium from its binding sites on the sarcoplasmic reticulum. In addition, postischemic calcium entry is further limited because magnesium prevents any entry of sodium into the cell, which is exchanged for calcium during the reperfusion period. Adding magnesium to hypocalcemic cardioplegic solutions allowed for complete recovery of metabolic and myocardial function.[5]

Customized Cardioplegia

Customized cardioplegia can be developed at any center based on protocols developed in each unit. This is usually delivered as a 4:1 solution (blood to crystalloid). The cardioplegia currently practiced at Amrita Institute of Medical Sciences (AIMS, Kochi) is mentioned in this article. Cold cardioplegia is used for induction. Multidose modified cardioplegia is used every 20–30 minutes. The crystalloid vehicle that is used to prepare the cardioplegia currently is Plasmalyte A (Baxter Healthcare Corporation, IL, USA), which has the following constituents: sodium 140 mEq/L, potassium 5 mEq/L, magnesium 3 mEq/L, chloride 98 mEq/L, acetate 27 mEq/L, and has an osmolarity of 280–310 mOsm/L.

The primary source of potassium is the St Thomas Cardioplegia solution. Mannitol is added to prevent myocardial cell edema whereas sodium bicarbonate functions as buffer. The typical induction dose is 20–30 mL/kg. The potassium concentration in the final reconstituted solution for induction dose ranges from 22 to 24 mEq/L. Blood to crystalloid ratio in this composition is 1:1. A suggested composition of induction dose cardioplegia is given in **Table 1**. Maintenance dose is 10–15 mL/kg repeated every 20–30 minutes.

St Thomas II Cardioplegia

This is probably the most commonly used commercially available cardioplegia. St Thomas cardioplegia solution contains a high potassium and magnesium concentration. The high potassium content ensures imme-

TABLE 1: A suggested composition of induction dose cardioplegia.

Constituents	Volume
Plasmalyte A	40 mL
Sodium bicarbonate	5 mL
Mannitol 20%	2.5 mL
St Thomas cardioplegia	2.5 mL
Blood	50 mL

TABLE 2: Composition of St Thomas II cardioplegia solution.

Constituents	Volume
NaCl	110 mmol/L
KCl	16 mmol/L
$CaCl_2$	16 mmol/L
pH	7.8
Osmolarity	285–300 mOsm/L

diate cardiac arrest. The solution also contains small amounts of procaine as a membrane stabilizer. The role of the small amount of calcium in the cardioplegia is controversial as some studies have shown that this is probably responsible for the incomplete myocardial protection seen with the solution. The composition of St Thomas II cardioplegia is given in **Table 2**.

St Thomas II solution does not contain procaine, which is an essential constituent of St Thomas I solution. Moreover, it is important to understand that the St Thomas solution locally available is slightly different from either St Thomas I or II solutions described in literature.

del Nido Cardioplegia

del Nido cardioplegia was developed by Pedro del Nido and his team from Pittsburgh University in 1990 and used primarily in pediatric cardiac surgery. del Nido is an extracellular type of cardioplegia, which is mixed with blood from the cardiopulmonary

TABLE 3: Components of del Nido cardioplegia.

Ingredient	Volume (mL)	Role
Plasmalyte A	1,000	Base solution. Na 140 mmol/L, K 5 mmol/L, Mg 3 mmol/L, Chloride 98 mmol/L, acetate 27 mEq/L, gluconate 23 mEq/L, pH 7.4
Mannitol	16.3	Free radical scavenger, oncotic pressure
$MgSO_4$ 50%	4	Calcium antagonist, improved myocardial recovery
$NaHCO_3$	13	pH buffer
KCl (2 mEq/L)	13	Immediate cardiac arrest
Lidocaine	13	Sodium channel blocker, hyperpolarizing agent

circuit and administered in a 1:4 ratio (blood: cardioplegia).

The basic components of del Nido cardioplegia is given in **Table 3**.

Plasmalyte A, the base solution is devoid of calcium, which minimizes the myocardial injury during ischemia and reperfusion. As blood constitutes only about 20% of the cardioplegia solution, it is likely to contribute to some degree of hemodilution on the cardiopulmonary bypass. However, this can be easily removed through conventional or modified ultrafiltration techniques. It is generally accepted that a single dose of del Nido cardioplegia can be used for aortic cross clamp times of up to 90 minutes without myocardial injury.

In a single center study of 34 patients undergoing complex cardiac surgery with cross clamp times >90 minutes, repeat customized blood cardioplegia (1:1 blood crystalloid ratio, repeated every 30 minutes) was compared to a single dose del Nido cardioplegia.[6] The study also included 8 patients where the duration of cross clamp times was >120 minutes. There was no significant difference in the outcome between the two groups although significantly lesser number of cardioplegia and lower blood sugar levels were noted in the del Nido group.

In another study of 100 children <12 years of age undergoing tetralogy of Fallot repair

or ventricular septal repair, single dose del Nido cardioplegia was compared to repeat dose of cold blood St Thomas cardioplegia.[7] The myocardial function, biomarkers of myocardial injury, and ultrastructural changes was assessed after surgery. The authors concluded that the cardiac index was on an average 0.5% $L/min/m_2$ higher in the del Nido group than in the blood cardioplegia group. They also noted that myocardial biomarkers were significantly lower in the del Nido group. Finally, duration of mechanical ventilation, intensive care unit, and hospital stays were shorter in the del Nido group. Electron microscopy showed greater myofibrillar damage in the St Thomas cardioplegia group.

Custodial Cardioplegia

Custodial cardioplegia is an intracellular type of cardioplegia by virtue of its low sodium and magnesium content. Also called *Bretschneider's solution* or *histidine-tryptophan-ketoglutarate (HTK) solution*, it induces hypopolarization of the myocardial membrane, which leads to diastolic cardiac arrest. Although first introduced into clinical practice as a cardioplegic agent, its role was later extended to organ preservation during transplant surgery. The components of Custodial solution are provided in **Table 4**.

The high histidine content neutralizes the acidemia that accrues from the anaerobic

TABLE 4: Components of Custodial solution.

Ingredient	Volume
Na$^+$	15 mmol/L
K$^+$	9 mmol/L
Mg^{2+}	4 mmol/L
Ca^{2+}	0.015 mmol/L
Histidine	198 mmol/L
Tryptophan	2 mmol/L
Ketoglutarate	1 mmol/L
Mannitol	30 mmol/L
pH	7.02–7.12

metabolism that occurs during the prolonged ischemic period. Ketoglutarate improves high-energy phosphate bond generation during the period of reperfusion and tryptophan stabilizes the cell membrane. Despite its widespread use in Europe there are considerable concerns regarding hyponatremia that can occur following rapid administration of appropriate doses of Custodial solution. Custodial cardioplegia is also more effective when vigorous topical cooling is used along with the technique.[8] Hyponatremia may be a major concern when Custodial solutions are used due to the low sodium content in the solution.[8]

A meta-analysis compared 14 studies where Custodial solution was compared with other cardioplegic techniques in adult cardiac surgical patients.[9] There was no difference in the incidence of death, which was the primary end point of the study, between patients who received Custodial versus conventional cardioplegia. There was no difference in the incidence of perioperative myocardial infarction or low output syndrome between the Custodial group and conventional cardioplegia group. There was a trend toward increased incidence of arrhythmias after release of cross clamp in the Custodial group, which however, did not reach statistical significance.

Kim et al. looked at the incidence of hyponatremia flowing HTK cardioplegia in pediatric cardiac surgery.[10] They found that >15 mmol/L change in serum sodium occurred in patients who were administered HTK cardioplegia. 3.2% of these children developed postoperative seizures. The authors concluded that wide fluctuations in serum sodium were associated with the use of HTK solution and this correlated strongly with postoperative seizures.

CARDIOPLEGIA DELIVERY

The delivery of cardioplegia may be divided into three phases—(1) induction, (2) maintenance, and (3) reperfusion.

Induction

In sick hearts, a warm cardioplegic induction has been suggested to restore the myocardial energy stores before shifting to cold cardioplegia. Normothermia optimizes the rate of cellular repair during the warm cardioplegia infusion. Enrichment of the cardioplegia with amino acids, aspartate, and glutamate, enhances recovery of high-energy phosphate stores, resulting in improvement in postoperative functional recovery and patient survival.[4,11] The induction temperature is not important in the unstressed neonatal heart because of the healthier energy stores.

Maintenance

All hearts receive some noncoronary collateral flow from pericardial connections and this may be more significant in infants with aortocoronary collateral flow. This collateral flow is at body temperature (significantly higher than the temperature of the cardioplegic arrested heart) and the flows may be sufficient to wash out the entire cardioplegia over a period of time. This collateral flow results in warming of the heart and return of electromechanical activity.

Periodic infusion of cardioplegia over 10–20 minutes counters this washout of the cardioplegia and prevents warming of the heart. Multidose cardioplegia is necessary even if electromechanical activity does not return because low level of electrical activity may precede mechanical activity and lead to delayed recovery, if cardioplegic replenishment is not provided. However, with the use of del Nido cardioplegia, a single dose has been shown to protect the myocardium up to 90 minutes and longer.

Reperfusion

No matter how "good" the method of cardioplegic delivery, some degree of ischemic damage is caused by a period of aortic cross clamp. Interestingly more myocardial damage is created during the period of reperfusion. Reperfusion injury is now considered as the primary cause of impaired myocardial performance in the immediate postbypass period and eventually to myocardial fibrosis that may follow surgical correction of congenital or acquired cardiac diseases.

Follette et al. were the first to show that postischemic reperfusion damage after global ischemia could be avoided in adult hearts by an initial reperfusion of the heart with a "hot shot" before exposing the myocardium to the unmodified blood after release of artic cross clamp.[12] Enriching the terminal warm blood cardioplegia with amino acid aspartate and glutamate vastly improved its efficacy, resulting in complete functional recovery. However, recent studies by Toyoda et al., have shown that a terminal warm blood cardioplegia, without amino acid enrichment, can still be beneficial in pediatric hearts.[13] They showed that a significantly larger number of hearts, which received terminal warm blood cardioplegia without enrichments, resumed normal sinus rhythm spontaneously and all

hearts could be weaned off cardiopulmonary bypass with no inotropic support.[13] The lactate extraction ratio was also significantly higher in the terminal warm blood cardioplegia group. Use of terminal warm blood cardioplegia confers the following advantages:

- Terminal warm blood accelerates recovery of enzymatic and metabolic functions and provides oxygen
- High potassium prolongs electromechanical arrest to decrease energy demands
- Low calcium prevents intracellular calcium overload, which is believed to be the major cause of ventricular contracture and reperfusion injury
- Alkalotic solution counteracts tissue acidosis and optimizes enzymatic and metabolic functions all areas of the myocardium
- High osmolarity counteracts tissue edema.

Use of a warm substrate enriched terminal cardioplegia is probably indicated in all infants.

CURRENT CARDIOPLEGIA CHOICE AND TECHNIQUES

A survey was conducted among cardiac surgeons of the Congenital Heart Surgeons Society on their choice and practice for pediatric myocardial protection.[8] Questions were based on the age of the children ranging from neonates to adolescents. 86% of the surgeons used a blood-based cardioplegic solution. del Nido cardioplegia was the most popular cardioplegia, being used by 43% of the surgeons followed by customized blood cardioplegia by 38% of surgeons. Custodial solution was used only by 7% of surgeons. 93% of surgeons preferred cold blood cardioplegia and this did not vary with the age of the child. 19% surgeons practiced deep hypothermia. "Hot shots" were used by 21%

of surgeons. Induction dose of cardioplegia was 30 mL/kg (46%) or 20 mL/kg (27%) while the maintenance dose was usually 10 mL.kg. Interval between two cardioplegia doses among those using customized cardioplegia was 20–30 minutes, while surgeons using del Nido cardioplegia used a single dose.

A similar survey was conducted among pediatric surgeons and perfusionists' in the United Kingdom and Ireland.[14] Similar to the previous study, 84.4% of surgeons preferred a blood cardioplegia with St Thomas solution being the most popular in 4:1 blood crystalloid ratio. 75% of surgeons were willing for a randomized controlled trial with del Nido cardioplegia, which is still not commercially available in UK. Most surgeons use their cardioplegia at 4–6°C irrespective of cardioplegia type, with an induction dose of 30 mL/kg and maintenance of 15 mL/kg. Interval between two doses was 20 and 25 minutes. Custodial cardioplegia was not popular with concerns raised about its myocardial protection, volume of crystalloid, and considered as a "backward step" from blood.

SUMMARY

- Surgeons and anaesthesiologists must refrain from using "simplistic cardioplegic solutions" for the reason that simplicity and safety are not synonymous.
- The immature neonatal myocardium has an increased tolerance to ischemia because of greater dependence on glucose for its metabolism, the abundant glycogen stores and low activity of 5' nucleotidase. However, a neonatal heart which is stressed and hypoxic shows similar intolerance to ischemia as an adult heart.
- Cardioplegic solutions should produce immediate arrest and have an appropriate pH, osmolarity and membrane stabilizing effect and should also prevent or reduce reperfusion injury.

- Blood cardioplegia has definite advantages over crystalloid cardioplegia in stressed hypoxic hearts.
- Magnesium is added to cardioplegia to counter the effects of calcium and potentiate the effects of potassium.
- Warm induction cardioplegia is a useful technique for resuscitating a sick myocardium before subjecting it to a period of ischemic arrest.
- Crystalloid cardioplegia can be either extracellular or intracellular type. St Thomas cardioplegia and del Nido are extra cellular types while Custodial cardioplegia is representative of intra cellular type.
- del Nido cardioplegia is very commonly used in pediatric cardiac surgery in North America and is rapidly gaining popularity in our country. A single dose can give myocardial protection lasting up to 90 minutes.
- Custodial cardioplegia is not very popular in pediatric cardiac surgery. Hyponatremia can be an issue with this type of myocardial protection.
- When using customized cardioplegia, repeat dosing is usually required to replenish the myocardial oxygen and energy stores as well as washout products of anaerobic metabolism. This should be given every 10–20 minutes.
- A terminal "hot shot" cardioplegia even if not enriched with amino acids can minimize reperfusion injury and result in near complete recovery of myocardial functions.

REFERENCES

1. Doenst T, Schlensak C, Beyersdorf F. Cardioplegia in pediatric cardiac surgery: do we believe in magic? Ann Thorac Surg. 2003;75:1668-77.
2. Teoh KH, Mickle DA, Weisel RD, Li RK, Tumiati LC, Coles JG, et al. Effect of oxygen tension and cardiovascular operations on the myocardial

antioxidant enzyme activities in patients with tetralogy of Fallot and aorta-coronary bypass. J Thorac Cardiovasc Surg. 1992;104:159-64.

3. Pridjian AK, Bove EL, Bolling SF, Childs KF, Brosamer KM, Lupinetti FM. Developmental differences in myocardial protection in response to 5'nucleotidase inhibitors. J Thorac Cardiovasc Surg. 1994;107: 520-6.

4. Aoki M, Nomura F, Kawata H, Mayer JE Jr. Effect of calcium and preischemic hypothermia on recovery of myocardial function after cardioplegic ischemia in neonatal lambs. J Thorac Cardiovasc Surg. 1993;105:207-13.

5. Kronon M, Allen BS, Hernan J, Halldorsson AO, Rahman S, Buckberg GD, et al. Superiority of magnesium cardioplegia in neonatal myocardial protection. Ann Thorac Surg. 1999;68:2285-95.

6. Charette K, Gerrah R, Quaegebeur J, Chen J, Riley D, Mongero L, et al. Single dose myocardial protection technique utilizing del Nido cardioplegia solution during congenital heart surgery procedures. Perfusion. 2012;27:98-103.

7. Talwar S, Bhoje A, Sreenivas V, Makhija N, Aarav S, Choudhary SK, et al. Comparison of del Nido and St Thomas Cardioplegia solutions in pediatric patients: a prospective randomized clinical trial. Semin Thorac Cardiovasc Surg. 2017;29(3):366-74.

8. Kotani Y, Tweddll J, Gruber P, Pizarro C, Austin EH 3rd, Woods RK, et al. Current cardioplegia practice in pediatric cardiac surgery: a North American multi-institutional survey. Ann Thor Surg. 2013;96:923-9.

9. Edelman JJB, Seco M, Dunne B, Matzelle SJ, Murphy M, Joshi P, et al. Custodial for myocardial protection and preservation: a systematic review. Ann Cardiothorac Surg. 2013;2:717-28.

10. Kim JT, Park YH, Chang YE, Byon HJ, Kim HS, Kim CS, et al. The effect of cardioplegic solution induced sodium concentration fluctuation on postoperative seizure in pediatric cardiac patients. Ann Thorac Surg. 2011;91:1943-8.

11. Kronon M, Allen BS, Bolling KS, Rahman S, Wang T, Maniar HS, et al. The role of cardioplegic induction temperature and amino acid enrichment in neonatal myocardial protection. Ann Thorac Surg. 2000;70:756-64.

12. Follette D, Fey K, Buckberg GD, Helly JJ Jr, Steed DL, Foglia RP, et al. Reducing post ischemic damage by temporary modifications of reperfusate calcium, potassium, pH and osmolarity. J Thorac Cardiovasc Surg. 1981;82:221-38.

13. Toyoda Y, Yamaguchi M, Yoshimura N, Oka S, Okita Y. Cardioprotective effects and the mechanisms of terminal warm blood cardioplegia in pediatric cardiac surgery. J Thorac Cardiovasc Surg. 2003;125:1242-51.

14. Drury NE, Horsburgh A, Bi R, Willetts RG, Jones TJ. Cardioplegia practice in paediatric cardiac surgery: a UK and Ireland survey. Perfusion. 2019;34:125-9.

Establishing a Pediatric Cardiac Intensive Care Unit: Special Considerations in a Limited Resource Environment

Rakhi Balachandran, Suresh G Nair, R Krishna Kumar

Reviewed by: R Krishna Kumar

◼ INTRODUCTION

Pediatric cardiac intensive care has evolved as a distinct discipline in well-established pediatric cardiac programs in developed nations.[1-3] The unique needs of critically ill patients with congenital heart disease (CHD) have necessitated establishment of dedicated pediatric cardiac intensive care units (PCICUs) with trained personnel for providing high-quality perioperative care.[4] With early diagnosis of CHD and increasing demand for pediatric heart surgery in emerging economies, a number of new pediatric heart programs have been established. A number of challenges need to be addressed while delivering pediatric cardiac intensive care in the developing world. Most programs encounter serious limitations with respect to infrastructure, human, and material resources. This calls for modification of existing models of pediatric cardiac intensive care, which are currently in place in established heart programs in the developed nations. In the absence of trained force in the specialty of pediatric cardiac intensive care, streamlining the expertise of available trained medical personnel in subspecialties such as cardiac surgery, cardiac anesthesia, pediatrics, and pediatric cardiology seems to be a reasonable alternative that is being currently pursued in emerging nations.[5] Focused strategies on minimizing perioperative costs while assuring

quality have also emerged as the need of the hour for ensuring the sustenance of pediatric cardiac programs in such resource limited environments. In this chapter, we have attempted to provide a brief overview of the strategies for establishing a dedicated pediatric cardiac intensive unit in a low-resource setting typical of the developing world.

◼ MODELS OF PEDIATRIC CARDIAC INTENSIVE CARE

The most common model of pediatric cardiac intensive care, particularly in the developed nations, is through a dedicated PCICU located in specialized children's hospitals. The clinical services are provided by a multidisciplinary team that includes pediatric cardiologists, pediatric cardiac surgeons, intensivists, critical care nurses, respiratory therapists, and other support personnel.[2] In a widely observed second model, pediatric cardiac patients are cared for in a general pediatric intensive care unit (PICU).[6] These two models are successfully used to deliver pediatric cardiac intensive care in several well established and large pediatric heart programs in the United States, Canada, Europe, and Australia. In addition to clinical services these units also offer focused pediatric cardiac intensive care training programs.[6]

In developing nations, due to the dearth of trained personnel and resource limitations, pediatric cardiac intensive care has not yet fully evolved as a distinctive discipline. Several patterns of pediatric cardiac intensive care have been observed. In India, the most desirable model is that of a dedicated pediatric cardiac intensive unit with specialized personnel, which has been successfully established in some states particularly in the private sector.[7] Some of the dedicated pediatric cardiac centers in developing nations have been supported by international collaboration and guidance from trained experts of established programs in the developed world.[8,9] These centers particularly focus on establishment of systems, protocols, local staff development, and quality improvement initiatives. Second model includes pediatric heart programs attached to well-established adult cardiology and cardiac surgery programs. Here the pediatric cardiac care is delivered in a common setting along with adult patients utilizing shared space, infrastructure and personnel. Thirdly, in small private establishments, which handle low-surgical volumes, pediatric cardiac care is delivered by a small group of professionals (mostly anesthesiologists) attached to the surgical unit.

WHY IS THERE A NEED FOR A DEDICATED PEDIATRIC CARDIAC INTENSIVE CARE UNIT?[5]

- The burden of pediatric heart disease in developing nations, particularly in India is overwhelming. With facilities for accurate diagnosis and surgical expertise, more and more children are undergoing corrective surgery for CHDs. Many of the tertiary heart care centers have been experiencing a parallel increase in surgical volumes every year.[10,11] This translates to an increased demand for trained personnel and dedicated space to care for these critically ill children.

- A dedicated team delivering specialized intensive care in a defined unit has translated into better outcomes in several centres.[12-14] In a high-volume pediatric cardiac center in South India, the establishment of a dedicated PCICU with specialized staff have resulted in shorter time to extubation, shorter intensive care unit (ICU) stay, early deintensification, and reduced bloodstream infection rates.[15] The team oriented focus allows members of the unit to possess an intellectual ownership of the program, which in turn reflects in the improved quality of care.

- The benefits of early primary surgical repair (during early infancy or newborn period) of many congenital heart lesions are now well-established.[16] In several centers, where pediatric cardiac care is linked to busy adult surgical programs, healthcare professionals trained in adult cardiac care may not be able to meet the unique healthcare needs of neonates and small infants. Hence, it becomes imperative to specially train a group of physicians, nurses, and supportive staff with expertise in the perioperative care of this vulnerable population.

REQUIREMENTS FOR AN IDEAL PCICU

Unit Design

The PCICU should be geographically distinct and equipped to receive children with congenital and acquired heart disease. The bed strength is typically decided on the basis of the center's expected surgical case volumes. It is reasonable to start with 6–10 beds with scope for future expansion as dictated by the projected case volumes.[5] The proximity of the unit to the operating rooms and cardiac catheterization laboratory is desirable for ease of patient transport and safety.

Easy accessibility to the elevators is mandatory to facilitate transport of patients from the ICU to other locations in the hospital. The access to the PCICU should be monitored to maintain patient and staff safety and confidentiality.[17] The on-call physician's room, staff rest rooms and family waiting areas should also be located close to the ICU. The unit design should also allow provision for at least two isolation rooms, clean and dirty utility rooms, nourishment preparation areas, medication station, narcotic locker, and a refrigerator. A conference room for staff education, conferences and case discussions is desirable.

Central Station

The central nursing station should offer good visibility to all patient beds and overhead monitors. Adequate space should be available for the physicians and nurses to write case details and order sheets. The central station should also have a central hemodynamic display monitor linked to individual patient monitors. At least two computers should be available for electronic data entry, clerical works and communication. Two telephone lines and intercom facilities should be available.

Bedside Facilities

Beds should be arranged in a manner, which allows visibility from a central care station. Patient area in the open PCICU should be 150–200 sq ft.[18] There should be adequate space around the bed for accommodating ventilators, syringe pumps, and IV poles. There should be easy accessibility to the head end of the bed/crib for emergency airway management. Bassinets with overhead radiant warmers are necessary for providing thermoneutral environments for neonates and small infants. There should be enough space for performing routine ICU procedures (e.g., central line placement, intercostal drain insertion, etc.). Due to space constraints monitoring equipment is typically wall-mounted in most settings. Electrical power from an uninterruptible power source (UPS), oxygen, medical compressed air and vacuum outlets sufficient in number to supply all necessary equipment should meet regulatory standards.[17] Backup power supply and medical gas supply should be ensured. If resources are available, it is desirable to have computers with transportable stands available at each bedside to facilitate electronic entry of patient data, and its transfer to remote locations as required.

Equipment

A list of basic equipment and utilities to support the needs of the pediatric cardiac patients under normal and emergency conditions is provided in **Tables 1 and 2**.[17,18] In addition, cardiac ICUs also need specialized equipment such as echocardiography machines and nitric oxide delivery systems.[19] Although ideally, paraphernalia for institution of mechanical circulatory support is desirable, there are specific concerns in procuring resource intensive extracorporeal membrane oxygenation (ECMO) services in many centers in the developing world. There are several programs that have achieved excellent outcomes without the availability of ECMO. It is perhaps reasonable to state that ECMO services should only be considered once a certain basic standard of care has been achieved with congenital heart surgery.

ADMINISTRATIVE STRUCTURE AND WORK PATTERN IN THE PCICU

PCICU should have a well-defined administrative structure and staff pattern of its own. There are no published recommendations,

TABLE 1: Essential equipment for the pediatric cardiac intensive care unit.

Monitoring equipment

- *Multichannel patient monitors:* Capable of continuous measurement of ECG, HR, CVP, ABP, SPO_2, $ETCO_2$, temperature, RR, should have facility for setting appropriate alarm limits, audible alarms, should have memory and display trends, print out feature should be available
- NIBP cuffs and hoses
- SPO_2 sensors-pediatric
- Temperature probes
- ECG leads and ECG cables
- Transport monitors

Procedural equipments

- Intravascular catheters
- Central venous catheters; 4 Fr, 5.5 Fr, 7 Fr
- Transducer assembly
- Pressure extension lines
- Disposable guidewires
- Dressing tray
- Suture removal set
- Central line tray
- Emergency sternotomy set
- Peritoneal dialysis catheters
- ICD insertion tray
- IV infusion sets
- Blood transfusion sets
- Three-way stopcocks
- Portable lights

Respiratory equipment

- Ventilators with waveform displays
- Noninvasive ventilators
- Breathing circuits
- Ambu bags
- Suction catheters
- Laryngoscopes
- Endotracheal tubes
- Stylet
- Bougie
- Suction catheters
- Humidifiers
- Nebulizer kit
- Oxygen masks
- Nasal cannulae
- Bi-level noninvasive ventilation
- Oxygen cylinders
- Vibrator
- Spirometers
- Continuous oxygen analyzers and alarms
- Tracheostomy set and tracheostomy tubes
- Flexible fiberoptic bronchoscope

Specialized equipments for cardiac ICU

- *Pacemaker:* Single chamber and dual chamber
- Pacing cables
- Transvenous pacing set
- Cardiac output monitor
- Internal paddles for defibrillator
- Nitric oxide delivery system
- Echocardiography machine
- ECG machine
- Ultrasound machine
- Hand-held Doppler

Portable equipment

- Crash cart
- Defibrillator
- Beds and bassinets
- Syringe pumps
- IV poles with wheels
- Suction machine
- Infant warmers
- Overhead warmers
- Warming blankets and Bair hugger
- Infant weighing machine
- Oxygen cylinders
- Bedside locker
- Bedside table
- Bedside chair
- Clocks and calendars

(ECG: electrocardiogram; CVP: central venous pressure; ABP: arterial blood pressure; RR: respiratory rate; ICD: intercostal drain; IV: intravenous; NIBP: noninvasive blood pressure; $ETCO_2$: end tidal carbon dioxide; HR: heart rate)

TABLE 2: Essential drugs in pediatric cardiac ICU.

Resuscitation drugs	Inotropes	Vasodilators
Adrenaline	Dopamine	Sodium nitroprusside
Atropine	Dobutamine	Nitroglycerine
		Phenoxybenzamine
Calcium chloride	Adrenaline	Enalapril
Calcium gluconate	Norepinephrine	Diuretics
Lignocaine	Isoprenaline	Frusemide
Sodium bicarbonate	Milrinone	Spironolactone
	Levosimendan	Acetazolamide
	Digoxin	Metolazone
Antiarrhythmics	Drugs affecting coagulation	Sedatives and analgesics
Adenosine	Heparin	Fentanyl
Amiodarone	Aspirin	Morphine
Bretylium	Warfarin	Midazolam
Lignocaine	Streptokinase	Paracetamol
Verapamil	Tranexamic acid	Ketamine
Magnesium sulphate	Protamine	Propofol
Ivabradine		Dexmedetomidine
Respiratory medicines	Miscellaneous	Muscle relaxants
Salbutamol respirator solution	Aminophylline	Vecuronium
Racemic epinephrine	Caffeine	Pancuronium
Budesonide respirator suspension	Dexamethasone, hydrocortisone	Atracurium
	Naloxone	
	Phenytoin	
	Phenobarbitone	
	Indomethacin	
	Prostaglandin E1	

but most of available evidence encourages developing a unit with a physician/intensivist as the leader/coordinator of the intensive care team.[1,6,15,17]

Leadership (Intensivist in-Charge) of the PCICU

The opportunities for obtaining pediatric cardiac intensive care training in established pediatric cardiac centers in the developed world seems to be a promising option for individuals aspiring to be pediatric cardiac intensivists. However, since a clear trajectory of pediatric cardiac intensive care training career is largely unavailable in most developing nations it is reasonable to delegate this responsibility to a physician trained in one of the pediatric subspecialties. Recognizing the paucity of dedicated pediatric cardiac surgeons as well as the intensity of their involvement for prolonged periods in the operating room, it is unrealistic to expect the surgeon to take up this role. A pragmatic approach is to enable a cardiac anesthesiologist or a pediatric cardiologist or a pediatric intensivist with focused interest to continuously engage in this role and over time, develop as a leader of the PCICU.

The intensivist in-charge is typically expected to assume the following responsibilities.[15,17]

- Act as a multidisciplinary team leader, coordinating care provided by the members of the team.
- Establishing policies and protocols in collaboration with members of other subspecialties in the team.
- Promote the implementation of the policies and protocols including admission and discharge criteria.
- Provide primary or consultative care for all the PCICU patients along with the physician on call in the ICU.
- Participate in quality improvement activities.
- Coordinate and participate in staff education and research.
- Maintain a database that describes unit experience and performance.
- Supervise cost containment measures in the ICU.
- Plan staffing requirements and work to ensure short-term and long-term adequacy of nursing and physician staff.

Other Physician Staff

An *in-house physician* (resident or fellow in pediatric cardiology or anesthesiology) skilled to provide emergency care to critically ill children with CHD should provide continuous cover for 12–24 hours shifts depending on the availability of personnel. He or she should not have any other simultaneous responsibilities while on clinical duty in the ICU.

Nursing Staff

The PCICU team should have a cadre of specially trained nurses of its own led by a senior nurse (Nurse-in-charge) with expertise in managing critically ill children with CHD.

The work pattern should be organized as 8 or 12 hours shifts based on the availability of staff nurses in the critical care team. There should preferably be a nurse leader for every shift (team leader). The ratio of nurses to patients is typically 1:1 or 1:2 depending on patient acuity and the number of staff available per shift.[20]

The *nurse-in-charge* should be responsible for the nursing program, delegation of roles and responsibilities to members of the nursing team, implementation of policies and procedures, quality assurance, the provision of supplies and equipment, and staff education and training.

The *bed-side nurse* is designated as the primary care giver of the patient. He or she should perform repeated clinical assessment of the patient, collect vital information, communicate relevant information to the physician staff and other members of the team, and provide compassionate care to the critically ill child. PCICU nurses should also interact with the family members and participate in patient and family education. A pediatric cardiac nurse is expected to possess reasonable knowledge and clinical practice skills to provide optimal perioperative care to a critically ill child with CHD. This includes a basic understanding of the anatomy and pathophysiology of common CHDs, the surgical treatment of CHD, cardiopulmonary bypass (CPB) and its effects on organ systems, hemodynamic monitoring of cardiac patients, essentials of pace makers and cardiac pacing, pharmacology of cardiovascular drugs, recognition, and management of the common postoperative complications, mechanical support of the heart, diagnosis, and management of cardiac arrhythmias and cardiopulmonary resuscitation techniques. However, in real life situations, this level of expertise is acquired over a considerable period of time. The value of experience merits special appreciation and should be adequately compensated for, by the administration.

Other Ancillary Staff

All PCICUs should be regularly supported by respiratory therapists, nutritionists, physiotherapists, medical social workers, and nursing assistants for comprehensive patient care.[21] Radiographers, ECG technicians, biomedical engineers, and electrical engineers should be easily accessible to meet emergencies/problems in the respective areas. A unit secretary should be appointed to carry out communication, electronic data entry, as well as paperwork involved in the smooth functioning of the unit.

◼ DAY-TO-DAY CARE IN THE PCICU

Once the necessary infrastructure and the manpower are in place, a system for the smooth functioning of the unit should be evolved. While initiating a new program on a collaborative approach of various subspecialties it would be logical to evolve a daily work pattern by discussion with senior members of each of the subspecialties of the team. There should be a forum where all the members of the care team can assemble together, present relevant clinical information, combine individual clinical expertise, conduct healthy discussions and formulate a care plan for each patient in the PCICU. In the pediatric cardiac unit this is best achieved at the bedside by conducting daily multidisciplinary rounds.[21,22]

A proposed pattern for workflow is described here.

The Daily Care Team

- The intensivist in charge
- Physician on call
- Pediatric cardiac surgeon/surgical fellow
- Pediatric cardiologist

- Nurse-in-charge
- Bedside nurse
- Respiratory therapist
- Nutrition specialist
- Medical social worker.

Prerounding Phase

The day starts with the nursing shift change over during which the night duty nurse hands over the patient details to the day duty staff. There should be minimal interruption of the nurses by physicians or other staff members to avoid communication errors. The morning blood draws should be completed early so that reports are ready for analysis during rounding. The physician staff collects information about the current status of the patient by communication with the night duty person, clinical assessment, review of flow sheets, and laboratory reports and issue any physician orders, as appropriate. After this, the primary care giver should synthesize data in a daily progress note and formulate a tentative plan for the day.

Multidisciplinary Rounds

The PCICU intensivist should lead the rounds. Interruptions during rounds should be avoided (except emergencies). The physician on call makes a comprehensive presentation of the patient data to the team in a uniformly structured format that summarizes the diagnosis, operation performed and most significant events till date. The past 24 hours is dealt with in greater detail and a complete *multisystem* assessment of the patient's current status is made. With practice, this presentation can be accomplished quite quickly. Once the data is presented, a group assessment of the child in the disease process (acute, plateau, and recovery phase) should be made and the child's greatest safety risk should be identified. Along with this, invasive catheters and drainage tubes, adequacy of pain control, sedation, ventilation, inotropic supports, current medications, and transfer or discharge needs should be reviewed. Based on the inputs of all the members of the team, the intensivist should formulate a care plan for the day. The care plan along with the daily medication orders should be written down by a member of the team and read back to the team. This facilitates closed-loop communication ensuring clarity and minimizing ambiguity in decision making. Incorporating a daily "goal chart" will help to keep the care team in focus and strive toward achieving the set goals for the day for each patient.[23] The variations in care plan from the set goal chart may sometimes be warranted due to evolving patient conditions. This should be clearly communicated to all the members of the care team as appropriate. In situations where the physician on call works on 12 hours shifts evening "sign-out" rounds would be appropriate to exchange clinical information and to identify short-term goals for the night shift.

COMMUNICATION WITH THE FAMILY

The concept of family centered care demands special emphasis in the pediatric intensive care setting.[24] Parental presence is encouraged at the time of decision making to enable transparency in patient care and to allay parental anxiety. Though, this concept is streamlined in developed nations, clear policies related to parental participation during multidisciplinary rounds do not exist in most centers in low-middle income countries. A reasonable alternative is to ensure daily communication to the patient's family by a trusted member of the critical care team. The current physical status of the patient, details of illness, major concerns in the next 24 hours, details of the care plan and the anticipated duration of ICU stay should be elaborated as appropriate. In resource limited settings, it is also appropriate to clearly communicate the economic implications of the major decisions taken in the care plan to the patient's family.

ESTABLISHING POLICIES AND PROTOCOLS

Controlling practice variation is a key variable in delivering quality patient care.[23] Typically, basic policies and protocols suited to each unit and its patient profile are derived from discussions with senior members of the multidisciplinary team based on available evidence and expertise, and is often used to streamline the repetitive procedures performed in the ICU (e.g., potassium correction, care of central venous line, pain management). Besides controlling practice variations and facilitating high quality care, established policies and protocols also serve as an educational tool to the junior members and trainees of the intensive care team. It is also desirable that these policies are periodically reviewed and updated according to the contemporary best practice evidence. It is worth stating that though guidelines and protocols serve as an initial reference point, one should have an open mind to critically evaluate each situation and provide an individualized approach to patient care.[21]

DATA COLLECTION SYSTEM

There should be a collective effort from all members of the team to maintain accuracy of records in the ICU. There should be a comprehensive and clear recording of the patient status and procedures by the primary caregivers (physician and nursing staff). Meticulous attention should be given to minimize errors in documentation. Introspection of the unit's data would help to evaluate the strengths and weaknesses of the system and further streamline the patient care. Electronic medical records system is becoming increasingly popular even in developing nations to minimize recording errors, to store a large data and allow easy retrieval for periodic review of performance.[22,23,25]

QUALITY CONTROL

Continuous quality improvement is a proactive process whereby all structures, processes and clinical activities occurring in critical care setting should be evaluated and considered for quality improvement initiatives.[26] The best variables for measuring quality are still unclear. However, conventional indicators of outcome after congenital heart surgery largely acceptable to most centers should be tracked. Readmission rates to ICU within 24 hours of transfer during a single hospital stay, reintubation rate, duration of mechanical ventilation, length of stay in ICU, frequency of catheter-related bloodstream infections are some of the variables that are frequently used as a measure of quality improvement.[23,27] Regular morbidity-mortality meetings allow performance analysis and help to define scope for future improvement.[21,23] Errors and adverse events occurring during patient care have been recognized as major concerns in intensive care.[27] These areas should be considered as potential targets for quality improvement in the ICU.

The International Quality Improvement Collaborative (IQIC) for congenital heart surgery was launched as a quality improvement project targeted at reducing mortality and major complications in children undergoing congenital heart surgery from the developing world.[28] The crux of this project is a robust international database on key outcomes after congenital heart surgery and nurse education on quality driven best practices using telemedicine platforms. This project allows benchmarking of data among the participating pediatric cardiac centers of the developing world, facilitate introspection of data and continuously explore the opportunities for quality improvement. In a large single center cohort of 1,702 patients undergoing congenital heart surgery, implementation of the IQIC project has facilitated a reduction in bacterial sepsis (15.1–9.6%, $p < 0.001$), surgical site infection (11.1–2.4%, $p < 0.001$), and median duration of ICU stay (114 hours to 72 hours, $p < 0.001$) over a period of 3 years.[28]

STAFF EDUCATION

The initiation of staff development and training should begin much before the actual implementation of the program. It would be beneficial for a senior member of each of the subspecialties to visit a well-established center and observe the day-to-day functioning of the unit. Arranging a short period of observer ship or overseas training can help substantially when a new program is being established with limited resources. After establishment, continuing "in-service" education programs should be implemented to provide ongoing training for all the medical and paramedical personnel in the unit. This can be accomplished in several ways. The *intensivist-in-charge* can coordinate the staff training program. All the senior members of the various subspecialties should engage in academic discussions and conduct formal lecture sessions for junior physician and nursing staff. Facilitated discussions of clinical case scenarios and critical care pathways of common congenital heart operations are particularly useful for junior trainees of the program. Special knowledge areas like single ventricle physiology, pulmonary hypertension, mechanical support, arrhythmia management, cardiopulmonary resuscitation, pacemaker use, etc., merits careful attention. The senior staff should encourage and guide trainees and nursing staff to pursue research projects. All members of the program should be encouraged to attend regional or national conferences with course content pertinent to the PCICU care on a regular basis to keep abreast of the current developments in the subspecialty.

SPECIAL CHALLENGES

Role of Leadership in the PCICU

When designing the organizational structure of the ICU the administrative hierarchy should be clearly delineated. The role of a leader is vital to streamline the multidisciplinary team work. The leader should be a well-accepted member of the team who has the confidence of other specialties and their consultants. The leader should also possess skills at management, organization, and mentorship.[21,29,30] The role of leader should incorporate the task behavior of delegating roles and responsibilities to the members of the team, and a relationship behavior through which team is held together.[29] In the initial phase of the unit, the leader should work along with the team participating directly in the task responsibilities. As the team becomes competent and mature the leader should engage in delegating responsibilities to other members of the team. However, in emergencies and crises (resuscitation in cardiac arrest) due to value of experience and command, the leader should be readily available to guide the team.

Ensuring Team Harmony and Managing Conflicts in the Unit

One of the requisites, particularly in the formative period of the PCICU is to establish a healthy working relationship among the team members who vary in their professional profile, clinical skills, knowledge, and managerial capacities. Conflicts and controversies are likely to arise when individuals with diverse ideas and profiles work together. There is no rule of thumb to avoid such situations. However, this can be minimized through conscious effort. First, each member of the team has to be cognizant of the common goal of facilitating the well-being of the patient. Second, standard operating procedures (e.g., policies and protocols) have to be developed to minimize diversities in practice. Third, concise and clear communication should be practiced between various members of the team at all levels.[29] The role of a leader in ensuring effective communication in the unit is crucial to win the trust of the team members and encourage close cooperation and cohesive team work.[31]

Dealing with Complications

Children undergoing congenital heart surgery are vulnerable to many complications and adverse events. These may be brought about by chance, due to the specific nature of the underlying illness, technical failures, or human errors.[27] When such an event occurs, attempts to blame individuals involved in the care pathway can generate unnecessary conflicts, upset the group morale, and add to the work stress of the team members. It would be ideal and in the best interest of the team to address these events through constructive criticism. The event or complication should be identified, root cause analysis should be performed, and changes made in the protocols and systems to prevent similar events in the future.

Decision Making in the ICU

Clinical decision making for a critical ill child requires physicians of various subspecialties to combine their clinical skills, past experiences and knowledge, to analyze the situation at hand, to decide the best course of action compatible with current practice guidelines and translate them into an action plan at the bedside.[25] The major decisions in the course of care delivery in a PCICU evolve after multidisciplinary rounds. These decisions should be clearly documented and communicated to the primary care givers who would then proceed to execute the plan. However, in acute care setting where changes in patient status from the expected course can occur at any time, the physician "on call" 24 hours should be authorized to make necessary alteration in the care plan to suit the situation. The changes and the reasons for change should be promptly communicated to the responsible senior members of the team. Decisions in relation to routine events and procedures (e.g., potassium replacement, changing an invasive line, administering a sedative) can be taken as and when required. In emergency situations, the primary care giver should have the full autonomy to take the best course of action, which he or she feels appropriate for the situation (e.g., cardioversion for a tachyarrhythmia, changing a blocked endotracheal tube).

In a limited resource environment, when the role of primary care taker is often vested upon junior members and trainees, inappropriate decisions might be taken in some instances due to lack of experience and the steep learning curve involved. In such instances, critical evaluation of the situation during a team huddle and guidance with respect to the most appropriate course of action should be provided through constructive criticism without jeopardizing the team morale. Allowing some degree of autonomy in clinical decision making to junior team members in appropriate areas can encourage creative thinking and motivate learning process.[30] However, senior members of the team should maintain a cautious supervision to compensate for the learning curve in the initial phase. A good decision, which has yielded a better outcome, should be appreciated by the senior members of the team. This will improve motivation, commitment to patient care and promote job satisfaction among the junior members of the care team.

Retention of Personnel

The field of pediatric cardiac care is consumed by an overwhelming need for more trained personnel at all levels of care in the ICU. This is especially relevant in the context of emerging nations where structured training programs and well-established ICUs are lacking.[32] There are very few trained pediatric cardiac intensivists. There is also a considerable attrition from already existing cadre due to migration to developed nations in pursuit of better remuneration.[33] One of the potential ways of addressing this manpower shortage is to utilize personnel from allied specialties of pediatric cardiology, cardiac anesthesiology and neonatology to share the responsibilities in delivering pediatric cardiac critical care.[34] Structured and accredited training programs have to be developed in emerging centers with the goal of training more health care professionals. Nurse residency programs facilitated by nongovernmental organizations along with international collaboration of nurse educators from overseas centers can provide training pathways for junior nurses improving their proficiency in pediatric critical care and facilitating nurse empowerment. Most of the physicians, nurses, and support staff working in cardiac programs in developing nations are underpaid for the amount of time and effort that they invest in executing the job. In a developing country, recognizing the monetary needs and offering better incentives can help to retain currently existing personnel.

The profession of pediatric cardiac intensive care is highly demanding in terms of efficiency, skills and long-working hours. Extremes of stress and emotional exhaustion can lead to premature burn outs, especially in the acute care setting of pediatric intensive care units.[35] Efforts to prevent such burnouts include facilitating career diversification in other areas of interest (e.g., research, administration, etc.), allowing sufficient time away from the ICU setting on a periodic basis and promoting better work-life balance on a daily basis.

Cost Containment

The large burden of CHD in low-middle income countries coupled with limited resources mandates the utilization of cost effective perioperative management strategies for sustenance of pediatric heart programs. In most developing nations, the cost for the ICU care constitutes one-tenth to one-sixth of the total costs of congenital heart surgery.[36] The goal of a successful intensive care team should be to reduce expenditures without compromising quality. Unless a conscious attempt is made toward this end, patient bills frequently get out of control, and the program will acquire the reputation of being very expensive with the attendant risk of premature collapse. Some of the cost containment measures worth considering in limited resource settings are discussed here.

Early Extubation

Fast tracking and early extubation has evolved as established strategies for facilitating early recovery and reducing healthcare-associated costs.[37] Fast tracking is not restricted to anesthetic management alone, but requires a multidisciplinary approach from anesthesia, surgery, perfusion, critical care nursing, and intensive care teams. Though, traditionally considered as extubation within 6–8 hours of surgery, wide variability in definitions exist

ranging from extubation in operating room to within first 24 hours of surgery, depending on institutional practices. The reported benefits of fast tracking include reduced duration of ventilation, reduced ICU stay, and decreased hospital stay.[37,38] Early extubation strategy can be adopted in uncomplicated cases by judicious selection of anesthetic agents and anesthetic techniques without compromising safety.[37]

Reduction of Laboratory Tests

There are no definite guidelines regarding the optimal frequency of postoperative laboratory tests or arterial blood gas estimations in the PCICU. However, the unit should evolve a policy suited to the patient profile. The tests should be done more frequently in the initial critical phase to ensure patient safety and should be scaled down when the child has been significantly deintensified. A proposed strategy for postoperative investigations is depicted in **Tables 3 and 4**. Alternative strategies such as continuous $ETCO_2$ monitoring and measuring blood sugar with glucostrips instead of laboratory blood testing should be tried whenever feasible. A conscious effort should be made by all stakeholders of the intensive care team to judiciously limit investigations to those essential for optimal perioperative care in an attempt to reduce cumulative expenditure. This is particularly relevant in patient subsets who are likely to have a prolonged postoperative course.

Medication Management

The management of a critically ill cardiac patient requires an armamentarium of drugs including inotropes, antibiotics, antiarrhythmic agents, vasodilators, opioids and sedative medications, and expensive gases such as nitric oxide. The choice of drugs and duration of treatment should be tailored to patient needs.

TABLE 3: A proposed strategy for frequency of arterial blood gas (ABG) sampling in the pediatric cardiac intensive care unit.

ABG timing in the postoperative course	Frequency of sampling
At admission/receiving from operation room	Immediate
After institution of initial ventilator change based on first ABG	Within 30 minutes
During the course of mechanical ventilation	Every 4–6 hours
Prior to extubation	Obtain sample on pressure support/volume support mode of ventilation
Postextubation	Within 30 minutes
In all extubated patients	6–8 hours
Reintubation	Immediate
Readmission into the ICU	Immediate
In case of hypo/hyperkalemia	1–2 hours based on severity of the electrolyte imbalance and hemodynamic disturbances

TABLE 4: A proposed strategy for laboratory tests in the postoperative period for typical open heart operations.*

Postoperative days/special situations	Suggested tests	Frequency
On admission into ICU (Day of surgery)	CBC, RFT, LFT, PT, APTT, INR, serum electrolytes, ECG	Immediate
	Chest X-ray	Immediate and after 6 hours
Postoperative Day (POD) 1	CBC, RFT Chest X-ray	Once daily Twice daily
POD 2 onward	CBC	Once daily
Patients on anticoagulants	PT, APTT, INR	Daily

(APTT: activated partial thromboplastin time; CBC: complete blood counts; ECG: electrocardiogram; INR: international normalized ratio; LFT: liver function tests; RFT: renal function tests; PT: prothrombin time)
*This can be modified to suit individual situations (e.g., operation for closure of atrial septal defects may require fewer tests).

Antibiotics and inotropes are the drugs most likely to be overused in the ICU unless there are guidelines. Limiting the duration of perioperative antibiotic prophylaxis to 24–48 hours and carefully choosing antibiotics based on hospital antibiogram can help to minimize irrational use of antibiotics and prevent development of multidrug-resistant microorganisms.[33,36] Inotropes should be selected to suit postoperative physiology and tapered off when they are no longer required. The introduction of inhaled nitric oxide (iNO) has added a new dimension to the treatment of pulmonary hypertension associated with CHD. However, the expenses involved are quite formidable. Efforts should be made to restrict the duration of use in "indispensable situations" such as weaning off CPB or managing pulmonary artery hypertensive crises in the postoperative period. While sildenafil may potentially substitute for iNO, its use in the early postoperative period needs to be studied and standardized.

Regulating Blood Product Usage

Unwarranted use of blood products can add to costs and increase transfusion related complications.[39] Strategies such as ultrafiltration during CPB, use of cell savers and antifibrinolytic drug therapy have been recognized as blood conservation strategies during pediatric cardiac surgery. Avoiding empirical use of blood products and determining transfusion needs based on point of care coagulation tests like thromboelastography are some of the suggested strategies for minimizing perioperative transfusions while managing postoperative bleeding after congenital heart surgery.

Reuse of Disposables and Developing Products Locally

Imported disposables from developed nations are being widely used in open heart surgery. With increasing demands the costs incurred upon most programs are substantial. It is important to promote development of indigenously manufactured alternatives at affordable prices. Reuse of selected disposables like cannulae for CPB, catheters and guidewires after appropriate sterilization is also an alternative option in a low-cost environment.[33,40]

Early Deintensification in the ICU

Once the patients are extubated and are hemodynamically stable without inotropic supports, invasive lines should be removed. Early removal of invasive lines can minimize the risk of catheter-related bloodstream infections and subsequent morbidity.[41] Early enteral feeding and ambulation can facilitate early transfer from the ICU and reduce ICU-related expenses.

Reducing ICU Stay

Sepsis, neurological complications, lung issues, pulmonary hypertension, diaphragm palsy, renal failure, and residual lesions can prolong ICU stay. All precautions should be taken to prevent or minimize these complications in the perioperative period. Infection control policies should be aggressively implemented to reduce perioperative sepsis, minimize expensive antibiotic usage, and reduce ICU stay.[42] Early deintensification at all levels of postoperative care ultimately aims at reduction in the total number of days spent in the ICU.

Critical Pathways

Recently, application of critical care pathways to postoperative management of children with CHD have been found to reduce resource utilization and costs of postoperative care.[43] This encompasses principles of early extubation, adequate pain control, early ambulation and alimentation, reducing ICU stays, discharge planning, and teaching. Implementing integrated clinical pathways in congenital heart programs have also been beneficial in improving teamwork and minimizing practice variations in pediatric critical care.[44]

■ SUMMARY

The growing burden of CHD and availability of treatment options emphasize the need for establishment of dedicated PCICU in developing economies. Establishing and sustaining a dedicated PCICU is extremely resource intensive and challenging. In the absence of well-established pediatric cardiac intensive care training programs, dedicated personnel from pediatric subspecialties remains the most important available workforce. The delivery of optimal care in the backdrop of limited resources mandates cohesive teamwork, perseverance and dedication. While awaiting the development of well-established quality institutions with robust training programs, emerging programs in developing nations need to be encouraged, and supported for facilitating optimal care of children with CHD.

■ ACKNOWLEDGMENT

Adapted with permission from Wolters Kluwer Health, Inc. [Balachandran R, Nair SG,

Kumar RK. Establishing a pediatric cardiac intensive care unit–Special considerations in a limited resource environment. Ann Pediatr Cardiol. 2010;3(1):40-9. (https://dx.doi.org/10.4103%2F0974-2069.64374)].

■ REFERENCES

1. Tchervenkov CI, Jacobs JP, Bernier PL, Stellin G, Kurosawa H, Mavroudis C, et al. The improvement of care for paediatric and congenital cardiac disease across the World: a challenge for the World Society for Pediatric and Congenital Heart Surgery. Cardiol Young. 2008;18 (Suppl 2):63-9.

2. Epstein D, Brill JE. A history of pediatric critical care medicine. Pediatr Res. 2005;58:987-96.

3. Downes J. Development of pediatric critical care medicine—How did we get here and why? In: Wheeler DS, Wong HR, Shanley TP (Eds). Pediatric Critical Care Medicine Basic Sciences and Clinical Evidence. London: Springer Verlag; 2007. pp. 3-30.

4. Chang AC. Pediatric cardiac intensive care: current state of the art and beyond the millennium. Curr Opin Pediatr. 2000;12:238-46.

5. Balachandran R, Nair SG, Kumar RK. Establishing a pediatric cardiac intensive care unit-Special considerations in a limited resource environment. Ann Pediatr Cardiol. 2010;3:40-9.

6. Stromberg D. Pediatric cardiac intensivists: are enough being trained? Pediatr Crit Care Med. 2004;5:391-2.

7. Kumar RK. Universal heart coverage for children with heart disease in India. Ann Pediatr Cardiol. 2015;8:177-83.

8. Liu J. Challenges and progress of the pediatric cardiac surgery in Shanghai Children's Medical Center: a 25-year solid collaboration with Project HOPE. Semin Thorac Cardiovasc Surg Pediatr Card Surg Annu. 2009;12-8.

9. Leon-Wyss JR, Veshti A, Veras O, Gaitan GA, O'Connell M, Mack RA, et al. Pediatric cardiac surgery: a challenge and outcome analysis of the Guatemala effort. Semin Thorac Cardiovasc Surg Pediatr Card Surg Annu. 2009:8-11.

10. Saxena A. Pediatric cardiac care in India: current status and the way forward. Future Cardiol. 2018;14:1-4.

11. Kumar RK. The nuts and bolts of pediatric cardiac care for the economically challenged. Ann Pediatr Cardiol. 2009;2(1):99-101.

12. Fuchs RJ, Berenholtz SM, Dorman T. Do intensivists in ICU improve outcome? Best Pract Res Clin Anaesthesiol. 2005;19:125-35.

13. Gajic O, Afessa B. Physician staffing models and patient safety in the ICU. Chest. 2009; 135:1038-44.

14. Baden HP, Zimmerman JJ, Brilli RJ, Wong H, Wetzel RC, Burns JP, et al. Intensivist-led team approach to critical care of children with heart disease. Pediatrics 2006;117:1854-6.

15. Balachandran R, Nair SG, Gopalraj SS, Vaidyanathan B, Kumar RK. Dedicated pediatric cardiac intensive care unit in a developing country: Does it improve outcome? Ann Pediatr Cardiol. 2011;4:122-6.

16. Jonas R. Why early primary repair? In: Jonas RA DJ, Laussen PC, Howe RD, LaPierre R, Matte G (Eds). Comprehensive Surgical Management of Congenital Heart Disease. London: Hodder Arnold Publishers; 2004. pp. 3-12.

17. Rosenberg DI, Moss MM. Guidelines and levels of care for pediatric intensive care units. Crit Care Med. 2004;32:2117-27.

18. Khilnani P. Consensus guidelines for pediatric intensive care units in India. Indian Pediatr. 2002;39:43-50.

19. Roth SJ. Postoperative care. In: Chang AC, Hanley FL, Wernovsky G, Wessel DL (Eds). Pediatric Cardiac Intensive Care. Baltimore: Williams & Wilkins; 1998. pp. 163-88.

20. Brilli RJ, Spevetz A, Branson RD, Campbell GM, Cohen H, Dasta JF, et al. Critical care delivery in the intensive care unit: defining clinical roles and the best practice model. Crit Care Med. 2001;29:2007-19.

21. Chang AC. How to start and sustain a successful pediatric cardiac intensive care program: a combined clinical and administrative strategy. Pediatr Crit Care Med. 2002;3:107-11.

22. Ho D, Xiao Y, Vaidya V, Hu P. Communication and sense-making in intensive care: an observation study of multi-disciplinary rounds to design computerized supporting tools. AMIA Annu Symp Proc. 2007;2007:329-33.

23. McMillan TR, Hyzy RC. Bringing quality improvement into the intensive care unit. Crit Care Med. 2007;35:S59-65.

24. Meert KL, Clark J, Eggly S. Family centered care in the paediatric intensive care unit. Pediatr Clin North Am. 2013;60:761-72.

25. Mack EH, Wheeler DS, Embi PJ. Clinical decision support systems in the pediatric intensive care unit. Pediatr Crit Care Med. 2009;10:23-8.

26. Garland A. Improving the ICU: part 2. Chest 2005;127:2165-79.

27. Gallesio AO. Improving quality and safety in the ICU: A challenge for the next years. Curr Opin Crit Care. 2008;14:700-7.

28. Balachandran R, Kappanayil M, Sen AC, Sudhakar A, Nair SG, Sunil GS, et al. Impact of the International Quality Improvement Collaborative on outcomes after congenital heart surgery: a single centre experience in a developing economy. Ann Card Anaesth. 2015;18:52-7.

29. Strack van Schijndel RJ, Burchardi H. Bench-to-bedside review: leadership and conflict management in the intensive care unit. Crit Care. 2007;11:234.

30. Kissoon N. Bench-to-bedside review: humanism in pediatric critical care medicine—a leadership challenge. Crit Care. 2005;9:371-5.

31. Kumar RK. Teamwork in pediatric heart care. Ann Pediatr Cardiol. 2009;2:140-5.

32. Kumar RK, Shrivastava S. Paediatric heart care in India. Heart. 2008;94:984-90.

33. Rao SG. Pediatric cardiac surgery in developing countries. Pediatr Cardiol. 2007;28:144-8.

34. Chang AC. Manpower shortage in pediatric cardiac intensive care: how can we undo this Gordian knot? Pediatr Crit Care Med. 2004;5:414-5.

35. Crowe S, Sullivant S, Miller-Smith L, Lantos JD. Grief and burnout in the PICU. Pediatrics. 2017;139:e20164041.

36. Talwar S, Choudhary SK, Airan B, Juneja R, Kothari SS, Saxena A, et al. Reducing the costs of surgical correction of congenitally malformed hearts in developing countries. Cardiol Young. 2008;18:363-71.

37. Mittnacht AJC, Thanjan M, Srivastava S, Joashi U, Bodian C, Hossain S, et al. Extubation in the operating room after congenital heart surgery in children. J Thorac Cardiovasc Surg. 2008;136:88-93.

38. Garg R, Rao S, John C, Reddy C, Hegde R, Murthy K, et al. Extubation in the operating room after cardiac surgery in children: a prospective observational study with multidisciplinary coordinated approach. J Cardiothorac Vasc Anesth. 2014;28:479-87.

39. Scott BH, Seifert FC, Grimson R. Blood trans-fusion is associated with increased resource utilisation, morbidity and mortality in cardiac surgery. Ann Card Anaesth. 2008; 11:15-9.

40. Kumar RK, Tynan M. Catheter interventions for congenital heart disease in the third World. Pediatr Cardiol. 2005;26:1-9.

41. O'Grady NP, Alexander M, Dellinger EP, Gerberding JL, Heard SO, Maki DG, et al. Guidelines for the prevention of intravascular catheter-related infections. The Hospital Infection Control Practices Advisory Committee, US Center for Disease Control and Prevention. Pediatrics. 2002;110:e51.

42. Bakshi KD, Vaidyanathan B, Sundaram KR, Roth SJ, Shivaprakasha K, Rao SG, et al. Determinants of early outcome after neonatal cardiac surgery in a developing country, J Thorac Cardiovasc Surg. 2007;134:765-71.

43. Price MB, Jones A, Hawkins JA, McGough EC, Lambert L, Dean JM. Critical pathways for postoperative care after simple congenital heart surgery. Am J Manag Care. 1999;5:185-92.

44. Willis TS, Yip T, Brown K, Buck S, Mill M. Improved teamwork and implementation of clinical pathways in a congenital heart surgery program. Pediatr Qual Saf. 2019;4:e126.

Index

Page numbers followed by *b* refer to box, *f* refer to figure,
fc refer to flowchart, and *t* refer to table.